HANDBOOK OF
ENDOCRINOLOGY
Second Edition
VOLUME I

EDITED BY
George H. Gass
Harold M. Kaplan

CRC Press
Boca Raton   New York   London   Tokyo

Publisher:	Robert B. Stern
Project Editor:	Albert W. Starkweather, Jr.
Marketing Manager:	Becky McEldowney
Cover Design:	Denise Craig
PrePress:	Carlos Esser
Manufacturing:	Sheri Schwartz

Library of Congress Cataloging-in-Publication Data

Handbook of endocrinology / edited by George H. Gass, Harold M. Kaplan. -- 2nd ed.
    p. cm.
    Rev. ed. of: CRC handbook of endocrinology / editors, George H. Gass and Harold M. Kaplan, c1982.
    Includes bibliographical references and index.
    ISBN 0-8493-9429-5 (v. 1 : alk. paper), -- ISBN 0-8493-9430-9 (V. 2 : alk. paper)
    1. Endocrinology--Handbooks, manuals, etc. I. Gass, George H. II. Kaplan, Harold Morris, 1908- . III. CRC handbook of endorcinology.
    [DNLM: 1. Endocrine Glands--physiology. 2. Hormones--physiology.
3. Endocrine Diseases. 4. Endocrinology. WK 100 H236 1996]
QP187.C73 1996
612′.4--dc20
DNLM/DLC
for Library of Congress

96-13983
CIP

This book contains information obtained from authentic and highly regarded sources. Reprinted material is quoted with permission, and sources are indicated. A wide variety of references are listed. Reasonable efforts have been made to publish reliable data and information, but the author and the publisher cannot assume responsibility for the validity of all materials or for the consequences of their use.

Neither this book nor any part may be reproduced or transmitted in any form or by any means, electronic or mechanical, including photocopying, microfilming, and recording, or by any information storage or retrieval system, without prior permission in writing from the publisher.

All rights reserved. Authorization to photocopy items for internal or personal use, or the personal or internal use of specific clients, may be granted by CRC Press, Inc., provided that $.50 per page photocopied is paid directly to Copyright Clearance Center, 27 Congress Street, Salem, MA 01970 USA. The fee code for users of the Transactional Reporting Service is ISBN 0-8493-9429-5/96/$0.00+$.50. The fee is subject to change without notice. For organizations that have been granted a photocopy license by the CCC, a separate system of payment has been arranged.

CRC Press, Inc.'s consent does not extend to copying for general distribution, for promotion, for creating new works, or for resale. Specific permission must be obtained in writing from CRC Press for such copying.

Direct all inquiries to CRC Press, Inc., 2000 Corporate Blvd., N.W., Boca Raton, Florida 33431.

PREFACE

This *Handbook of Endocrinology, Volumes I and II,* presents a review of selected topics by 36 authors. Each topic is broad in scope and intensive in approach. The endocrine literature is now so extensive that it would take several volumes to encompass it.

The present book is a general reference source for the academic endocrinologist, teacher, and researcher, for graduate students working in current areas of the field, and for biologists interested in the chemical control of bodily systems, adjunctive to neural regulation. Physicians with special interests in endocrinology will find chapters that have considerable relevance to their work. The references provided herein are numerous and updated. The descriptions of the endocrine processes provide data in the fields of anatomy, histology, physiology, and pathophysiology.

Overall, the reader will have access to a comprehensive survey of the chemical nature of hormones, their synthesis, secretion and transport, their actions and mechanisms of action, and their degradation and excretion, in mammals and man.

The editors fully appreciate the expertise and the large amount of time spent by the contributors. This book is their work.

George H. Gass
Harold M. Kaplan

THE EDITORS

George H. Gass, M.D., is the retired Chairman of the Department of Basic Medical Sciences of the Oklahoma State University College of Osteopathic Medicine (formerly the Oklahoma College of Osteopathic Medicine and Surgery). Previously he held the position of Director, Endocrinologic Pharmacology Research Laboratory at Southern Illinois University, during which time he also held the positions of Professor of Physiology and Professor of Medicine. He has had a very diverse career, including industry (Lederle Laboratories) and government (Food and Drug Administration).

Dr. Gass was awarded his doctorate at The Ohio State University. Following graduation Dr. Gass served in the Endocrine Branch of the Food and Drug Administration in Washington, D.C., where he performed biological assay procedures, biostatistics, and endocrine research for four years before leaving to enter higher education. Dr. Gass' best known work in the Food and Drug Administration was in the co-development of the uterine weight method for estrogen assay and detection. Dr. Gass assumed his duties at Southern Illinois University, Department of Physiology, in the fall of 1959 and immediately upon arrival set up the Endocrinologic Pharmacology Research Laboratory. A number of students obtained their research experience under Dr. Gass in that laboratory, where it was first discovered that a quantitative measure of a chemical carcinogen (diethylstilbestrol)-dose response of mammary tumors existed. This research has become a classic and, although published in 1964, has more recently been repeated by the Center for Toxicological Research with Dr. Gass consulting.

Dr. Gass, as a member of the staff of Southern Illinois University, received a number of honors and served on numerous occasions as a consultant for government and industry. Dr. Gass is a fellow of the American Association of Science, an Alexander von Humboldt fellow, and a Fullbright alumnus.

He was requested to serve as a consultant for the National Center for Toxicology, Food Administration, to help determine the carcinogenicity and estrogenicity of female sex hormones, both naturally occurring and synthetic. During his 18 years at Southern Illinois University he taught physiology and pharmacology. His last position as Chairman of the Department of Basic Medical Sciences allowed him intimate contact with the basic scientists in the college, including those in human anatomy, histology, pharmacology, physiology, behavior, and biochemistry.

Harold M. Kaplan, Ph.D., is Visiting Professor in the Medical Preparatory Program in the School of Medicine at Southern Illinois University (SIU) at Carbondale. Dr. Kaplan received the A.B. degree at Dartmouth College in 1930, the A.M. degree at Harvard University in 1931, and the Ph.D. degree at Harvard in 1933. He was an Assistant Instructor at Harvard, 1933–1934, and Instructor to Professor of Physiology at Middlesex University Medical School in Massachusetts, 1934–1945, as well as Department Chairman for many years. He was Professor of Veterinary Physiology and Department Chairman at Brandeis University from 1945 to 1947. He was Associate Professor of Physiology at the University of Massachusetts at Fort Devens from 1947 to 1949, serving as Department Chairman in 1948–1949. Dr. Kaplan was Associate Professor at SIU in 1949 and became Professor of Physiology and Department Chairman in 1971. He was simultaneously a professor in the SIU School of Medicine from 1974 to the present. He was Director of the SIU Animal Quarters (Vivarium) intermittently from 1950 to 1982.

Dr. Kaplan was President of the Illinois State Academy of Science, 1969–1970, and is both a life member and honorary member. He was President of the American Association for Laboratory Animal Science, 1966–1967, and is a life member and honorary member. He was on the Board of Directors of the Institute of Laboratory Animal Resources, 1965–1969, and the Illinois Society for Medical Research, 1962–1986. He was on the Science Advisory Committee at Illinois Wesleyan University, 1970–1976. He was President of Sigma Xi (National Honor Society) SIU chapter, 1989–1990, as well as Phi Kappa Phi (National Honor Society), SIU chapter, 1976–1977 and 1983–1984. He was an editorial advisor for the National Forum, 1986–1989. He was President of the Emeritus Faculty Organization at SIU, 1993–1995. Dr. Kaplan has served as Science Consultant for the Applied Research and Development Laboratory in Mt. Vernon, IL, since 1983. He is a fellow of the AAAS. He was Chairman of the Editorial Board, Laboratory Animal Science, 1963–1974.

Dr. Kaplan is the co-author of about 200 research papers and has written 10 books. He is a contributor to five chapters in an accepted biological laboratory text.

CONTRIBUTORS

Nancy A. M. Alexiuk
Department of Anatomy
University of Manitoba
Winnipeg, Manitoba, Canada

Rebecca S. Bahn
Mayo Clinic
Rochester, Minnesota

Andrzej Bartke
Department of Physiology
Southern Illinois University
School of Medicine
Carbondale, Illinois

John B. Buse
Diabetes Care Center
Chapel Hill, North Carolina

Monica E. Doerr
Division of Endocrinology
University of North Carolina
School of Medicine
Chapel Hill, North Carolina

Warren E. Finn
Department of Physiology & Pharmacology
College of Osteopathic Medicine
Oklahoma State University
Tulsa, Oklahoma

Milton D. Gross
Department of Internal Medicine
University of Michigan Medical Center
Ann Arbor, Michigan

Charles A. Hodson
Department of Obstetrics & Gynecology
East Carolina University
Greenville, North Carolina

Abby Solomon Hollander
Pediatric Endocrinology
St. Louis Children's Hospital
St. Louis, Missouri

Kathleen A. Jones
School of Medicine—MEDPREP
Southern Illinois University
Carbondale, Illinois

Bess Adkins Marshall
Pediatric Endocrinology
St. Louis Children's Hospital
St. Louis, Missouri

Brahm Shapiro
Department of Internal & Nuclear Medicine
University of Michigan Medical Center
Ann Arbor, Michigan

William E. Sonntag
Department of Physiology & Pharmacology
Gray School of Medicine at Wake Forest
Winston-Salem, North Carolina

Richard W. Steger
Southern Illinois University
School of Medicine
Carbondale, Illinois

Jerry Vriend
Department of Anatomy
University of Manitoba
Winnipeg, Manitoba, Canada

Hing-Sing Yu
Institute of Environmental Science
  & Technology
San Antonio, Texas

TABLE OF CONTENTS

Chapter 1

SUMMATION OF BASIC ENDOCRINE DATA

Kathleen A. Jones

CONTENTS

0-8493-9429-5/96/$0.00+$.50
© 1996 by CRC Press, Inc.

THYROID GLAND

TRIIODOTHYRONINE AND THYROXINE
Structure, Development, and Aging

The thyroid is present in all vertebrates. In humans, it has two lobes, connected by an isthmus, on either side of the trachea. It is enervated by parasympathetic and sympathetic fibers, which control only the diameter of the blood vessels they are in. Histologically it is composed mostly of follicles, containing colloid, which is thyroglobulin. There are also parafollicular cells, which produce calcitonin.

The gland begins to develop in the third embryonic week as an evagination of the pharynx and is clearly differentiated in the 15th week, producing thyroxine. The ultimobranchial body from endoderm cells of the sixth pharyngeal pouch is incorporated into the thyroid and produces the parafollicular or C cells. Thyroid tissue is present in all vertebrates.

Marked changes occur in the thyroid with age. Its structure then resembles the gland when it is in a state of hypothyroidism. Connective tissue increases and many follicles are obliterated. The gland is not essential to life, but its functions are.

Classification

The two chief hormones are L-thyroxine (T_4) and 3,5,3'-1-triiodothyronine (T_3). Another is reverse T_3 (rT_3). Thyroglobulin is the storage form and has no hormonal properties per se. Very little thyroglobulin enters the circulation. Calcitonin, secreted by the C cells, will be considered separately. The hormones T_3 and T_4 are glycoproteins.

Biosynthesis

The synthesis starts with iodide, which the thyroid follicles actively take up. The iodide is oxidized to active iodine, which is incorporated into tyrosine. This is followed by peptide linkages, which are glycoproteins called thyroglobulin. Monoiodotyrosine (MIT) and diiodotyrosine then develop. These couple to form T_3 and T_4, although very little rT_3. An enzyme called thyroid peroxidase catalyzes the whole sequence of reactions.

Release

To obtain the release of T_3 and T_4, there is proteolysis of thyroglobulin followed by endocytosis. Thyrotropin-releasing hormone (TRH), which is hypothalamic in origin, stimulates the pituitary to synthesize and release the thyroid-stimulating hormone (TSH). This promotes the uptake of iodide by the thyroid.

Normal Bodily Effects

The effects vary with the specific hormone that is circulating to the cells of the body. The material stored in colloid as thyroglobulin is translocated to the lumen of each thyroid follicle. T_4, which is necessary for life, is the dominant circulatory form and gives rise to most of T_3 and just about all of rT_3. The hormones circulate almost totally bound to proteins. Thyroxine-binding globulin is the major binding protein; it is a glycoprotein-α-globulin. Other binding proteins are albumin and a thyroid-binding albumin.

A major effect is to increase protein synthesis in all bodily tissues. T_3 is about four times as active metabolically as T_4; T_3 has about two-thirds of the biologic activity of the thyroid hormones. There are effects on thermoregulation, food metabolism, growth and development, reproduction, water and electrolyte activities, and neural behavior.

Basis of Bodily Effects

Thyroid-stimulating hormone is involved, from the anterior pituitary. It binds to the membranes of the follicles and stimulates adenylate cyclase. cAMP is produced, but its control over T_3 and T_4 release needs further study. T_3 and T_4 can enter virtually all body cells when unbound.

CALCITONIN (THYROCALCITONIN)

Structure, Development, Aging

Since calcitonin is produced in the thyroid gland, refer to relevant data for the thyroid. The parafollicular cells of the thyroid are the secretory elements for calcitonin. These originate in the neural crest in the fetus. In vertebrate animals there is an origin in the ultimobranchial body. Calcitonin concentration in the plasma reduces with age and is generally lower in women than in men.

Classification

Calcitonin is a single-chain polypeptide, containing 32 amino acids, with a molecular weight of about 3500. There are species differences in the amino acid sequence. This suggests that the specific sequence order determines the characteristic action. Human calcitonin has been synthesized.

Biosynthesis

Calcitonin is produced in the human thyroid gland in parafollicular cells that lie in the interstitial tissue among the thyroid follicles. The precursor of calcitonin is preprocalcitonin, which hydrolyzes to calcitonin and other polypeptides. The gene for calcitonin is transcribed and changed to a different mRNA in the brain, a peptide called calcitonin-gene-related peptide, whose function other than vasodilation is unknown.

Release

Calcitonin secretion and release increase when the thyroid gland is normally perfused with high plasma concentrations of calcium. Potent natural stimulants include gastrin, dopamine, estrogen, β-adrenergic agonists, and other substances. In man, the thymus and parathyroid may secrete some calcitonin. Hypercalcemia may be the major stimulus for calcitonin secretion.

Normal Bodily Effects

Calcitonin decreases circulating calcium and phosphate levels by inhibiting release of these substances from bone to plasma. This is opposite to the action of the parathyroid hormone (PTH; parathormone). Calcitonin is a short-term regulator of calcium ion concentration, whereas PTH is a long-term regulator that more than offsets the calcitonin effects. Thus, overall, the calcitonin control in the human adult is weak. The hormone has a half-life less than one hour and is excreted by the kidneys. Its peak effect is less than one hour. Calcitonin may be effective against hypercalcemia caused by excessive calcium intake. Whether it is essential for development and maintenance of the skeleton is not clear.

Basis of Bodily Effects

The mechanism underlying the effects involves calcitonin receptors in bones and kidneys. The action permitting the decreasing of calcium in plasma is the inhibition of bone resorption induced by cAMP. There is an increase in osteoblastic activity, but this lasts only a few days. The prolonged effect is in preventing the formation of osteoclasts. In the long run, the parathyroids regulate the level of extracellular calcium.

PARATHYROID GLAND

PARATHYROID HORMONE
Structure, Development, and Aging

There are two pairs of parathyroid glands in man. Each is close to the posterior wall of the thyroid glands. The parathyroids are present only in vertebrates. They secrete PTH.

In the fetus at the fifth week the endoderm of the third pharyngeal pouch differentiates into the inferior aspect of the parathyroids. The endoderm of the fourth pharyngeal pouch is the superior aspect.

The parathyroid glands in the adult human are composed mainly of chief and oxyphil cells. The chief cells secrete PTH and persist throughout life.

Classification

The hormone, PTH, is a single-chain polypeptide containing 84 amino acids.

Biosynthesis

PTH is synthesized as a large precursor molecule on the ribosomes. The precursor is transported to the endoplasmic reticulum in which preproparathyroid hormone is enzymatically changed to proparathyroid hormone and the latter is sent to the Golgi apparatus. The resulting definitive hormone is encapsulated into granules, which are released as the ionized calcium in the extracellular fluids is decreased.

Release

It is the level of ionic calcium in the blood that controls hormonal secretion by way of a negative feedback system. The volume of secretion varies inversely with the calcium level.

Normal Bodily Effects

The major effect is to increase the plasma calcium level. About 90% of the calcium in the body is sent to bone, as a calcium phosphate compound. The hormone degrades the bone matrix. Many other hormones are also involved in bone activity, mostly for growth (e.g., growth hormone and sex hormones) and bone catabolism (e.g., thyroid and glucocorticoids).

PTH promotes calcium resorption by the renal tubules as well as by the renal excretion of phosphates. Still another area of activity is absorption of calcium from the small intestine to the blood, but this involves the adjunctive action of vitamin D.

Basis of Biological Effects

PTH activates adenylate cyclase in bone and kidney, resulting in cAMP production. Since all varieties of bone cells have PTH receptors, the cAMP levels are responsive to PTH. The first effects of PTH occur in minutes, but the subsequent events take days to weeks and involve proliferation and resorption of bone.

PTH increases plasma calcium by decreasing its absorption through the kidney. It augments calcium absorption from the alimentary canal and brings calcium from bone to plasma.

VITAMIN D

RELATIONSHIP TO PARATHYROID HORMONE
Structure

Vitamin D is a general term for a variety of related compounds which are determined by the chemical pathway of their formation. The one of interest herein is vitamin D_3 (cholecalciferol). Other forms will not be discussed. Vitamin D_3 is synthesized in the skin by the action of sunlight.

Classification

Vitamin D is a sterol.

Biosynthesis

The most important member of the group of related sterols comprising vitamin D is D_3. The ultraviolet light of the sun produces it in the skin of mammals. The light activates certain provitamins, e.g., 7-dehydrocholesterol.

Vitamin D is not per se the active chemical that causes the effects once ascribed to the compound. It has to be changed in the liver to cholecalciferol, which is then converted in the liver to 25-hydroxycholecalciferol. The latter conserves D_3 by allowing it to be stored in the liver for several months.

The final conversion is from 25-hydroxycholecalciferol to 1,25-dihydroxycholecalciferol, which is the most potent form of vitamin D. This conversion occurs in the kidneys and cannot proceed in the absence of the kidneys or the parathyroid hormone. The hormone secretion is itself controlled greatly by plasma calcium ion concentration and the same is the case for 1,25-dihydroxycholecalciferol.

Release

The vitamin D_3 is transported in the plasma bound to a globulin which is called vitamin-D-binding protein (DBP). It is this form that transports vitamin D_3 from the skin to the blood. Some vitamin D_3, which travels in the blood, is exogenous.

Normal Bodily Effects

Vitamin D, generally considered to be a hormone, acts with PTH as the chief regulators of calcium and phosphorus activities. It is antirachitic and is an essential cofactor for PTH. The PTH promotes formation of the active metabolite of vitamin D.

Vitamin D_3 causes resorption of bone much like PTH does. Small amounts of the vitamin can calcify bone, by increasing the absorption of calcium and phosphate from the intestine.

Vitamin D_3 is more important than PTH in maintaining skeletal structure and function. The targets of the vitamin's active metabolites are bone and intestine. D_3 is a potent stimulator of calcium absorption from the intestine and it facilitates the rate of formation of bone. Pharmacologic doses stimulate resorption of calcium from bone into the blood.

Biochemical Basis of Bodily Effects

The mode of action of vitamin D_3 may involve a metabolite of D called 1,25-dihydroxy-cholecalciferol; this metabolite increases the transport of calcium across cell membranes, acting as a hormone, and it also aids formation of calcium-binding protein in the intestinal cells, as well as causing formation of ATPase in the lining cells affected. The same metabolite also aids phosphate absorption, acting perhaps through a calcium-absorption mediator.

Bone contains exchangeable calcium that is in equilibrium with calcium in the extracellular fluids. This provides a quick buffering system which keeps extracellular calcium ions from rising or falling excessively.

THYMUS GLAND

Structure, Development, and Aging

The thymus is a lymphoepithelial endocrine gland located in the mediastinum, and it extends from the thyroid in the neck into the thoracic cavity. It is well developed before birth. It reaches maximum size at about two years of age and then gradually regresses, especially after puberty. Only about 15% of its structure remains at age 50. The gland is replaced by fatty tissue, which decreases its capacity to provide T cells in later life. The origin of the gland in the fetus is mainly the third but also the fourth pharyngeal pouches. The earliest origins of the thymus, thyroid, and parathyroids are virtually common. Thymic tissue is present in every vertebrate.

The thymus is involved in T-lymphocyte activity. The precursor cells of these lymphocytes start their development in the fetus, and the process continues from the neonate throughout life. The cell production eventually passes from the bone marrow to the thymus and thence to the peripheral lymph tissues. The thymus can produce T cells independently of the bone marrow. For B-lymphocytes, the bone marrow is the area of maturation, and the cells migrate to the lymphoid organs. Both B and T cells can undergo mitosis in the peripheral lymphoid structures. Among the lymphoid structures, the thymus has the highest rate of cell proliferation.

Classification

The earliest thymic factor, extracted from animals, was called thymosin (thymic hormone). This is the best characterized of the thymic humoral factors. Thymosin α-1 (molecular weight 3,100) and β-4 (molecular weight 5,250) are both peptides. Thymopoietin (molecular weight 5,500), thymic humoral factor (molecular weight 3,200), and protein human thymic factor (molecular weight 56,700) are polypeptides. Serum thymic factor (molecular weight 847) is a nonapeptide.

Biosynthesis

Because the thymic hormones are virtually all polypeptides, their synthesis is the same as that of proteic substances in general.

Release

The thymus is very sensitive to other hormonal influences. Nonhormonal agents also influence the rates of synthesis and secretion, and their identification and chemical changes require more information and definition.

Normal Bodily Effects

The thymus is involved in producing lymphoid cells that travel to organs such as the lymph nodes and the spleen. The T-lymphocytes are important in thymic function. They are active in cellular immunity. Some, called helper cells, secrete lymphokines, the most important being interleukin-1 (IL-1) and interleukin-2 (IL-2). IL-1 is a polypeptide whose chief origin is the macrophage. This substance stimulates production of IL-2 as well as B-lymphocytes. IL-2 activates the hypothalamus in the production of fever. IL-2 also acts as a growth factor that stimulates proliferation of B and T cells, suppressor T cells, and also natural killer cells which are not thymic in origin.

T-lymphocytes secrete not only the lymphokines mentioned above, but also interferon (for antiviral and antitumor function), macrophage-activating factor (which promotes phagocytosis), chemotactic factors (which attract leukocytes to an infected region), and a macrophage-migration inhibiting factor (which prevents phagocytes from leaving an infected area). T-lymphocytes, unlike B-lymphocytes, do not form plasma cells or antibodies.

The thymus is involved as a site of origin in autoimmune disease. In myasthenia gravis, where there is great muscular weakness and fatigue, acetylcholine receptors at neuromuscular junctions are significantly decreased in number. The B-lymphocytes that function specifically for the production of acetylcholine receptor antibodies play a major part in the autoantibody response. T cells also produce acetylcholine antibodies and are numerous in the thymus of patients with myasthenia gravis.[1]

Basis of Bodily Effects

All the thymic hormones interact with specific cell receptors, leading to the production of cAMP or gAMP. This eventuates in the expression of the T cell actions.

PINEAL GLAND

Structure, Development, and Aging

The pineal gland (epiphysis) originates in the brain. The caudal diencephalic roof plate gives rise to the midline diverticulum which becomes the gland. Proliferation of cells in its walls converts the gland into a solid pine cone-shaped organ, about 8 mm long.

The exact importance of the pineal gland is unknown; its position suggests that it is at least in part the homologue of the third or parietal eye of lower vertebrates. In these vertebrates it has both nerve cells and light receptors, but there are no light-sensitive structures in the human pineal gland.

The gland starts to involute just prior to puberty. It is large in human infants. In the adult, calcium often deposits, allowing the gland to be a landmark on an x-ray of the skull. The pineal gland may retain its production and activity throughout life.

Classification

The major active secretion of the pineal gland is melatonin. This is an indole, *N*-acetyl-5-methoxytryptamine. Melatonin is also known as melanocyte-stimulating hormone.

Biosynthesis

Melatonin is derived from tryptophan through a cascade of stages. The tryptophan is converted enzymatically (tryptophan hydroxylase) to 5-hydroxytryptophan, which changes to 5-hydroxytryptamine (serotonin) by aromatic L-amino decarboxylase. Serotonin *N*-acetyl transferase then changes serotonin to *N*-acetyl serotonin plus hydroxyindole-*O*-methyl transferase. The transfer of a methyl group from *S*-adenosylmethionine to the 5-hydroxyl of *N*-acetyl serotonin yields melatonin.

Release

The pineal gland transduces neural signals into the hormonal melatonin output. The secretion has a circadian rhythm associated with the 24-hour light-dark cycle. Light taken in by the eyes and sent to the brain through the optic nerve radiates to the sympathetic nerves that supply the pineal gland. The light reduces the output of norepinephrine from the nerve endings. Darkness, on the contrary, increases the output.

Normal Bodily Effects

Melatonin lightens the skin of frog tadpoles by an action on melanophores. In mammals its functions are still uncertain. It does not appear to control skin color in man.

In animals, melatonin may detect seasonal changes. It inhibits gonadal function in both sexes by blocking the production of pituitary gonadotropins. It is thought to regulate the onset of puberty, because it drops in concentration as puberty progresses.

The pineal gland is outside the blood-brain barrier because it has fenestrated capillaries and high cell permeability.

Basis of Bodily Effects

Stress activates the sympathetic nervous system to release catecholamines from the nerve endings. The release is increased in darkness and the pineal gland becomes involved. The gland is stimulated by adrenal medullary or neural hormones in that their secretions bind to β-adrenergic receptors. This activates adenylate cyclase and leads to the production of cAMP, then protein kinases, and finally the involvement of enzymes essential to the synthesis of melatonin. Most of the melatonin secretion occurs at night as part of a circadian cycle.

CIRCUMVENTRICULAR ORGANS

The circumventricular organs are sets of neurons situated around the borders of the ventricles of the brain. They include the subfornical organ, organum vasculosum, median eminence, area postrema, and pineal gland.

Their importance is that they lack a blood-brain barrier and contain fenestrated capillaries which permit neurons to receive substances, including certain hormones, to pass directly between the blood and the brain. Thus, the subfornical organ monitors angiotensin-II levels and projects into the hypothalamus. The area postrema monitors cholecystokinin and projects by lower nuclei to the hypothalamus. The organum vasculosum of the lamina terminalis monitors cytokines in the blood and projects to the brain stem and hypothalamus. The median eminence, pineal gland, and pituitary gland, all of which lack a blood-brain barrier, secrete their own hormones from the central nervous system into the general circulation. Some brain circumventricular organs recognize cytokines in the blood, and if the cytokines are transmitted to the brain, they contribute to the production of fever.[2]

ADRENAL GLAND

MEDULLA
Structure, Development, and Aging

The paired adrenal glands are located at the upper pole of each kidney. The adrenal medulla is a sympathetic postganglionic fiber in the fetus and it modifies to a gland. It is supplied only by preganglionic fibers. In the seventh or eighth fetal week, neural crest cells penetrate the adrenal cortex and become the adrenal medulla. The whole gland grows rapidly, peaking at midgestation, after which it grows more slowly and reaches the size found at birth.

Classification

The medulla produces two major hormones, epinephrine and norepinephrine. These are called catecholamines and are biogenic amines. The term "catecholamine" stems from the fact that these substances contain catechol (ortho-dihydroxybenzene) and a side chain with an amino group.

The compound called dopamine is another catecholamine which is in the intermediate synthetic chain in the synthesis of this group of hormones.

Biosynthesis

Catecholamines are produced from the amino acids phenylalanine and tyrosine. The catalysts for them, which are hydroxylases, are in the liver.

Tyrosine enters the adrenal medulla and also into those neurons where it can convert to L-dopa and then to dopamine; these changes utilize tyrosine hydroxylase and dopa decarboxylase. Dopamine is placed into granulated vesicles and changed to norepinephrine by the dopamine-β-hydroxylase.

Some neurons and cells of the medulla release norepinephrine from the vesicles and convert it by the action of phenolethynolamine-*N*-methyl transferase to epinephrine. The transferase is absent in early fetal development.

Release

In the adrenal gland, the medulla secretes norepinephrine and its derivative, epinephrine. Norepinephrine is also secreted by neurons of the hypothalamus and brain stem, and it is put out peripherally by postganglionic sympathetic neurons; some of the receptors affected cause excitation in the cells and others cause inhibition. Both compounds are released probably by exocytosis and are differentially bound to α or β receptors in the target organs.

The compound called dopamine is secreted by neurons of the substantia nigra. Upon release, it acts by way of dopamine receptors. The D_1 receptor activates adenylate cyclase whereas the D_2 receptor inhibits adenylate cyclase. In this process, hydrolysis of guanosine triphosphate is involved as a regulatory subunit for the adenylate cyclase activity. Epinephrine is typically a hormone whereas norepinephrine acts more as a neurotransmitter.

Normal Bodily Effects

Norepinephrine and epinephrine stimulate the nervous system. Their metabolic actions include glycogenolysis in liver and muscle and control over the metabolic rate. Norepinephrine constricts blood vessels via α receptors. Epinephrine dilates vessels via β_2 receptors and regulates cardiac muscle contraction via β_1 receptors.

Dopamine causes renal vasodilation, but vasoconstriction elsewhere. It forms a β_1 receptor complex which increases the cardiac force. Dopamine is also a precursor of norepinephrine. In the basal ganglia it may be a neurotransmitter.

Basis of Bodily Effects

The medulla for the most part releases epinephrine and norepinephrine simultaneously with their comparable neural stimulation. This provides a generalized, supportive action which is widespread. This activity requires only a low frequency of stimulation and a basal energetic tone. If the autonomic neurons are denervated, the tone may be restored by the intrinsic activity of the bodily structures involved.

Stimulation of parasympathetic or sympathetic nerves may cause either excitation or inhibition, depending upon the target organ, and this must be kept in mind for any autonomic effector under study. Norepinephrine excites chiefly α receptors, although β receptors to a lesser degree. Epinephrine excites α and β receptors about equally.

The catecholamines tend to act as first messengers, reacting in the target membranes with specific receptors. These in turn activate the second messengers within the target cells and a cascade of the observable events follows.

CORTEX
Structure, Development, and Aging

The cortex is the outer region of the retroperitoneal adrenal gland. All regions of the cortex secrete hormones, possibly 50 in number, but only a few are of major clinical importance.

The cortex forms in the sixth fetal week by condensation of mesoderm between the root of the dorsal mesentery and the gonad. The adrenocorticoid hormones of the cortex maintain their production and secretion throughout life.

Classification

The cortical hormones are steroids. These have a cyclopentane-hydrophenanthrene nucleus. Most but not all are called 17-ketosteroids because they have a keto group at position 17 on the molecule. Corticosterone does not form a 17-ketosteroid. Both glucocorticoids and mineralocorticoids have 21 carbon atoms.

Biosynthesis of Cortisol and Aldosterone

Cholesterol is the precursor of the cortical steroids. It is cleaved in the adrenal mitochondria to produce a 21-carbon molecule called pregnenolone. To produce cortisol, the pregnenolone is transformed in the mitochondria and forms the cortisol.

To produce aldosterone, pathways involving deoxycorticosterone and corticosterone (both originating from progesterone) occur. The corticosterone is enzymatically changed to 18-hydroxycorticosterone within the mitochondria. The enzyme called 18-hydroxysteroid dehydrogenase activates the chemical changes that produce aldosterone.

Release

The cortex can release any of the five varieties of hormones: (1) glucocorticoids (e.g., cortisol, corticosterone), whose primary action is to elevate blood sugar levels, (2) mineralocorticoids (e.g., aldosterone), which regulate ionic plasma sodium and potassium, (3) androgens, (4) progestins, and (5) estradiol. Groups 3, 4, and 5 are unimportant outputs of the cortex.

The release of aldosterone is regulated by (1) renin, (2) adrenocorticotropic hormone (ACTH; corticotropin) from the anterior pituitary, and (3) a direct effect of plasma sodium and potassium ion levels on the cortex. For cortisol, most that is released is bound to an α globulin and some to albumin. The bound cortisol serves as a reservoir. The free cortisol inhibits the release of ACTH. The latter is a more potent stimulus for the release of cortisol than for aldosterone. Cortisol secretion, like that of ACTH, exhibits diurnal variations in its output. There is little plasma level change with age.

Normal Bodily Effects

Glucocorticoids have many functions. Cortisol is the prime example and it is essential to life. It has a weak effect on electrolyte and water metabolism. It releases liver glucose, increases gluconeogenesis, stimulates protein metabolism in the liver, releases fatty acids from adipose tissue, inhibits fibroblasts and epithelial cell proliferation, lowers serum calcium, and has other effects. The net effect is catabolic.

Mineralocorticoids, aldosterone being the prime example, affect the distal tubules of the kidney, and thus promote resorption of sodium from the urine and excretion of potassium into the urine. These hormones are also antiinflammatory.

Basis of Bodily Effects

Aldosterone secretion is regulated chiefly by angiotensin and potassium, which directly stimulate the adrenocortical cells. Aldosterone exerts most of its effects by occupying a type 1 mineralocorticoid receptor which then binds to DNA and influences the transcription of various genes. Aldosterone may also react with a membrane-bound receptor.

Cortisol secretion is regulated for the most part by ACTH controlled from the anterior pituitary. The ACTH, in turn, is regulated by the corticotropin-releasing hormone (CRH) carried from the hypothalamus in its portal system to the pituitary gland where ACTH is stored and released.

ACTH acts on specific receptors in the adrenal cortex, whereupon adenylate cyclase, acting as a second messenger, induces the formation of cAMP inside the cytoplasm of the cells. In the cascade that follows, phosphoprotein kinases phosphorylate proteins. An important step is the subsequent activation of desmolase; this converts cholesterol esters to pregnenolone, upon which all later steps depend.

PITUITARY GLAND (HYPOPHYSIS)

POSTERIOR LOBE (NEUROHYPOPHYSIS)
Structure and Development
The pituitary gland is at the base of the brain, in a depression called the sella turcica. It is connected to the hypothalamus above by a hypophyseal stalk. The gland is divided into an anterior lobe (adenohypophysis) and a posterior lobe (neurohypophysis), and between them a small structure called the pars intermedia. The posterior lobe hormones are manufactured first in the hypothalamus and then transported through a neurosecretory pathway to the posterior lobe where they are stored.

The pituitary develops from two distinctly different areas. For the posterior lobe, a neuroectodermal thickening called the infundibulum in the floor of the diencephalon, and which is composed of neuroglia cells, develops as the stalk and the pars nervosa (posterior lobe) of the neurohypophysis. The hypothalamus sends into the stalk a number of nerve fibers. Then, pituicytes resembling neuroglia cells proliferate in the distal end of the infundibulum.

Classification
The hormones stored in the neurohypophysis are vasopressin (antidiuretic hormone) and oxytocin. Both are polypeptides, with a sulfide link between two cysteines. The arginine vasopressin in man is essential for maximal activity. Both hormones contain eight amino acids; six of them are identical, but oxytocin has leucine and isoleucine instead of arginine and phenylalanine.

Biosynthesis
Both posterior pituitary hormones have been synthesized. The natural compounds are derived from precursor proteins within the hypothalamus. A protein carrier transports them down the axons in membrane vesicles to the neurohypophysis. Appropriate stimuli produce the action potentials within the hypothalamus all the way down the system to the neurohypophysis. There they discharge from nerve terminals.

Release
Vasopressin is synthesized mostly in the supraoptic nucleus of the hypothalamus whereas oxytocin is synthesized primarily in the paraventricular nuclei. Both hormones while still in the hypothalamus are packaged in neurosecretory granules, bound with a protein called neurophysin.

Several factors influence release from the posterior pituitary to the plasma. The hormones dissociate from neurophysin after their secretion. The hypothalamus responds first to any one or more of a great diversity of stimuli and in turn controls the hormonal release. As one example, the release is influenced by extracellular fluid osmolarity. Ingestion of water inhibits release.

Normal Bodily Effects
Vasopressin
The chief effect of this hormone is to maintain the osmolarity of the blood. This is accomplished by a marked antidiuretic effect. Water reabsorption by the kidney distal tubules and collecting ducts is activated.

Vasopressin stimulates smooth muscles of blood vessels, intestine, and uterus. This is a pressor effect. There is peripheral vasoconstriction, but the effect on blood pressure is weak.

Oxytocin

The effects are chiefly on reproductive functions in the female, although it is present in the male in whom the functions are obscure or nonexistent. Oxytocin is a marked stimulant of the pregnant uterus at term and also postpartum. It does not affect blood vessels, water diuresis, coronary arteries, or intestinal smooth muscle.

Basis of Bodily Effects
Vasopressin

Pores for the flow of water along osmotic gradients increase in size. The adenylate cyclase system is activated and the concentration of cAMP is increased.

The hormone promotes water conservation by the renal collecting ducts. In high concentration it causes vasoconstriction. The osmotic pressure of body water is the chief stimulus regulating hormonal secretion. The osmoreceptor cells of the hypothalamus sense the stimuli. This mechanism is the first line of defense in water balance control.

Oxytocin

This hormone causes smooth muscle cells surrounding the alveoli of the mammary glands to contract. Milk then flows from the alveoli to the large sinuses when the milk is to be expressed. The hormonal release is a response to impulses from the nipples during suckling.

For the uterus, the contraction of its smooth muscle cells is highly dependent on estrogen, although the mechanism of action of oxytocin is uncertain.

ANTERIOR LOBE
Structure and Development

The pituitary gland is divided into three parts: (1) anterior lobe, (2) posterior lobe, and (3) infundibulum. The anterior lobe is in turn divided into the pars distalis and pars tuberalis. These two sections plus a pars intermedia are usually termed the adenohypophysis. In the human infant, the pars intermedia can be seen between the pars distalis and the pars nervosa (neurohypophysis), but in adults fusion occurs between the greater lobes and the intermediate lobe becomes obscure.

The anterior lobe in the fetus forms from an ectodermal evagination of the stomodeum (primordial mouth) just anterior to the buccopharyngeal membrane (Rathke's pouch). At the third fetal week, this grows toward the infundibulum, which is a downward extension of the diencephalon. At the close of the second month, Rathke's pouch loses its connection with the mouth and comes into contact with the infundibulum. Cells in the pouch proliferate and form the anterior lobe of the pituitary gland. The pars intermedia develops from the posterior wall of Rathke's pouch. The infundibulum produces the stalk and the pars nervosa.

The hypothalamus develops a portal venous system to transmit its regulatory factors into the anterior lobe of the pituitary gland. The portal secretions are pulsatile. They induce effects through calcium, cAMP, and membrane phospholipid mediators.

Classification

Hormones secreted by the anterior pituitary are generally large proteins or glycoproteins. They include human growth hormone (hGH; somatotropin), ACTH, TSH, gonadotropic hormones (follicle-stimulating hormone [FSH] and luteinizing hormone [LH]), and prolactin (PRL).

In addition to the above, the hypothalamus produces releasing and inhibitory hormones (or factors) which regulate the anterior pituitary hormonal secretions. These include TRH,

CRH, growth hormone-releasing hormone (GHRH), growth hormone-inhibiting hormone (GHIH), gonadotropin-releasing hormone (GnRH), prolactin-releasing hormone (PRH), and prolactin-inhibiting hormone (PIH), which is probably dopamine.

Biosynthesis

FSH, LH, and PRL originate from basophilic cells of the anterior pituitary. Growth hormone (GH) comes from acidophilic cells. ACTH also comes from basophilic cells and it is classified as a polypeptide called β-lipoprotein (β-lipotropic hormone; β-LPH). The β-lipoproteins produce the endorphins and enkephalins, which are opioids which simulate narcotics such as morphine.

Although the hormones of the neurohypophysis are synthesized in the hypothalamus with their binding proteins, from which they are later separated, the situation for the anterior pituitary hormones is less well known. Being larger molecules, they probably do not need binding for the transport process.

Release

On the afferent aspect the hypothalamus receives its signals from various areas of the cerebral cortex and also from the lower brain and spinal cord. This releases the neurotransmitters, which link visceral and intellectual stimuli acting by way of the hypothalamus and from there to the anterior pituitary and finally to target organs. Stimulating the release of anterior lobe hormones is the major function of the hypothalamus in its relation to the anterior lobe of the pituitary. The hypothalamic control of releasing factors is a result of both humoral and neural afferent stimuli.

Normal Bodily Effects of the Hormones Produced Within the Anterior Pituitary
Growth Hormone

GH regulates bodily growth, including the skeleton, connective tissue, and visceral organs. This requires synthesis of nucleic acid and proteins. GH lipolyses fat cells and regulates the homeostasis of glucose. GH is inhibited by somatostatin, which comes from the delta cells of the pancreas and from the hypothalamus as GHIH.

Adrenocorticotropin

ACTH stimulates secretion of cortisol and adrenal androgens, stimulates utilization of glucose and release of fatty acids, and enhances release of insulin from the pancreas. It may also have an effect on behavior.

Thyroid-Stimulating Hormone

TSH is a polypeptide glycoprotein produced and released by the anterior pituitary gland. Its function is to produce and release T_3 and T_4 within the thyroid gland. The thyroid hormones are essential for bodily growth, development, and metabolism. The hypothalamus controls the TSH level through its TRH.

Gonadotropins (FSH and LH)

FSH activates the proliferation of ovarian follicles during the follicular phase of the ovarian cycle. In the male, it increases the activity of the seminiferous tubules.

LH is involved in the maturation of the ovarian follicles and their transformation to corpora lutea in the luteal phase of the nonpregnant ovarian cycle. In the male it stimulates the Leydig cells and the output of testosterone.

Prolactin

PRL is a peptide hormone stimulated mostly by pregnancy, nursing, sleep, and stress. It is produced in both sexes. In the female, its lactogenic and mammotropic effects involve ovarian and adrenal steroids, insulin, and probably the thyroid hormones. It can produce an antigonadal action, such as the absence of the menses. Some effects are similar to those of GH.

Basis of Bodily Effects of Hormones Produced Within the Anterior Pituitary
Growth Hormone (GH)

GH is regulated by the GHRH and the GHIH, both originating in the hypothalamus. The ventromedial nucleus of the hypothalamus releases GHRH. The nutritional status of the body tissues may be a prime regulator of this release.

GH increases transport of amino acids through cell membranes. It enhances protein synthesis through RNA translation on the ribosomes and the transcription of DNA in the nuclei of cells. It also has a diabetogenic effect.

An adjunctive substance called somatostatin may act by inhibiting secretion of thyrotropin and other substances. It induces liver synthesis of peptide factors called somatomedins, which mediate the effects of GH on skeletal tissues.

Adrenocorticotropin

The activation of the rate of synthesis of adrenal cortical steroids by ACTH is by its stimulation of cholesterol to pregnenolone. ACTH brings about skin darkening by dispersing skin melanin. It has a lipolytic action by activating triglyceride lipase. It stimulates adenylate cyclase, producing a cascade of reactions.

Thyroid-Stimulating Hormone

TSH acts by binding to its specific receptor in cell membranes within the thyroid gland. Adenylate cyclase is activated and cAMP is increased, followed by the stages leading to thyroid development and functions.

Although TSH secretion is stimulated by TRH from the hypothalamus, it is inhibited by somatostatin and by T_3 and T_4 levels in the thyroid gland.

Gonadotropins (FSH and LH)

One of the substances in this category called human chorionic gonadotropin (hCG) produces effects similar to those of LH, but it is a placental hormone and will not be discussed at this point.

The receptors for FSH and LH are distinct. FSH activates adenylate cyclase in the membranes of the Sertoli cells of the testes and in the granulosa cells of the ovaries. LH activates adenylate cyclase, with the subsequent generation of cAMP followed by the appropriate cellular cascade of events.

Prolactin

PRL exerts its actions by binding to glycoprotein receptors, followed by augmented synthesis of mRNA for casein and α-lactalbumin. The lactogenic and mammotropic effects involve the adjunctive action of the hormones that follow. Estrogen and progesterone in the postpubertal ovary enhance proliferation of the mammary glands and this is facilitated by thyroid hormones and adrenal cortical steroids. Placental output of estrogens, progesterones, and gonadotropins is the final stage in the maturation of the mammary glands. Suckling is the mechanism in the production of milk. Suckling causes the release of oxytocin, thus producing contraction of the mammary myoepithelial cells.

Although secretion of most anterior pituitary hormones is controlled chiefly by stimulating hormones, PRL secretion is tonically inhibited by dopamine.

KIDNEY HORMONES

RENIN-ANGIOTENSIN SYSTEM

The renin-angiotensin system, along with aldosterone from the adrenal cortex, is the prime regulator of sodium and potassium balance and of blood pressure-fluid volume homeostasis. Renin is the enzyme that initiates the synthetic processes leading to the formation of the active hormone, angiotensin-II (AT-II). In this synthesis, the release of aldosterone occurs. In turn, aldosterone acts on the renal distal tubules to bring about sodium resorption from tubules to plasma. In the process, plasma potassium levels become stabilized. The regulation of aldosterone output is controlled to a lesser degree by ACTH from the anterior pituitary.

Structure of the Kidney for Renin Output

Most renal nephrons lie close to the surface of the kidney and are called cortical nephrons. Those nephrons extending from the glomeruli that lie deep in the cortex are called juxtamedullary; these extend far down into the medulla of the kidney and then return to the cortex. Their epithelial cells in the distal tubule are called the macula densa; these send secretions toward the arterioles. Thus arterioles in close contact with the epithelial cells are packed with renin and are called juxtaglomerular cells. These cells plus the macula densa are called the juxtaglomerular complex. A paucity of sodium and chloride ions at the macula densa stimulates the juxtaglomerular cells to release active renin. This catalyzes angiotensin to increase the glomerular filtration rate. The ion concentrations may then return to normal levels and thus provide a feedback mechanism for constancy in renal function.

Classification

Renin is a proteolytic enzyme produced when the juxtaglomerular cells of the kidney are stimulated by reduction in (1) sodium concentration or (2) blood volume.

Angiotensin is an octapeptide hormone containing eight amino acids.

Biosynthesis

The enzyme renin is synthesized in the juxtaglomerular cells where it is stored as an inactive form called prorenin. A drop in arterial pressure plus other factors stimulate renin release. The ensuing cascade involves splitting of angiotensinogen to angiotensin-I (AT-I), a decapeptide, and then to AT-II by an enzyme in the lung and also in the brain and kidney.

AT-II does not remain long in the body. It is converted by aminopeptidases to des-Asp-heptapeptide (AT-III), and this is changed to inactive substances by angiotensinases.

Release of Renin and Angiotensin

Renin

One mechanism of renin release may involve pressure or stretch-sensitive receptors in the renal afferent arterioles. A second mechanism may be the macula densa receptors responding to changing sodium concentrations. Disturbances in potassium balance may be a stimulus. Plasma angiotensin levels act as another feedback mechanism. Even autonomic nerves can take part in the mechanisms of action.

Angiotensin

Renin in the blood reacts with a protein that is an α_2 globulin protein fraction. This fraction is produced in the liver and is called angiotensinogen. This substance is hydrolyzed by renin to release AT-I, a decapeptide. A converting enzyme in the vascular epithelium, primarily in the lungs and called depeptidyl carboxypeptidase, changes AT-I to AT-II. AT-III, along with AT-II, is released into the plasma.

Normal Bodily Effects of Angiotensin-II

AT-II is a powerful vasoconstrictor for systemic arterioles. It affects the vasomotor centers in the medulla, involving the sympathetic postganglionics to release catecholamines. This elevates both systolic and diastolic blood pressures. Thus, it is an extremely potent pressor compound. It has a minor stimulating action on the heart. Its potency on the vessels is much greater than that of AT-III.

The compound stimulates aldosterone synthesis by the adrenal cortex. Renal tubular sodium ion resorption is increased. Aldosterone-III may have a similar effect.

AT-II induces platelet aggregation, inhibits plasminogen activity, and is chemotactic to mononuclear cells. It activates the circumventricular organs to increase water input, vasopressin secretion, and ACTH action. This compound may be a central transmitter because all its components are also found in the brain.

Basis of Angiotensin-II Bodily Effects

AT-II actions are mediated by specific receptors located on the cell surface of target organs such as arterioles, adrenal cortices, kidneys, and sympathetic nerve endings. Its binding to arterial smooth muscle cells activates cellular phopholipase C. This produces second messengers, e.g., inositol phosphate and diacylglycerol. Calcium ions increase and muscle contractile force is enhanced.

The compound has a growth promoting effect due to activation of protein kinase C; this accelerates gene transcription and protein synthesis in cells.

The action of the compound to produce retention of salt and water is to constrict kidney blood vessels and to activate tubular resorption. By increasing the rate of aldosterone secretion, sodium resorption is increased greatly.

The arteriole pressure increases because of the osmotic effects in the blood vessels from salt and water retention.

ERYTHROPOIETIN (HEMOPOIETIN)
Structure, Development, and Aging

Red blood cells, platelets, and white blood cells after birth are produced in the bone marrow. Erythropoietin is a hormone that acts in the bone marrow to increase the rate of red blood cell production in response to hypoxia. Lymphocytes can also form in the thymus and lymph organs after birth. In the third fetal week, the blood cells appear in the splanchnic mesoderm of the yolk sac and this region is called the angioblast. About the same time, blood cells develop in the extraembryonic mesoderm of the placental villi and in the connecting stalk (basis of the future placenta) of the mother. In late fetal life, blood cell production is transferred to the liver, spleen, and lymph nodes. About 25% of the blood cells manufactured by the marrow are red cells in the process of maturing to their final erythrocyte stage. At about 20 years of age the marrow is no longer active, except for the vertebrae, sternum, ribs, pelvis, calvaria, and the ends of the long bones. The yellow marrow, which accumulates fat, becomes inactive, but it can regain function in certain hematologic disorders.

The average life of the mature erythrocytes in a person's circulation is about 120 days. There is an endocrine control of the production and release of the erythrocytes that maintains the constancy of these processes. The hormone is erythropoietin, produced in the kidneys, but the liver is the chief site in the first few weeks of life.

Classification

Erythropoietin is a glycoprotein having a molecular weight of about 34,000.

Biosynthesis

Erythropoietin is produced chiefly in the kidneys, although the liver may be a source. In the kidney, the glomerular epithelium is one probable site of formation. Another site is the juxtaglomerular cells. Nephrectomy, however, does not always abolish the formation of the hormone.

There is a substance called renal erythropoietic factor (erythrogenin), secreted by the kidneys from a precursor plasma globulin, that may have originated in the liver or kidneys; this is involved in the synthesis of erythropoietin.

Release

In bleeding, very high elevation, or any disorder causing hypoxia, synthesis and output of red blood cells from the bone marrow is increased. If the red cells increase considerably, as in certain polycythemias, then the natural production and release may be variably lowered. The mechanism involves erythropoietin. A polycythemia can occur if a malignant tumor, usually renal, is overproducing the hormone. The condition called polycythemia vera may occur when red cell precursor cells arise from regulatory failures during cell-line maturation.

Normal Bodily Effects

The rate of red cell production is not regulated directly by the red cell concentration but indirectly by the capacity to transport sufficient oxygen to tissue cells. Red cell production must be significantly involved as a mechanism of adaptation. Erythropoietin does respond to oxygen lack from any cause by increasing red cell production in the bone marrow. In the absence of the hormone, the marrow does not respond. Hypoxia in that case does not display a stimulating effect.

The half-life of erythropoietin is about five hours in the circulation, but its effects on obtaining maximal red cell numbers in the blood may take several days.

There is a growing literature on the role of extracellular factors in the proliferation and differentiation of hemopoietic cells. The mechanisms involve hemopoietic growth factors, cytokines, and oncogenes.[3]

Basis of Bodily Effects

Erythropoietin stimulates the stem cells in the bone marrow to convert to proerythroblasts. This requires mRNA synthesis. The hormone increases the rate of cell division of the stem cells and hastens differentiation of these cells through a line of successive cells that end as mature erythrocytes. The entire process is closely coordinated with iron metabolism, which is essential for hemoglobin production. Lipoproteins are also needed for the construction of the red cell membranes.

CARDIAC HORMONES

ATRIAL NATRIURETIC FACTOR
Site of Origin

Although there may be other cardiac hormones, the atrial natriuretic factor (ANF) is the one most completely defined. The ANF is located in cells in both the right and left cardiac atria but chiefly in the right atrium. It is produced within the myocardial cells. The ANF, in contributing to blood volume control, acts as a set of stretch receptors in the atrial muscles.

Classification

ANF in the human is a polypeptide derived from a molecule with 151 amino acid residues. ANF is probably only one of several natriuretic factors.

Biosynthesis

ANF is produced in both atria of the heart under conditions when it is necessary to increase water excretion because of high blood volume.

Release

ANF is released when an increase in blood volume stretches the atrial wall; this occurs, for example, when blood enters the right atrium from the venae cavae. The hormonal release is a response to augmentation of extracellular fluid volume and to sodium loading.

Normal Bodily Effects

ANF produces an increased rate of glomerular filtration, thus causing both salt and water excretion at the outset of kidney function.

ANF inhibits the release of renin, vasopressin, and aldosterone. Blood pressure and volume are decreased. It exerts a marked inhibition of vessel contraction that may have been caused by epinephrine and AT-II. It is an important regulator of sodium chloride and water distribution in tissues. Overall, ANF is an important regulating agency for blood volume.

Sodium ion excretion is one of its major effects. It does not affect sodium transport mechanisms across cell membranes. It stimulates guanylase cyclase activity, particularly in kidney glomeruli. This enzyme helps form guanosine monophosphate (GMP), a second messenger that inhibits smooth muscle contraction. The inhibition involves changing the degree of phosphorylation of several enzymes. Intracellular calcium ion concentration is reduced.

Basis of Bodily Effects

There are ANF-containing neurons in the brain, with a pathway from the hypothalamus to the medullary area of the brain that regulates blood vessel diameters. If the blood volume increases, so do cardiac output, blood pressure, and urinary flow, although only over the first few hours. The concomitant elevated pressure in the right atrium causes pressure augmentation within that atrium. This becomes the stimulus for afferent impulse transmission to the brain. On the efferent side, nerves to the kidney exert an effect on the vessels, which results in elevated urine flow.

When ANF dilates renal blood vessels, sodium output is increased. ANF inhibits tubular resorption and the ADH of the posterior pituitary, adding to the increased urine output. These adjustments may not be long term.

Another adjunctive mechanism involves the simultaneous responsiveness of the carotid sinus baroceptor; this adds to the effects of the atrial volume receptors.

Overall, the right side of the heart has adaptive reactions to the volume flow of blood through it. Because of the local mechanisms that exist, the cardiac chambers pump out a volume of blood equal to the venous input.

GASTROINTESTINAL HORMONES

The gastrointestinal hormones considered herein are cholecystokinin (CCK; pancreozymin), gastric inhibitory peptide (GIP), gastrin, motilin, secretin, substance P, and vasoactive intestinal peptide (VIP). These are manufactured and released from the mucosa of the stomach and/or small intestine.

CHOLECYSTOKININ (PANCREOZYMIN)
Structure

The lining of the small intestine secretes CCK. The hormone is put out in the duodenum and jejunum.

Classification

CCK is a polypeptide containing 33 amino acids. This is its physiologic form in the gastrointestinal tract. It has the same C-terminal tetrapeptide as gastrin. A sulfate group on the seventh C-terminal amino acid is important for its biologic activity. CCK is found in certain neurons of the central nervous system.

Biosynthesis

The formation of CCK involves the usual steps in the synthesis of proteins.

Release

The alimentary form of CCK is released in response to the presence of certain fatty acids, but other foodstuffs are also stimuli. These include some single amino acids, proteoses, and peptones. Undigested protein is an ineffective releaser whereas phenylalanine is a potent releaser.

The chyme in the intestine evokes the secretion of CCK. The hormone directly stimulates the acinar cells of the pancreas to release its contents of zymogen granules, but there is very little activation of the pancreatic duct epithelium.

Normal Bodily Effects

CCK is the chief endocrine stimulus of enzyme secretion from the acinar cells of the pancreas. Large amounts of pancreatic enzymes and the aqueous components of pancreatic juice are secreted. This simulates vagal nerve action. CCK importantly promotes the emptying of bile from the gallbladder, the presence of fats being essential in the meal. CCK diminishes secretory activity of the stomach when gastric emptying is taking place. The endocrine effect on emptying is aided by the enterogastric reflex in which duodenal acidity activates vagal afferents to decrease gastric motility and emptying. CCK stimulates glucagon release as well as the release of insulin.

Basis of Bodily Effects

CCK is the most important mediator of the pancreatic exocrine response to the digestive products of certain lipids and proteins. CCK may produce its effects by increasing intracellular calcium efflux from pancreatic acinar cells.

CCK competes with gastrin for receptor sites on target cells, thus blocking the action of gastrin. CCK inhibits the parietal cells that produce stomach acid secretion. In general, hormones that stimulate pancreatic acinar cells do so by raising cAMP or the ionic calcium levels.

GASTRIC INHIBITORY PEPTIDE
Structure

GIP is produced by the mucosal cells of the duodenum and jejunum. It was once considered to be a hypothetical hormone called enterogastrone.

Classification

GIP is a peptide containing 43 amino acids. Chemically, it resembles secretin.

Biosynthesis

The synthesis of proteins in general holds for GIP.

Release

Carbohydrates such as glucose in the duodenum and proximal jejunum are prime stimulants for the release of GIP. There is also a stimulating effect of fat and protein products in the duodenum and upper jejunum. The vagus nerve may secrete GIP as a final transmitter to the target cells.

Normal Bodily Effects

GIP is an inhibitor of stomach acid secretion, motility, and emptying. It also regulates the release of insulin from the pancreas.

Basis of Bodily Effects

The hormone acts directly on the islet cells of the pancreas. It inhibits gastric acid secretion by preventing gastrin release and also by inhibiting parietal cell acid secretion.

GASTRIN
Structure

There are several types of productive cells in the gut. The G cells secrete gastrin in the duodenum and proximal jejunum.

Classification

Gastrin is a polypeptide. One form, G-34, contains 34 amino acids. A second form, G-17, has 17 amino acids and is the more abundant species; G-17 is also called gastrin I or little gastrin. G-34 is called big gastrin and is much less important than gastrin I.

Biosynthesis

Gastrin is not only produced by G cells in the pyloric stomach and in the intestinal mucosa, but is also found in the pituitary gland and in some peripheral nerves.

Release

Gastrin secretion is regulated by food in the stomach and small intestine. Mechanical wall distention activates stretch receptors, which in turn increase motility and secretion. The chemical stimuli are chiefly the peptides of protein hydrolysis. These act on the G cells and release gastrin in the very active or second (gastric) phase of stomach digestion. Stimulation of the vagal nerve fibers also helps to release gastrin.

Normal Bodily Effects

Gastrin has a positive motor effect on the stomach muscles. Whether the hormone plays a part in the early cephalic phase of gastric digestion is uncertain.

The upper intestine, which contains G cells, releases gastrin upon stimulation by amino acids and peptides. The hormone can stimulate the stomach parietal cells to increase their secretion of hydrochloric acid; the acid is built from the reaction of hydrogen ions and chloride ions, both compounds having entered the mucosa from the blood.

Basis of Bodily Effects

The activity of gastrin lies in its terminal four amino acids. Also, the pH of the gastric juice importantly determines the ability of gastrin to stimulate secretion. A pH of 2.0 blocks the exit of gastrin from the mucosa to the lumen. A low acidity inhibits the neurally active secretion which is a regulatory feedback system.

MOTILIN
Structure

The cells in the lining of the upper small intestine produce and release motilin.

Classification

Motilin is a polypeptide containing 22 amino acids. It is classified as a neuroactive, gut-brain peptide.

Biosynthesis

In general, neuropeptides may be produced in the cell bodies of neurons. Following encoding by DNA, they are transcribed to mRNA and this is translated on polyribosomes bound to the endoplasmic reticulum. Transport to the Golgi complex then occurs.

Neurohormones may be produced as preprohormones and then converted to prohormones, after which they are cleaved to peptide sequences.

Release

Secretory vesicles pass from the Golgi complex to axon terminals. The stimulus for hormonal release is uncertain. The cleavage of the substance within the vesicles as a neuro-humor is followed by its release to an active peptide.

Normal Bodily Effects

Motilin acts as both a hormone and a neurotransmitter. It is widely distributed in the body, as seen by its presence in the central nervous system where it excites most corticospinal neurons. In animal experiments, the hormone increases the motility of the stomach and intestine and it activates contraction of the lower esophageal sphincter.

Motilin may be the hormone that initiates the migrating myoelectric complexes that travel intermittently from the stomach through the ileum and which, as electrical outbursts, clean the intestine down as far as the cecum. During feeding, motilin is not released.

Basis of Bodily Effects

There is much uncertainty in this category. Whatever stimuli cause the glands to secrete motilin, it is the release from the vesicles that produces the target effects.

SECRETIN
Structure and Development

Secretin is a hormone derived from the mucosa of the duodenum and also from the jejunum. It is among the gut compounds that originate in the ectoblast of the embryo.

Classification

Secretin is a hormone containing 27 amino acids, all of which are needed for adequate activity. The compound exists in more than one form.

Biosynthesis

The synthesis of secretin follows the usual sequence for that of proteins in general.

Release

The hormone is contained in granules concentrated close to capillaries. It is released chiefly in response to the low pH of the gastric contents entering the small intestine. The release from the small intestinal mucosa is especially great when the pH drops below 4.5. Fatty acids are another set of releasing stimuli.

Normal Bodily Effects

The primary action of secretin is to stimulate in the duodenum a copious secretion of pancreatic fluid and bicarbonate. It also stimulates the growth of the exocrine pancreas. In these functions, it is assisted by CCK. Secretin stimulates secretion of biliary fluid and bicarbonate, an activity also complemented by CCK. Secretin and CCK stimulate the chief cells to secrete pepsinogens.

Basis of Bodily Effects

The activity of secretin requires its binding with a specific receptor on the membranes of appropriate digestive cells. This involves the activation of adenylate cyclase and the conversion of ATP to cAMP. The cascade of target events follows.

SUBSTANCE P
Structure
Substance P is produced and released in several areas of the body. Its hormonal status is uncertain. It occurs both in the brain and the digestive tract mucosa.

Classification
Substance P is a polypeptide containing 11 amino acids. Its name comes from the fact that it was originally extracted and stored as a powder. It is a neuroactive gut-brain peptide.

Biosynthesis
The basis of formation of substance P is the general synthesis of proteins.

Release
Substance P can be released in the salivary glands by nerve terminals in the mouth. It is also present in the intestine. Additionally, substance P is found in the nervous system, in the brain and spinal nerves. It is released peripherally by nerve pain fibers situated in the dorsal horns of the spinal cord, from which it travels contralaterally to the brain.

Normal Bodily Effects
Substance P is generally excitatory in the body. It may mediate the myenteric reflex and increase the motility of the small intestine. It stimulates gallbladder contraction. It is a potent salivary secretagogue. It may bring about axon reflexes. It causes vasodilation, thus lowering the blood pressure. It may act as a neurotransmitter in the central and peripheral nervous system. In the brain, it may cause neurons in the substantia nigra to release dopamine.

Basis of Bodily Effects
Substance P exerts its effects by increasing intracellular calcium levels along an inositol phosphate pathway. The release of calcium increases cyclic gAMP, which activates the subsequent cascade of events to the target. Substance P, acting as a neuropeptide, may produce its effects as a hormone or as a neurotransmitter.

VASOACTIVE INTESTINAL PEPTIDE
Structure
The endocrine glands throughout the GI tract include VIP in their secretions. Nerve endings in the gut also contain the hormone.

Classification
VIP is a polypeptide chemically related to secretin and GIP. It contains 28 amino acids.

Biosynthesis
VIP is widely distributed in the central nervous system and in the intrinsic gut neurons. Its synthesis is essentially that for proteins in general.

Release
Stimulation of the vagus nerve, apparently acting as a neurotransmitter, releases VIP from the gut. Other sources of release are uncertain.

Normal Bodily Effects
VIP vasodilates certain blood vessels during secretory activity. It stimulates the release of pancreatic bicarbonate and inhibits the secretion of gastric juice. It also stimulates secretion of intestinal enzymes, pancreatic hormones, glycogen breakdown in the liver, and fat metabolism.

Basis of Bodily Effects

Although VIP is classified as a neuroactive, gut-brain peptide, it is uncertain whether it acts as a true neurotransmitter, a hormone, or a neuromodulator (which regulates synaptic transmission). It may be an inhibitory transmitter to smooth muscle and an excitatory transmitter to glandular epithelial cells.

The hormone appears to be a potent activator of the adenylate cyclase complex in liver, fat cells, and pancreas. The usual cascade of events succeeds the enzyme activity.

PANCREATIC HORMONES

INSULIN

Structure and Development

The pancreas is both an endocrine and exocrine organ. The endocrine aspects, secreted by the islets of Langerhans, are the more prominent. The principal hormones are insulin and glucagon. Other hormones are somatostatin and pancreatic polypeptide. The endocrine cells develop from the endodermal pancreatic ducts. Insulin secretion begins significantly at about the fifth fetal month although the islets develop as early as the 60th to the 90th day.

Classification

Insulin contains two straight chains of polypeptides joined by two disulfide linkages. One chain contains 21 amino acids and the other 30. The molecule is originally a monomer that forms dimers (molecular weight 12,000).

Biosynthesis

Insulin is synthesized in a gene in islet β cells and is transcribed by mRNA to preproinsulin, after which proinsulin is formed. The synthesis occurs in the ribosomes of the endoplasmic reticulum. The proinsulin is cleaved by a protease in the β cells. The insulin formed is stored in granules within the Golgi apparatus. Another fragment that is formed is called C-peptide, but this lacks biologic activity. The granules upon demand travel to the β cell membranes and release their contents into the extracellular spaces. The insulin reaches the tissues by way of the blood. Most of the hormone is inactivated as it passes through the liver.

Release

The release of insulin is by exocytosis. After a meal, insulin blood levels may increase markedly because of the excess of food. The most important stimulus for release is glucose. Protein digestive products are significant stimuli, especially arginine and lysine.

Insulin is normally transported unbound. Carbohydrates cause its dissociation from any protein carrier. The half-life in the plasma is 5 to 8 min. Release does not appear to involve any regulating factor such as the pituitary or any direct feedback mechanism. However, insulin synthesis and release are increased by the growth hormone, glucose levels, glucagon, secretin, and pancreozymin. Release is inhibited by epinephrine and α-adrenergic receptors, whereas it is stimulated by interaction with β-adrenergic receptors. Insulin is metabolized chiefly in the kidney and liver by a specific protease and a transhydrogenase.

Normal Bodily Effects

Insulin is the prime regulator of metabolic processes which are anabolic. It influences the metabolism of carbohydrates, fats, and proteins. The organs affected most are adipose tissues, liver, and muscles. In the liver, insulin increases glucose uptake and its storage as glycogen. In muscle, insulin is necessary to transport glucose from plasma to cells, and it has a similar action in adipose tissues. Insulin facilitates transport of magnesium, phosphate, and potassium into muscle, and phosphate and potassium into liver, all for the purposes of glycogen and protein storage.

The metabolism of fat from all sources is greatly affected. Storage is increased. Both mobilization and oxidation of fatty acids are inhibited. Insulin induces the enzymatic secretion of lipoproteins from capillaries to tissues by lipoprotein lipase, thus facilitating fatty acid entrance to the tissues.

Recombinant insulin-like growth factor I (IGF-I) appears to be a potent stimulator of bone growth. It may accomplish this by influencing bone remodeling. Insulin is necessary for the normal liver production of IGF-I.

Basis of Bodily Effects

Insulin action is initiated at the plasma membrane receptors before the hormone enters the cells. Uptake of glucose across the membranes and into cells is increased, thus lowering sugar in the blood. The hormone apparently hastens the activity of a carrier molecule in the membranes. Pyruvate and lactate increase because of greater utilization of glucose. Organic phosphate decreases as glucose is phosphorylated. Plasma potassium decreases because the liver storage of glycogen is accompanied by potassium entrance to the liver. The actions of insulin on fat and protein metabolism are independent of the actions on glucose. The storage of foodstuffs is a major function of insulin.

Glucose is continually released from its storage in the liver, a process which importantly involves glucose-6-phosphatase. Glucose is convertible to α-glycerophosphate, which changes in turn to free fatty acids and triglycerides. Overall, insulin is active in many of the processes occurring in the intermediate metabolism of foodstuffs. Receptors for insulin have been identified in osteoblasts.

GLUCAGON
Structure and Development

There are several types of cells in the pancreas. The acinar cells contain the zymogen granules for exocrine secretion. The islets of Langerhans produce the endocrine secretion. The islet β cells manufacture insulin, whereas the islet α cells manufacture glucagon. The islets also have γ and δ cells whose functions are uncertain.

Classification

Glucagon is a polypeptide. It is composed of a single straight chain of 29 amino acid residues. The molecular weight is about 3500.

Biosynthesis

Glucagon in humans is synthesized on chromosome 2 by α cells in the islets. A prepro-hormone is converted to a prohormone called glycentin, which is localized to the peripheral area of the secretory granules whereas glucagon is in the core of the granules. In several animal species, glucagon is synthesized in the GI tract.

Release

Glucagon is synthesized and released from secretory storage granules by exocytosis in the α cells of the islets of Langerhans. In humans, the release occurs mostly if glucose is low in the circulation. This contrasts with the effect of glucose on insulin secretion. Glucagon is also secreted in response to a protein meal, especially if it contains alanine and arginine.

The secretion of glucagon is increased by generalized stress and by autonomic nerve stimulation. High levels of circulating fatty acids inhibit glucagon secretion. The hormone circulates mostly unbound in the plasma.

Normal Bodily Effects

Glucagon actions are for the most part opposite to insulin actions. Thus, it makes energy available to tissues, especially between meals. It promotes mobilization but not storage of energy sources, e.g., glucose. It is called the hyperglycemic factor, protecting against hypoglycemia.

The primary target organ of glucagon is the liver in which it maintains the ouput of glucose. This is its most important effect. It influences the rates of hepatic glycogenolysis, glycolysis, lipolysis, and gluconeogenesis. Epinephrine, in particular, is a similar promoter of liver glycogenolysis. Glucagon may not stimulate glycogenolysis in muscle and it does not appear to nave an effect on the peripheral tissue utilization of glucose.

Glucagon is ketogenic as well as hyperglycemic. It also activates adipose tissue lipase. It inhibits sodium resorption by the kidney tubules. It activates adenylate cyclase in the cardiocytes and increases both cardiac contractility and rate.

The hormone is degraded mostly in the liver and kidney. The half-life of pancreatic glucagon is about 6 min.

Basis of Bodily Effects

Glucagon initiates metabolic processes by binding in the liver to a specific receptor, which couples to adenylate cyclase by a guanine nucleotide binding protein. There also appears to be an inhibitory guanine nucleotide binding regulatory protein whose functions are unclear. Cyclic AMP in the liver quickly increases. Protein kinases are activated, which in turn lead to the formation of phosphorylase b and then phosphorylase a kinases. The end result is the enhancement of glycogenolysis. Glucagon can also elevate liver gluconeogenesis and inhibit glycolysis. These actions involve cAMP and an increase in protein kinase activity.

Glucoreceptors in the hypothalamus respond to rapidly falling glucose concentration. It may be that stimulation of glucagon involves the activation of the sympathetic nervous system through fibers descending from the hypothalamus and ending in the pancreas. There may be an effect of glucose deprivation in the α cells, or even an effect secondary to circulating epinephrine.

MALE SEX HORMONES

ANDROGENS
Structure, Development, and Aging

All male sex hormones are called androgens. The testes are the principle source for their syntheses. The important androgen produced in the testis is testosterone. A second, less potent hormone is androsterone. In certain states, the adrenal cortex may secrete significant amounts of androgens.

The testes are composed mainly of seminiferous tubules wherein the sperm are produced by a succession of maturing germ cells. Interstitial cells of Leydig are located between the tubules and they produce the hormonal secretions of the testes. Sertoli cells are supporting epithelial cells in the tubule system. They gain contact with the developing sperm and provide or exclude nutrients to and from the fluid surrounding the germ cells and the tubules, thus acting as a blood-testis barrier.

The fetal testes produce androgens, which stimulate growth of the penis, formation of the penile urethra, and development of the prostate gland and seminal vesicles. Although the Y chromosome of the sperm is male-determining, all developing structures pass through an indifferent stage and may differentiate in either a male or a female direction.

The testicular production of androgen is low before age 10 and increases greatly at male puberty. The hormonal secretion is fairly constant throughout the life of the adult male and sexual development and its functions are maintained under the control of the pituitary gonadotropins. The hormone production declines in very old age.

Classification

The precursor for all adrenocortical hormones is cholesterol, a 27-carbon molecule. The androgens are C-19 steroids and testosterone is the prototype. The androgens are excreted in the urine as 17-ketosteroids, whose origin is chiefly the testis and adrenal cortex in the male and the ovary and adrenal cortex in the female.

Biosynthesis

Testosterone synthesis and release by Leydig cells are regulated by LH, which is controlled by LHRH. The synthesis of gonadal steroids closely resembles that in the adrenal cortex, and this is true in both sexes. The initial precursor is cholesterol, delivered by plasma lipoproteins. LH stimulates the gonads to secrete androgens. In this process, LH binds to membrane receptors, which activate adenylate cyclase, resulting in elevated cAMP levels. There is a subsequent activation of protein kinases, and protein steroidogenesis occurs.

Within the mitochondria, the following scheme of steroid forming events occurs: acetyl coenzyme A produces cholesterol in the Leydig cells and these convert to Δ^5-pregnenolone. The following chain of successive compounds are 17-α-OH-pregnenolone, dehydroepiandrosterone, androstenedione, and testosterone.

In the above steps within the testes, the cholesterol is synthesized and stored as esters in the Leydig cells. Some cholesterol is sent to the endoplasmic reticulum for chemical completion to testosterone.

Release

The release of testosterone by the interstitial cells of Leydig requires that these cells be activated. This is accomplished by a feedback system to the anterior pituitary gland. The pituitary secretes the gonadotropin, LH, also known as the interstitial cell stimulating hormone. The response of the cells of Leydig to the LH action catalyzes spermatogenesis. Other hormones, including FSH, and probably estradiol, prolactin, and growth hormone, are mutually interactive in the control of spermatogenesis.

The hypothalamus is involved in a regulatory manner because it transports releasing factors to the anterior pituitary, which in turn releases its gonadotropins that are transported in the blood to the testes. The action of FSH is to stimulate the germinal epithelium of the seminiferous tubules. The androgen feedback exerts a negative effect on the central centers and this in turn regulates the synthesis of FSH.

Normal Bodily Effects

Testosterone develops and maintains male secondary sexual characteristics that have been markedly activated at the time of puberty. Even in the fetus, the hormone has already initiated differentiation of the male phenotype.

Testosterone, by feedback, regulates pituitary gonadotropin secretion. It has an anabolic action on proteins. It favors growth of epiphyseal cartilage and closure of the bone epiphyses; closure is also regulated by androgens in the female.

The Sertoli cells of the testes are important. In the fetus, they control the development and descent of the testes, the germ cells, and the cells that secrete hormones responsible for masculinization. In adulthood they nourish the early germ cells as they mature into sperm. Also in the fetus, a hormone named mullerian inhibiting substance is produced by Sertoli cells and is claimed to cause the regression in the male of the fetal structures called the mullerian ducts at about eight weeks. These ducts in the female differentiate into the fallopian tubes.

The androgens of the adrenal gland are not important in males, because testosterone is produced chiefly in the testes.

Basis of Bodily Effects

Activation of protein synthesis results from an effect of testosterone on microsomal ribonucleic acid. Testosterone from the Leydig cells stimulates the epithelium of the seminiferous tubules, thus providing the androgens needed for sperm production. In prostate gland chemistry, testosterone converts to dihydrotestosterone, the active compound in the prostate gland. The enzyme involved is 5-α-reductase. The mechanism of testosterone control of Leydig cells involves cAMP and its sequelae of chemical changes.

FEMALE SEX HORMONES

ESTROGENS
Structure, Development, and Aging

Estrogens are synthesized in the ovaries, placenta, and adrenal cortex. In the male, synthesis is in the testes, liver, and other tissues. The ovary in the nongravid female is the primary source. Its follicles in the first half of the ovarian cycle secrete estrogens by its granulosa cells. The estrogens include β-estradiol, estrone, and estriol. Estradiol is the most important for development of the female phenotype. At ovulation, the second half of the cycle begins and the empty follicle becomes a new endocrine producer called the corpus luteum; this secretes progesterone and some β-estradiol. The growth of the follicles as well as its estrogen secretions are stimulated by FSH from the anterior pituitary. Toward the close of the follicular phase, two to three days before ovulation occurs, LH is stimulated to secretion by way of positive feedback on the hypothalamus but mainly on the anterior pituitary. Between ovulation and menstruation, the hormones exert a negative effect on the hypothalamus and pituitary and this suppresses FSH and LH; these will increase again beginning with menstruation.

FSH causes growth of the follicle and its production of estrogens. LH stimulates interstitial cells in the ovary and thus the corpus luteum. Ovulation is stimulated and FSH secretion is inhibited. In pregnancy the placenta becomes the source of progesterone.

The primordial germ cells develop in the walls of the yolk sac at about the fourth embryonic week. They proliferate and migrate to the ovaries in which they convert to oogonia and some to primary oocytes. Further development ceases until puberty. During menopause the follicles and their eggs begin to disappear.

Classification

All estrogens and progesterone are steroids. A controlling hormone from the hypothalamus, LHRH or GnRH, is a decapeptide. The anterior pituitary FSH and LH are proteins. LHRH controls the release of FSH and LH. In turn, FSH is the major control of the follicular phase of the ovarian cycle and LH is the major regulator of the luteal phase.

Biosynthesis

In the nongravid female, in the production of estrogens, the precursor is cholesterol, brought in from the plasma. Under the influence of LH, pregnenolone is synthesized. From there, one pathway will lead to the formation of progesterone. The other can convert to 17-hydroxyprogesterone, then androstenedione. This last compound can convert to estrone, estradiol, and estriol.

In pregnancy, estrogen precursors are formed in the adrenal glands and transported to the placenta where they are built to estradiol, estrone, and estriol. The female also produces testosterone. To do this, the ovary and adrenal cortex utilize steroid prohormones such as androstenedione and dehydroepiandrosterone; these are finally converted to testosterone in the liver and peripheral tissues.

Release

Estrogens are secreted by precursors of the follicular cells called granulosa cells and by another layer of follicular cells called the theca interna. Another source, of lesser importance, is the adrenal cortex.

Normal Bodily Effects

In the nongravid female, estrogens are essential for the growth and development of the sex organs. They aid uterine development and promote cyclic changes in the endometrium. They are necessary for maturation of secondary sexual characteristics. In pregnancy, they stimulate development of the mammary glands and uterine enlargement and relax pelvic ligaments. They promote deposition of fat in subcutaneous tissues. They regulate bone growth in length, more so than androgens do in males.

Basis of Bodily Effects

The estrogens bind to specific receptors that are present in the target organs. There are nuclear receptor sites in which the initial complexes are transferred to the nucleus. Processes occur such as the production and utilization of rRNA and this becomes involved in the synthesis of enzymes and proteins. DNA is activated. The overall processes that are essential for the action of progesterone are similar to those for estrogens.

The normal cyclic regulation of ovarian activity, characteristically beginning with puberty, involves first the hypothalamus and its LHRH, the subsequent production of FSH and LH from the pituitary, and the ovarian secretion of female and male hormones.

PROGESTERONE

Elements of the preceding discussion primarily on estrogens apply to the progestins, the major one being progesterone. This hormone is a 21-carbon steroid that is a precursor to other steroids. It is secreted cyclically in nonpregnant women under the influence of LH. In this process, cAMP synthesis in the corpus luteum increases. The testes and the adrenal cortex may be additional sites of progesterone formation. The corpus luteum, which is the chief source of progesterone, develops and its endocrine output in pregnancy is increased by hCG, which starts to be secreted by trophoblast cells of the embryo. At about the 80th day, hCG secretion falls rapidly and remains at a low level throughout pregnancy. However, the placenta takes over and secretes large quantities of estrogen and progesterone. The corpus luteum involutes gradually after the 13th to the 17th week of gestation and its endocrine output is small.

Progesterone is to a great extent a hormone of pregnancy. It prepares the uterus for the implantation of an ovum and maintains the uterus during pregnancy. It inhibits FSH and LH, and this suppresses ovulation during gestation. The hypothalamus is a primary, central, suppressive center because it keeps all the gonadotropins in check until puberty.

Progesterone stimulates maturation of the mammary glands in preparation for lactation. It depresses uterine contractility in pregnancy until a late phase when estrogens dominate and increase the excitability which favors birth at parturition. Progesterone stimulates the decidual cells of the pregnant uterus to synthesize prolactin. Whereas estrogens prime the target tissues, progesterone decreases the number of estrogen receptors, thus favoring anti-estrogen actions. In the nonpregnant female it promotes the changing phases within the uterine cycles.

RELAXIN

The functions of relaxin are limited to the period of pregnancy, at which time the ovaries secrete this peptide hormone. Its actions are to loosen the ligaments of the pubic symphysis and to soften the cervix. These activities importantly assist the delivery of the fetus at parturition.

INHIBIN

Structure, Development, and Aging

Inhibin is a hormone that inhibits the secretion of FSH. The origin of the hormone is most likely the Sertoli cells and probably the seminiferous tubules in males and the ovarian follicles in females.

At the time of birth in males, germ cells have developed in the sex cords of the testes, surrounded by supporting cells which become the Sertoli cells. The sex cords also develop a lumen and become the seminiferous tubules.

Circulating levels of FSH and LH in males increase with aging. After age 40, gonadotropin levels are increasing. Seminiferous tubule degeneration with a decreased inhibin production occurs to a greater extent than decreases in Leydig cell function.

In women, a loss in the secretion of inhibin could explain the higher follicular-phase levels of FSH in the perimenopausal state. In general, inhibin may provide a mechanism to regulate the number of follicles that are maturing during each cycle.

Classification

Inhibin is a polypeptide hormone and a glycoprotein. The compound that has been extracted from ovarian follicular fluid contains three polypeptide subunits. One is an alpha compound with a molecular weight of 18,000. There are two beta subunits, $beta_A$ and $beta_B$, both with molecular weights of 14,000. Subunit alpha can form dimers with $beta_A$ or $beta_B$.

Both inhibin$_A$ (alpha beta$_A$) and inhibin$_B$ (alpha beta$_B$) inhibit FSH secretion. There are other subunits that may stimulate FSH secretion.

Biosynthesis

In the male, inhibin is produced most likely by the Sertoli cells of the testes, although there is a view that the seminiferous tubules can be regions of production. In the female, inhibin is produced by the ovarian follicles and perhaps by the corpus luteum.

Release

The hormone in the male that was produced by the Sertoli cells is also secreted by them. In the female, granulosa cells of the follicles secrete the hormone.

Normal Bodily Effects

Inhibin inhibits FSH secretion in response to GnRH stimulation, without influencing to any marked degree the secretion of LH. The FSH effect is the major function of inhibin. In males the FSH produced acts in turn on the Sertoli cells. LH, however, acts on Leydig cells. It is probable that inhibin is also a factor in the functioning of the seminiferous tubules.

In females, inhibin decreases secretion particularly of the FSH of the anterior pituitary and even LH (controversially). The action is complemented by estrogen and to a lesser degree by progesterone. The inhibition is a negative feedback process. It occurs during the luteal phase of the ovarian cycle, at about the 12th day of the life phase of the corpus luteum. The resultant loss of gonadotropic maintenance from the hypothalamus and pituitary, a short number of days prior to the start of a menstrual cycle, removes the pituitary feedback, whereupon the pituitary again secretes FSH (and LH); the next ovarian cycle then begins.

Basis of Bodily Effects

FSH is inhibited in both males and females by estradiol and testosterone; both block the pituitary response to LHRH. Inhibin is the third blocker. The inhibition is produced in males particularly in the Sertoli cells and in females in the ovarian follicles.

FSH increases the synthesis of inhibin, which produces a feedback loop that helps regulate the availability of FSH according to the demands of specific aspects and stages of gametogenesis. In the male, if the seminiferous tubules do not produce sperm, then the anterior pituitary increases its secretion of FSH. However, if the rate of spermatogenesis increases greatly, FSH secretion decreases. These actions result from activation of the Sertoli secretion of inhibin. There appears to be a simultaneous, although weaker secretion of the hypothalamus.

PLACENTAL HORMONES

The placenta takes care of the food and waste exchange between fetus and mother. It is also an endocrine gland. The hormones secreted are estrogens, progesterone, and the anterior pituitary polypeptide and protein hormones, which include hCG and human chorionic somatomammotropin (hCS; also called placental lactogen [hPL]); hCS consists of a single polypeptide chain containing 191 to 199 amino acid residues. Other placental hormones are also produced.

Human Chorionic Gonadotropin

hCG is a glycoprotein with two subunits. An alpha subunit is identical to that of TSH, FSH, and LH. A beta subunit closely resembles that of LH and has a molecular weight of about 28,000.

hCG is produced and secreted by the syncytiotrophoblast cells of the embryo. These cells are the forerunners of the placenta. The biochemical steps in producing hCG follow that of general protein synthesis.

hCG is detectable in the plasma and urine of pregnant women when the trophoblast structure is well developed. Urine testing about the seventh day measures the beta subunit and is a test for pregnancy. The hCG levels reach a peak at 9 to 12 weeks and decline to a constant level thereafter.

The hCG in pregnancy maintains the growth of the corpus luteum and its secretions and prevents its involution before the 13th to 17th week of pregnancy. The placenta then takes over, secreting estrogen and progesterone.

There is a normal stimulating effect of hCG on the thyroid glands, resulting in an increased production of thyroid hormones. This is reinforced by another TSH secreted by the placenta called human chorionic thyrotropin. Still another hormone called relaxin is secreted by the placenta and also within the corpus luteum under the influence of hCG. Relaxin is a polypeptide whose molecular weight is about 9,000. In certain animals it is claimed to relax the ligaments of the symphysis pubis during the estrous cycle. This effect is weak or missing in pregnant women.

Placental hCG stimulates ovarian functions in the female fetus. When there is reproductive immaturity after birth, hCG no longer acts as a stimulating agent.

hCG is sometimes used clinically to correct failure of ovulation that results from hyposecretion of pituitary gonadotropic hormones. hCG maintains the functions of the corpus luteum in pregnancy for most of its gestation period.

hCG stimulates testosterone production and secretion in the male fetus by activating the production of Leydig cells. These effects are similar to those of LH, which also stimulates Leydig cells to produce testosterone. Another testosterone-producing hormone is PRL, which potentiates the effects of LH.

Human Chorionic Somatomammotropin

hCS (or hPL) is a hormone unique to pregnancy. hCS is a protein with a molecular weight of about 30,000. It is structurally similar to hGH and PRL.

The hormone is formed in the placental syncytiotrophoblast in the fourth or fifth week after ovulation and fertilization. It can be detected in the serum of pregnant women at about six weeks of gestation. Its levels increase progressively to about the 35th week of pregnancy after which they plateau. The levels of hCS in the plasma of the fetus are far less than those in the plasma of the pregnant mother. After delivery of the fetus the hormone disappears quickly from the maternal blood.

In normal function hCS in lower animals, such as sheep and goats, helps stimulate their mammary development, partly supporting the action of PRL. hCS also stimulates milk secretion in these animals. The human female appears to be far less responsive in these actions.

hCS has properties similar to those of hGH, adding protein mass to the body. However, it is much weaker in potency.

hCS probably plays a role in the nutrition of the fetus, particularly in regard to fat and glucose metabolism. Glucose is diverted to the fetus in pregnancy by decreasing the mother's capacity to utilize this sugar. Fatty acids in the maternal adipose tissue are lipolyzed and released, providing the mother with an important store of bioenergetic fuel. The hormone thus directs the metabolic traffic in the fetus, but with special importance in the mother so that she may maintain an appropriate flow of nutrients to the fetus.

APPENDIX I: QUANTITATIVE ASPECTS OF RECEPTOR BINDING

Drugs, including hormones, interact with receptors in the body, and these complexes include a wide variety of structures. Not all drug actions are mediated by receptors, however.

In hormone-receptor interactions the selective nature of the effect on the target organ depends not only on the hormonal messenger but also on the specific receptor involved. A drug acts by triggering a response via an action on that part of the cell called a receptor. A deficiency of receptors or hormones may explain a pathologic effect. The nature of the response may also be determined by a changed concentration of elements in the hormone-receptor complex or by the rate of the drug-receptor events.

The binding forces in a drug-receptor complex are covalent, ionic, hydrogen bonds, and van der Waals forces.[4] In covalent bonds the electrons are shared between atoms. The high-energy covalent bonds are irreversible. Antagonistic drugs with covalent binding produce a noncompetitive antagonism. Ionic bonds are important because many drugs have an anion and cation content with attractive forces. For hydrogen bonds, a hydrogen atom is shared between two reacting polar groups, which strengthens the bond. In van der Waals bonding, the interaction occurs weakly between any two atoms or groups of atoms, but it is effective only over a very short distance.

The reactions occurring in a hormone-receptor system may be quantitatively expressed by dose-response curves. These can show the magnitude of the response as a function of the concentration of the constituents of the complex at the receptor sites. The log of the dose is plotted against the effect, if the dose and the effect are known.

In drug effects, the terms *affinity* and *efficacy* are used frequently and can be differentiated in graphs. Affinity expresses the tendency of a drug to combine with receptors. The magnitude of the response is determined by the number of receptors that react and this is expressed as efficacy, i.e., intrinsic activity or power. The term *power* indicates the amount of transformation in a given time or place. A drug that has both affinity and efficacy is called an agonist. A drug that is called a competitive antagonist has affinity but not efficacy; such a drug competes with another for space on the same receptor.

One can show quantitatively the binding of a drug (D) with the available receptors (R) where there is continual occupation by the drug.[5] The effect of (D) is a function of the concentration of the drug-receptor complex.

In the following equation, R^* is an activated receptor and $\underline{R}$ is an unavailable receptor.

$$[D]+[R]\xrightarrow[k_2]{k_1}[DR]\xrightarrow{k_3}DR^*\xrightarrow{k_4}[D]+[\underline{R}];[\underline{R}]\xrightarrow{k_5}R \qquad [1.1]$$

The ratio k_1/k_2 expresses the affinity of the receptor for a drug. The ratio k_3/k_2 expresses the efficacy.

Where the response is thought to be proportional to the number of receptors occupied, this is called an occupation theory.[5,6] In a view called the rate theory, the response is directly proportional to the rate of association of the drug with the receptor.[7]

$$\text{Drug} + \text{Receptor} \xrightarrow[k_2]{k_1} \text{Complex} \longrightarrow \text{Response} \qquad [1.2]$$

For an antagonist, in the rate theory, this type of drug may dissociate slowly from the complex. This explains the persistence of effect for such drugs.

A graphic treatment can be used to illustrate the difference between efficacy and potency (degree of biologic activity). Potency can be expressed by the site along an X-axis, in relation to an intensity effect along a Y-axis. To elaborate, two different drugs may have maximal effects that appear to be equal. However, it is possible for one of these drugs (A) to have a larger peak effect than the other (B) does. In this instance, A has both greater potency and efficacy. Thus, drug A in a dose of 0.1 g may have the same effect as 1.0 g of drug B.[6]

Drugs may display a competitive or noncompetitive antagonism. A competitive antagonist combines with a receptor similar to the way that an agonist drug does. However, the formation of the complex is weak or ineffective. Increasing the concentration of the agonist usually breaks through the blockade, making the blockade reversible.

There are other types of antagonism. A response to a drug may be variably reduced by another drug with a reverse effect, or abolished by inducing a chemical alteration of a drug's molecular structure.

In noncompetitive antagonism, the antagonist combines irreversibly with a receptor. This produces an inhibition, which prevents any concentration of a drug from exerting a maximum effect. This can be illustrated in log-dose response curves, in which the number of drug-receptor interactions is seen to be decreased. The reader is referred to Schild,[8] who introduced a scale to measure drug antagonism in relation to potency. In this scale, the term potency refers to the concentration of a substance that effectively competes for a target site. Another term, IC_{50}, is used to denote the concentration that inhibits binding by 50%.

The effects of a drug involve its absorption, distribution, metabolism, and excretion. Membrane interactions are highly involved at all stages of these processes. A discussion of the binding problems in the drug-receptor interactions at membranes can be found in many texts. The reader is referred to a succinct review in Neubig.[9]

In models relating drug concentration to effect, the law of mass action is useful to analyze the factors determining receptor occupation. This is because with most drugs the binding to receptors is not absolutely tight so that a reversible dissociation may occur. This means that drugs may not have excessively long persistence and duration of activity.

A Scratchard plot is useful in drug-receptor studies. It is a method to determine values for the binding of drugs to independent sites in which all have the same K_D for the drug, the K_D being the free drug concentration at which DR is 50% of the $(DR)_{max}$. The Scratchard plot converts curves of linear or semilogarithmic plots of binding data into straight lines.[9]

Following a positive interaction between a drug and its receptor, the drug is absorbed and distributed to target organs. The volume of distribution (V_D) is used to describe the relationship between the dose given and the concentration of the drug reached in the blood.

$$V_D = \text{Amount of drug in the body/concentration of drug in plasma} \qquad [1.3]$$

In determining the distribution of a drug in the body, a single compartment model involving drug kinetics has been a promising device. However, it oversimplifies conclusions drawn from it because it assumes that there is a homogeneous and instantaneous distribution of a drug. A two-compartment model is better in that it considers the phase in which the decrease of drug concentration in the body is reflecting the gradual distribution of a substance from the plasma to the tissues.[10]

Drugs are eventually cleared (excreted) from the body. This is an important process in that it determines the quantity of a drug needed to maintain a steady-state drug concentration in the tissues. There are many interacting factors; among them, the rate of elimination determines the regimen of the dose. In the period of disappearance of a drug from the body, exponential decay curves and the so-called half-life of a drug are productive methods of visualizing the internal persistence in time of the drug in the body (see Figure 1).[6]

In the temporal phases of the passage of drugs through the body, cell membranes are involved at each transfer area and their importance cannot be overemphasized. In the case where a drug ionizes, the Henderson-Hasselbalch equation is a measure of the capacity for passage; this is a function of the pH of a cell's interior and the so-called pK_a of the drug. The pK_a, or negative log of the acid dissociation constant, is the pH at which numerator and denominator quantities (seen in the following equation) are equal.

$$\text{pH, negative log}\left[H^+\right] = pK_a + \log \text{base/acid} \qquad [1.4]$$

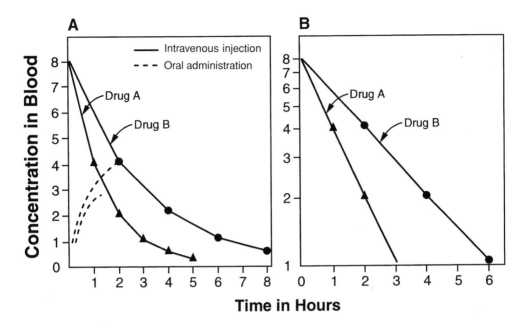

FIGURE 1. Schematic representation of drug disappearance curves and biologic half-life. The Y-axis is on the arithmetic scale in **A** and on the logarithmic scale in **B**. Drug A has a biologic half-life of one hour. The biologic half-life of drug B is two hours. *(Reprinted with permission. Data from Clark, W. G., Brater, D. C., and Johnson, A. R., Eds., Goth's Medical Pharmacology, 13th ed., Mosby-YearBook, St. Louis, 1992, 28.)*

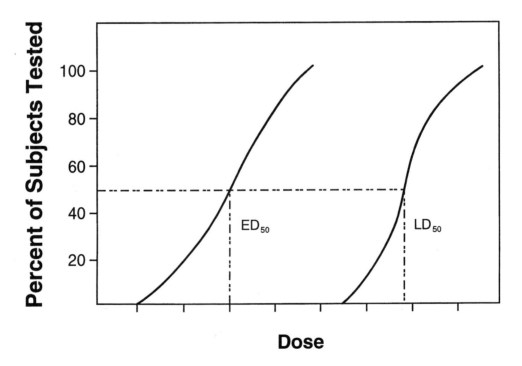

FIGURE 2. Therapeutic index. *(Reprinted with permission. Data from Clark, W. G., Brater, D. C., and Johnson, A. R., Eds., Goth's Medical Pharmacology, 12th ed., C. V. Mosby, St. Louis, 1988, 40.)*

Acids with low pK_a are absorbed well from the stomach and bases with high pK_a have to reach the more alkaline small intestine to be absorbed well.

Another process to be considered is that after a drug passes through cell membranes, a concern arises about how much of a therapeutic dose should have been given before toxicity is a likely possibility. This can be evaluated by the use of a concept called the therapeutic index (TI_{50}), a ratio between the median lethal dose (LD_{50}) and the median effective dose (ED_{50}).

$$TI_{50} = LD_{50} / ED_{50} \qquad [1.5]$$

where the numerator is the median lethal dose and the denominator is the dose required to produce a specified effect, whereas the lethal dose is the dose that kills 50% of animals in a given population of experimental animals.[6] The graph herein (Figure 2) illustrates this modality. It is noted that no drug produces a single effect. Several TIs can be calculated for each effect. The TI is thus a measure of selectivity or margin of safety.

Only a few concepts have been discussed herein relevant to the quantitation of receptor binding. An abundant literature exists, however, on the applications of mathematics to the problems at hand. Many of these data were published between 1950 and 1960 and emphasize the use of quantitative models. The problem with models is that they need to correspond to the facts. The model is a hypothesis and it can be tested by perturbations in a system to find if it truly applies. Also, it acts as an economical condensation of the observations.

Because pharmacokinetics is drawn upon in many quantitative studies, the reader is referred to a useful chronological bibliography listing literature prior to 1963 and ending in 1971.[10]

APPENDIX II: TABLE OF NORMAL REFERENCE LABORATORY VALUES

The reference values herein are for endocrine chemistry tests commonly ordered at the Massachusetts General Hospital (MGH) and recorded in the case records of the MGH.

TABLE 1
Endocrine Chemistry

Analyte	Fluid	MGH Units	SI Units	Method or Machine	Factor to Convert to SI Units
Aldosterone					
Standing (normal-salt diet)	S, P	4–31 ng/dl	111–860 pmol/L	Immunoassay	27.74
Recumbent (normal-salt diet)	S, P	<16 ng/dl	<444 pmol/L	Immunoassay	27.74
Normal-salt diet (100–180 meq of Na)	U	6–25 μg/day	17–69 nmol/day	Immunoassay	2.774
Low-salt diet (10 meq of Na)	U	17–44 μg/day	47–122 nmol/day	Immunoassay	2.774
High-salt diet	U	0–6 μg/day	0–17 nmol/day	Immunoassay	2.774
Androstenedione	S	60–260 ng/dl	2.1–9.1 nmol/L	Immunoassay	0.0349
Antidiuretic hormone	P	1.0–13.3 pg/ml	1.0–13.3 ng/L	Immunoassay	1
Calcitonin	S			Immunoassay	
Female		0–20 pg/ml	0–20 ng/L		
Male		0–28 pg/ml	0–28 ng/L		
Catecholamines					
Dopamine	U	65–400 μg/day	424–2612 nmol/day	Liquid chromatography	6.53
	P	0–30 pg/ml	0–196 nmol/L	Liquid chromatography	6.53
Epinephrine	U	1.7–22.4 μg/day	9.3–122 nmol/day	Liquid chromatography	5.458
Supine	P	0–110 pg/ml	0–600 pmol/L	Liquid chromatography	5.458
Standing	P	0–140 pg/ml	0–764 pmol/L	Liquid chromatography	5.458
Norepinephrine	U	12.1–85.5 μg/day	72–505 nmol/day	Liquid chromatography	5.991
Supine	P	70–750 pg/ml	0.41–4.43 nmol/L	Liquid chromatography	0.005911
Standing	P	200–1700 pg/ml	1.18–10.0 nmol/L	Liquid chromatography	0.005911
Chorionic gonadotropin (hCG) (nonpregnant)	S	<10 mIU/ml	<10 mIU/ml	Immunoassay	1
Corticotropin (ACTH)	P	6.0–76.0 pg/ml	1.3–16.7 pmol/L	Immunoassay	0.2202
Cortisol	P			Immunoassay	27.59
Fasting, 8 a.m.–noon		5.0–25.0 μg/dl	138–690 nmol/L		
noon–8 p.m.		5.0–15.0 μg/dl	138–410 nmol/L		
8 p.m.–8 a.m.		0.0–10.0 μg/dl	0–276 nmol/L		
Cortisol, free	U	20–70 μg/day	55–193 nmol/day	Immunoassay	2.759

TABLE 1 (continued)
Endocrine Chemistry

Analyte	Fluid	MGH Units	SI Units	Method or Machine	Factor to Convert to SI Units
C-Peptide	S	0.30–3.70 µg/L	0.10–1.22 nmol/L	Immunoassay	0.33
11-Deoxycortisol (after metyrapone)	P	>7.5 µg/dl	>216 nmol/L	Immunoassay	28.86
1,25-Dihydroxy-vitamin D	S	16–42 pg/ml	38–101 pmol/L	Immunoassay	2.4
Erythropoietin	S	<19 mU/ml	≤19 U/L	Immunoassay	1
Estradiol	S, P			Immunoassay	3.671
Female					
Premenopausalj		23–361 pg/ml	84–1325 pmol/L		
Postmenopausal		<30 pg/ml	<110 pmol/L		
Prepubertal		<20 pg/ml	<73 pmol/L		
Male		<50 pg/ml	<184 pmol/L		
Gastrin	P	0–200 pg/ml	0–200 ng/L	Immunoassay	1
Growth hormone	P	2.0–6.0 ng/ml	2.0–6.0µg/L	Immunoassay	1
Hemoglobin A	P	3.8–6.4%	0.038–0.064	Liquid chromatography	0.01
Homovanillic acid	U	0.0–15.0 mg/day	0–82 µmol/day	Liquid chromatography	5.489
17-Hydroxycortico-steroids	U			Colorimetry	2.759
Female		2.0–6.0 mg/day	5.5–17 µmol/day		
Male		3.0–10.0 mg/day	8–28 µmol/day		
5-Hydroxyindole-acetic acid (lower in women)	U	2–9 mg/day	10–47 µmol/day	Colorimetry	5.23
17-Hydroxypro-gesterone	S			Immunoassay	3.026
Female					
Prepubertal		0.20–0.54 µg/L	0.61–1.63 nmol/L		
Follicular		0.02–0.80 µg/L	0.61–2.42 nmol/L		
Luteal		0.90–3.04 µg/L	2.72–9.20 nmol/L		
Postmenopausal		<0.45 µg/L	<1.36 nmol/L		
Male					
Prepubertal		0.12–0.30 µg/L	0.36–0.91 nmol/L		
Adult		0.20–1.80 µg/L	0.61–5.45 nmol/L		
25-Hydroxyvitamin D	S	8–55 ng/ml	20–137 nmol/L	Immunoassay	2.496
Insulin	S	0–29 µU/ml	0–208 pmol/L	Immunoassay	7.175
17-Ketogenic steroids	U			Colorimetry	3.467
Female		3.0–15.0 mg/day	15–52 µmol/day		
Male		5.0–23.0 mg/day	17–80 µmol/day		
17-Ketosteroids	U			Colorimetry	3.467
Female and male ≤10 years old		0.1–3.0 mg/day	0.4–10.4 µmol/day		
Female and male 11–14 years old		2.0–7.0 mg/day	6.9–24.2 µmol/day		
Female ≥15 years old		5.0–15.0 mg/day	17.3–52.0 µmol/day		
Male ≥15 years old		9.0–22.0 mg/day	31.2–76.3 µmol/day		
Metanephrines, total	U	0.0–0.90 mg/day	0.0–4.9 µmol/day	Spectro-photometry	5.458

TABLE 1 (continued)
Endocrine Chemistry

Analyte	Fluid	MGH Units	SI Units	Method or Machine	Factor to Convert to SI Units
Parathyroid hormone	P	10–60 pg/ml	10–60 ng/L	Immunoassay	1
Parathyroid-related protein	P	>1.5 pmol/L	>1.5 pmol/L	Immunoassay	1
Pregnanediol	U			Gas chromatography	3.12
Female		0.2–6.0 mg/day	0.6–18.7 μmol/day		
Follicular phase		0.1–1.3 mg/day	0.3–5.3 μmol/day		
Luteal phase		1.2–9.5 mg/day	3.7–29.6 μmol/day		
Pregnancy		Gestation period dependent	Gestation period dependent		
Male		0.2–1.2 mg/day	0.6–3.7 μmol/day		
Pregnanetriol	U	0.5–2.0 mg/day	1.5–6.0 μmol/day	Gas chromatography	2.972
Prolactin	S			Immunoassay	1
Female		0–15 ng/ml	0–15 μg/L		
Male		0–10 ng/ml	0–10 μg/L		
Renin activity	P			Immunoassay	0.2778
Normal salt intake					
Recumbent 6 hr		0.5–1.6 ng/ml/h	0.14–0.44 ng/(L · s)		
Upright 4 hr		1.9–3.6 ng/ml/h	0.53–1.00 ng/(L · s)		
Low salt intake					
Recumbent 6 hr		2.2–4.4 ng/ml/h	0.61–1.22 ng/(L · s)		
Upright 4 hr		4.0–8.1 ng/ml/h	1.11–2.25 ng/(L · s)		
Upright 4 hr, with diuretic		6.8–15.0 ng/ml/h	1.89–4.17 ng/(L · s)		
Somatomedin C	P			Immunoassay	1
Female					
Preadolescent		60.8–724.5 ng/ml	60.8–724.5 μg/L		
Adolescent		112.5–450.0 ng/ml	112.5–450.0 μg/L		
Adult		141.8–389.3 ng/ml	141.8–389.3 μg/L		
Male					
Preadolescent		65.5–841.5 ng/ml	65.5–841.5 μg/L		
Adolescent		83.3–378.0 ng/ml	83.3–378.0 μg/L		
Adult		54.0–328.5 ng/ml	54.0–328.5 μg/L		
Testosterone, total, morning sample	P			Immunoassay	0.03467
Female		20–90 ng/dl	0.7–3.1 nmol/L		
Male, adult		300–1100 ng/dl	10.4–38.1 nmol/L		
Testosterone, unbound, morning sample	P			Equilibrium dialysis	34.67
Female, adult		0.09–1.29 ng/dl	3–45 pmol/L		
Male, adult		3.06–24.0 ng/dl	106–832 pmol/L		
Thyroglobulin	S	0–60 ng/ml	0–60 μg/L	Immunoassay	1
Thyroid-hormone-binding index		0.83–1.17	0.83–1.17	Charcoal resin	1
Thyroid-stimulating hormone	S	0.5–5.0 μU/ml	0.5–5.0 mU/L	Immunoassay	1

TABLE 1 (continued)
Endocrine Chemistry

Analyte	Fluid	MGH Units	SI Units	Method or Machine	Factor to Convert to SI Units
Thyroxine, free	S	0.8–2.7 ng/dl	10–35 pmol/L	Direct equilibrium dialysis	12.87
Thyroxine-binding globulin	S	Age and sex dependent	Age and sex dependent	Immunoassay	
Thyroxine, free, index		4.6–11.2	4.6–11.2	Calculation	1
Thyroxine, total (T_4)	S	4–12 µg/dl	51–154 nmol/L	Immunoassay 12.87	
Triiodothyronine, total (T_3)	S	75–195 ng/dl	1.2–3.0 nmol/L	Immunoassay 0.01536	

Jordan, C. Diana, Flood, James G., Laposata, Michael, and Lewandrowski, Kent B., *N. Engl. J. Med.,* 327 (10), 720, 1992. With permission.

APPENDIX III: SMITHKLINE BEECHAM CLINICAL LABORATORIES PERFORMING ENDOCRINE DIAGNOSTIC TESTS

The editors and chapter author wish to thank Ms. Barbara Wickersham, Quality Assurance Manager at SmithKline Beecham Clinical Laboratory in St. Louis, for providing a geographic list of the major SKB diagnostic laboratories.

ATLANTA
1777 Montreal Circle
Tucker, GA 30084
(404) 934-9205
(800) 877-8805

Drugs of Abuse Testing
3175 Presidential Drive
Atlanta, GA 30340
(800) 729-6432

BALTIMORE
11425 Cronhill Drive
Owings Mills, MD 21117
(301) 581-2400
(800) 729-7525

BOSTON
343 Winter Street
Waltham, MA 02154
(617) 890-6161
(800) 669-4566

CHICAGO
506 East State Parkway
Schaumburg, IL 60173
(708) 885-2010
(800) 669-6995

CLEVELAND
6180 Halle Drive
Valley View, OH 44125
(216) 328-7500
(800) 854-1774 (OH only)

DALLAS
8000 Sovereign Row
Dallas, TX 75247
(214) 638-1301
(800) 442-2102

DETROIT
24469 Indoplex Circle
Farmington Hills, MI 48335
(313) 478-4414
(800) 356-2142

HONOLULU
4400 Kalanianole Highway
Honolulu, HI 96821
(808) 735-9855

HOUSTON
8933 Interchange Drive
Houston, TX 77054
(713) 667-5829
(800) 669-6605

LEXINGTON
2277 Charleston Drive
Lexington, KY 40505
(606) 299-3866
(800) 366-7522

LOS ANGELES
7600 Tyrone Avenue
Van Nuys, CA 91405
(818) 989-2520
(800) 877-2520

LOUISVILLE
2307 Greene Way
Louisville, KY 40220
(502) 491-3484
(800) 877-8570

MIAMI
5601 Northwest 159th Street
Hialeah, FL 33014
(305) 620-0650
(800) 745-7225 (FL only)

MINNEAPOLIS
600 W. County Road D
New Brighton, MN 55112
(612) 635-1500
(800) 882-7012

NASHVILLE
2545 Park Plaza
Nashville, TN 37203
(615) 327-1855
(800) 342-2113 (in TN)
(800) 251-2633 (outside TN)

NEW ORLEANS
4648 S. I-10 Service Road West
Metairie, LA 70001
(504) 889-2307
(800) 452-7669

NEW YORK CITY
575 Underhill Blvd.
Syosset, NY 11791
(516) 677-3800
(800) 877-7530

PHILADELPHIA
400 Egypt Road
Norristown, PA 19403
(215) 631-4200
(800) 523-5447

PHOENIX
2727 West Baseline, #8 and #9
Tempe, AZ 85283
(602) 438-8477
(800) 829-7225 (AZ only)

SAN ANTONIO
601 North Frio Street
San Antonio, TX 78207
(512) 225-5101
(800) 292-7466

SAN DIEGO
9530 Padgett Street, #101
San Diego, CA 92126
(619) 536-1338
(800) 479-2121 (within San Diego Co.)

SAN FRANCISCO
6511 Golden Gate Drive
Dublin, CA 94568
(415) 828-2500
(800) 228-3008 (Northern California)

SEATTLE
1737 Airport Way South
Suite 200
Seattle, WA 98134
(206) 623-8100
(800) 877-0051

ST. LOUIS
11636 Administration Drive
St. Louis, MO 63146
(314) 567-3905
(800) 669-7525
(800) 669-8077 (client response)

TALLAHASSEE
1892 Professional Park Circle
Tallahassee, FL 32308
(904) 877-5171

TAMPA
4225 East Fowler Avenue
Tampa, FL 33617
(813) 972-7100
(800) 282-6613 (FL only)

AFFILIATED LABORATORIES
Scripps Immunology Reference Laboratory
11107 Roselle Street
Suite A
San Diego, CA 92121
(619) 453-7155

REFERENCES

1. **Drachman, D. B.,** Myasthenia gravis, *N. Engl. J. Med.,* 330(25), 1797, 1994.
2. **Sapir, C. B. and Breder, C. D.,** The neurologic basis of fever, *N. Engl. J. Med.,* 330(26), 1880, 1994.
3. **Cacciola, E., Deisseroth, A. B., and Guistolisi, R., Eds.,** *Hemopoietic Growth Factors, Oncogenes and Cytokines in Clinical Hematology,* S. Karger, Farmington, CT, 1994.
4. **Bowman, W. C., Rand, M. J., and West, G. B.,** *Textbook of Pharmacology,* Blackwell Scientific, Oxford, 1968.
5. **Goth, A.,** *Medical Pharmacology,* 9th ed., C. V. Mosby, St. Louis, 1978, 8.
6. **Clark, W. G., Brater, D. C., and Johnson, A. R., Eds.,** *Goth's Medical Pharmacology,* 12th ed., C. V. Mosby, St. Louis, 1988, 40, and 13th ed., Mosby-YearBook, St. Louis, 1992, 28.
7. **Ross, E. M. and Gilman, A. G.,** in *Goodman and Gilman's The Pharmacological Basis of Therapeutics,* 7th ed., Gilman, A. G., Goodman, L. S., Rall, T. W., and Murad, F., Eds., Macmillan, New York, 1985, 35–48.
8. **Schild, H. O.,** A new scale for the measurement of drug antagonism, *Br. J. Pharmacol. Chemother.,* 2, 189, 1947.
9. **Neubig, R. R.,** The time course of drug action, in *Principles of Drug Action,* 3rd ed., Pratt, W. B. and Taylor, P., Eds., Churchill Livingstone, New York, 1990, 297.
10. **Wagner, J. G. and Pernarowski, M.,** *Biopharmaceutics and Relevant Pharmacokinetics,* Drug Intelligence Publications, Hamilton, IL, 1971, 331.

Chapter 2

EFFECTS OF ENVIRONMENTAL FACTORS ON THE ENDOCRINE SYSTEM

Hing-Sing Yu

CONTENTS

INTRODUCTION

The endocrine system plays a crucial regulatory role in the internal environment of an organism. Some of its components had evolved to merge with the nervous system that possesses sensory detectors for external stimuli such as light and temperature. This integration of neural and endocrine tissues created a neuroendocrine interface capable of accepting neural signal inputs and secreting hormones into the blood circulation. It can transduce information from the external environment into endocrine signals.[1] With the ability to receive and interpret environmental cues through the neuroendocrine system, the endocrine system is enhanced in its adaptability to the environment. In response to external environmental changes, proper endocrine adjustments can be evoked in the internal environment. The neuroendocrine system, as its name implies, is an integrated control system of both neural and endocrine functions. In this chapter, the neuroendocrine system is discussed as a part of the endocrine system, though it can be considered as a system on its own.[2]

The endocrine portion of the neuroendocrine component may also be derived from the nervous system developmentally. For example, the adrenal medulla is the oldest known endocrine gland secreting norepinephrine (NE) differentiated from postganglionic cells of the sympathetic nervous system. Evidently, such an integration of endocrine and neural functions is favored by natural selection. It provides the gateway for interactions between the external and internal environments. The evolutionary success of a species depends on how well the individuals can predict daily and seasonal changes in environmental factors and make necessary metabolic adjustments to cope with the fluctuations. Because reproductive success is the major measure of the fitness for survival, most of these metabolic adjustments are ultimately associated with reproductive physiology. We should, however, be aware of the involvement of the endocrine system in other environmentally related processes such as thermoregulation and ionic homeostasis.

During the past three decades, our understanding of the interactions between the endocrine system and the environment has been increasing exponentially. The pituitary gland, or hypophysis, is still considered the central component of the endocrine system. This gland is also an integral part of the hypothalamo-hypophyseal complex, which is under constant influence by neuroendocrine signals from the higher centers in the brain. The pineal gland, or epiphysis, is another neuroendocrine organ located centrally between the two cerebral hemispheres and in front of the cerebellum at the posterodorsal area of the diencephalon. The pineal gland plays a role in the transduction of environmental cues into neuroendocrine signals, possibly through its neural hormone called melatonin. Through a series of melatonin signals, the pineal gland conveys all necessary environmental information to the endocrine system, in which an orchestra of biorhythms has to perform in harmony with the external environment.

In this chapter, the organization of the endocrine orchestra is first described with an emphasis on its ability to use biorhythmicity as a time-keeping mechanism for interpreting environmental cues. The environment is apparently a powerful driving force in regulating biorhythmicity if all environmental factors are fluctuating rhythmically with a set of parameters optimal for the organism. In seasonal animals, circadian and circannual rhythms are two evolutionary products of this relationship. If an environmental factor deviates outside the optimal range, it may become "toxic" to the organism. Therefore, endocrine toxicology, discussed later in this chapter, is essential for understanding the dual roles of the environment in affecting the endocrine system.

THE ENDOCRINE ORCHESTRA

Endocrine glands exert their effects on target tissues by secreting hormones into the circulatory system. The pancreas, for instance, secretes insulin and glucagon for regulating carbohydrate metabolism, say, in brain cells. This is only one example of the many endocrine glands and tissues, all of which must be orchestrated with other endocrine components and be integrated with neuroendocrine systems to function holistically in regulating the internal environment. To understand the interactions among different components, an analogy of an orchestra is used to visualize this complicated coordination.[2] The pituitary gland has long been considered the master gland of all endocrine subsystems and is certainly appropriate to be named the conductor of the endocrine orchestra. The conductor is, in turn, under the higher hierarchy of the neuroendocrine systems, the hypothalamus and pineal gland. The main players are the gonads, which help coordinate other players to respond to the signals from the conductor.

THE CONDUCTOR AND PLAYERS

The pituitary gland consists mainly of three portions: adenohypophysis, neurohypophysis, and the pars intermedia between the two (see Figure 1). The adenohypophysis is the glandular lobe including the pars tuberalis, pars distalis, and pars intermedia. All these structures are derived from the Rathke's pouch during embryonic development. It is part of the developmental oral cavity and is not of neural origin. In contrast, the neurohypophysis is neural, consisting of the infundibulum, infundibular stem, and infundibular process (or the neural lobe).

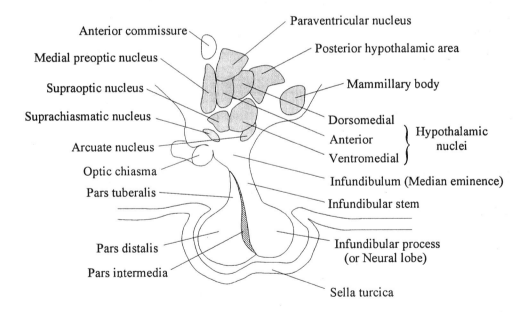

FIGURE 1. The hypothalamo-hypophyseal complex and associated nuclei. (*From Yu, H.S.,* Human Reproductive Biology, *CRC Press, Boca Raton, FL, 1994, 47. With permission.*)

As an endocrine organ, the pituitary gland secretes hormones into the blood circulation to exert its effects on the target tissues; they are adrenocorticotropic hormone (ACTH), growth hormone (GH), luteinizing hormone (LH), follicle-stimulating hormone (FSH), thyroid-stimulating hormone (TSH), melanocyte-stimulating hormone (MSH), prolactin, vasopressin, and oxytocin. As a conductor, the pituitary gland uses these hormones as signals to the players in the endocrine orchestra. It also responds to commands from the higher hierarchy in the brain and to feedback from the players.

Target reproductive organs are the players, including the gonad, accessory sexual structures, and structures associated with secondary sex characteristics. In the female, the ovary is the main player although the uterine structures and mammary glands are also being targeted. In addition, estrogen and progesterone secreted by the ovary influence fat distribution, bone maturation and turnover, and other physiological processes leading to feminine sex characteristics. In the male, the testis is the main player. The penis, prostate gland, and seminal vesicles are the other reproductive structures involved. It should be emphasized that the testis, being the main player, also participates in regulating other players through testosterone.

The thyroid gland is another endocrine organ conducted directly by the anterior pituitary gland. TSH is secreted by thyrotropin cells into the blood circulation. As a player, the thyroid gland secretes thyroxine and triiodothyronine in response to TSH stimulation. A feedback mechanism exists for TSH secretion when the plasma concentration of thyroid hormones becomes high. Similarly, the adrenal cortex is regulated by ACTH in its corticosteroid secretion, whereas some other tissues are responsive to pituitary hormones such as GH and MSH. GH regulates cellular growth and MSH plays a role in melanin production in melanocytes of skin.

THE HIGHER HIERARCHY

The hypophysis is under the influence of higher brain centers in the hypothalamus, the gonad, and possibly the pineal gland. The hypothalamus is a collection of nuclei in an area at the base of the brain above the hypophysis but below the thalamus (see Figure 1). Each nucleus is a bundle of nerve cell bodies and they are mostly bilaterally symmetrical about the third ventricle except the suprachiasmatic nucleus (SCN) and arcuate nucleus (see Figure 2). The preoptic nucleus (PON), arcuate nucleus, and anterior hypothalamic nucleus are involved in reproduction. The SCN is a circadian generator responsible for maintaining endogenous rhythms.

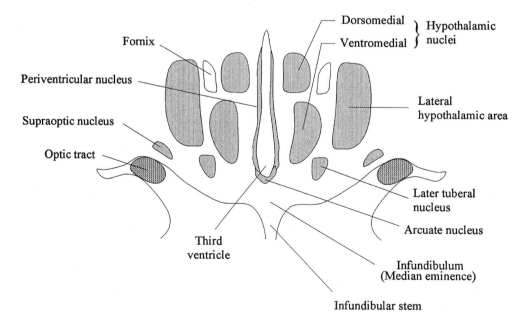

FIGURE 2. Bilateral symmetry of hypothalamic nuclei. (*From Yu, H.S.,* Human Reproductive Biology, *CRC Press, Boca Raton, FL, 1994, 47. With permission.*)

Hypophysiotropic hormones are signals given to the hypophysis by hypothalamic nuclei; they are releasing or inhibiting factors. They are thyrotropin-releasing hormone (TRH), corticotropin-releasing hormone (CRH), gonadotropin-releasing hormone (GnRH), growth hormone-releasing hormone (GHRH), somatostatin (or growth hormone-inhibiting hormone [GHIH]), prolactin-releasing factor (PRF), and dopamine (or prolactin-inhibiting factor [PIF]). As shown in Figure 3, an elaborate vascular system extending from the median eminence and infundibular stem to the adenohypophysis is present for the secretion of these hormones. It is the vascular portal system of the pituitary with a characteristic portal blood vessel having capillaries at both ends. This portion system is important for transporting hypothalamic factors to the hypophysis.

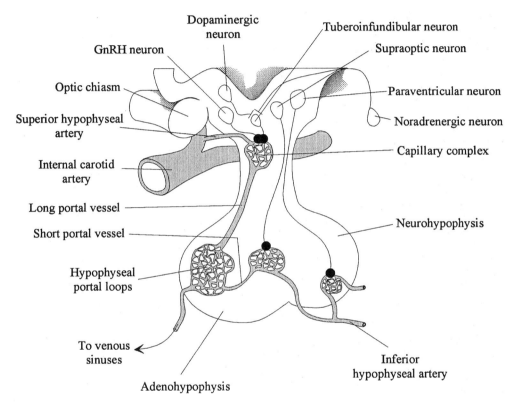

FIGURE 3. Vascular portal system of the pituitary and associated neurons. (*From Yu, H.S.,* Human Reproductive Biology, *CRC Press, Boca Raton, FL, 1994, 47. With permission.*)

PVN is an important hypothalamic center. It has magnocellular neurons, 20% of which project to the neural lobe for neuropeptide secretion. Another pathway of the magnocellular neuron is to the median eminence. Parvicellular neurons in PVN also project to the brainstem. Interestingly, most of these neurons contain oxytocin and vasopressin, though they are not the same neuronal type. PVN is also a source of TRH, a tripeptide (p-Glu-His-Pro-NH$_2$) derived from a 30-kDa peptide.[3] The TRH-producing neurons terminate at the arcuate nucleus and median eminence. TRH is primarily responsible for stimulating TSH release from thyrotropes in adenohypophysis. However, it also enhances prolactin and GH release. There are other effects such as increased NE turnover leading to the possible antidepressive action of TRH. Interestingly, TRH has also been postulated to play a role, with serotonin, in the control of male sexual behavior in rats.[4]

Corticotropin-releasing factor (CRF) is also produced in PVN; it is mainly found in parvicellular neurons and is colocalized with oxytocin and vasopressin. It is a peptide with

41 amino acids and is derived from a precursor molecule of 196 amino acids. The major function of CRH is to induce the release of hormones derived from proopiomelanocortin (POMC). POMC is the precursor for ACTH and β-lipotropin produced in corticotropes of adenohypophysis. PVN is also a relay station for the signals from the retina to the pineal gland. PVN also has a pathway to the third ventricle, secreting into cerebral spinal fluid.

The supraoptic nucleus (SON) has magnocellular neurons, up to 90% of which project to the neural lobe, as in PVN, for the secretion of oxytocin and vasopressin. As the name implies, SON is above the optic tract on both sides. There are two nuclei laterally symmetrical to each other at approximately the same level as the floor of the third ventricle.

The arcuate nucleus is situated in the mediobasal hypothalamus just beneath the floor of the third ventricle. It is an important nucleus for reproductive functions such as menstrual cyclicity,[5] primarily responsible for GnRH and dopamine. This is a neuronal oscillator responsive to many endogenous factors; one of them has been shown to be estrogen.[6] As demonstrated in the rat brain, estrogen is possibly involved in fetal neurogenesis, shaping sex differences in synaptology, postsynaptic membranes, and glia within the arcuate nucleus.

The gonad and the pineal gland are the two ends of this hypothalamo-hypophyseal-gonadal axis. Environmental light-dark information is fed to the pineal gland, mostly through the retina, and is transduced into neuroendocrine signals acting at various levels. The gonad, as the ultimate target organ, responds to a set of these signals from the entire hierarchy. The ultimate effect expressed holistically is simply a timed developmental program of the gonad. In this way, the events during gonadal development are well orchestrated with environmental changes.

THE SIGNALS

There are specialized cell types responsible for producing the signals from the pituitary gland. Known signals from the conductor include ACTH, prolactin, dopamine, oxytocin, vasopressin, and gonadotropins. Although it is generally thought that most endocrine signals originate from the pituitary, recent data suggest signals generated by the hypothalamus and pineal gland may directly affect reproductive target organs.

ACTH is secreted by chromophobe cells in the pars distalis of the adenohypophysis. The release is regulated by CRH from PVN in the hypothalamus. ACTH is a signal to the adrenal gland, regulating androgen and corticosteroid production. As part of ACTH molecule in the precursor POMC, α-MSH is also secreted with a function in regulating skin pigmentation. As MSH, β-endorphin or enkephalin is also found in POMC with an inhibitory effect on LH release but a stimulatory effect on prolactin secretion.[7]

Prolactin is secreted by lactotrophs found in the pars distalis and the release is regulated by a factor called PHI27 from PVN. Enkephalin is also produced in PVN and inhibits dopamine release in neighboring neurons. Dopamine is PIF that down-regulates the production of prolactin, which is a signal to the mammary gland for milk production. In association with oxytocin, prolactin is secreted by the anterior pituitary to stimulate milk secretion by alveolar epithelial cells.

Oxytocin is secreted by oxytocin neurons originated from both PVN and SON. It is a signal to the uterus to induce smooth muscle contraction (oxytocic effect) and also to the mammary gland for milk ejection (galactogogic effect). The oxytocic effect of neurohypophyseal extracts on mammalian uteri was first discovered and confirmed by Dale nearly a century ago.[8,9] The oxytocic effect is important for the induction of labor, and the neuropeptide was named oxytocin with reference to this effect.

Vasopressin is secreted by vasopressin neurons originated from both PVN and SON. It is an antidiuretic hormone with two main effects: pressor effect (V_1 receptor-linked) and antidiuresis (V_2 receptor-linked). The pressor effect is the induction of vascular smooth muscle contraction, and the antidiuresis is the enhanced water retention in the kidney. There are membrane-bound V_2 receptors on epithelial cells lining the lumen of distal tubules and collecting ducts. The receptor is linked with adenylate cyclase that converts ATP to cAMP, leading to an activation of a protein kinase. The protein kinase phosphorylates some membrane proteins, causing an increase in water permeability. Because the lumen of tubules and ducts is hypotonic to the extracellular fluid, water flows from lumen to the blood. V_1 receptors, mediating a different effect, are less defined; they are linked to Ca^{2+} instead of cAMP. Vasopressin is crucial for osmoregulation. Its secretory process is regulated by the neuron with osmoreceptors responsive to blood osmolality.

Recently, a new protein called pituitary adenylate cyclase activating polypeptide (PACAP) has been found in a high concentration in the central nervous system (CNS), adrenal medulla, and testis.[10] cDNAs encoding its precursor have also been cloned in the sheep, human, and rat. Immunohistochemical localization has shown PACAP-containing neural fibers in the median eminence, SON, and PVN. In addition, there are four types of high-affinity PACAP receptors demonstrated in CNS, pituitary, adrenal medulla, and germ cells. A recent study has shown that PACAP stimulates cAMP accumulation in cultured Sertoli cells of the rat.[11] It also stimulates the secretion of lactate, estradiol, and inhibin in a dose-response fashion. Therefore, PACAP may be a new member of hypothalamic signals with a direct action on the gonad.

The ultimate function of the endocrine orchestra is to provide a balanced control of all physiological processes in harmony with the nervous system. The pineal gland acts as a neurotransducer to interpret light-dark signals through the visual system and sends a series of melatonin signals into the blood circulation. The plasma melatonin rhythm regulates diversely expressed biorhythms in various tissues at different levels.[1] Such an orchestrated effort allows the internal environment to be adjusted dynamically according to the cues from the changing external environment.

LIGHT-DARK CYCLE AND BIORHYTHM

The light-dark cycle is a periodic fluctuation of light intensity because of the earth's axial rotation. There is a continually changing duration of exposure to sunlight throughout a year. Accompanying this change, temperature also fluctuates generally with a higher temperature when the day length is longer. These changes pose a difficult problem for living organisms. To cope with these changes, these organisms have to schedule their activities accordingly. A timing mechanism is therefore an important part of the system to generate these well-orchestrated biorhythms. Endocrinologists begin to understand how these endocrine biorhythms can function in their individual subsystems and yet in a harmonious way holistically. It is feasible to define the biorhythmic algorithm mathematically and to underscore the commonality among diversified biorhythms under the light-dark cycle imposed by the environment.

BIORHYTHMS

Biorhythms (or biological rhythms) are endogenous to living organisms evolved to cope with the varying length of the light-dark cycle each year. These endogenous biorhythms are synchronized and closely associated with the light-dark cycle or temperature fluctuations.

What Is a Rhythm?

A rhythm is a regular recurrence of a characteristic that can be measured in a system. When the change in the expression of the characteristic is measured as a response variable against time, the regularity can be defined mathematically by three basic parameters: amplitude, period, and displacement. The amplitude is the height of the peak response, and the period is the interval between two adjacent peaks. Displacement is the interval between a reference timepoint and the first peak that follows (see Figure 4).

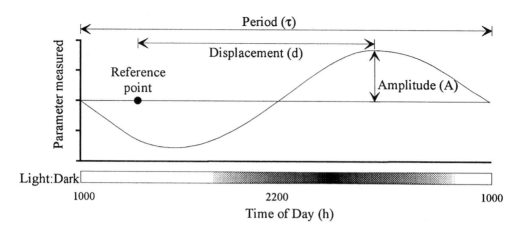

FIGURE 4. A hypothetical diurnal rhythm represented as a chronogram. (*From Yu, H.S.*, Human Reproductive Biology, *CRC Press, Boca Raton, FL, 1994, 221. With permission.*)

Definitions of Biorhythms

Circadian rhythm is a free-running, endogenous rhythm that persists in constant darkness with a period of slightly longer than 24 h. Daily rhythm is a biorhythm with a period of exactly 24 h after synchronization and a light-dark cycle environment of 24-h periodicity.

Diurnal rhythm is a biorhythm of biological activity with observable differences during the day between sunrise and sunset or during the illuminated portion of an artificial light-dark cycle. Nocturnal rhythm is a biorhythm of biological activity with observable differences during the night between sunset and sunrise or during the dark portion of an artificial light-dark cycle.

Time-Series Analysis of a Biorhythm

The period governs the frequency of the rhythm; shorter periods are found in rhythms of higher frequencies and vice versa. The displacement is the position of the peak relative to a reference timepoint. The hypothetical rhythm shown in Figure 4 is a chronogram showing the diurnal rhythm of a parameter measured and can be represented by the following equation.

$$Y(t) = \beta_0 + \beta_1 t + \beta_2 \cos\left(\frac{2\pi t}{\tau}\right) + \beta_3 \sin\left(\frac{2\pi t}{\tau}\right) \qquad [2.1]$$

The first two terms are components of the long-term trend, which is the axis of the rhythm, and is often called the secular trend line. The third and fourth terms are components contributing to the cyclic effect varying according to the time (t) and period (τ). The amplitude (A) and displacement (d) are determined by the coefficients (β_0, β_1, β_2, and β_3). These are only basic terms for this simple mathematical model. Additional terms can be added to the equation to model an actual biorhythm that deviates from this basic pattern. These terms can also be combined to simplify the equation. If we take $\omega = 2\pi/\tau$ as the angular frequency, we have $Y(t) = M + A\cos(\omega t + \phi)$, where M is the rhythm-adjusted mean called mesor and ϕ is the acrophase. With this equation, a chronogram can be transformed into another rhythmic representation called a cosinor if the time of day on the X-axis is converted to degrees (see Figure 5).

Cosinor representation is very useful for comparing peaks of different rhythms. In Figure 5, two peaks P_1 and P_2 with amplitudes A_1 and A_2 occur at different timepoints. If midnight is taken as 0° at the origin of the chronogram, the positions of the peaks can be

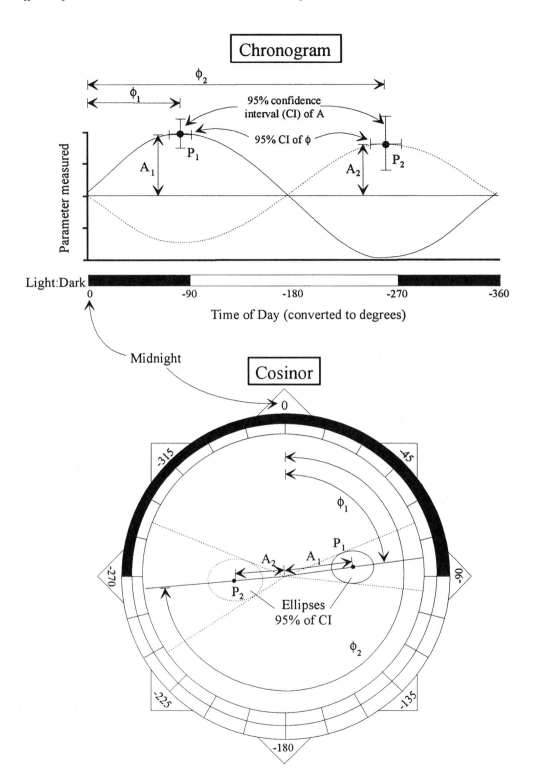

FIGURE 5. Transformation of a chronogram into a cosinor. (*From Yu, H.S.,* Human Reproductive Biology, *CRC Press, Boca Raton, FL, 1994, 221. With permission.*)

defined as ϕ_1 and ϕ_2 in the unit of degrees. The entire 24-h period is 360°. These parameters can be conveniently shown in a cosinor diagram. Besides, the 95% confidence intervals of A and ϕ are transformed into an ellipse for each peak. The sizes and positions of the ellipses can easily be compared. Although the cosinor method is a very useful tool for quantifying these parameters, there are cases where the representation is inadequate. Information is lost during transformation from a chronogram to a cosinor, such as the asymmetry of the peak or plateau.

Time-series analysis is a general statistical procedure to model the changes in a response variable with time.[12] Although the technique is widely used in seasonal trends in econometrics and physical sciences, it is seldom applied in annual rhythms. Boklage et al.[13] studied the annual and subannual rhythms in human conception rates by time-series analyses. They demonstrated statistically significant annual and weekday but not monthly rhythms in human conception rates. This statistical procedure is an appropriate test for data taken at multiple timepoints.

In the analysis of daily rhythms, time-series analysis may not be adequate if the experimental design is limited only to four sampling timepoints within one 24-h cycle. For example, in studying the daily rhythm of hormonal concentrations such as melatonin,[14] a minimum number of timepoints with small sample sizes is necessary to reduce the number of animals used. The animals at each timepoint are considered a treatment group exposed to a unique time of day. Analysis of variance (ANOVA) is applied to test whether there is a difference among groups at different timepoints. The peak is then located by pairwise comparisons. Because the timepoints are selected by the experimenter before the experiment, the amplitude and displacement may vary from one report to another if the data are analyzed by ANOVA.

The ANOVA method does have its drawbacks. For example, the treatment groups at different timepoints are essentially separate experiments performed within 24 h. In contrast to time-series analysis, ANOVA provides no analysis on the trend from one timepoint to another with the assumption that the variances are homogeneous across different groups. Therefore, prior to ANOVA, it is recommended to run Bartlett's tests for homogeneity of variances.

A 1990 report described a computer program, written in BASIC and called COSIFIT, for biorhythm analysis.[15] It is an interactive nonlinear least-squares analysis for simultaneous multioscillator cosinor analysis of time-series data. The program computes optimal frequency, mesor, amplitude, and phase, with standard errors of measurement and both parametric and nonparametric estimates of goodness-of-fit. In addition, ANOVA was also employed to show statistical differences between parameter values of selected curves.

Types of Biorhythms

The period of biorhythms varies greatly from several seconds to many years. For example, in the smooth muscle of the digestive tract in humans and other mammals, there are rhythms in mechanical and electrical activity with periods ranging from 2 s to 2.5 h.[16] Based on period length, there are four common classes of reproductive rhythms: annual, daily, infradian, and ultradian.

The infradian and ultradian rhythms are those with periods longer or shorter than 24 h, respectively. When the period length is much more than 24 h but less than a year, the rhythms are called subannual. There are weekly and monthly rhythms found in human activities. There are ultimate and proximate causes but both are external. Some rhythms are apparently driven by external causes, whereas others may have endogenous cyclicity. The menstrual cycle is an excellent example of an endogenous monthly cycle altered by extrinsic factors.

If the period length is about one year, it is known as circannual rhythm. Although the circannual rhythm is endogenous and persists in a constant environment, it needs to be synchronized, in the real world, with the annual cycle in seasonal animals. Seasonality in humans is controversial. Details will be discussed in the next section.

It should be noted that there are true periodic and pseudoperiodic biorhythms. Periodic biorhythms are rhythms with regular cycles such as estrous cycles and many hormonal rhythms. These are said to be generated by "accurate pacemakers." Some biorhythms such as serum LH are not well defined in their periodicity and are called pseudoperiodic biorhythms. The irregular patterns may be produced by "sloppy pacemakers."[17] Although time-series analysis has been used to describe these biorhythms as random fluctuations with a mean frequency, a well-defined mathematical model is necessary to accomplish more reliable analyses.

CIRCADIAN RHYTHMS

As defined rigorously earlier, a circadian rhythm is an endogenous rhythm that persists in constant darkness. If it is synchronized with the light-dark cycle, it becomes indistinguishable from a diurnal rhythm. If a diurnal rhythm does not persist in constant darkness, it is not circadian. Because most well-defined diurnal rhythms are normally circadian, the term circadian is often used, though less accurately, to describe diurnal rhythms observed under natural or artificial light-dark cycles.

Circadian rhythms can be demonstrated in most biochemical, physiological, and behavioral processes related to reproduction. The ultimate purpose of these rhythms is to provide a time-sensitive regulatory mechanism for temporal organization of reproductive events. It is a clock mechanism interacting with the light-dark cycle that provides cues or *Zeitgeber* (time sense) for resetting the clock. Such a mechanism is probably a prerequisite for all plants and animals to survive on earth,[16] including humans.

The circadian system consists of multiple oscillators operating at different levels and frequencies. They couple with each other in response to the ambient light-dark cycle and other physical factors such as temperature. As discussed earlier, the universal pacemaker SCN located in the hypothalamus orchestrates the rhythmicity of the neuroendocrine system. In humans, hormonal biorhythms may play crucial roles in reproductive functions, despite the lack of a true physiological seasonality. Some features of the human circadian system may be clinically significant.[18] For example, the responsiveness to drug treatment fluctuates with the light-dark cycle. Also, the characteristics of physiological events and hormonal biorhythms have diagnostic values. A healthy person usually has a high degree of temporal sequence.

Gonadotropins

LH and FSH are pseudoperiodic with no clear-cut diurnal property, though rhythms of serum gonadotropin levels have been reported in some mammalian species. In humans, there is no marked diurnal fluctuation of LH and FSH in men, and the plasma LH rhythm is modulated by the menstrual cycle in women (see Figure 6). Diurnal changes in gonadotropin release have weak rhythmicity and the nocturnal rise may be sleep related.[19]

Prolactin

Serum prolactin level exhibits a distinct diurnal rhythm in many species, including humans. The diurnal rhythm in humans is bimodal with a trough occurring at noon, followed by increased secretion in the afternoon and a major peak at the onset of sleep. Studies on "jet-lag" subjects with delayed sleep-wake cycles have shown that sleep onset did not induce a sustained elevation of prolactin level, suggesting that the rhythm is not driven by the sleep-wake cycle. However, the true circadian rhythmicity of serum prolactin level in humans can be confirmed only if the rhythm persists in constant darkness.

Steroids

Diurnal rhythms of testosterone in young men and of estrogen and progesterone in women have been observed. The testosterone rhythm in old men is lower than that in young men (see Figure 7). Aging probably induces a loss of diurnal rhythmicity. These rhythms become

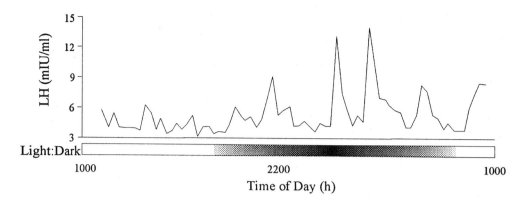

FIGURE 6. A diurnal rhythm of luteinizing hormone (LH). (*Modified from Kapen, S., et al., J. Clin. Endocrinol. Metab., 39, 293, 1974. With permission.*)

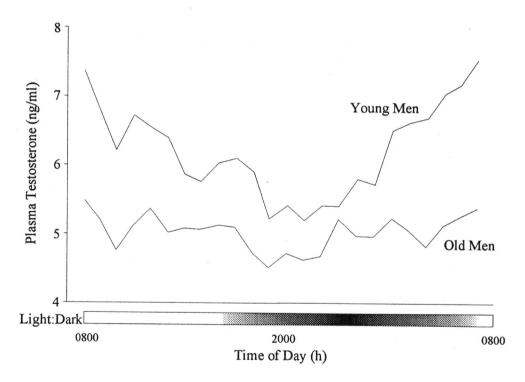

FIGURE 7. Diurnal rhythms of plasma testosterone in young and old men. (*Modified from Bremner, W.J., Vitiello, M.V., and Prinz, P.N., J. Clin. Endocrinol. Metab., 56, 1278, 1983. With permission.*)

less conspicuous in aged individuals.[20] In women, the diurnal fluctuations of estrogen and progesterone are more pronounced around the time of ovulation. Some reports show variable fluctuations during other phases of the menstrual cycle. In addition, it has been suggested that the steroid rhythms may be associated with the cortisol rhythm, which exhibits a well-defined diurnal rhythm.[17]

Melatonin

The most well-defined circadian rhythmicity is the melatonin rhythm. Melatonin is a neural hormone secreted by the pineal gland into the general blood circulation. It is also synthesized in extrapineal tissues such as the retina.[14] Figure 8 shows a well-defined diurnal rhythm of retinal melatonin that is endogenous to the eye. Although melatonin function is still uncertain in humans, its role in the reproductive physiology of seasonal breeders is well documented. The melatonin rhythm plays an important role in the time-keeping mechanism for the hypothalamo-hypophyseal-gonadal axis. This rhythm is a major component for internal signaling of photoperiodic changes, leading to the expression of the seasonality of the physiological state.[21]

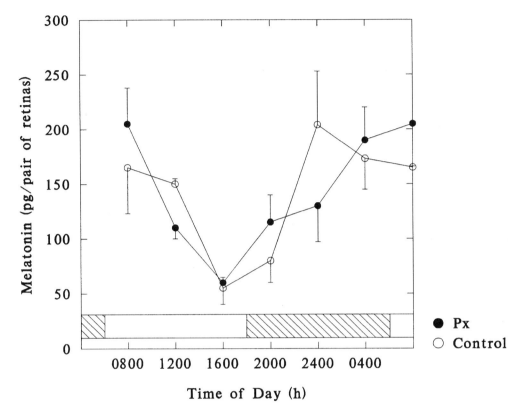

FIGURE 8. Diurnal rhythms of retinal melatonin in normal and pinealectomized (Px) rats. (*From Yu, H.S., Melatonin: Biosynthesis, Physiological Effects, and Clinical Applications, Yu, H.S. and Reiter, R.J., Eds., CRC Press, Boca Raton, FL, 1993, 365. With permission.*)

Other Hormones

Circadian and ultradian rhythms of plasma thyroid hormones have been analyzed in lactating dairy cows.[22] Triiodothyronine and thyroxine exhibited circadian rhythms with minima between 1500 and 1300 h and maxima at 1700 and 0200 h (lights on from 0700 h to 2300 h). The thyroxine rhythm preceded the body temperature rhythm by 2 h. Because thyroid hormones are associated with thermoregulation, these circadian rhythms are likely to play a role in the process. Circadian rhythms are also observed in other hormones, such as NE, corticosteroids, secreted by other tissues in many species.

ANNUAL CYCLE AND SEASONALITY

In contrast to circadian rhythm, circannual rhythm depends very much on external factors, although the oscillator is known to be endogenous. Two possible origins of this circannual oscillator in mammals become apparent. First, it was established in response to the annual cycle during mammalian evolution. Second, it had to be present before the emergence of mammals. Because nonmammalian animals also possess a circannual oscillator, the second possibility is favored. On the other hand, the first possibility is also reasonable because the circannual rhythm is very sensitive to proximate and ultimate factors. Perhaps, both are possible. Early mammals 65 million years ago might have inherited a primitive circannual oscillator from their nonmammalian ancestors. In response to environmental changes, this primitive system might have evolved into a wide range of circannual rhythms in today's mammals.

There are now more than 4000 mammalian species. They occupy different niches in different habitats with unique sets of proximate and ultimate factors. Seasonal fluctuations of these factors vary from one niche to another. The reproductive process must be finely tuned in harmony with the microenvironment. With an appropriate neuroendocrine pathway, they evolved to adapt these factors with unique patterns of seasonal reproductive physiology. The ultimate control is located in the brain. The circannual oscillator is an extremely complex system involving the pineal gland, SCN, and GnRH pulse generator.[23] These enable seasonal animals to detect changes in food availability, ambient temperature, photoperiod, pheromonal cues, nonspecific aversive emotional stimuli, etc.

CIRCANNUAL AND SEASONAL RHYTHMS

Circannual rhythms are endogenous biorhythms with a period of about one year. Like circadian rhythms, circannual rhythms will be free-running without environmental cues. The annual cycle of environmental cues on earth varies because its orbit around the sun provides a resetting mechanism for circannual rhythms. In mammals, there are different environmental cues used as signals for seasonal changes. The major ones are the changing light-dark cycle, temperature, and food availability. When a circannual rhythm is synchronized with the annual cycle, the reproduction of the animal is seasonal. This feature is known as seasonality.

Similar to the difference between the definitions of "diurnal" and "circadian," "seasonal" is not equivalent to "circannual." Seasonality refers to the seasonal responses of animals to the annual cycle. In most seasonal mammalian species, their annual reproductive cycles are truly driven by the endogenous circannual rhythm synchronized with the annual cycle. Natural selection favors such a synchrony because it provides a mechanism to time an appropriate set of environmental conditions for reproduction. It has been suggested that all different forms of mammalian seasonality evolved from a single ancestral mechanism for annual time-keeping.[21] Because it is regulated mostly by a photoperiodic mechanism, this annual time-keeping mechanism is linked with the circadian oscillator.

INTEGRATIVE MODEL OF SEASONALITY

For seasonality in mammals, Bronson[23] has proposed an integrative model in which most environmental factors are considered. The interaction among the factors produces the resultant effect. The GnRH pulse generator, which regulates the secretion of LH and FSH, is the central core of the mechanism. Photoperiod, temperature, food availability, social primers, and nonspecific emotional stimuli are the major external factors affecting the pulse generator directly or indirectly via negative-feedback sensitivity. Social primers are those associated with pheromones and stress related to social status found in rodents and primates. Nonspecific emotional stimuli refer to those factors evoking physiological responses that alter the hormonal secretion.

To study the possible seasonality in human reproduction, we must understand the mechanisms involved in seasonal breeders with clear annual rhythmicity. Seasonality is closely linked to photoperiodism with a strong genetic basis. There are significant species differences in photoperiodic responsiveness with a varying degree of seasonality. Exposure to different environmental conditions is the main driving force for the evolution of seasonality. Domestication, for example, is known to reduce seasonality.

In humans, seasonality is probably diminished by domestication. In developed countries, food supply and environmental conditions can almost be controlled with high constancy. Seasonal reproduction in such an environment becomes less important and humans are apparently sexually active throughout the year. The seasonality observed is likely to be residual responses to environmental factors associated with some endogenous behavioral rhythms. It is unlikely that seasonality in human reproduction can be eliminated because we are still responsive to the light-dark cycle.

CIRCANNUAL RHYTHMICITY OF STEROIDS

Both the light-dark cycle and temperature are important factors affecting events regulated by steroidal hormones such as ovulation and endometrial receptivity. It is well known in the poultry industry that extra light exposure at night during winter enhances egg production in hens.[24] During the winter season, there is a higher incidence of anovulation, leading to endometrial hyperplasia. This is thought to be caused by exposure to short light periods.

As shown in the ewe, estrogen acts on the hypothalamus to exert both negative and positive feedback effects on GnRH secretion. Because GnRH cells do not possess estrogen receptors, estrogen effects are mediated through other systems. NE is involved in the negative feedback regulation of GnRH secretion during the anestrous period, and γ-aminobutyric acid (GABA) agonists and antagonists injected into the medial preoptic region of the hypothalamus inhibit LH secretion in ovariectomized ewes. The inhibitory effects of GABA agonists and antagonists can be observed both in the presence and absence of estrogen.[25] The authors also reported that a seasonal shift in the responsiveness to the negative feedback effects of estrogen involves a shift in the function of GABA receptor subtypes.

In another recent study on ewes, the authors suggested some season-specific time cues for photoperiodic synchronization of a circannual reproductive rhythm.[26] In pinealectomized ewes reproductively nonresponsive to changes in day length, circannual LH cycles became free-running; that is, they were not in synchrony with the seasonal changes. When exogenous melatonin was administered in a pattern similar to the natural melatonin rhythm in ewes with intact pineals, the LH cycles were synchronized with the annual cycle.

According to epidemiological studies on humans in several geographical areas, seasonality exists in natural conception and birth rates. It is well documented that the rate of natural conception in women varies annually, with a peak during winter in warm areas worldwide.[27] In the United States, two significant decreases in births occur in early spring and early autumn (see Figure 9). The bimodal trend has been explained by the changes in sperm quality, ovulation, and conception rates throughout the year. During the hot summer, the sperm quality is poor, resulting in low conception rates. Thus, the birth rate is low in spring, and this is especially pronounced in southern areas such as San Antonio, TX.[28] On the other hand, if the temperature is too low during winter, the ovulation and conception rates may be reduced.[29] Therefore, the birth rate is low in autumn, about 10 months after the month with low temperature records. The most pronounced effect of temperature is on semen quality. It seems to occur in many mammalian species including humans.[27] Sperm production may be reduced in areas with higher temperature and relative humidity. It is well known that spermatogenesis is inhibited when scrotal temperature is raised to body temperature.

In third world countries where food availability varies seasonally, seasonality in natural conception is probably associated with food supply, seasonal employment, sociocultural factors, and health conditions. It may not be similar to the circannual rhythm of seasonal breeders where the highest birth rate occurs at the time of high food availability. The factors involved are less complicated than in developed countries, where the practice of contraception, variable lifestyles, modern diets, stress-induced physiological changes, etc., are additional factors.

In correlation with its effect on the ovulation rate, the light-dark cycle also influences the menstrual cycle. Continuous nocturnal light has been shown to reduce the cycle length in

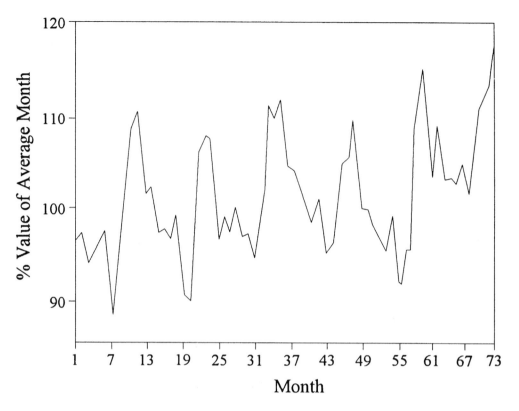

FIGURE 9. Seasonality of birth in humans. The study was performed for 72 consecutive months in North Carolina. "% value of average month" is the percentage of each monthly last menstrual period (LMP) count relative to the average LMP count of all the months. (*Modified from Boklage, C.E., Zincone, L.H., and Kirby, C.F., Jr.,* Hum. Reprod., *7, 899, 1992. With permission.*)

women having irregular menstrual cycles. Seasonality of the human menstrual cycle exists with longer cycle periods in winter,[30] and seasonality in endometrial receptivity may be associated with endogenous rhythms of steroids. The menstrual cycle is certainly an endogenous rhythm. Oocyte maturation, ovulation rate, and endometrial receptivity are parts of the menstrual cycle.

ENDOCRINE TOXICOLOGY

Under specific conditions, some environmental factors may evoke toxic responses from the organism. In a recent review by Iatropoulos,[31] the role of the endocrine system was emphasized in toxicological pathology. The toxic response may involve multiple endocrine malfunctions detrimental to the internal environment of the organism. The mechanism of the endocrine toxic response is often difficult to determine. One hormone may act on a wide variety of tissues, and one target tissue can be affected by several hormones. Also, the intimate relationship of the endocrine system with the neural and immune systems has further created complications in studying these toxic responses. As suggested by Iatropoulos, knowledge of comparable endocrinology across different species, biochemistry, and hormonal rhythmicity and secretion patterns is imperative. Endocrine toxicology thus encompasses broad research areas including the regulation of general energy metabolism, the maintenance of the internal environment, and the coordination of growth and reproduction. The ultimate goal is to establish the causality link between a specific toxic dose and the effect of a toxic substance with corresponding endocrine responses in most species studied including humans.

Toxic substances, or toxicants, can act at different levels. For example, brain intoxication by alcohol may alter brain activities at the behavioral level, whereas testicular damage by cadmium may be caused by disruption of energy metabolism at the mitochondrial level. In most cases, however, causal links with the endocrine system can be identified. The toxicity of a substance is most detrimental if its endocrine effects are associated with reproductive physiology. When they cause endocrine deficiencies or hormonal imbalances, these reproductive toxins may damage the gonad directly, resulting in reduced fertility or even infertility. Mutations may occur in oocytes or sperms exposed to them, leading to fetal anomalies or subsequent birth defects. Suppressed postnatal development may also reduce the reproductive capacity of the adult. Apart from naturally occurring toxic factors such as radiation, gases, and chemicals, some organisms may produce substances that are toxic to other species. In humans, there are many hazardous industrial chemicals with widespread effects on both humans and animals. Studies on lead toxicity was one of the early examples of reproductive toxicology in the late 19th century. It was found that women working in industries where lead was involved had a much higher rate of infertility, spontaneous abortions, neonatal deaths, and malformations. Despite these early reports about lead toxicity in workers, actions were not taken to protect workers.

In recent years, there are more concerns about fertile or pregnant women in an environment associated with high reproductive and teratogenic risks. Although endocrine malfunctions resulting in reproductive failure are emphasized, other abnormal endocrine changes such as thyroid and adrenal malfunctions also affect the survival of individuals. Despite the apparent success of the reproductive process, deficiencies in these systems also lead to high mortality of the offspring. According to some recent studies, there are many risk factors, such as solvents, different types of pollution, anesthetic agents, and even video display terminals.[32] Special attention is necessary in clinical uses of hormonally related drugs. They include synthetic hormones or hormonal extracts as well as their agonists and antagonists. Because they have profound effects on the endocrine system, the use of these drugs requires stringent screening tests. Toxicological testings with higher sensitivities are necessary.[33]

WHAT IS A TOXIN?

Despite the simplicity of this question, it is difficult to define a toxin in general terms. A toxin is a substance interfering with the normal physiology of a cell, tissue, organ, or the entire organism. Without specifying necessary conditions such as concentration and treatment duration, almost anything can be a toxin. Distilled water, for example, is toxic to living cells and tissues in culture. On the other hand, an extremely poisonous toxin from a venomous snake may not harm its predator. For toxicity of a substance, its expression depends on conditions, species, and the testing methodology.

Since the establishment of the causal link between thalidomide and limb abnormalities,[34] there has been an extensive search for systemic methods for screening new compounds, and rules have been implemented for drugs and other chemicals in many countries. According to the U.S. Food and Drug Administration (FDA) guidelines,[35] there are three basic types of investigations: general reproductive studies, teratological studies, and perinatal/postnatal studies. These guidelines are still widely accepted. For a new chemical without previous teratological evaluation, there are variations between countries in their guidelines, such as the number of treatment groups, sample number per treatment, duration of treatment, selection of doses, and number of different species used.

Perhaps because of the thalidomide catastrophe, the FDA became extremely cautious in drug approval. It may now take several years for a drug to pass through the evaluation process. The recent issue of mifepristone (RU486) not being approved by FDA is possibly caused by, in addition to the political issue, the fear of a situation similar to the thalidomide disaster. RU486 is a synthetic derivative of norethisterone with antagonist activities against progesterone. It competes with progesterone at the receptor level and possibly alters the endocrine state of the mother. In combination with prostaglandins, RU486 terminates postimplantation development in 95–99% of the cases. Those fetuses that failed to be aborted should be thoroughly studied to identify possible teratogenic effects.

MECHANISMS OF TOXICITY

There is no general mechanism of toxicity; a toxin may act at a single site or multiple sites. There are only two types of actions: direct and indirect. A toxin with direct effects may have a chemical structure similar to an endogenous compound specifically involved in a process. These toxins are commonly agonists or antagonists of hormones such as diethylstilbestrol, a nonsteroidal estrogen. In other words, these toxins interact with receptors directly responsible for the process being affected. Direct actions may also include other levels such as levels of gene expression and protein synthesis. These compounds may be simple molecules (e.g., cadmium) or complex proteins (e.g., mitomycin C). They can be mutagenic, carcinogenic, or chemically reactive.

Toxins with indirect effects may require metabolic activation after entering the organism or may alter physiological control governing some steps in the reproductive process. There are different types of indirect actions. The toxin may be metabolized into a compound with direct toxic effects. Cyclophosphamide (Cytoxan), a therapeutic agent for kidney diseases, is metabolized by microsomal monoxygenases to active toxic metabolites. The toxin may alter steroid synthesis, secretion, or degradation. Pesticides, such as dichlorodiphenyltrichloroethane (DDT), are good examples of these indirect toxins.

Oxidative damage is another toxic mechanism associated with light toxicity. Exposure to light is the major cause of free-radical generation in tissues. This is an inevitable risk that organisms on earth must cope with in their adaptation to the light-dark cycle. In a recent review, Reiter[36] has suggested that melatonin is involved in protecting free-radical damage in tissues. Its primary action may not depend on membrane receptors, as previously suggested, in association with the rhythmicity of reproductive physiology. Melatonin may be a more powerful free-radical scavenger relative to the two well-known scavengers, glutathione and mannitol. Melatonin may have two ways to protect the cell from oxidative damage. It breaks down hydrogen peroxide to water and scavenges any hydroxyl radicals generated. From an evolutionary point of view, it is advantageous for melatonin, a molecule of biorhythm regulation, to offer an extra protection against oxidative damage. A high level of melatonin in the circulation and retinal tissues at night allows the tissues to remove devastating free radicals accumulated to prepare for the next period of light exposure.

TOXICITY ON GONADS

The ovary and testis are vulnerable to many toxic substances, directly or indirectly. Direct toxins alter the process of gametogenesis whereas indirect toxins induce changes in endocrine functions of gonads. In both cases, if gametogenesis is altered, the reproductive potential of the individual is affected.

Ovarian Toxicity

The ovary is central to the control of the female reproductive cycle. The normal running of the ovarian cycle is essential for timely supply of Graafian follicles for ovulation. Reproductive toxins may act on different locations of the ovary at different times. Indirect toxicity may be through actions on blood supply, affecting the follicular development. For direct effects on follicles, there is a differential follicle complex toxicity.[37]

Different toxins may act on follicles of different stages. If a toxin destroys matured follicles specifically, fertility is reduced immediately until the removal of the toxin. If a toxin kills primary and secondary follicles specifically, reduced fertility will not be observed immediately. After the removal of the toxin, it will take a much longer time to restore the fertility. Obviously, if primary follicles are affected, there will be an increased rate of atresia.

Because there is a fixed number of follicles after birth, the loss of primary follicles will lead to premature ovarian failure or early menopause. This results in a reduction of the female reproductive lifespan.

Testicular Toxicity

In contrast to oogenesis, the entire process of spermatogenesis occurs in the adult testis. Spermatogonia lying along the basement membrane of the seminiferous tubule mitose to maintain the stem cell population. Whereas type A spermatogonia continue to divide mitotically, type B spermatogonia derived from some of their daughter cells, intermediate spermatogonia, further divide into primary spermatocytes. Each primary spermatocyte undergoes meiosis and differentiates into a sperm. Because it takes about 64 days for a spermatogonium to form a matured sperm, spermatogenesis can easily be disrupted at any point by toxins.

If the toxin does not wipe out all spermatogonia and the exposure time is short, the damage is often reversible. There is only a temporary loss of fertility if the remaining spermatogonia can resume normal mitosis. Ionizing radiation and alkylating agents (e.g., cyclophosphamide, nitrogen mustards) are toxic to dividing spermatogonia but nontoxic to resting spermatogonia, resulting in transient infertility. The male reproductive lifespan is seldom affected if the resting spermatogonia are not permanently damaged.

It should be noted that the time required for spermatogenesis is apparently a constant.[38] Almost all toxic agents tested failed to alter the rate of differentiation of individual spermatogonia. The toxic response of each spermatogonium is all-or-none; it may continue to differentiate on schedule or degenerate. With millions of differentiating sperms having a varying degree of toxic response to the same treatment, the overall toxic response is a decreased rate of sperm production.

Although spermatogenesis is a process more sensitive to reproductive toxic agents, matured sperms before and after ejaculation are also vulnerable to environmental insults. As an explanation for the seasonality of human reproduction discussed earlier, sperms during the hot summer have lower fertilizing capability. A hostile environment in the vagina or uterus can create a barrier to fertilization. Spermicidal contraceptives are good examples.

There are many chemicals known to induce testicular toxicity either directly or indirectly. They include analgesics such as indomethacin and morphine, androgens and their antagonists, antibiotics such as amphotericin B, insecticides such as DDT and parathion, some food additives such as cyclamates, metanil yellow, and caffeine, heavy metals, etc.

TOXICITY ON UTERUS AND FETUSES

The uterine cavity is the external environment for the zygote. The uterus is, in turn, governed by the endocrine environment of the mother. It is obvious that toxicants altering maternal physiology can affect the subsequent development of the zygote. After fertilization, the zygote enters the stage of preimplantation development leading to another stringent screening checkpoint, implantation. It has been estimated that only about 40% of preimplantation zygotes can implant successfully in a normal female.[39]

Implantation is a crucial step in eliminating possible abnormal zygotes to avoid babies with birth defects later. There are numerous chemicals that interfere with implantation.[40] After fertilization, the zygote needs to be properly transported down to the uterus by the oviduct while it continues to cleave. In addition to the oviduct-driven egg transport, the intraoviductal environment must be maintained optimal for preimplantation development. A reproductive toxin upsetting this maternal environment inhibits implantation. On the other hand, if the toxicant is embryotoxic, the abnormal development of preimplantation zygotes also leads to implantation failure.

The process of implantation requires proper interactions between progesterone and estrogen. Analogs of LHRH and steroids or other compounds interfering with progesterone or estrogen are found to affect implantation. For example, DDT analogs and polychlorinated biphenyl (PCB) compounds are insecticides with estrogenic properties. In mice, they have been shown to prolong pregnancy or reduce the number of implantation sites. Ions of heavy or transition metals such as cadmium, copper, and zinc inhibit the binding of estrogen, leading to implantation failure.

If the toxicant does not lead to implantation failure, there are three possibilities for the fate of the implanted zygote. First, in spite of the damage, the embryo continues to develop and restore the damaged parts of the zygote. If the toxicant is removed or not toxic to postimplantation zygotes, the embryo may succeed in developing into a normal fetus. Second, the toxicant may not be toxic to postimplantation zygotes. The damage to the zygote before or during implantation was so extensive that the subsequent embryonic development is abnormal. A malformed fetus may be formed and later resorbed or become a newborn with congenital abnormalities.

For the third possibility, the toxicant may also be toxic to the postimplantation zygote. Depending on the specificity of its toxic action, malformation may occur at any point during postimplantation development. If the toxicant leads to a newborn with birth defects, it is teratogenic. If it kills the embryo eventually, it is embryotoxic. The developmental system fails to eliminate malformed embryos exposed to teratogenic toxicants. Perhaps, these malformed embryos eventually die shortly after birth. Some newborns may survive but are burdened with congenital anomalies.

TOXICITY ON OTHER ENDOCRINE STRUCTURES

Although some toxicants directly or indirectly toxic to the gonad are reproductive toxins, other toxicants benign to the gonad may also be reproductive toxins if they are toxic to structures associated with the reproductive process. Alternatively, they may be toxic to both the gonad and related structures. For example, a number of xenobiotic chemicals, such as pesticides, heavy metals, antibiotics, and alcohol, have been found in the human seminal plasma, indicating that accessory genital glands are also susceptible to environmental insults. Even if the gametes produced are normal, the presence of toxicants in the seminal plasma imposes risks on the reproductive process.

It should be mentioned that prostate cancer is the second leading cause of cancer mortality in men.[41] About 10% of American men will develop prostate cancer with an annual incidence of 20,000 prostate cancer cases in men under the age of 65. In addition to possible predisposed genetic factors for prostate cancer, environmental factors are suspected to play a role. Early diagnosis is imperative when the disease is still pathologically organ-confined so that treatment is possible.[42] The prostate function is at least partially lost. This may become a factor leading to sexual dysfunction.

Because sexual behavior plays a crucial role in mating, some drugs affecting the brain are known to induce reproductive failure. For example, drugs inhibitory to steroid biosynthesis such as alcohol and narcotics or those that block steroid receptors such as cyproterone acetate and spironolactone are found to lower libido and sexual performance.[43] Drugs including alcohol have detrimental effects both prenatally and postnatally.[44] Besides morphological anomalies, damages to the CNS not discernible immediately during sexual differentiation and development may occur. If the damages are irreversible, the affected individual may suffer from abnormal permanent sexual behavior that may jeopardize reproductive capability. Drugs may also induce transient change in the sexual behavior. Although the change is transient, the change in sexuality does affect the reproductive outcome. For example, the effects of alcohol on human sexuality have been demonstrated in psychological studies.[45]

Other endocrine structures such as the adrenal and thyroid glands are also susceptible to influences by environmental factors. Chemicals, radiation, and other physical factors can drastically alter these endocrine organs. These effects are ultimately expressed as abnormal endocrine functions and possibly changes in behavior. In some cases, the toxicity of a substance is attributed to its bioactivation in the endocrine gland. For example, a recent study has shown that an environmental pollutant, 3-methylsulphonyl-2,2-bis(4-chlorophenyl)-1,1-dichloroethene, is activated and may become toxic in the adrenal gland.[46] Because the entire endocrine system works holistically to maintain an optimal internal environment, any disruptions of one component can be detrimental. If the organism fails to adjust accordingly, its toxic responses may become fatal.

SPECIES AND GENDER DIFFERENCES IN TOXIC RESPONSES

Since the endocrine environment is substantially different even among related species, the toxic response varies from one species to another. Species differences in toxic responses pose complex problems in toxicity assessment. Depending on specific mechanisms, a reproductive toxin may be extremely safe in one species but a powerful toxicant in another. Thalidomide is an excellent example.[34] Because differences between rats and mice and even among different strains of mice can be observed, toxicological tests using animal models do not provide a reliable extrapolation to humans. Therefore, multiple toxicological tests across different species including nonhuman primates and *in vitro* tests using human cell lines are necessary prior to clinical trials.

Another concern is the gender difference in toxic responses. This is especially true for the endocrine system, because there are considerable differences between males and females in their endocrine characteristics. In humans, differences in immune responses between men and women have also been established. Although it is still uncertain whether there is a gender difference in toxic responses, it is always beneficial to take the sex of the subject into consideration during studies. In addition, there are other important variables such as developmental stages, or age. For some toxicants, their actions may be more effective at a certain time of the reproductive process. For example, galactose or azathioprine are toxic to the developing ovary before birth but are nontoxic to postnatal ovaries.[47]

TOXICITY OF SELECTED COMPOUNDS
Steroids and Related Compounds

Hormonal contraceptives are steroid analogs that alter gonadotropin release. The risk of voluntarily taking oral contraceptives has frequently been discussed.[48] The dosage used for contraception is maintained at a low daily level (e.g., 50 μg). However, occupational exposure to these preparations for female workers is hazardous to their reproductive health. Impaired ovarian function is often observed in women exposed to dust containing mestranol or ethinylestradiol, leading to reduced fertility.[49] Occupational exposure to androgens is also a concern for women. Exposed individuals may develop an enlarged clitoris, increased hair growth, and masculinization.

Obviously, steroids and their analogs also have pronounced effects on men. In the sporting world, the use of anabolic-androgenic steroids has become epidemic,[50] although their use is prohibited by the International Olympic Committee. Because their use is more popular even among recreational and adolescent athletes, the problem is now a public health issue. If the use of steroids is supervised correctly with supplements at optimal dosages, the treatment may improve muscular performance. Because steroids are easily available, with misleading promotional materials even through the mail,[51] the control of abuse is difficult. Some health risks associated with overdosage may be irreversible and life-threatening, especially when they are used in combination with other drugs.

Heavy Metals

Lead, mercury, and cadmium are common heavy metals known to impair the reproductive process. Both prenatal and postnatal exposure to these heavy metals are detrimental. They can be presented in various forms such as chloride, sulfates, or organic complexes. The toxicity of the metal depends on its form. For example, their chlorides vary greatly in aqueous solubility; lead chloride is sparingly soluble whereas cadmium chloride is highly soluble in aqueous solutions. Lead is more toxic in the form of acetate or organic complexes such as tetramethyl or tetraethyl lead because these forms are highly soluble in lipid. Cadmium chloride, on the other hand, is highly toxic in aqueous solutions but the inorganic cadmium ion has difficulty crossing the cell membrane.

The source of these heavy metals is usually industrial.[52] For example, organic lead is a component of antiknock mix, and inorganic mercury is used in barometers and other electrical machinery. Cadmium is found in batteries, electroplating, and as an amalgam in dentistry. A recent study on workers exposed to cadmium in smelters or to lead in a battery factory in Belgian showed that fertility of these workers was reduced.[53] In another study on women in areas with high lead and cadmium content in soil, there were fewer women with three or more pregnancies and the number of preterm deliveries was higher in comparison to women in control areas with low lead and cadmium content in the soil.[54]

Both prenatal and postnatal exposure to these heavy metals are detrimental, as shown in studies on rodents. Prenatal exposure often results in birth defects such as ancephaly, and in mild situations, as with cadmium, gonadal formation is impaired. During the postnatal development establishment of the hypothalamic-hypophyseal-ovarian-uterine axis, treatment of these heavy metals results in ovarian atrophy, decreased fertility, and altered cycles.

Pesticides

Common pesticides used are dibromochloropropane (DBCP), DDT, and the once popular chlordecone. There are many different pesticides and herbicides used in agriculture. They are mostly organic compounds. In 1977, DBCP was the first pesticide reported to have reproductive toxicity.[55] It is associated with occupational exposure in manufacturing workers. Male workers report impotence or decreased libido with elevated FSH levels. There is a loss of germ cells, leading to azoospermia or oligospermia and eventually to reduced fertility.

In laboratory animals, DBCP has also been shown to induce severe testicular degeneration in males and irregular estrous cycles in females. DDT also causes a marked reduction in fertility in mice with its possible estrogenic actions. However, in contrast to DBCP, the reproductive toxicity of DDT on humans has not been clearly demonstrated. Chlordecone (Kepone) is also associated with reduced sperm count and motility and with an increased number of abnormal sperm in humans. Workers exposed to high levels of this pesticide have symptoms such as nervousness, tremor, and visual problems.[52] Interestingly, this pesticide can also be found in breast milk, indicating that it may also affect the infant.

Organic Compounds

In contrast to pesticides, organic solvents are simpler molecules. Examples are ethylene glycol, toluene, benzene, and hexane. Almost all organic solvents studied have reproductive toxicity; they either reduce gonadal function or interfere with embryonic development. Because organic molecules are lipophilic, they can pass through the cell membrane easily. They diffuse readily through the uterine wall, placenta, and blood-gonadal barrier. In highly industrialized countries, there are numerous types of organic solvents used. It becomes a health concern not only for workers involved in the industrial process but also for the public.

Ethylene glycol ethers are commonly used as antifreeze in automobile coolant. They have been shown to induce testicular degeneration in rats, but there has been no documented reproductive toxicity in humans. Toluene is a common solvent in paints. Some women exposed to toluene occupationally suffer from menstrual disorders. In pregnant women, there is a decrease in fetal growth and newborn weight among those exposed to toluene which is embryotoxic rather than teratogenic.

Recently, PCBs and dioxins, which are similar to thyroid hormones in chemical structure, have been shown to affect fetal development at doses nontoxic to the mother.[56] Children and animals exposed to these compounds pre- or postnatally exhibit behavioral disorders. As recently reviewed, PCB toxicity may depend on its involvement at the receptor level as thyroid and steroidal hormones.[57]

Alcohol and Nicotine

In a study on prepubertal female rats, alcohol induced an increase in the hypothalamic content of GHRH and LHRH with a concomitant decrease in serum GH and LH.[58] These results support earlier studies showing that alcohol causes a delayed onset of puberty in female rats.[59] The alcohol-treated rats had a delay in vaginal opening, decreased uterine weight, and abnormal ovarian functions. A clinical study on pregnant women who drink twice a week or more showed that about 50% of cases of spontaneous abortions may be attributed to alcohol consumption.[60] The mean alcohol intake per drink was 0.72 to 2.50 oz in absolute amount, but a chronic consumption of 6 oz per day is agreed to constitute a high risk.[61] Also, spontaneous abortion is a natural screening mechanism to eliminate malformed fetuses.

A fetus may not be aborted if the pregnant woman starts to drink late in her pregnancy. Some fetuses may develop to apparently normal babies, whereas others may develop fetal alcohol syndrome (FAS). At least several hundred children each year are born with full FAS and thousands more with some alcohol-induced defects.[61] FAS includes microcephaly, mental retardation, cardiac abnormalities, and other neural defects. Alcohol possibly induces fetal growth retardation and neural tube defects.

In addition to its possible effects on the reproductive system, alcohol may also alter sexual behavior, as shown in some psychological studies in humans.[45] Alcohol at low doses disinhibits psychological sexual arousal and at higher doses suppresses physiological responses to sexual stimulation. It may affect sexual behavior indirectly through altering the cognitive function transiently and may possibly evoke these changes through its effects on the endocrine and nervous systems.

Alcoholic mothers very often smoke or even take illegal drugs during pregnancy. The teratogenic effect of alcohol is compounded by the endocrine changes induced by smoking. Nicotine in tobacco plants is thought to be the main causative agent. As a potent vasoconstrictor, nicotine reduces uteroplacental blood flow and causes fetal growth retardation.[62] It is not surprising to find a lower mean birth weight among infants of smoking mothers. Mediated through nicotinic receptors, this drug stimulates uterotubal motility. It also enhances norepinephrine release and oxytocin secretion from the pituitary gland.[47] Nicotine is known to increase the rate of spontaneous abortion and suppress fetal tissue growth directly.[62] Therefore, it is now difficult to dispute the harmful effects of alcohol drinking and smoking on our endocrine and nervous systems.

DUAL ROLES OF THE ENVIRONMENT

Environmental factors can be abiotic or biotic. Temperature, humidity, atmospheric pressure, and electromagnetic waves including ultraviolet and visible lights are abiotic factors. Biotic factors are attributed to the activities of living organisms. The characteristics of these factors depend on the interactions among individuals of the same or other species. Living organisms may also change the characteristics of abiotic factors. Pollution is an example of the impact of human activities on abiotic factors. To survive and pass their genes to the next generation, all existing species must cope with these factors in their habitats.

Biotic and abiotic factors interact with one another dynamically; they may change in concentration or intensity and their effects may vary in specificity or severity under different conditions. For example, light intensity and temperature fluctuate daily, and the concentration and nature of pollutants alter with changes in human activities at different locations. If the fluctuation of a factor is rhythmic and predictable, the species may develop an ability to detect and predict the changes. During evolution, many species had acquired a time-keeping mechanism to determine the optimal time for feeding or reproduction. Seasonal animals have been using circadian and circannual rhythms as time-keeping mechanisms to schedule their annual activities.

The characteristics of some abiotic factors may vary and become unfavorable to the species. Light, for instance, is both a biorhythm regulator and a phototoxic agent. In many species, prolonged exposure to strong sunlight leads to retinal damage, although the tolerance to phototoxicity varies from one species to another. Under the normal light-dark cycle with predictable changes in light intensity, seasonal breeders evolved to adopt light as a regulatory factor for their biorhythms. This regulatory mechanism is driven by the balance between optimal and hostile environmental conditions encountered by the species. Although the environment plays a regulatory role in biorhythms, it can also disrupt the physiology of the organism. These two contradictory roles of the environment are the engine of the natural selection mechanism, helping one species to eliminate its competitors if this species can adapt to these changes successfully.

Biorhythmicity is apparently a key mechanism employed by most species, from protozoa to humans, in facing this environmental challenge throughout evolution. The evolutionary success of a species depends on its biorhythmic algorithm to compute and predict environmental changes and its ability to cope with the duality of the environment. The recent emergence of the human species has altered the ecosystem dramatically; pollution and habitat destruction are the two most notorious environmental changes induced by us. If our restorative effort fails to rectify the possible environmental catastrophe, many species including ourselves may not have the appropriate mechanism to combat these hostile conditions. As an intelligent species, we should be able to anticipate these consequences. Hopefully, we can devise some ways in time to solve this new environmental challenge.

REFERENCES

1. **Yu, H.S., Tsin, A.T.C., and Reiter, R.J.,** Melatonin: history, biosynthesis, and assay methodology, in *Melatonin: Biosynthesis, Physiological Effects, and Clinical Applications*, Yu, H.S. and Reiter, R.J., Eds., CRC Press, Boca Raton, FL, 1993, 1.
2. **Yu, H.S.,** Reproductive neuroendocrinology, in *Human Reproductive Biology*, CRC Press, Boca Raton, FL, 1994, 47.
3. **Weiner, R.I., Findell, P.R., and Kordon, C.,** Role of classic and peptideneuromediators in the neuroendocrine regulation of LH and prolactin, in *The Physiology of Reproduction,* Knobil, E. and Neill, J., Eds., Raven Press, New York, 1988, 1235.
4. **Hansen, S., Svensson, L., Hökfelt, T., and Everitt, B.J.,** 5-Hydroxytryptamine-thyrotropin releasing hormone interactions in the spinal cord: effects on parameters of sexual behavior in the male rat, *Neurosci. Lett.,* 42, 299, 1983.
5. **Krause, B. and Moller, S.,** Menstrual cycle, opioids and hypothalamic amenorrhea: from physiology to pathology, *Zentralbl. Gynaekol.,* 112, 725, 1990 (in German).
6. **Naftolin, F., Garcia-Segura, L.M., Keefe, D., Leranth, C., Maclusky, N.J., Brawer, J.R.,** Estrogen effects on the synaptology and neural membranes of the rat hypothalamic arcuate nucleus, *Biol. Reprod.,* 42, 21, 1990.
7. **Mastroianni, L., Jr. and Coutifaris, C.,** Reproductive physiology, in *The F.I.G.O. Manual of Human Reproduction,* Vol. 1, Rosenfield, A. and Fathalla, M.F., Eds., Parthenon, Park Ridge, NJ, 1990.
8. **Dale, H.H.,** On some physiological actions of ergot, *J. Physiol. (London),* 34, 165, 1906.
9. **Dale, H.H.,** The action of extracts of the pituitary body, *Biochem. J.,* 4, 427, 1909.
10. **Arimura, A.** Pituitary adenylate cyclase activating polypeptide (PACAP): discovery and current status of research, *Regulatory Peptides,* 37, 287, 1992.
11. **Heindel, J.J., Powell, C.J., Paschall, C.S., Arimura, A., and Culler, M.D.,** A novel hypothalamic peptide, pituitary adenylate cyclase activating peptide, modulates Sertoli cell function *in vitro, Biol. Reprod.,* 47, 800, 1992.
12. **Wei, W.W.S.,** *Time Series Analysis: Univariate and Multivariate Methods,* Addison-Wesley, Reading, CA, 1990.

13. **Boklage, C.E., Zincone, L.H., and Kirby, C.F., Jr.,** Annual and sub-annual rhythms in human conception rates: time-series analyses show annual and weekday but no monthly rhythms in daily counts for last normal menses, *Hum. Reprod.*, 7, 899, 1992.

14. **Yu, H.S.,** Melatonin in the eye: functional implications, in *Melatonin: Biosynthesis, Physiological Effects, and Clinical Applications*, Yu, H.S. and Reiter, R.J., Eds., CRC Press, Boca Raton, FL, 1993, 365.

15. **Teicher, M.H. and Barber, N.I.,** COSIFIT: an interactive program for simultaneous multioscillator cosinor analysis of time-series data, *Comput. Biomed. Res.*, 23, 283, 1990.

16. **Edmunds, L.N., Jr.,** Cellular and molecular bases of biological clocks: models and mechanisms for circadian timekeeping, Springer-Verlag, New York, 1988.

17. **Turek, F.W. and van Cauter, E.,** Rhythms in reproduction, in *The Physiology of Reproduction,* Knobil, E. and Neill, J., Eds., Raven Press, New York, 1988, 1789.

18. **Aschoff, J.,** Circadian rhythms in man, in *Biological Timekeeping,* Brady, J., Ed., Cambridge University Press, Cambridge, 1984, 143.

19. **Kapen, S., Boyar, R.M., Finkelstein, J.W., Hellman, L., and Weitzman, E.D.,** Effect of sleep-wake cycle reversal on luteinizing hormone secretory pattern in puberty, *J. Clin. Endocrinol. Metabol.*, 39, 293, 1974.

20. **Bremner, W.J., Vitiello, M.V., and Prinz, P.N.,** Loss of circadian rhythmicity in blood testosterone levels with aging in normal men, *J. Clin. Endocrinol. Metabol.*, 56, 1278, 1983.

21. **Goldman, B.D. and Nelson, R.J..,** Melatonin and seasonality in mammals, in *Melatonin: Biosynthesis, Physiological Effects, and Clinical Applications*, Yu, H.S. and Reiter, R.J., Eds., CRC Press, Boca Raton, FL, 1993, 225.

22. **Bitman, J., Kahl, S., Wood, D.L., and Lefcourt, A.M.,** Circadian and ultradian rhythms of plasma thyroid hormone concentrations in lactating dairy cows, *Am. J. Physiol.*, 266, R1797, 1994.

23. **Bronson, F.H.,** Seasonal regulation of reproduction in mammals, in *The Physiology of Reproduction,* Knobil, E. and Neill, J., Eds., Raven Press, New York, 1988, 1831.

24. **Warren, D.C. and Scott, H.M.,** Influence of light on ovulation in the fowl, *J. Exp. Zool.*, 74, 137, 1936.

25. **Clarke, I.J. and Scott, C.J.,** Studies on the neuronal systems involved in the estrogen-negative feedback effect on gonadotrophin releasing hormone neurons in the ewe, *Hum. Reprod.*, 8 (Suppl. 2), 2, 1993.

26. **Woodfill, C.J., Wayne, N.L., Moenter, S.M., and Karsch, F.J.,** Photoperiodic synchronization of a circan-nual reproductive rhythm in sheep: identification of season-specific time cues, *Biol. Reprod.*, 50, 965, 1994.

27. **Rojansky, N., Brzezinski, A., and Schenker, J.G.,** Seasonality in human reproduction: an update, *Hum. Reprod.*, 7, 735, 1992.

28. **Levine, J.R., Matthew, R.W., Chenault, B.C., Brown, M.H., Hurtt, M.E., and Bently, K.S.,** Differences in the quality of semen in outdoor workers during summer and winter, *N. Engl. J. Med.*, 323, 12, 1990.

29. **Kauppila, A., Kivela, A., Pakarinen, A., and Vakkuri, O.,** Inverse seasonal relationship between melatonin and ovarian activity in humans in a region with a strong seasonal contrast in luminosity, *J. Clin. Endocrinol. Metab.*, 65, 823, 1987.

30. **Sundararaj, N., Chern, M., Gatewood, L., Hichman, L., and McHugh, R.,** Seasonal behavior of human menstrual cycles: a biometric investigation, *Hum. Biol.*, 50, 15, 1978.

31. **Iatropoulos, M.J.,** Endocrine considerations in toxicologic pathology, *Exp. Toxicol. Pathol.*, 45, 391, 1994.

32. **Persaud, T.V.,** The pregnant woman in the work place: potential embryopathic risks, *Anat. Anz.*, 170, 295, 1990.

33. **Sullivan, F.M.,** Reproductive toxicity tests: retrospect and prospect, *Hum. Toxicol.*, 7, 423, 1988.

34. **McBride, W.G.,** Thalidomide and congenital abnormalities, *Lancet,* 2, 1358, 1961.

35. **U.S. Food and Drug Administration,** Guidelines for reproduction studies for safety evaluation of drugs for human use, U.S. Food and Drug Administration, Washington, D.C., 1966.

36. **Reiter, R.J.,** Interactions of the pineal hormone melatonin with oxygen-centered free radicals: a brief review, *Braz. J. Med. Biol. Res.*, 26, 1141, 1993.

37. **Mattison, D.R.,** Clinical manifestations of ovarian toxicity, in *Reproductive Toxicology*, Dixon, R.L., Ed., Raven Press, New York, 1985, 109.

38. **Desjardins, C.,** Morphological, physiological, and biochemical aspects of male reproduction, in *Reproductive Toxicology*, Dixon, R.L., Ed., Raven Press, New York, 1985, 131.

39. **Kline, J. and Stein, Z.,** Very early pregnancy, in *Reproductive Toxicology*, Dixon, R.L., Ed., Raven Press, New York, 1985, 251.

40. **Wu, J.T.,** Chemicals affecting implantation, in *Reproductive Toxicology*, Dixon, R.L., Ed., Raven Press, New York, 1985, 239.

41. **Carter, B.S., Carter, H.B., and Isaacs, J.T.,** Epidemiologic evidence regarding predisposing factors to prostate cancer, *Prostate*, 16, 187, 1990.

42. **Scardino, P.T., Weaver, R., and Hudson, M.A.,** Early detection of prostate cancer, *Hum. Pathol.*, 23, 211, 1992.

43. **Eliasson, R.,** Clinical effects of chemicals on male reproduction, in *Reproductive Toxicology*, Dixon, R.L., Ed., Raven Press, New York, 1985, 161.

44. **Hoegerman, G., Wilson, C.A., Thurmond, E., and Schnoll, S.H.,** Drug-exposed neonates, *West. J. Med.,* 152, 559, 1990.

45. **Crowe, L.C. and George, W.H.,** Alcohol and human sexuality: review and integration, *Psychol. Bull.,* 105, 374, 1989.

46. **Jonsson, C.J. and Lund, B.O.,** In vitro bioactivation of the environmental pollutant 3-methylsulphonyl-2,2-bis(4-chlorophenyl)-1,1-dichloroethene in the human adrenal gland, *Toxicol. Lett.,* 71, 169, 1994.

47. **Mattison, D.R. and Thomford, P.J.,** Mechanisms of action of reproductive toxicants, in *Toxicology of the Male and Female Reproductive Systems,* Working, P.K., Ed., Hemisphere, New York, 1989, 101.

48. **Yu, H.S.,** Contraception and assisted conception, in *Human Reproductive Biology,* CRC Press, Boca Raton, FL, 1994, 196.

49. **DeMorales, A.V., Rivera, R.O., Harrington, J.M., and Stein, G.F.,** The occupational hazards of formulating oral contraceptives: a survey of plant employees, *Arch. Environ. Health,* 33, 12, 1978.

50. **Kleiner, S.M.,** Performance-enhancing aids in sport: health consequences and nutritional alternatives, *J. Am. Coll. Nutr.,* 10, 163, 1991.

51. **DiPasquale, M.G.,** Beyond anabolic steroids, in *Drugs in Sports Series,* M.G.D. Press, Warkworth, ON, 1990.

52. **Barlow, S.M. and Sullivan, F.M.,** *Reproductive Hazards of Industrial Chemicals,* Academic Press, London, 1982.

53. **Gennart, J.P., Buchet, J.P., Roels, H., Ghyselen, P., Ceulemans, E., and Lauwerys, R.,** Fertility of male workers exposed to cadmium, lead, or manganese, *Am. J. Epidemiol.,* 135, 1208, 1992.

54. **Laudanski, T., Sipowicz, M., Modzelewski, P., Bolinski, J., Szamatowicz, J., Razniewska, G., and Akerlund, M.,** Influence of high lead and cadmium soil content on human reproductive outcome, *Int. J. Gynaecol. Obstet.,* 36, 309, 1991.

55. **Whorton, D., Krauss, R.M., Marshall, S., and Milby, T.H.,** Infertility in male pesticide workers, *Lancet,* ii, 1259, 1977.

56. **Porterfield, S.P.,** Vulnerability of the developing brain to thyroid abnormalities: environmental insults to the thyroid system, *Environ. Health Persp.,* 102 (Suppl. 2), 125, 1994.

57. **McKinney, J.D. and Waller, C.L.,** Polychlorinated biphenyls as hormonally active structural analogues, *Environ. Health Persp.,* 102, 290, 1994.

58. **Les Dees, W., Skelley, C.W., Hiney, J.K., and Johnston, C.A.,** Actions of ethanol on hypothalamic and pituitary hormones in prepubertal female rats, *Alcohol,* 7, 21, 1990.

59. **Bo, W.J., Krueger, W.A., Rudeen, P.K., and Symmes, S.K.,** Ethanol-induced alterations in the morphology and function of the rat ovary, *Anat. Rec.,* 202, 255, 1982.

60. **Kline, J., Shrout, P., Stein, Z., Susser, M., and Warbuton, D.,** Drinking during pregnancy and spontaneous abortion, *Lancet,* ii, 176, 1980.

61. **Brent, R.L. and Beckman, D.A.,** Principles of teratology, in *Reproductive Risks and Prenatal Diagnosis,* Appleton & Lange, Norwalk, CT, 1992, 43.

62. **Werler, M.M., Pober, B.R., and Holmes, L.B.,** Smoking and pregnancy, *Teratology,* 32, 473, 1985.

Chapter 3

THE PINEAL GLAND AND MELATONIN

Jerry Vriend and Nancy A. M. Alexiuk

CONTENTS

0-8493-9429-5/96/$0.00+$.50
© 1996 by CRC Press, Inc.

INTRODUCTION

The inclusion of a chapter on the pineal gland suggests that the pineal gland has a kinship with the other classical endocrine glands. Like other glands that deposit hormones into the blood vascular system, the pineal gland is a highly vascular structure. It is now well documented that the pineal gland secretes at least one active substance, *N*-acetyl-5-methoxy-tryptamine, commonly known as melatonin. This indole has been detected both in the pineal gland, from which it was originally isolated,[1,2] and in the circulation of amphibians,[3] birds,[4] fish,[5,6] and a large number of mammalian species including man.[7-16] A definitive demonstration of a physiological action of melatonin at a site distant from the pineal gland is required before melatonin can be regarded as meeting the requirements for classification as a classical hormone. An increasing number of researchers regard the central nervous system (CNS) as a site of action of melatonin. However, general agreement on one or more specific CNS locations at which melatonin acts is lacking. Furthermore, reports of the diverse actions of melatonin put in doubt the view that the various effects of melatonin can be accounted for by an action at a single CNS site. Identification of the mechanism of action of melatonin would be a major landmark in this field of research.

Research on the pineal gland has become extremely diversified in the last two decades. Basic scientists from a growing list of disciplines, as well as clinicians, have contributed to the literature. The current chapter is intended to present some of the diversity of pineal research, but focuses on basic aspects of structure and function, with emphasis on the mammalian pineal gland. While the literature in this field portrays a dynamic area of research, it also reflects an area of research in which fundamental questions concerning the pineal gland remain unanswered. The paradoxical biological actions of melatonin suggest that this substance may give new meaning to our definition of a classical hormone.

ANATOMY

PHYLOGENETIC CONSIDERATIONS

On a phylogenetic scale, a pineal organ can be found in all classes of vertebrates ranging from primitive fish (including lampreys) to amphibians, reptiles, birds, and mammals (including man).[17] The vertebrate pineal gland, or epiphysis, develops as an evagination of the roof of the diencephalon. The lumen of the epiphyseal primordium is continuous with the third ventricle. In phylogenetic studies, a distinction is made between the diencephalic primordium, which develops into the pineal gland, and a more rostral primordium, which, in lower species, develops into a parapineal organ, such as the extracranial, subcutaneous frontal organ of anurans or the parietal eye (third eye) of lacertilian and sphenodon lizards.[18] Some authors regard the pineal gland and the parapineal organs as originating from a common primordium and use the term "pineal complex" to include pineal and parapineal derivatives.[19] Already before the turn of the century, the pineal anlage of fish, amphibians, and reptiles was recognized as developing into a photosensory organ[18,20] similar to the retina of the eye. In the pineal gland of these species, photoreceptor cells can be distinguished from supportive cells and sensory nerve cells, all of which originate from the neuroepithelial cell layer of the pineal primordium.[21] A phylogenetic relationship between the pineal gland and retina is further suggested by the presence of proteins in the pineal gland that are associated with phototransduction in the retina; these include the retinal protein referred to as S antigen, a protein which reportedly regulates light-dependent phosphodiesterase in rod outer segments,[22,23] interphotoreceptor retinol-binding protein (IRBP),[24,25] and transducin, a GTP-binding protein also found in rod outer segments. Evidence for the presence of transducin in pineal glands of submammalian (but not mammalian) vertebrates has been presented.[26] Two additional proteins that bind to transducin, phosducin[27] and MEKA[28]—a protein named after the letter symbols for the N-terminal amino acids—have been found in rat and sheep pineal glands. It has been suggested that photoreceptors of the retina and pinealocytes share common components of signal transduction.[29] It has been proposed that phosducin modulates synthesis of cAMP by regulating the amount of G protein units available for activating adenyl cyclase. Cases of concurrent uveoretinitis and pineal gland tumors in children[30] could be related to an abnormal response to an excess of one or more of these antigens. Pineal tumors may express protein antigens usually detected only during retinal development.[31]

Evidence for the presence of melatonin in the retina of amphibians, reptiles, fish, and birds is accumulating,[32] whereas convincing data for its presence in mammalian species is not available. A recent study suggests that melatonin is either very low or absent in the bovine eye.[33]

Although the pineal gland has been reported to be absent in several species (including crocodiles, anteaters, sloths, and armadillos), this has been questioned from an embryological point of view.[34] Early histological studies suggested that in addition to a photoreceptor function, photosensory cells in the pineal also had a secretory function.[18] Dense-core, secretory-type vesicles were observed in fish, amphibian, and reptilian pineal cells, supporting this view.[35-40] Phylogenetic variation in the pineal is well illustrated in birds, in which photoreceptor elements are rudimentry,[41-46] but secretory vesicles are relatively abundant.[47-49]

A pineal nerve, or tract, homologous to the optic nerve, has been described in studies of a variety of fish, amphibian, reptile, and avian pineals. Descriptions of synaptic connection of photoreceptor cells with fibers of the pineal tract are well documented,[50] but the central projections of the pineal tract have been studied in detail by few investigators. The central projections of the pineal tract reported for these species include the lateral habenular nucleus, pretectal area, and brainstem tegmentum.[50-52] In the lamprey, most of the fibers of the pineal tract enter the brain through the posterior commissure. In this species, projections of this tract include the subcommissural organ, pretectal area, thalamus, dorsal hypothalamus, optic tectum, and midbrain tegmentum.[53] These central projections of the pineal organ appear to be associated with photosensory (and possibly olfactory) functions in lower species, rather than with the phylogenetic progression to neuroendocrine functions in higher vertebrates.

THE MAMMALIAN PINEAL GLAND

The mammalian pineal gland appears to have no direct photosensory function. In pineal glands of some mammalian species, rudimentary photoreceptor cells and cells intermediate between photoreceptor and secretory cells have been described.[54] This raises the question of whether the pinealocyte comprises a heterogeneous population of cells, only some of which are derived from a rudimentary photoreceptor cell.

Although the mammalian pineal gland does not appear to be directly photosensitive, it does respond to changes in environmental lighting, via a rather circuitous route involving the visual system (see below). Dense-core secretory vesicles, which have been observed in pinealocytes of a number of mammalian species,[55,56] increase in number in blind mice and decrease in number in mice subjected to constant light.[57,58] Interruption of the dark phase of the light-dark cycle of rats by 30 min of light was sufficient to decrease the number of secretory vesicles.[59] These observations provided anatomical evidence that light restriction increased the secretion of the pineal gland.

Anatomy

The mammalian pineal gland (Figure 1) is a solid parenchymal structure (in contrast to the pineal of submammalian species, which may be saccular or follicular in structure) surrounded by a capsule of connective tissue and pia mater. In many mammals, including humans, it is located under the splenium of the corpus callosum; rodents are an exception, having a more superficial pineal gland, which is embedded in the dura of the confluens of sinuses. The mammalian pineal gland is connected to the brain via a stalk which is attached dorsally to the habenular commissure and ventrally to the posterior commissure. The functional significance, if any, of these connections to the brain, are not known. The pineal stalk contains both neural and vascular elements, but these are currently not considered to have any major significance, unlike those that connect the hypothalamus and pituitary gland. The cavity between the dorsal and ventral roots of the pineal stalk is the pineal recess of the third ventricle. A suprapineal recess also extends from the third ventricle. The close association of the pineal and the third ventricle has led to the classification of this gland as a circumventricular organ.

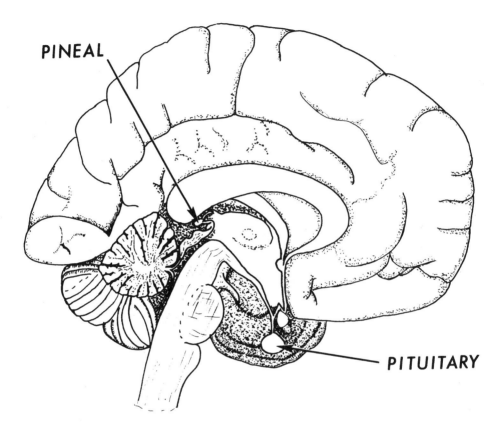

FIGURE 1. Location of the human pineal gland.

In the developing pineal of mammals, modified ependymal cells may be found, not only lining the pineal recess, but also, in some species, forming follicular-like structures with cilia and microvilli on the apical surface.[55] The pineal anlage becomes invaded by connective tissue and blood vessels, forming a highly vascular structure that has been likened to the capillary glomerulus of the kidney.[55] Because the pineal recess retains its lining of ependymal cells, there is apparently no direct contact of pineal parenchymal cells with cerebrospinal fluid (CSF); the CSF can, however, be found in the subarachnoid space surrounding the gland.

Considerable variability exists in the morphology of the pineal gland of mammals. Vollrath[60] has classified pineals as to their proximity to the habenular and posterior commissures, and to the site of the pineal anlage during ontogenesis. Thus, the pineal gland may be superficial, deep, or extend the entire distance from the commissures to the confluens of sinuses. In laboratory rodents, such as the rat and Syrian hamster (*Mesocricetus auratus*), the gland is located deep to the confluens of sinuses and is attached by a stalk to the brain stem close to the third ventricle. Some parenchymal tissue may be found in the stalk as well as at the site of attachment to the brain stem;[61] this has led to the description of a superficial and a (smaller) deep pineal for these species. The anatomical significance of these differences is not clear. Considerable variation in relative size of the pineal gland also exists. Animals with a large pineal gland, relative to brain size, include the walrus, seal, and sea lion;[62,63] the pineal of the horseshoe bat is also comparatively large.[64] Animals with a small pineal include the anteater, sloth, and armadillo.[19,65] Ralph[65] related the size of the pineal gland of mammals to the seasonal reproductive pattern; many species with a highly restricted seasonal pattern of breeding were observed to have well-developed pineal glands.

A pineal nerve has been described in studies of sheep, rabbit, and human fetuses.[66,67] This nerve was described as extending from the pineal gland to a group of nerve-cell bodies dorsal to the subcommissural organ. Similar pineal nerves have not been reported in adult mammals.

Ultrastructure of Mammalian Pinealocytes

The mammalian pinealocyte is difficult to classify. Although the pineal gland is attached to the brain, it is not typical neural tissue; nerve cells are not commonly found in the pineal glands of adult mammals. In spite of the apparent endocrine role of the mammalian pineal gland, pinealocytes do not have the appearance of cells that secrete either peptide or steroid hormones. The pinealocyte must be considered a unique derivative of ependymal cells,[68] a cell type in its own right. Classifying pinealocytes as paraneurons may, however, add to an understanding of these cells. Synaptophysin and synapsin I, usually considered to be specific for synaptic vesicles of neurons, have been found concentrated in microvesicles in pinealocyte terminals.[69]

Ultrastructural studies have shown that the mammalian pinealocyte characteristically possesses one or more cytoplasmic processes.[70-72] These cellular processes possess expanded endings which terminate in pericapillary spaces or between other pinealocytes. Pevet and Collin[54] have compared the shape of the mammalian pinealocyte to that of the photoreceptor cells in pineals of lower vertebrates; their work suggests that the mammalian pinealocyte retains characteristics of the basal part of submammalian photoreceptor cells.

Most of the organelles of the mammalian pinealocyte do not differ substantially from those of other mammalian cells. The nucleus may be irregular in shape with indentations of the surface. A prominent nucleolus is present. Both smooth and rough endoplasmic reticulum are consistently reported;[72] but Wolfe[70] pointed out that in the rat the endoplasmic reticulum is not typical and has referred to it as intergrade endoplasmic reticulum. Clusters of ribosomes, not associated with membranes, are found throughout the cytoplasm. Although mitochondria are generally reported as normal in mammalian pinealocytes, considerable variation in size and shape have been documented.[70,73-75] They are relatively numerous in most pinealocytes. Centrioles, although not present in great numbers, have been reported to differentiate into structures called microtubular sheaves (microtubules arranged in sheaves).[70-76] The presence of cilia depends on the species studied and on the developmental stage examined. Clabough[77] observed cilia in pinealocytes of fetal and neonatal rats, but cilia were absent or very rare in pinealocytes of adult rats.[70,78] In some species, such as the mole, cilia may be a characteristic feature of each pinealocyte.[54] In this species, the cilia were reported as having filaments in a 9 + 0 arrangement in the shaft, an arrangement also found in photoreceptor cells.

An organelle found in pinealocytes, but not usually found in other mammalian cells, is the synaptic ribbon,[79] which consists of an electron-dense rod surrounded by vesicles. These structures, which may occur singly or in groups, are usually associated with the cell membrane. It has been suggested that this structure is involved in cell-to-cell communication between adjacent pinealocytes.[80] One hypothesis is that synaptic ribbons function to regulate the number of β-adrenergic receptors on the pinealocyte cell membrane. Similar structures have been found in the retina.[81] Although the precise function of synaptic ribbons is not known, they are present in all mammalian pineal glands studied.

Secretory granules are much rarer in mammalian pinealocytes than would be expected of an organ considered to be primarily secretory in function. Dense-core vesicles, presumably secretory vesicles, have been observed in many species both in perikarya and in pinealocyte processes. Dense-core vesicles have been reported in pineal glands of many mammals including rat, mouse, hamster, cat, sheep, cow, monkey, and seal pinealocytes.[55,72,82-86] *In vitro* evidence that the dense-core vesicles represent a secretory product was provided by Romijn and Gelsema,[87] who found that norepinephrine (NE), which stimulates melatonin production, also produces a great increase in the number of dense-core vesicles in rabbit pinealocytes. Thyrotropin-releasing hormone (TRH) administration in rats was also reported to increase the number of dense-core vesicles in pinealocytes.[88] *In vivo* studies have shown that there is a 24-h rhythm in number of dense-core vesicles of several species.[89,90] This rhythm appears to be regulated by environmental lighting conditions.[91] Athough researchers have interpreted the dense-core vesicles as a packaged form of secretory product, a second type of secretory processes has been postulated from ultrastructural studies of the rat pineal; this process has been described as release of flocculent material from the endoplasmic reticulum.[92] Intracellular vacuoles containing this material have been described.[72] The chemical nature of either the dense-core vesicles or the flocculent material remains to be determined. Lysosomes are also typically found in pinealocytes; their role in the secretory process, if any, is also unknown. The sensitivity of lysosomal enzymes to photoperiod suggests the possibility that lysosomes are involved in pinealocyte function.[93]

Unlike other endocrine glands, the pineal gland shows little ultrastructural evidence that it is storing a hormonal product. Its known secretory product, melatonin, appears to be released almost immediately after it is synthesized. Storage mechanisms for melatonin, if they exist, are short term.

Other well-known structures found in the pineal are the corpora arenacea, calcium containing concretions[94] that increase in number with age. Although at one time thought to be characteristic of human pineals, similar structures have been reported in an increasing number of species including the monkey, horse, gerbil, aged rat, and mink.[95-98] Functionally these structures are not well understood. Their function may be associated with a high demand of calcium exchange of pinealocytes.[99]

Although the pinealocyte is the most numerous and most extensively studied cell type in the mammalian pineal, other cell types have been observed. Glial cells have been estimated to account for up to 12% of the total number of cells in the rat pineal.[100] Immunocytochemical studies of glial cells in the rat pineal provide evidence that the glial cells are primarily astrocytes.[101] Astrocyte-specific glial antigens, vimenten, glial fibrillary acid protein (GFAP) and S-100 were localized in the pineal gland of rats, hamsters, and gerbils.[23,102] Glial processes were also found in the pineal stalk, where they are described as encircling neural and vascular elements of the stalk.[103]

Blood Supply

The pineal gland is supplied by branches of the posterior choroidal arteries,[104-106] which are derived from the posterior cerebral arteries. It has been estimated that the mammalian pineal gland has a blood flow (per gram of tissue) that is exceeded only by the kidney.[107] The pineal is drained by venules which join the great cerebral vein of Galen and the internal cerebral veins.[107] The perivascular spaces of the mammalian pineal are the site of termination of pinealocyte processes as well as of sympathetic nerve fibers. The extent of the relationship between pinealocyte processes and perivascular spaces may vary considerably from species to species, but is considered to be of basic structural and functional importance.[71] Melatonin is thought to be secreted into the perivascular spaces prior to being distributed by the venous system into the general circulation.

Innervation

Although the pineal gland is attached to the brain, the functional significance of this attachment is not known. The primary innervation of the mammalian pineal is via peripheral sympathetics. The sympathetic innervation was definitively demonstrated in the albino rat,[107-109] and was since demonstrated in many other mammalian species by a variety of methods. Both anatomically and functionally, the pineal gland is an end-organ of the sympathetic nervous system. Kappers[107] showed that after surgical removal of the superior cervical ganglia, the sympathetic nerve fibers in the rat pineal disappeared. The sympathetic nerves release NE into pericapillary spaces; norepinephrine in turn, via β-receptors on pinealocyte membranes, stimulates the synthesis of melatonin from serotonin.[110-112] This mechanism is mediated by an adenylate cyclase system in the pinealocyte.[113-114]

The inhibitory effects of light on pineal secretion of melatonin depend on intact postganglionic sympathetics to the pineal gland. The pathway by which light information reaches the pineal gland has been partially demonstrated by experimental methods: light information is converted to neural information in the retina and travels via the optic nerve through the optic chiasm. Following the decussation, the fibers involved in the photoregulation of melatonin leave the neural pathway involved in vision. Impulses are transmitted by a direct retinohypothalamic pathway to the suprachiasmatic nuclei (SCN).[115-117] The SCN project caudally into the hypothalamus, reach the lateral hypothalamus via one or more neurons, and synapse with central sympathetic fibers running through the medial forebrain bundle.[115,116] These fibers project to the intermediolateral cell column of the thoracic cord, the source of preganglionic fibers to the superior cervical ganglia. The preganglionic neurons travel up the sympathetic trunk to synapse with postganglionic neurons in the superior cervical ganglia. These fibers reach the pineal gland via the tentorium cerebelli and enter the pineal gland as the nervi conarii.[107] Sympathetic fibers enter the pineal with blood vessels distributing themselves in the gland to terminate among pinealocytes or in pericapillary spaces.

The retinohypothalamic tract to the SCN is important in the entrainment of visually dependent circadian rhythms. Another tract, with terminations in the SCN, is the geniculohypothalamic tract (GHT), a secondary visual projection which may participate in entrainment of circadian rhythms.[118,119] The intergeniculate leaflet, which is the source of the GHT, also, according to recent reports, projects directly to the pineal gland in the rat and gerbil.[120,121] However, any functional role it may have in providing light information to the pineal gland does not appear to have been investigated. Parasympathetic innervation of pinealocytes is not considered to be of major importance in mammals.[107] Parasympathetic fibers, however, have been reported in the monkey and in the rabbit.[122,123] The parasympathetic innervation of the pineal in mammals originates from perikarya in the pterygopalatine ganglia.[124] Cholinergic receptors have been demonstrated in the rat pineal.[125] Pharmacological studies have shown parasympathetic effects on indole metabolism in the pineal but little influence on melatonin production.[126] Ganglion cells have been observed in primates,[127] rabbits,[123,128] and the ferret.[129,130] The relationship of the ganglion cells to other autonomic fibers is not clear.

Although the sympathetic innervation of the pineal gland appears to be the major innervation of the gland, central innervation of the pineal has been postulated from immunocytochemical and electrophysiological studies. Nerve fibers entering the pineal from the habenular area have been noted in several species;[107,131-133] these findings, however, have been put in question by horse-radish peroxidase (HRP) tracing studies in the rat.[134] Electrophysiological studies were also interpreted as evidence for a habenular-pineal connection.[135,136] It has been suggested the the habenular nuclei play a role in functionally linking pinealocytes with the olfactory system.[107,137,138] Immunocytochemical studies have shown nerve fibers or neurosecretory fibers entering the deep pineal or the pineal stalk from the habenular area; thus substance P-immunoreactive nerve fibers were reported to enter the bovine pineal gland[139] from the habenular region, serotonin-immunoreactive nerve fibers reported to enter the deep pineal of the Syrian hamster from the habenula,[140] and S-antigen-immunoreactive nerve fibers reported to enter the mouse pineal region from the medial habenular nucleus.[141] Although most neuropeptide Y (NPY)-immunoreactive nerve fibers in the pineal gland were found to originate from the superior cervical ganglia, some of these fibers originated centrally from the habenula to enter the deep pineal.[142] Functional studies suggest that NPY may inhibit noradrenergic-stimulated cAMP acccumulation[143] and noradrenergic-stimulated melatonin secretion in the rat.[144] NPY neurons are reported to be colocalized with NE in sympathetic neurons entering the pineal gland from the superior cervical ganglia.[145] Nerve fibers entering the pineal gland from the posterior commissure have been reported in studies of the dog and rat pineal.[146-148]

Oxytocin and vasopressin neurosecretory axons have been reported in the mammalian pineal gland. These peptidergic fibers, demonstrated by immunocytochemistry of oxytocin and vasopressin in hedgehog brains, have been reported to enter the pineal gland via the habenular commissure.[148] In both the guinea pig and hedgehog, such fibers have been reported to originate in the paraventricular nuclei (PVN) of the hypothalamus, a conclusion based on HRP tracing methods.[149,150] The presence of vasopressin and oxytocin in the mammalian pineal has been confirmed by radioimmunoassay.[151] Results demonstrating the presence of oxytocin and vasopressin in the mammalian pineal suggest more attention should be given to the possible functional role of these peptides in the pineal gland.

BIOCHEMISTRY

PURIFICATION AND IDENTIFICATION OF MELATONIN

In 1917, McCord and Allen[152] reported that cattle pineal glands contained a substance that was very effective in causing melanin concentration in tadpole melanophores. This substance was isolated in 1958 from extracts of bovine pineals by Lerner, a melanin biochemist.[1] It was subsequently identified as *N*-acetyl-5-methoxytryptamine, a derivative of serotonin.[2] Because of its skin-blanching effects on tadpole skin it was termed melatonin. Of the substances found in the mammalian pineal gland, melatonin is the most highly investigated. Soon after it was isolated and identified, Wurtman and Axelrod[153] stimulated interest in melatonin by proposing that the endocrine effects of the mammalian pineal gland were attributable to melatonin. According to this hypothesis, the pineal was considered an endocrine organ, secreting a substance, melatonin, into the blood to effect an action at a distant site.

PEPTIDES IN THE PINEAL GLAND

An alternative to the melatonin hypothesis of pineal function is the hypothesis that the pineal gland produces one or more proteins or polypeptides which are responsible for the endocrine-like actions of the pineal gland. A variation of this view is that melatonin acts via a pineal polypeptide. Much of the research on peptides in the pineal gland arose out of the search for a natural antigonadotropic substance. Despite numerous preliminary reports of pineal peptide and polypeptide "factors," the hypothesis that the pineal synthesizes and secretes a unique physiologically active peptide hormone is one that currently lacks critical evidence to support it.

One substance that received considerable attention some years ago as a putative pineal hormone was arginine vasotocin (AVT), a nonapeptide that occurs naturally in the neurohypophysis of nonmammalian vertebrates. Although AVT was reported as present in the mammalian pineal gland[154-158] and accepted as a pineal hormone by a number of researchers,[159,160] subsequent studies with more rigorous controls reported that this substance is not present in the mammalian pineal gland.[151,161-164] AVT was found to cross-react, in radioimmunoassay and immunocytochemistry, with antibodies to vasopressin and oxytocin, nonapeptides that are present in the mammalian pineal gland and are structurally similar to AVT. This would account for the preliminary reports of AVT in extracts and in tissue sections of pineal glands. Although AVT may have some interesting endocrine actions when administered to laboratory mammals,[165,166] the available evidence suggests that it is not a hormone of the mammalian pineal gland.[163,164] A 1992 review by Goldstein,[167] however, appears to be an attempt to revive the AVT hypothesis of pineal function.

Studies of partially purified fractions of pineal extracts have led to a large number of reports of hormonally active factors in the mammalian pineal. Although techniques similar to those used to purify hypothalamic hormones have been used on pineal extracts, these studies have not been as successful. In fact, many of the peptide factors reported from *in vitro* and *in vivo* testing of fractions of pineal extracts appear to be laboratory artifacts. We include as probable artifacts anestrina,[168] anovulin,[169] Crinofizin,[170] the Milcu extract,[171] the Orts factor,[172,173] the pineal antigonadotropin (PAG) of Ebels and co-workers,[174-176] the Ota factor,[177] the Cheesman extract,[178] a prolactin inhibitory factor,[179,180] a TRH inhibitor,[181] and a luteinizing hormone-releasing hormone (LHRH) inhibitor.[182]

The laboratory of Benson and Ebels[183] appears to be the only one to attempt large scale purification of pineal peptides. They have published the amino acid sequence of a decapeptide which they describe as the bovine pineal gland-derived antigonadotropic decapeptide (AGD).[183] When injected into rats at a dose of 10 mg, the extracted decapeptide, as well as its synthetic analog, significantly reduced blood levels of prolactin and LH. The amino acid sequence of this peptide, as the authors noted, revealed a homology with a fragment of the α-chain of bovine hemoglobin. This report leaves unanswered the question of whether AGD is merely a fragment of hemoglobin purified from bovine pineal glands (i.e., a laboratory artifact) or indeed a physiologically important antigonadotropic peptide. The authors presented the ad hoc hypothesis that the pineal gland has enzymes specifically designed for cleavage of AGD from hemoglobin. However, considering the high blood flow to the pineal gland, this hypothesis seems worth testing.

Small amounts of hypothalamic releasing (and release inhibiting) hormones have been found in pineal extracts; these hormones could account for some of the reported biological actions of the partially purified extracts. Convincing evidence for the presence of small amounts of TRH and LHRH in extracts of mammalian pineal gland has been reported.[184-186] Studies of extracts of bovine pineal glands separated on Sephadex columns indicated the presence of LHRH as determined by radioimmunoassay and confirmed by bioassay (release of LH from pituitary cells in culture).[181] Unpublished data from the authors' laboratory, show that in methanol extracts of 600 rat pineal glands, LHRH could be detected by radioimmunoassay (slightly more than 1 pg LHRH per gland). Compared to the levels in the rat hypothalamus (3000 to 8000 pg), the levels in the pineal gland are so small as to be of questionable physiological significance.

Oxytocin, vasopressin, and their neurophysins also have been reported as present in extracts of pineal glands of a number of mammalian species.[151,187-190] Vasopressin and oxytocin have been isolated and purified from bovine pineal glands.[164] Vasopressin mRNA has been detected in substantial quantities in the rat pineal gland.[191] One estimate of oxytocin concentrations in the human pineal is 200 times less than that of the neurohypophysis.[192]

SYNTHESIS AND REGULATION OF MELATONIN SECRETION

Melatonin is synthesized in the pineal gland from serotonin via a two-step procedure (Figure 2). Acetylation of serotonin is the first step. This requires the enzyme serotonin *N*-acetyl transferase (NAT) and an acetyl donor, acetyl-coenzyme A (CoA).[193] The second step is the transfer of a methyl group to *N*-acetyl serotonin from S-adenosylmethionine, using the enzyme 5-hydroxyindole-*O*-methyltransferase (HIOMT).[194,195] HIOMT was initially purified from extracts of bovine pineal glands.[196] It has been found in the pineal glands of all mammalian species studied. The enzyme NAT has been reported in brain regions other than the pineal gland.[197,198] Initial studies with the enzyme HIOMT suggested that it was present only in the pineal gland,[199] but subsequent studies provided reports that in many vertebrates, HIOMT was also found, in lower concentrations, in the retina.[200,201] *In situ* hybridization has been used to localize mRNA for HIOMT to the chicken pineal and retina.[202] The activity of this enzyme has been reported to be higher in the hen retina than in rabbit

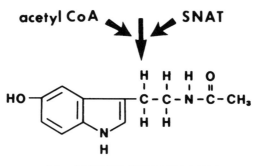

SEROTONIN

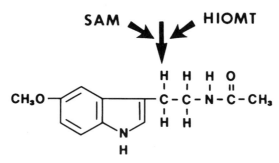

N - ACETYLSEROTONIN

MELATONIN   (N-acetyl-5-methoxytryptamine)

FIGURE 2.   Synthesis of melatonin.

retina.[203] Immunocytochemical studies report HIOMT immunoreactivity in rod and cone photoreceptors and in bipolar cells of the inner nuclear layer of rats.[204]

Serotonin is produced in pinealocytes from circulating tryptophan, which is hydroxylated by tryptophan hydroxylase to produce 5-hydroxytryptophan (5-HTP); 5-HTP, in turn, is converted to serotonin by the enzyme 5-HTP decarboxylase.[196,205] The pineal gland contains a higher concentration of serotonin than other brain tissue.[206] Other methoxyindoles found in the pineal gland include 5-methoxytryptophol, 5-methoxyindole acetic acid, and 5-methoxytryptamine.[207] Melatonin synthesis from serotonin is stimulated by sympathetic input via the nervi conarii.[107-109] In both plasma and pineal gland, melatonin levels follow a distinct circadian pattern cued to the daily light-dark cycle. In all mammals studied to date, the photoperiodic rhythm in melatonin is characterized by a nighttime rise. This has been reported in species including rat, hamster, squirrel, sheep, cattle, donkey, pig, camel, monkey, and humans.[208-215] In the rat, a 60-fold increase in NAT was measured during the dark phase of the daily light-dark cycle of the rat.[216] If lights are turned on during the dark phase a rapid decrease in NAT and melatonin occurs.[217,218] The nighttime rise in melatonin has been extensively studied since melatonin was first identified in the mammalian pineal and continues to stimulate research interest.

In organ culture, NE stimulates the secretion of NAT (and to a lesser extent, HIOMT) and melatonin.[219,220] In humans, administration of propranolol, a β-adrenergic blocker, inhibits or prevents melatonin secretion.[221-223] Thus, it is clear that melatonin secretion in mammals, including man, is under noradrenergic control. The β-adrenergic stimulation of NAT and melatonin is regulated by cyclic AMP.[224-226] To produce maximal stimulation of cAMP and NAT, both α_1 and β-adrenergic receptors must be occupied. This mechanism has been referred to as a biochemical "AND GATE."[227,228] β-Adrenergic activation alone will increase cAMP and cGMP levels as much as 10-fold, whereas concurrent stimulation of α_1 and β-adrenergic receptors by NE can increase cAMP and cGMP levels more than 100-fold.[229] β-Adrenergic activation is mediated by GTP binding proteins.[230] The postreceptor mechanisms in the α_1 potentiation of β-adrenergic response involve activation of a protein kinase and elevation of intracellular calcium.[231,232]

Investigators have suggested that the output of melatonin by the pineal may be significantly influenced by peripheral hormones. The hormones of the adrenals, thyroid, and gonads have all been studied for their effects on pineal secretion of melatonin. Studies of endocrine organ ablation showed that hypophysectomy, thyroidectomy, and adrenalectomy resulted only in small, or no, reductions in the nighttime rise in pineal secretion of melatonin.[233-235] Insulin-induced hypoglycemia may increase NAT activity and pineal melatonin content.[236] Small variations in the nighttime secretion of melatonin have also been reported to occur during the estrous cycle of the rat.[237] In male rats, castration is reported to reduce the ability of pineal glands in organ culture to synthesize 5-methoxyindoles, whereas testosterone administration restored this ability to control levels.[238]

Thyroid hormones would be expected to increase noradrenergic sensitivity of the pineal gland by increasing the density of β-adrenergic receptors. Thyroxine (T_4) and triiodothyronine (T_3) have been reported to stimulate noradrenalin-induced increases in melatonin secretion.[239] This effect could be investigated as a feedback loop because the pineal gland, under the influence of variations in the daily light-dark cycle, influences circulating levels of thyroid hormones in photosensitive species (see below).

The mammalian pineal gland appears to have a mechanism to prevent circulating levels of NE and other catecholamines from stimulating melatonin secretion to any significant degree. In the rat, circulating NE was reported as being taken up by sympathetic nerve terminals during the day.[240] This may be a mechanism to prevent adrenal-mediated stress from having any great influence on melatonin secretion.

DISTRIBUTION AND METABOLISM OF MELATONIN

Studies with tritiated melatonin have shown that this indoleamine binds to plasma proteins.[201] Presumably, this facilitates the distribution of melatonin by inhibiting metabolism. Melatonin has a biphasic (or possibly multiphasic) disappearance curve from plasma. When injected into rats, the first phase is a distribution and binding phase; this is followed by an elimination phase.[241] The distribution phase has a half-life in the order of 2 min, and the elimination phase, a half-life of 20 to 40 min.[241,242] Although most tissues of the body take up melatonin, the pineal gland has been reported to be more effective than any other tissue in the uptake of injected melatonin.[243]

Pineal secretion of melatonin is strongly influenced by the light-dark cycle. On exposure of a laboratory animal to light (during its normal dark period), melatonin in the pineal gland decreases rapidly; the half-life of disappearance has been estimated to be 10 min or less in the Syrian hamster.[244] Exposure of the rat to l min of light, at night, inhibits dramatically the activity of pineal NAT and reduces the secretion of melatonin.[245]

It has been estimated that during a single pass through the liver, 90% of blood melatonin is cleared.[246] Melatonin is metabolized in the liver to 6-hydroxymelatonin; this metabolite is conjugated primarily with sulfate (but a small percentage is also conjugated to glucuronide) and excreted in the urine.[242,247,248] In rats 6-sulfatoxymelatonin levels increase in urine 2 to

5 h after the onset of darkness.[249] In the mammalian brain melatonin may be converted to *N*-acetyl-5-methoxykynurenamine.[250]

ASSAYS FOR MELATONIN

Melatonin was isolated using bioassay.[251] This particular assay depended on skin blanching of frog tadpoles. A fluorometric assay for melatonin was developed soon after[252] and used to study a circadian rhythm in the pineal content of the indole.[253] A number of laboratories have used radioimmunoassay (RIA) to measure melatonin levels under various physiological conditions.[254-258] Although convenient and sensitive, RIAs of melatonin were not without problems. Different RIAs, although "validated," gave somewhat different results, suggesting that the antibodies used had varying specificities. Furthermore, various extraction procedures were used to prepare tissue and serum or plasma for assay. The different procedures varied in their success in removing substances that interfered in the assay. These problems resulted in conflicting data on some issues. For example, melatonin was reported as present in plasma of pinealectomized rats,[259] but was later reported to be absent in another laboratory using improved techniques.[260] Some of the best validated assays include those of Grota and Brown,[254] Wetterberg et al.,[258,261] and Kennaway.[262] Others may also be reasonably accurate if used with an appropriate extraction procedure. For RIA of melatonin in serum or plasma, melatonin is extracted into a nonpolar organic solvent such as chloroform or dichloromethane. Various procedures differ in the extent to which the organic phase is washed and separated from the aqueous phase. Additional steps may be required for extracts of tissue samples. Although thin-layer chromatography (TLC) adds considerably to the purification of the extract to be assayed, it is not convenient to do this on a routine basis if many samples are to be processed.

The development of a RIA for 6-hydroxymelatonin by various laboratories has also proved useful in providing an index of pineal activity in experiments requiring noninvasive sampling. This RIA is often used to measure the 6-hydroxy metabolite of melatonin in urine.[263]

Another method used for measuring melatonin levels is high-performance liquid chromatography (HPLC) with electrochemical or fluorescence detection. Although in the past these procedures have not had the sensitivity of RIA, recent reports show that some of the newer HPLC systems can compete in sensitivity with melatonin RIAs. Sensitivities as low as 6 pg have been reported using HPLC with fluorescence detection[264] and 8 pg using HPLC with electrochemical detection.[265]

Melatonin has also been assayed using gas chromatography and electron-capture mass spectroscopy (GC-MS).[207,266,267] The sensitivity of GC-MS was increased by negative chemical ionization; a sensitivity of 1 pg was reported by this method.[268] This technique has resulted in some very convincing melatonin data.[260,268,269] Serum and plasma levels reported with this method tend to be somewhat lower than values reported with the RIAs. For most laboratories, however, this technology is prohibitively expensive.

PHYSIOLOGICAL EFFECTS OF THE PINEAL AND MELATONIN IN CONTROL OF ENDOCRINE SYSTEMS

EFFECTS ON THE HORMONES OF REPRODUCTION IN MALES

Although the melatonin hypothesis of pineal function was proposed on the basis of results obtained with female rats,[270,271] the pineal and melatonin have a modulatory effect on the hormones of reproduction in male mammals as well. The regulatory effects of the pineal and melatonin on gonadal function are most marked in seasonal breeders. Research with laboratory species such as the Syrian hamster, or domestic species such as the sheep has contributed extensively to our knowledge in this area. The pineal gland mediates the effects of changing photoperiods on gonadal hormones in these species and thus is thought to be an important factor regulating seasonal breeding.[272,273]

Exposure of male Syrian hamsters, under laboratory conditions, to darkness, short photoperiod, or blindness results in a dramatic involution of the testes.[274] By 8 to 10 weeks of such exposure, the testes may be reduced to as little as one tenth their original size and lack mature spermatozoa.[274-277] The role of the pineal gland in this phenomenon was demonstrated and confirmed many times by Reiter and co-workers in experiments showing that pinealectomized hamsters subjected to conditions of light restriction had gonads that did not differ in size or structure from normal controls.[274,278,279] The pineal gland thus mediates the effects of variations in the photoperiodic environment on the endocrine system.[280] If hamsters whose superior cervical ganglia had been removed surgically were subjected to short photoperiod or darkness, their gonads similarly did not differ significantly from normal controls.[281,282] These identical results of pinealectomy and superior cervical ganglionectomy demonstrate that the sympathetic innervation of the pineal gland is functionally necessary for the inhibitory effect of the pineal gland on the gonads; pineal glands transplanted under the kidney capsule were not effective in this regard.[283] In intact Syrian hamsters, short photoperiod induces testicular regression through neural pathways involving hypothalamic regulation of sympathetic control of melatonin production in the pineal. Destruction of the PVN blocks the short photoperiod response.[284,285] The PVN may also control melatonin production in animals such as the rat, which do not have dramatic photoperiodically induced changes in testicular size or in circulating levels of gonadotropic hormones.[286]

Studies of hormonal levels in Syrian hamsters subjected to short photoperiod, darkness, or blindness, have consistently shown a marked decrease in pituitary prolactin;[287-289] a depression of plasma prolactin, LH, and FSH may also be observed, especially in the period preceding gonadal involution.[290,291] These effects were not observed in hamsters that were pinealectomized. These studies provided strong evidence that the pineal gland had a major role in regulating circulating levels of adenohypophyseal hormones associated with reproduction.

Increases in hypothalamic content of LHRH have also been reported to be associated with short photoperiod-induced gonadal involution.[291] This could account for the reduced secretion of LH and FSH in light-restricted hamsters—assuming that increased tissue content of LHRH reflected decreased release. Changes in prolactin secretion in these animals could be related to reduced release of TRH from the PVN,[292] reduced release of another (as yet unidentified) prolactin releasing factor or increased release of the major prolactin inhibiting factor, dopamine.

Hamsters with involuted gonads induced by short photoperiod, do not remain in this condition indefinitely. After about 20 weeks, spontaneous return (recrudescence) of gonadal size and function occurs.[278,293] Such animals (in which regeneration of gonads had occurred), after an exposure to long photoperiod for at least 20 weeks,[294,295] could again undergo gonadal involution in response to light restriction, provided their pineal glands were intact. The duration of time during which hamsters did not respond to light restriction was termed a "refractory period."[294] Observations from such experiments were fundamental to the conclusion that the pineal gland was involved in regulation of seasonal breeding in the hamster[292] and gave credibility to similar studies with other species.

Injections of microgram amounts of melatonin daily can result in gonadal involution in the male hamster, provided that the injections are administered in the evening, shortly before the onset of the dark phase of a 14L/10D photoperiod.[296] These results indicated that the effects of melatonin administration were similar to those of short photoperiod and led to the view that melatonin was a substance involved in regulation of seasonal breeding.[272] The findings showing a daily period of sensitivity to melatonin injections was confirmed by several groups of investigators.[297,298] Elevated temperatures (30°C) in the animal rooms was found to inhibit the rate of gondal involution in response to melatonin injections or to short photoperiod.[299]

Evening injections of melatonin were thought to be effective (whereas similar morning injections were not) because they increase the duration that blood levels are increased in a 24-h daily light-dark cycle, or alternatively, because they coincided with a restricted period of receptor sensitivity.[300] Recent experiments in which pinealectomized hamsters received timed infusions of melatonin via implanted cannula confirmed that the duration of elevated blood levels of melatonin was an important factor in the gonadal response. Hamsters receiving 14 h of melatonin infusions daily, underwent gonadal regression, whereas those receiving two daily infusions of 5 h separated by a 4-h break did not undergo gonadal regression.[301] Studies in sheep[302] and Djungarian hamsters[303] confirmed that the duration of the melatonin signal was a critical factor. Also important was the interval between melatonin infusions. In the Syrian hamster, for melatonin infusions to be effective there must be a daily period when melatonin is absent.[301]

Paradoxically, subcutaneous implants of large amounts of melatonin, injections of milligram amounts, or melatonin in the drinking water prevented the effects of light restriction.[292,304,305] Such effects, termed "counterantigonadal," were demonstrated in both the Syrian and Djungarian hamster.[292,305,306] These results support the view that melatonin may play a role in gonadal recrudescence as well as in gonadal involution. In seasonal breeders, the physiolgoical role of melatonin may depend on the season of the year.

Changes in sensitivity of gonadotropin secretion to testosterone feedback occur with pineal-mediated changes in gonadal status. In adult hamsters, there is an increase in sensitivity to negative feedback in hamsters maintained in short days.[307] This effect was duplicated by late afternoon injections of melatonin.[308] Short days do not cause gonadal atrophy before puberty, at which time a decrease in feedback sensitivity to testosterone occurs.[307] In humans, melatonin administration is also reported to increase sensitivity to testosterone-induced suppression of LH secretion in adult males.[309]

In sheep, the annual rhythm in reproduction includes changes in testis size, as well as changes in circulating hormone levels. The breeding season, in the fall and early winter, is characterized by increases in testes weight, increases in circulating LH, and decreases in circulating levels of prolactin.[310] Reverse changes occur during the nonbreeding season. Pinealectomized rams, or rams without superior cervical ganglia, do not respond to seasonal changes in photoperiod.[311] Lincoln[312,313] has described changes in sensitivity to testosterone feedback during different photoperiod. The testosterone effect may be due to estrogen, because testosterone is aromatized to estrogen in peripheral tissues. During the breeding season there is, according to this view, an escape from testosterone suppression of LH.[312,313]

EFFECTS ON THE HORMONES OF REPRODUCTION IN FEMALES

The variation of photoperiod has a dominant role in regulating reproductive function in the female hamster. In a stimulatory photoperiod (>12.5 h of light per day) females exhibit normal 4-day ovulatory cycles.[314] Light deprivation via orbital enucleation or exposure to short photoperiods (<12.5 h of light per day) for several weeks disrupts estrous cyclicity and renders the females acyclic and anovulatory.[288,291,314-318] This is accompanied by morphological changes in the reproductive organs. The uteri undergo atrophy and the number of endometrial glands in the uteri are reduced; the ovaries are characterized by few preantral follicles, rare corpora lutea, and increases in weight due to hypertrophy of ovarian interstitium.[288,291,315,316] The sympathetic nervous system and the pineal gland mediate the photosensitivity of the female hamster gonads.[291,318,319] Because pinealectomy or superior cervical ganglionectomy reversed the effects of light restriction, the physiological effects of decreases in light exposure were considered to be the result of an activated pineal gland.[291,320] Hamsters blinded and pinealectomized had regular estrous cycles and reproductive organs that were indistinguishable from females maintained in stimulatory light conditions.[288,291,317] Neither pinealectomy nor superior cervical ganglionectomy influenced the estrous cycles or reproductive organs of hamsters maintained in a long photoperiod.[291] Thus, as in the male, a pineal gland activated by light restriction has a strong inhibitory effect on reproductive status in the female hamster.

Regardless of how gonadal atrophy was induced (by prolonged exposure to reduced lighting conditions, light deprivation, or orbital enucleation), the gonads began to regenerate between 20 and 27 weeks.[294,314] Hamsters remain refractory until they are exposed to long photoperiod for at least 10 weeks.[294,321] In hamsters with intact eyes and optic nerves, the refractory state is broken during this period and the animals can again respond to reduced lighting conditions.

The work of Tamarkin et al.[296] showed that the effectiveness of melatonin depended on the time of administration. Tamarkin, and subsequently other investigators, reported that daily subcutaneous injections of melatonin (25 μg/day), late in the afternoon, duplicated the effects of short photoperiod or light deprivation.[296,322,323] Hamsters receiving the same melatonin treatment early in the morning (3 h after lights on) maintained reproductive competency.[296] Melatonin injected during the middle of the dark period had little or no influence on the hamster's reproductive capacity.[324] Tamarkin and co-workers suggested that melatonin administered to pineal-intact hamsters prior to onset of darkness was temporally adding to the endogenous melatonin secreted by the pineal gland to induce gonadal involution. Reiter[325] regarded melatonin as the hormone that mediated gonadal regression following exposure of female hamsters to inhibitory photoperiods. This view is supported by the similarities in the results of daily melatonin injections and reduced lighting conditions; both resulted in acyclicity in three to six weeks.

Continuously available melatonin in silastic capsules, or in beeswax pellets implanted subcutaneously in female hamsters, counteracted the reproductive effects following light deprivation, short photoperiod, or daily afternoon melatonin injections.[326,327] This counterantigonadal effect is similar to that observed in males. A mechanism postulated to explain this counterantigonadal effect is that continuously available melatonin in large amounts may down-regulate melatonin receptors.[272]

The changes in serum gonadotropin levels during the 4-day cycle of the female hamster are characterized by a gonadotropin surge on the day of proestrus.[328,329] Exposure to short photoperiods, or light deprivation, results in a daily surge of gonadotropin secretion, rather than a 4-day cycle,[314,322,323,327,330,331] with increased concentrations of LH and FSH and decreased concentrations of prolactin within the anterior pituitary.[315,327,332] Daily afternoon injections of melatonin for several weeks in female hamsters also resulted in an afternoon surge of LH and FSH every day.[296]

The ovarian feedback system is functional in hamsters between 20 and 26 days of age.[333] In the absence of ovarian feedback in ovariectomized hamsters, the pituitary content of LH and FSH are elevated and prolactin levels are depressed in animals maintained under a stimulatory (14L/10D) photoperiod.[334-336] Blood levels of LH and FSH are increased whereas circulating levels of prolactin are decreased.[314,335,337] Following ovariectomy, daily surges in LH and FSH were observed.[314,330,331,338] In hamsters rendered acyclic by short photoperiod, ovariectomy eliminated the abnormal diurnal pattern of progesterone secretion,[338] but did not eliminate the daily surge of gonadotropin secretion.[314,330]

The results of experiments with female hamsters are consistent with the view that the pineal gland, via melatonin, acts on the brain. It has been suggested that the neural mechanism utilized in triggering the daily surges of gonadotropins in light-deprived hamsters is similar to the mechanism utilized in initiation of the preovulatory gonadotropin release in hamsters undergoing normal cycles.[329] The time of day of the gonadotropin surges in hamsters under the two conditions coincides.

In sheep, ovaries are active during short days because ewes are short day breeders. They mate during seasons of decreasing daylength. Under the influence of short days (and long nights) the frequency of gonadotropin-releasing hormone (GnRH) pulses increases and stimulates LH secretion. It has been suggested that a change in sensitivity to estrogen feedback is responsible for the seasonal changes in LH secretion and reproductive competence.[273] This is supported by experiments showing a seasonal escape from estrogen suppression in ovariectomized ewes receiving estrogen replacement.[339] In ewes that were pinealectomized, changes in reproductive competence were no longer synchronized to variations in day-length.[273] In estradiol-treated ovariectomized ewes, pinealectomy prevented the expected increase in LH in response to short days; pinealectomy also prevented the inhibitory effects of long photoperiods. The pineal gland, therefore, appears to be necessary for the reproductive response to photoperiod of sheep.

Melatonin administration has been used to induce early onset of the breeding seasons in ewes.[340] The duration of the nighttime elevation of circulating melatonin of sheep is proportional to the length of the dark phase of the daily light-dark cycle. The daily rhythm of melatonin secretion determines the reproductive response to photoperiod. Melatonin is thought to modulate the frequency of LHRH secretory pulses from the hypothalamus; a short day pattern of melatonin secretion apparently stimulates LHRH pulse frequency and LH secretion, whereas a long day pattern of melatonin secretion inhibits LHRH pulse frequency and LH secretion.[273] The site of action of melatonin in the reproductive response of the ewe has been postulated to be a CNS location important in the neural regulation of LH secretion. Malpaux and colleagues[341] studied the effects of melatonin implants in the brains of ewes on the secretion of LH. They concluded that the mediobasal hypothalamus could be the site of action of melatonin in the control of seasonal reproduction.

In women nocturnal hyperprolactinemia has been reported to be associated with elevated secretion of nighttime melatonin.[342] Evening administration of melatonin reportedly enhances the pulsatile secretion of prolactin in normally cycling women.[343] Single doses of melatonin (100 mg) may also amplify pulsatile LH secretion,[344] whereas melatonin (300 mg) administration for 4 months were reported to significantly decrease circulating LH levels in women.[345] Wetterberg and co-workers[346] reported a variation in serum melatonin during the menstrual cycles of Swedish women. He suggested that low melatonin secretion by the pineal gland at midcycle was permissive for ovulation. Data showing marked augmentation of nocturnal melatonin secretion in amenorrheic athletes[347] provide further indication that melatonin may contribute to gonadotropin regulation in women. Although melatonin cannot be used as a contraceptive by itself, it has been suggested that melatonin could be a useful addition to progestin preparations.[345]

The Pineal and Thyroid Hormones

Considerable evidence is available for a role of the pineal gland in regulating circulating levels of thyroid hormones in mammals. These effects tend to be most significant in seasonal breeders and tend to parallel the effects on reproduction; experimental protocols that result in pineal-mediated inhibition of reproduction tend to result in inhibiton of circulating levels of thyroid hormones. Both pineal-gonadal and pineal-thyroid interactions depend on the availability of melatonin.

Enlargement of the thyroid gland after pinealectomy has been noted in rats and mice;[348-353] increased mitotic activity of the follicular epithelial cells and increased height of these cells have also been reported.[354] The data showing mild hypertrophy of the thyroid gland after pinealectomy suggested increased activity of the thyroid after pinealectomy. Thyroid function tests supported this view. Increased iodine uptake by the thyroid and increased thyroid secretion rate were observed in pinealectomized rats.[355,356] Relkin[357,358] found that prepubertal rats kept in constant darkness had significantly lower plasma TSH and protein-bound iodine than rats kept in standard 12L/12D lighting conditions. Pinealectomy was reported to prevent the effects of constant darkness on a short-term basis, but had no lasting effect. Niles and co-workers,[359] however, in a more extensive study, showed long-term effects of pinealectomy in rats. They found a highly significant increase in plasma concentrations of thyroid-stimulating hormone (TSH) in pinealectomized rats kept under short photoperiod (1L/23D) for 72 days compared to controls with intact pineals. In male hamsters, reducing the length of the photoperiod to less than 12 h of light per day, or blinding hamsters, resulted in reduced plasma levels of total T_4, as well as reduced free thyroxine index (FTI), a reliable indicator of free thyroxine.[360] The role of the pineal gland in this phenomenon was demonstrated in experiments in which pinealectomy or surgical removal of the superior cervical ganglia prevented the depression of plasma T_4 and FTI observed in blinded male hamsters.[361] These data were interpreted as evidence for an inhibitory effect of the pineal on the neuroendocrine-thyroid axis.

Female hamsters that were placed in short photoperiod or blinded also had reduced plasma levels of T_4 and FTI.[362,363] This reduction in circulating T_4 and FTI was prevented by pinealectomy as well.[362] Circulating TSH was reported to be depressed by short photoperiod.[363] Short photoperiod (1L/23D) was found to attenuate the thyroid weight increase observed in animals treated with the goitrogen thiourea.[364] TRH content of the hypothalamus was found to be increased by blinding, an effect that was again prevented by pinealectomy.[365] The interpretation of this work was that an intact pineal gland had an inhibitory influence on TRH release in hamsters, an interpretation shared by several laboratories.[292,358,359]

Melatonin administration has been reported to inhibit thyroid weight in rats and mice and to prevent the mild hypertrophy obtained after pinealectomy.[366-368] Administration of melatonin was found to inhibit iodine uptake by the thyroid gland[367,369-372] and to decrease the thyroid hormone secretion rate.[356,373,374] On the other hand, rats bearing melatonin antibodies had plasma levels of TSH that were significantly higher than controls.[359] DeProspo and co-workers[372] found that rats maintained in constant darkness had iodine uptake values of less than 50% of control values of rats kept in 12L/12D laboratory lighting conditions. The inhibition of iodine uptake in rats in constant darkness was interpreted to be causally related to increased production of endogenous melatonin by the pineal glands under these conditions.

In the hamster, the endocrine effects of melatonin injections depend on the dose and mode of administration. Subcutaneous administration of melatonin (50 to 100 µg/day for 10 days) inhibited thyroid secretion rate.[374] Injections of melatonin (25 µg/day) for periods of 3 to 10 weeks inhibited plasma levels of T_4 and the plasma FTI in both male and female hamsters.[360,363,375,376] Removal of the pineal gland, or the superior cervical ganglia, attenuated or prevented melatonin-induced reductions in plasma T_4.[375,376] Presumably, a synergy of injected and endogenous melatonin from the pineal gland was required to inhibit T_4 levels in hamsters under laboratory photoperiods of 14L/10D. Melatonin injections were more effective in inhibiting T_4 levels if administered in the evening (prior to lights out) than if administered in the morning after lights on.[363,375] Reduction of circulating T_4 and FTI was not prevented by gonadectomy in males or by ovariectomy in females.[360,363]

Reductions of plasma TSH levels by melatonin injections have also been reported;[363] however, the RIA used in this study, was a rat TSH RIA, an assay that may not be suitable for measuring resting levels of TSH in the hamster. Melatonin administration can inhibit some of the effects of thyroid blocking agents such as thiourea or methylthiouracil, including the rise in TSH that occurs in hamsters treated with these substances.[367,377] TRH concentrations in the hypothalamus of male hamsters receiving melatonin injections were increased.[377] These results support the view that the pineal gland, via melatonin, has a modulatory effect on the neuroendocrine-thyroid axis, an effect which in most laboratory protocols is inhibitory.

Paradoxical effects of pharmacological doses of melatonin have been reported. Maintaining high blood levels of melatonin continuously, by high-dose injections, by implants, or by placing melatonin in the drinking water, did not result in inhibitory effects on T_4, FTI, or TSH levels in the hamster.[363,378]

One aspect that has received little attention is the potential interaction of T_4 in the regulation of prolactin secretion. Because TRH releases prolactin, as well as TSH, the number of TRH receptors in the pituitary is a major factor regulating TRH-induced prolactin release. Regulation of TRH receptors by thyroid hormones has been demonstrated both *in vitro* and *in vivo.*[379-382] Changes in sensitivity of TSH secretion to T_4 feedback, as a result of melatonin administration, can be predicted but such alterations have not yet been demonstrated. In such experiments, one would expect changes in prolactin secretion concomitantly with changes in sensitivity to T_4 feedback. Although major alterations in prolactin secretion do occur in hamsters under short photoperiod and in hamsters injected with melatonin, the relationship of these changes to TRH and T_4 feedback has not been determined.

Thyroid investigators interested in deiodinase enzymes have provided an additional area of research relating thyroid function and the pineal gland. Tanaka and colleagues[383] found high levels of type II T_4 5′-deiodinase (T_4D) activity in rat pineal glands. This enzyme is considered to be important in providing adequate levels of intracellular T_3 by deiodination of T_4 in selected body tissues, including the brain. Subsequent investigation showed that the activity of this enzyme in the pineal gland had a daily rhythm greater in amplitude than in any other tissue investigated.[384] Similar to the activity of NAT in the rat pineal gland, type II T_4D activity was elevated at night, during the dark phase of the daily light-dark cycle.[384] Its activity was influenced by β-adrenergic agonists and antagonists in intact rats[384] and was blocked by surgical removal of the superior cervical ganglia.[385] The β-adrenergic activation of this enzyme was potentiated by α-adrenergic activation. The rhythm in type II T_4D activity was found to precede by approximately 1 h, the rhythm in pineal NAT and was not as sensitive to light-induced inhibition as NAT.[387] Thus this area of research suggests that the pineal gland is a tissue in which intracellular levels of T_3 are elevated at night, under the influence of postganglionic sympathetics entering the pineal gland. The relationship of pineal T_4D to circulating levels of thyroid hormones, if any, remains undetermined. Pinealectomy of rats does interfere with circadian rhythms of circulating T_4 and T_3.[388]

Pineal-Thyroid and Pineal-Gonadal Axes: Are They Independent?

There are many similarities between the effects of the pineal on the neuroendocrine-gonadal axis and the neuroendocrine-thyroid axis. The inhibitory effects of an active pineal gland, or of melatonin injections, on gonadal and thyroid axes occur simultaneously in the hamster under a variety of experimental conditions.[389] These effects have a time course of 3 to 10 weeks depending on the experimental conditions. Pinealectomy prevents both the antithyroid and the antigonadal effects of light restriction (see above). Surgical removal of the superior cervical ganglia also prevents both the antithyroid and antigonadal effects of light restriction. Both the gonadal and thyroid axes respond similarly to melatonin administration. Because the antithyroid and antigonadal actions of an active pineal gland make use of the same neural pathways and occur simultaneously, they appear to be different aspects of a syndrome produced by melatonin at a single CNS site.[389]

Experiments demonstrating effects of melatonin and the pineal gland on thyroid function and on circulating levels of thyroid hormones raised the question of the role of thyroid hormones in sensitivity of the reproductive system to melatonin. In sheep (ewes), thyroidec-tomy blocks the seasonal suppression of reproductive activity.[390] Secretion of T_4 is required for neuroendocrine changes that lead to an increase in sensitivity to estradiol negative feed-back on LH and an end of the breeding season.[391] In thyroidectomized sheep that fail to go into seasonal anestrous, the pulsatile secretion of GnRH is increased, leading to the hypothesis that T_4 is required to switch GnRH secretion to a pattern that ends the breeding season. Pulsatile GnRH secretion was generally not observed in thyroid-intact sheep that had become anestrous.[391] In hamsters whose thyroid hormone levels had been reduced by elevated environmental temperatures (32°C), melatonin injections were less effective in inhibiting gonadal weights in males, and inducing anestrous in females, than in controls maintained at 22°C.[392] Melatonin was also less effective in inducing gonadal involution in hamsters made hypothyroid with thiourea.[393] In the natural environment, seasonal temperature cycles may influence reproductive cycles via changes in circulating levels of thyroid hormones. Thus, in seasonal breeders, both light and temperature may interact to regulate hormonal levels to produce a functional cycle of reproductive and metabolic hormones.

EFFECTS ON THE ADRENAL GLAND

The pineal gland has been interpreted as having an inhibitory action on secretion of the adrenal cortex via melatonin. Early studies making this claim were based on changes in adrenal gland weight. Pinealectomy was found to increase adrenal weight, particularly in light-deprived rats.[254,394-396] Light deprivation was found to reduce adrenal weight in rats.[397,398] In hamsters, pinealectomy prevented the reduction in adrenal weight resulting from light deprivation.[281] Melatonin administration was found to decrease adrenal weight in mice and to decrease compensatory adrenal hypertrophy after unilateral adrenalectomy.[399]

Light deprivation reduced circulating levels of corticosterone in rats.[397,400] Pinealectomy has been reported to increase corticosterone levels[401,402] or prevent the effects of light deprivation.[397] Melatonin administration has been reported to inhibit corticosterone secretion in rats.[403,404] Daily injection of 30 mg/kg for 10 days decreased levels of corticosterone in both adrenals and plasma.[405] An inhibitory effect of the pineal on the secretion of aldosterone has been concluded from studies in which plasma aldosterone was increased in pinealectomized rats.[406,407]

Although studies of the effects of pinealectomy and melatonin administration on adrenal hormone levels vary in the extent to which hormones were sampled over a 24-h period, the data seem to support the view that the pineal has an inhibitory effect on the secretion of adrenal hormones. Melatonin may play a role in regulating circadian rhythms of corticosterone in rats; Laakso and colleagues[408] suggested that the decrease in corticosterone that occurs during darkness in rats is causally related to the increase in secretion of melatonin at this time. Only at high doses do pineal indoles inhibit corticosterone output *in vitro*,[409] suggesting that the effect of melatonin on adrenal activity must lie in the brain and/or the pituitary. Indirect evidence that the effect of the pineal on adrenal hormones in rats is mediated by adrenocorticotropic hormone (ACTH) comes from studies with compensatory adrenal hypertrophy.[399] Direct evidence was provided in a study in which ACTH was assayed.[410] It has been recently suggested that the effect of melatonin on pituitary-adrenal hormone secretion may depend on an effect of melatonin on vasopressin secretion.[411] In humans, little evidence exists for an effect of melatonin on circulating levels of adrenal hormones.

An interesting report of hypertrophy of rat adrenal medullary cells after pinealectomy stimulated interest in a possible connection between the adrenal medulla and the pineal gland.[412] This effect could be mediated by glucocorticoid hormones, which are known to stimulate conversion of norepinephrine to epinephrine. Changes in secretion of the enzyme regulating the conversion of dopamine to norepinephrine, dopamine-β-hydroxylase (DBH), have also been studied in relation to changes in lighting and pineal activity. DBH concentrations in the adrenal have been reported to increase several-fold soon after darkness in the rat. This rise in DBH was inhibited by pinealectomy.[413,414]

Although there may be a mechanism to protect the pineal from responding to circulating catecholamines,[240] there are reports of increased melatonin secretion by the pineal gland following immobilization stress in rats.[415] The increases in melatonin secretion following stress could be modified by adrenergic blockade.[416,417] In humans, the pineal gland has been shown to be unresponsive to stress-induced sympathetic activation during the day; however, physical exercise at night is reported to blunt the nocturnal increase of plasma melatonin.[418,419] Exercise training was found to modify the melatonin response to physical activity at night. With training, melatonin secretion eventually increased in response to physical activity at night.[420] Thus, any effect of "stress" on melatonin secretion is not a simple one. In the context of experiments on the pineal gland the word "stress" covers a variety of physiological conditions.

EFFECTS ON GROWTH HORMONE SECRETION

The evidence for an effect of the mammalian pineal gland or melatonin on the modulation of growth hormone secretion is not extensive. Constant darkness was reported to inhibit plasma and pituitary growth hormone levels in rats;[421] these effects were reversed by pinealectomy. Similar results were obtained in blinded rats.[422,423] Light deprivation, by blinding, was found to depress pituitary growth hormone content in hamsters;[424] this was also prevented by pinealectomy. In this study, the investigators failed to show an effect of pinealectomy on plasma growth hormone levels. Other reports of no effect of pinealectomy on plasma growth hormone in rats and hamsters have appeared.[425-427] Because daily evening melatonin injections increase body weight in hamsters, an increase in circulating GH might be expected. An increase in serum GH of male hamsters treated with melatonin for 10 weeks was reported; in addition, a highly significant increase in serum levels of insulin-like growth factor I (IGF-I) was reported.[428,429] The increase in serum levels of GH and IGF-1 could account for the increased body weight in these experiments. The effect of melatonin on GH is complicated by data suggesting that this interaction may depend on thyroid status.[430] Because melatonin administration influences circulating levels of thyroid hormones, the interpretation of these experiments must take into consideration the fact that variations in circulating levels of thyroid hormones influence GH secretion.

In humans, melatonin administration was reported to cause a rise in plasma GH levels.[431] The melatonin-induced stimulation of GH secretion was thought to occur through pathways not involving GH-releasing hormone.[432]

OTHER EFFECTS OF THE PINEAL GLAND

Other effects of the pineal may be directly or indirectly related to the effects of the pineal on the endocrine systems.

Some interest has arisen in research relating the pineal to temperature regulation. Although most of this work provided evidence relating light and the pineal complex to temperature regulation in amphibians and reptiles,[433] reports of avian and mammalian studies have also appeared. A depression of body temperature of sparrows after injection of melatonin was reported by Binkley.[434] In rats, the effect of melatonin on body temperature was reported to be dependent on ambient temperature; in warm-adapted rats, melatonin lowered body temperature, but in cold-adapted rats, melatonin elevated body temperature.[435] The interaction of photoperiod and ambient temperature may prepare the pineal for modulating metabolic responses.[436] A role for the pineal gland in temperature regulation in the hamster has also been suggested.[437]

Secretion of melanocyte-stimulating hormone (MSH) in rats has been reported to be increased after pinealectomy.[438] Melatonin administration, on the other hand, decreased pigmentation in cats.[439]

The pineal and melatonin may influence the endocrine pancreas of the rat. Whereas blinding rats resulted in elevated blood glucose,[440] pinealectomy reduced glucose levels and increased circulating insulin after a glucose challenge.[441,442] These results suggested that the pineal gland, via melatonin, had a diabetogenic effect when activated by darkness. This hypothesis has not yet been critically tested.

Also interesting are reports that melatonin administration has an antihypercholesterolemic effect in rats.[443] Another potentially important finding is that melatonin administration reduces blood pressure in rats.[444]

The Pineal Gland and the Central Nervous System

The site(s) and mechanism(s) of action of melatonin continue to elude researchers. Using the assumption that melatonin is the active pineal hormone, we may restate the question of the site(s) of action of pineal products in terms of the site(s) of action of melatonin. It should be noted, however, that a considerable amount of research, during the 1970s and 1980s, dealt with attempts to identify, isolate, purify, and synthesize a pineal peptide hormone. Unlike the research resulting in the isolation and synthesis of hypothalamic hormones, attempts at identifying a specific pineal peptide hormone were remarkably unsuccessful. Many of these studies were attempts to isolate a specific pineal antigonadotropic hormone.[161,177,445-447]

An increasing number of researchers assume that melatonin is sequestered by the brain after it is secreted into the peripheral circulation.[448,449] If radioactive melatonin is injected into the venous system, it can be detected in all tissues, including the brain. Regional CNS uptake of tritiated melatonin was first reported by Anton-Tay and Wurtman.[450] Evidence for a brain site of action for the antigonadotropic effect of melatonin in the Syrian hamster was obtained by Reiter and colleagues,[451] from experiments in which melatonin was administered to hamsters with hypothalamic cuts made with Halasz-type instruments. Because anterior hypothalamic cuts prevented the antigonadal effects of melatonin, the authors considered the SCN as a possible site of action of melatonin. The PVN, however, also appear to play a role in hamster photoperiodic responses mediated by melatonin.[285] Studies in which melatonin was implanted into mouse brain also led Glass and Lynch[452] to conclude that the hypothalamus was the site of the antigonadal action in the mouse. Melatonin binding studies of the past several years (see below), however, are not consistent with the view that melatonin has a single site of action in the brain.

Melatonin Binding Sites

Early studies, in the late 1970s, made use of tritiated melatonin to localize melatonin binding sites[453,454] throughout the brain (as well as outside the CNS); however, these findings were not consistent and proved difficult to reproduce in other laboratories. The radioiodination of melatonin in the laboratory of Vakkuri and colleagues[455] provided a tool that enabled investigators to study binding of high affinity and low density. The radioligand, 2-^{125}I-melatonin, that they synthesized facilitated the use of radioautography to study the CNS distribution of melatonin binding. Extensive investigation with 2-^{125}I-melatonin since 1984 has provided a substantial amount of information on the characteristics and distribution of high-affinity melatonin binding sites. A key question arising out of this work is the nature of the relationship of melatonin binding to biologically active melatonin receptors.

Although the most directly suitable model for studying the cellular mechanism of action of melatonin is the ability of this indole to aggregate melanin granules of amphibian melanophores, this model is not used to study melatonin binding per se. There is, however, a good correlation between the ability of melatonin agonists to aggregate pigment granules and their affinity in ^{125}I-melatonin binding assays in chicken brain.[456]

In mammals, high-affinity melatonin binding sites have been consistently demonstrated in two CNS locations: the pars tuberalis (PT) of the pituitary and the SCN of the hypothalamus.[457-463] Binding originally reported as in the median eminence of the hypothalamus[464] has been attributed by others to the PT. Morgan and co-workers[465] have submitted the hypothesis that the PT is stimulated by melatonin to secrete a PT-specific product which acts on the CNS to mediate seasonal photoperiodic reproductive effects. Species in which ^{125}I-melatonin binding has been localized to the PT include the rat, mouse, hamster, rabbit, sheep, goat, deer, and ferret.[466] The SCN, however, have also been hypothesized to be a site of melatonin action. This is consistent with the demonstration of high-affinity binding sites in this region across several vertebrate classes. An important association between the CNS and melatonin's role in the synchronization of biological rhythms has been made by several investigators.[460,467,468] Such an association could account for a role of melatonin in synchronization of activity cycles, sleep cycles, and various hormonal and neurotransmitter rhythms to the daily photoperiod.

Although the SCN and PT areas of the mammalian brain have received more recent attention than other areas of the brain as possible sites of action of melatonin, results of radioautography studies have provided evidence for ^{125}I-melatonin binding in a variety of brain regions. Specific binding sites in brain regions including the cortex, anterior hypothalamus, and the paraventricular nucleus of the thalamus have been reported in at least five different mammalian species.[466] Less consistent, from species to species, were reports of binding to other areas of the brain including the amygdala, various nuclei of the thalamus, the habenular nuclei, the superior and inferior colliculi, ventral tegmentum, substantia gelantinosa of the spinal cord, area postrema of the rhombencephalon, choroid plexus, pars distalis of pituitary, and the arteries of the circle of Willis. Membrane-binding assays have identified ^{125}I-melatonin binding sites in spleen of mice, guinea pigs, and hamsters,[469] in rat thymus,[470] in guinea pig kidney,[471] and in rat liver.[472] There is even a report of ^{125}I-melatonin binding to human spermatozoa.[473]

In lower vertebrates, specific ^{125}I-melatonin binding is much more extensive than in mammals. In the chick (*Gallus domesticus*), goldfish (*Carassius auratus*), frog (*Rana pipiens*), and lizard (*Anolis carolinensis*), I-melatonin binding can be found throughout the brain. The most intense labeling in radioautographic preparations occurs in areas that receive primary or secondary visual input (optic tectum, lateral thalamic nuclei, SCN, corpus geniculatum, and interpeduncular nuclei) and in tracts associated with the visual system (optic nerve, optic chiasm, optic tract).[474-477] These findings have led to the conclusion that melatonin binding sites may be associated with visual processing. Specific ^{125}I-melatonin binding has also been reported in the inner plexiform layer of the retina in chicks,[478] as well as in rabbits.[479] In the chicken retina, there appears to be a correlation between melatonin binding and the ability of melatonin to reduce calcium-dependent dopamine release.[480]

Characteristics of the melatonin binding sites are important in considering their relevance as physiological melatonin "receptors." Although some inconsistency appears to exist in the literature concerning the affinity states of melatonin binding sites, recent reviews[466,481] have put much of this work in an understandable perspective. High-affinity (picomolar) binding sites are reported in a number of laboratories as having K_d's between 20 and 400 pM. Evidence has accumulated suggesting that these high-affinity binding sites exist in two affinity states. The first has a K_d of approximately 40 pM and is thought to be associated with a guanine nucleotide binding protein (G protein). The second has a K_d of approximately 400 pM and is considered to be a melatonin receptor that has dissociated from the G protein. This melatonin receptor can be dissociated from the G protein by physiological as well as laboratory conditions. The G protein apparently has a cellular role in modulating the affinity state of melatonin receptors.

In addition to the picomolar binding sites identified in many different species, low-affinity, nanomolar binding sites have been reported in hamster brain.[462]

The inconsistencies in the melatonin binding studies have led some investigators to question whether melatonin actually acts through a classical membrane-bound receptor to produce its physiological and/or pharmacological effects.[482] Because melatonin is characteristically highly lipophilic, it could diffuse readily into cell nuclei to modify DNA transcription. Supporting this hypothesis are recent studies that have demonstrated nuclear melatonin binding.[472,483] Another consideration is that melatonin may bind to calmodulin, a calcium binding protein.[484] Benitez-King and co-workers,[484] based on experiments with tritiated melatonin, have suggested that calmodulin meets the requirements for a melatonin receptor. This question has not been addressed in binding studies with 2-iodomelatonin.

Melatonin and Second Messenger Systems

The precise relationship between melatonin and signal transduction pathways has not been clearly established. Several groups of researchers have demonstrated melatonin-induced inhibition of cAMP levels.[485-487] This inhibition involves a pertussis toxin-sensitive G inhibitory protein in various tissues including hypothalamus and PT of the pituitary.[486,488,489] Experiments with PT preparations suggest that this melatonin- induced inhibition may require intact cells. Data showing a lack of melatonin-induced inhibition of forskolin-stimulated cAMP in membrane homogenates of ovine PT cells suggested that melatonin was inhibiting the production of cAMP via an indirect mechanism.[490] One such mechanism could involve calcium and calmodulin.[484] Paradoxically, higher doses of melatonin (nanomolar concentrations) did not inhibit adenylate cyclase activity,[486] suggesting that the low melatonin binding sites were positively coupled to this enzyme.

Melatonin and Neurotransmitters

Melatonin administration in laboratory animals reportedly influences the turnover of several CNS neurotransmitters. Studies to date, generally have not been able to distinguish the direct effects of melatonin on neurotransmitter turnover, from indirect effects resulting from neurotransmitter interactions—or those resulting from hormone-neurotransmitter interactions. The conclusions from these studies reflect the uncertainty concerning the mechanism and site(s) of action of melatonin.

It has been suggested that the neuroendocrine and neurochemical effects of a pineal gland activated by darkness are similar to those of late afternoon melatonin administration.[272] According to this hypothesis, melatonin injections late in the day would be expected to influence neurotransmitter turnover and release in a manner identical to, or, at least very similar to, that resulting from maintaining animals in a short photoperiod.

Based on experiments that showed increased serotonin content of the midbrain and hypothalamus of rats after acute melatonin administration, the hypothesis was proposed that melatonin acts on serotoninergic neurons to produce its neuroendocrine effects.[491] Although originally postulated to account for antigonadal influences of melatonin, the hypothesis could also apply to antithyroidal influences of the indole. Serotoninergic axons from raphe neurons could influence hypothalamic neuroendocrine centers via input to the medial forebrain bundle.[492] Ruzsas and co-workers[493] have postulated a role of the serotoninergic raphe nuclei in the modulation of ovulation by melatonin in rats. Serotonin has been reported to modulate secretion of several hormones in mammals including most of the pituitary hormones; gonadotropins,[494] adrenocorticotropin,[495] TSH, prolactin, and growth hormone.[496-498] Although binding data do not strongly support the concept that melatonin acts on the raphe nuclei, this hypothesis has not yet been disproved.

Evidence in support of the serotonin hypothesis comes from a number of studies using the Syrian hamster. Melatonin administration was found to increase tissue content of the serotonin (5-HT) metabolite, 5-HIAA (hydroxyindoleacetic acid), or the 5-HIAA/5-HT ratio, in both the hypothalamus and the brain stem (pons-medulla).[499] Maintaining hamsters under short photoperiod, or blinding hamsters by orbital enucleation, increased the 5-HIAA/5-HT ratio in mediobasal hypothalamus (MBH).[500] The *in situ* activity of tryptophan hydroxylase, the rate-limiting enzyme in 5-HT synthesis, was elevated in the MBH of hamsters kept under short photoperiod,[501] suggesting increased 5-HT synthesis under these conditions. In female hamsters chronically treated with daily melatonin injections, 5-HT synthesis (as determined by the accumulation of 5-HT after administration of pargyline) was increased in the pontine brain stem of intact as well as gonadectomized hamsters.[502] In the amygdala, however, 5-HT synthesis was significantly decreased by melatonin administration only in ovariectomized hamsters.[502] It appears from these studies that melatonin, or a pineal gland activated to secrete melatonin, does influence either the synthesis or oxidative metabolism of 5-HT in some brain regions.[502,503]

Evidence has also accumulated that melatonin may modulate catecholamine turnover and/or metabolism in the MBH. Although investigators interested in the neuroendocrine-reproductive effects of melatonin have focused on the MBH as a site of melatonin action, effects of this indole on catecholamine turnover in extrahypothalamic regions may be of more functional significance in nonseasonal breeders.

Melatonin treatment for several weeks in the Syrian hamster—a long-day seasonal breeder—has been consistently found to decrease dopamine (DA) content in the median eminence-arcuate region of the MBH.[503,504] These results are similar to DA content data obtained with short photoperiod.[505-508] Melatonin-induced inhibition of DA content in the neurointermediate lobe of the pituitary,[504] concurrently with inhibition in the median eminence-arcuate region of the MBH, suggests the possibility that this indole may be acting (directly or indirectly) on the arcuate nuclei, the origin of tuberoinfundibular and tuberohypophyseal DA fibers to the median eminence and posterior pituitary. In support of this view are data from the authors' laboratory showing substantial (and highly significant) melatonin-induced increases in the *in situ* activity of MBH tyrosine hydroxylase (TH), the rate-limiting enzyme in catecholamine synthesis (Figure 3). These elevations in TH were consistently observed over a 24-h period, compared to levels in saline-injected controls. The increase in TH occurred concurrently with decreased DA. The greatest difference in DA content between controls and melatonin-treated hamsters occurred at 2 am, during the dark phase of the light-dark cycle (Figure 4). These data, showing melatonin-induced increases in TH activity, are consistent with the interpretation that melatonin stimulates DA synthesis and release. This conclusion, however, is not in agreement with conclusions made from DA "turnover data" in studies of the effects of short photoperiod in male hamsters.[505-507]

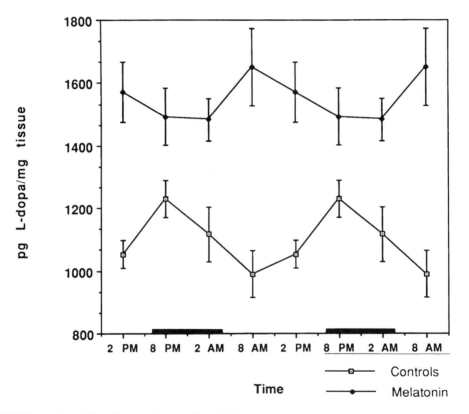

FIGURE 3. *In situ* activity of tyrosine hydroxylase (l-DOPA accumulation after NSD-1015, 100 mg/kg), over a 24-h period, in the median eminence-arcuate region of the mediobasal hypothalamus of male Syrian hamsters treated with saline or melatonin for 9 weeks. Data points (means ± SE) are *double plotted*. Dark horizontal bars indicate the 10-h dark period of the daily light-dark cycle (6 pm–4 am). By analysis of variance, a highly significant effect of treatment was observed ($F = 57.8, p < .001$). Differences due to treatment were significant by t-test at all timepoints.

Further studies are necessary to determine the temporal effects of melatonin on TH, as well as the, technically more difficult, effects of melatonin on DA release. Melatonin may act by shifting daily rhythms in DA synthesis and/or release. Although DA is an important

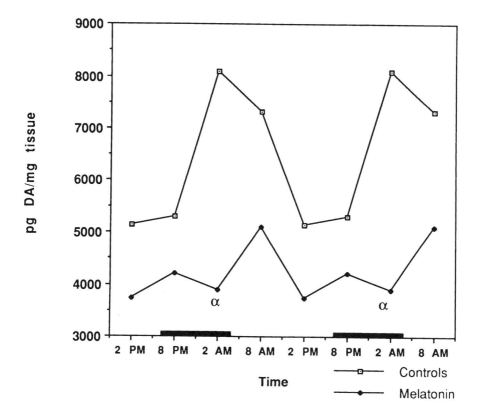

FIGURE 4. Dopamine concentrations, over a 24-h period, in the median eminence-arcuate region of the medio-basal hypothalamus of male hamsters treated with saline or melatonin for 9 weeks. Because these animals were used to obtain the tyrosine hydroxylase data of Figure 3, all animals received an injection of NSD-1015, 100 mg/kg, 40 min prior to sacrifice. Data points (means) are *double plotted*. Dark horizontal bars indicate the 10-h dark period of the light-dark cycle (6 pm–4 am). By analysis of variance, a highly significant effect of treatment was observed ($F = 19.19$, $p < .001$). Differences due to treatment were significant by t-test only at 2 am (indicated by α).

prolactin-inhibitory factor, a cause-effect relationship of melatonin-induced changes in DA release and prolactin secretion has not been established.

In several studies, short photoperiod was reported to decrease NE turnover (by the α-mpt method) in the median eminence and MBH[505,507-509] of male Syrian hamsters. These data should be interpreted with caution because the α-mpt method for determining catecholamine (NE and DA) turnover makes the assumption of steady-state, a condition that may not be met in long-term studies dealing with changes in photoperiod,[505,507,509] or in long-term studies dealing with chronic daily melatonin injections.[429] The content of NE in the median eminence-arcuate region was found to be increased by melatonin injections, with peak levels obtained approximately 15 h after the last injection (Figure 5), suggesting a melatonin-induced phar-macological effect on noradrenergic neurons. Because tissue content reflects primarily intra-cellular NE, these data could be interpreted as indirect evidence for melatonin-induced inhibition of NE release. The melatonin-agonist, 6-chloromelatonin, was reported to decrease NE turnover the in hypothalamus of mice 30 and 60 min after administration of a single dose.[510]

Early studies showing a dose-dependent effect of acute melatonin administration on γ-aminobutyric acid (GABA) content of the rabbit brain[511,512] led to the hypothesis that indole is capable of modifying the activity of the major CNS inhibitory system—GABAergic neurons. Data from the authors' laboratory show that chronic daily melatonin administration

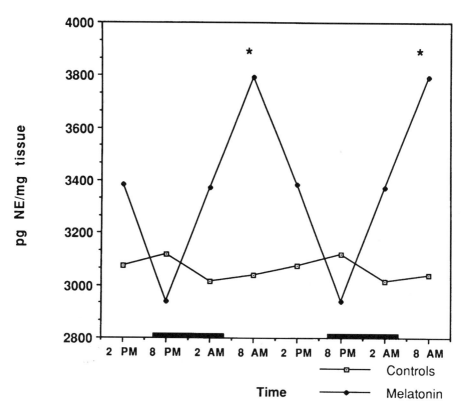

FIGURE 5. Norepinephrine concentrations, over a 24-h period, in the median eminence-arcuate region of the mediobasal hypothalamus of male hamsters treated with saline or melatonin for 9 weeks (see Figures 3 and 4). Data points (means) are *double plotted*. Dark bars indicate the 10-h dark period of the daily light-dark cycle (6 pm–4 am). By analysis of variance, a significant effect of treatment was observed ($F = 5.61, p < .05$). Differences were significant by *t*-test only at the 8 am timepoint (indicated by asterisks).

reduced MBH tissue content of GABA (Figure 6) and glutamine. These data suggest that melatonin does, indeed, have marked effects on GABAergic activity and/or metabolism in the MBH. Other studies show that melatonin significantly increases GABA turnover in rat hypothalamus, cerebellum, cortex, and pineal gland,[513] possibly via an increase in the activity of the rate-limiting enzyme in GABA synthesis, glutamic acid decarboxylase.[514,515] Other studies reported melatonin-induced increases in benzodiazepine, GABA, and GABA agonist (muscimol) binding to the GABA "A" receptor sites.[516,517] These data led to the hypothesis that melatonin may produce its primary effects on GABAergic neurons. According to this model, melatonin-induced modulation of serotoninergic and catecholaminergic neurons would occur secondarily to melatonin-induced changes in GABAergic neurons synapsing on monoaminergic neurons. Melatonin-induced increases in chloride ion influx in rat brain[514] could also occur secondarily to increased release of GABA.

PINEAL RESEARCH AND CIRCADIAN RHYTHMS

The SCN are considered to be the CNS regions generating endogenous, genetically determined circadian rhythms. These rhythms are synchronized to exogenous environmental cues. The 24-h light-dark cycle is the primary cue (*zeitgeber*) regulating melatonin secretion by the pineal gland. Melatonin, has been appropriately described as the chemical expression of darkness,[518] a substance which acts as an internal *zeitgeber*.

The sensitivity of the brain to melatonin injections depends on the time of day relative to the onset of darkness.[296] Lesions of the SCN blocked the gonad-inhibiting effect of short photoperiod[519,520] as well as the gonadal involution caused by daily afternoon melatonin

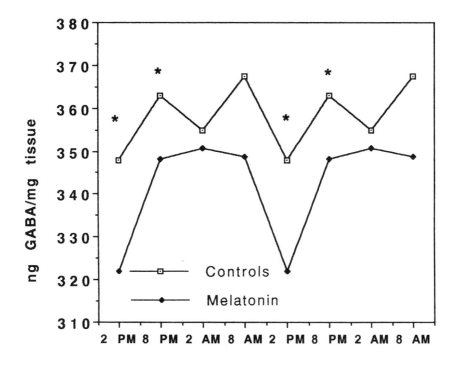

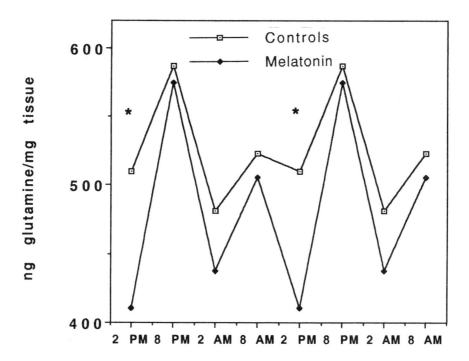

FIGURE 6. GABA and glutamine concentrations, over a 24-h period, in the median eminence-arcuate region of the mediobasal hypothalamus of male hamsters treated with saline or melatonin for 9 weeks (see Figures 3–5). Data points (means) are *double plotted*. The dark period of the daily light-dark cycle was from 6 pm to 4 am. By analysis of variance, significant effects of treatment were observed for GABA (F = 16.33, p < .001) and for glutamine (F = 8.12, p < .01). Differences were significant by t-test at 2 and 8 pm for GABA and at 2 pm for glutamine (indicated by asterisks).

injections.[521] These studies led to the concept that the SCN were a site of action of the pineal product, melatonin.

In rodents the preovulatory surge of gonadotropins and LHRH occurs at specific times of day.[328,522-524] Melatonin injections appear to disrupt a neural or neuroendocrine system responsible for regulating gonadotropin release.[313,323] Changes in concentrations of circulating thyroid hormones also occur on a daily basis in rodents. In hamsters maintained on a 14L/10D photoperiod, highest levels of circulating T_4 and T_3 occur at the end of the light phase of the light-dark cycle, during the time when hamsters are most sensitive to melatonin injections.[525] The interaction of melatonin with rhythms in secretion of adrenal hormones, growth hormone, and prolactin has not been adequately clarified.

Activity rhythms may also be influenced by melatonin. Early studies using pinealectomized birds and lizards[526,527] demonstrated that removal of the pineal glands resulted in desynchronization of locomotor activity rhythms. Similar results were obtained in studies using high-dose constant infusions of melatonin. Initial findings in mammals, however, suggested that the mammalian pineal gland was not involved in the expression of circadian rhythms. Later, investigators demonstrated that administration of picomolar concentrations of melatonin could, in fact, synchronize locomotor patterns in the rat and in the Djungarian hamster,[528,529] suggesting that the indole was capable of rhythm entrainment in mammals as well. Evidence that melatonin is involved in synchronization of feeding/drinking rhythms, of temperature rhythms, and of the sleep-wake cycle has also been reported.[530-533] Although the role of melatonin in mammalian circadian rhythm synchronization is not completely clear, Cassone[533] suggested that this pineal indole may act as temporal feedback within the SCN, modulating circadian phase and sustaining rhythm stability.

MELATONIN: PSYCHOPHARMACOLOGICAL EFFECTS AND CLINICAL IMPLICATIONS

The psychopharmacological effects and mechanism(s) of action of melatonin have been compared to those of the major groups of sedative/hypnotic drugs, the benzodiazepines and barbiturates.[534] These drugs also have anxiolytic, anticonvulsive, and muscle-relaxant properties. Melatonin's sedative/hypnotic potential has been recognized for many years and has been demonstrated in laboratory animals and in humans.[535-538] Anxiolytic effects of melatonin in rats and mice have been reported.[539,540] Melatonin may offer a pharmaceutical alternative to the existing, widely used sedative/hypnotic drugs.

Studies of circulating melatonin rhythms in humans suggest that melatonin may be useful in treating disorders of biological rhythms.[541] Following the report of Marczynski and coworkers[542] that it induced sleep in cats, melatonin has been linked to sleep mechanisms. Melatonin administration may result in sleep in humans[543] and has been reported to synchronize sleep cycles in a patient lacking a pineal gland[544] and in a blind individual.[545] A melatonin-induced alleviation of "jet lag" and "shift workers" syndrome has been confirmed in several recent studies,[546-549] however, it has been questioned whether this effect will eventually have any practical significance.[550] Melatonin administration could be useful in the treatment of delayed sleep phase syndrome, particularly in older individuals in whom the secretion of melatonin is reduced.[551]

Many studies have examined circulating melatonin rhythms in humans in an attempt to discern a causal relationship between various clinical conditions and pineal function. Decreased melatonin levels have been reported in paranoid schizophrenic patients[552] and in individuals with certain depressive subtypes.[553,554] Elevations in serum melatonin have been reported in hypothalamic amenorrhea,[555,556] anorexia nervosa,[557-559] late luteal phase dysphoric disorder,[560] hypogonadotropic hypogonadism,[561] and mania.[562] Abnormalities in the amplitude, duration, or timing of melatonin rhythms have also been associated with premenstrual and seasonally related depressions, oligospermia, aspermia, delayed or advanced puberty, and excessive exercise.[280,541]

The evidence to support a direct involvement of the pineal or melatonin, in the etiology/pathophysiology of all of these clinical conditions, however, is circumstantial, at best.

Considerable attention has been given by psychiatrists to the possible role of environmental lighting and melatonin in seasonal affective disorder (SAD).[563,564] In some individuals with SAD, daily treatment with high-intensity fluorescent light appears to offer alleviation of some of the symptoms.[565,566]

PINEAL GLAND AND SEIZURES

The induction of seizures by pinealectomy in gerbils or by pinealectomy plus parathyroidectomy of rats [567-569] led to studies testing melatonin for anticonvulsive activity. Later investigations did, in fact, provide evidence for a modest inhibitory effect on seizure activity in a variety of animal seizure models including pentylenetetrazol-kindled seizures in rats and gerbils,[570] light-induced seizures in baboons,[571] and oubain-induced seizures in rats.[572] Data on the most effective time course of melatonin administration for anticonvulsive effects have been reported for the hamster.[573,574]

Data showing that pargyline, a monoamine oxidase inhibitor, prevented the severe seizures that occurred after pinealectomy in parathyroidectomized rats[575] suggested that pinealectomy-induced seizures resulted from changes in one or more of the aminergic systems of the brain. In different strains of rats, the telencephalic content of serotonin was depressed in one strain after pinealectomy-induced seizures; NE content was reduced in another strain after similar seizures.[576] Melatonin may be modulating the activity of neurotransmitters involved in the induction of seizure activity.

PINEAL AND MELATONIN: ONCOLOGY AND IMMUNOLOGY

MELATONIN AND IMMUNE RESPONSE

As early as 1970, a report of pinealectomy influencing the immune reponse of rodents appeared.[577] Removal of the pineal gland of rats was reported to inhibit the immune response (Arthus reactivity) to bovine serum albumin. Melatonin administration was later found to stimulate the humoral immune response to T cell-dependent antigens.[578] Melatonin was effective only in antigen-primed mice.[579] An anti-stress effect of melatonin was concluded from studies showing that melatonin administration counteracted the effects of corticosteroids on thymus weight and antibody production.[580] Studies by Maestroni and Conti[578] indicated that melatonin stimulated activated T cells to release peptides of the opioid family, which in turn acted to enhance the immune response. Studies in humans led to the suggestion that the immunostimulatory action of melatonin requires the presence of the lymphokine, interleukin-2 (IL-2).[581] The studies of Maestroni and Conti[578-580] led to the concept that the pineal gland, via its "hormone" melatonin, acts to enhance humoral immune response. Seasonal effects on the immune response may be related to seasonal changes in melatonin secretion.[582]

Although melatonin binding sites have been reported in the spleens of birds and mammals,[583] evidence that melatonin binds directly to a specific population of lymphocytes appears to be lacking.

Melatonin administration has been reported to inhibit solid tumor growth. Melatonin administration, alone or in combination with the lymphokine, IL-2, has been tested for its antitumor effect in humans.[584] Tumor regression rate was reported to be significantly greater in patients treated with both melatonin and IL-2 than with IL-2 alone. Melatonin was also reported to inhibit estrogen-stimulated proliferation of human breast cancer cells *in vitro*.[585] Although the available data suggest a rather modest antitumor effect of melatonin, they are sufficient to warrant further testing of this effect in patients with selected tumor types.

Data providing evidence for melatonin inhibition of free radical formation has stimulated interest in the role of melatonin in the development of cancer. Reiter[586,587] has suggested that melatonin provides DNA protection against oxidative damage, protection that may be important in preventing chromosomal damage leading to carcinogenesis. This interpretation suggests that melatonin may be more important in preventing the initiation of tumors than in inhibiting tumor growth.

PINEAL TUMORS

Frequently tumors of the pineal region have been referred to simply as "pinealomas." However, this term has been used to describe more than one histological tumor type and, therefore, may now be useful only to describe the general location of the tumor. Pineal tumors are rare—they have been estimated at less than 1% of brain tumors.[588] Tumors of pineal origin include germ cell tumors, glial tumors, and parenchymal tumors.

Parenchymal tumors make up less than one third of this number.[589] A 1993 estimate is that 10 to 50 cases of pineal parenchymal tumors will be diagnosed annually in the United States.[588] These tumors have microscopic features of pineal parenchymal cells in various stages of development. Tumors of mature-appearing pinealocytes are referred to as pinealocytomas, whereas those of more primitive appearance are referred to as pineoblastomas.[590-592] Parenchymal tumors of intermediate differentiation, or mixed types, are also described. Pineoblastomas with retinoblastoma-like structures have been reported.[593] The development of pineoblastoma-like pineal tumors in some patients with retinoblastoma (bilateral or trilateral retinoblastoma) has been well documented.[593,594] Hypogenitalism has been reported to occur among male patients with pineal parenchymal tumors.[595]

The most common type of pineal region tumor are the germinomas.[596] This tumor may also be found in the anterior part of the third ventricle, in which case it may be referred to as an ectopic pinealoma. Morphologically pineal germinomas are similar to germinoma and seminoma occurring in the gonads and in extragonadal sites.[597,598] The cells of origin of these tumors have not been definitively identified. Magnetic resonance imaging reportedly is able to distinguish germinomas from pineoblastomas.[599]

Some pineal tumors (germinomas as well as nongerminomatous tumors) secrete human chorionic gonadotropin (hCG)[600,601] and may be responsible for the association of precocious puberty and pineal tumors. RIA of hCG in serum or CSF has become a routine part of diagnosis of pineal tumors. Several cases of pineal tumors that secrete the tumor marker, α-fetoprotein, have also been reported.[602] These tumor markers may contribute to diagnosis as well as provide information on the response to therapy. Melatonin, on the other hand, has not proven to be a useful tumor marker.

Teratomas and astrocytomas of the pineal gland have also been described.[603,604] Diagnosis of the various pineal tumor types is important in selection of treatment, be it surgical resection, local radiotherapy, chemotherapy, or a combination of chemotherapy and aggressive radiotherapy extending beyond the pineal gland.

REFERENCES

1. **Lerner, A. B., Case, J. D., Takahashi, Y., Lee, Y., and Mori, W.,** Isolation of melatonin, the pineal gland factor that lightens melanocytes, *J. Am. Chem. Soc.,* 80, 2587, 1958.
2. **Lerner, A. B., Case, J. D., and Heinzelman, R. V.,** Structure of melatonin, *J. Am. Chem. Soc.,* 81, 684, 1959.
3. **Baker, P. C.,** Melatonin levels in developing *Xenopus laevis, Comp. Biochem. Physiol.,* 28, 1387, 1969.
4. **Ralph, C. L.,** Correlations of melatonin content in pineal gland, blood and brain of some birds and mammals, *Am. Zool.,* 16, 13, 1976.
5. **Fenwick, J. C.,** Demonstration and effect of melatonin in fish, *Gen. Comp. Endocrinol.,* 14, 86, 1970.
6. **Gern, W. A., Owens, D. W., and Ralph, C. L.,** Plasma melatonin in the trout: day-night changes demonstrated by radioimmunoassay, *Gen. Comp. Endocrinol.,* 34, 453, 1978.

7. **Pang, S. F. and Ralph, C. L.,** Pineal and serum melatonin at midday and midnight following pinealectomy or castration in male rats, *J. Exp. Zool.,* 193, 275, 1975.

8. **Reiter, R. J., Trakulrungsi, W. K., Trakulrungsi, C., Vriend, J., Morgan, W. W., Vaughan, M. K., Johnson, L. Y., and Richardson, B. A.,** Pineal melatonin production: endocrine and age effects, in *Melatonin Rhythm Generating System,* Klein, D. C., Ed., S. Karger, Basel, 1982, 143.

9. **Reiter, R. J., Vriend, J., Brainard, G. C., Matthews, S. A., and Craft, C. M.,** Reduced pineal and plasma melatonin levels and gonadal atrophy in old hamsters kept under winter photoperiods, *Exp. Aging Res.,* 8, 27, 1982.

10. **Kennaway, D. J., Sanford, L. M., Godrey, B., and Friesen, H. G.,** Patterns of progesterone, melatonin and prolactin secretion in ewes maintained in 4 different photoperiods, *J. Endocrinol.,* 97, 229, 1983.

11. **Kennaway, D. J., Gilmore, T. A., and Seamark, R. F.,** Effects of melatonin implants on the circadian rhythm of plasma melatonin and prolactin in sheep, *Endocrinology,* 110, 2186, 1982.

12. **Reppert, S. M., Perlow, M. J., Tamarkin, L., and Klein, D. C.,** A diurnal melatonin rhythm in primate cerebrospinal fluid, *Endocrinology,* 104, 295, 1979.

13. **Vaughan, G. M., Pelham, R. W., Pang, S. F., Laughlin, L. L., Wilson, K. M., Sandock, K. L., Vaughan, M. K., Koslow, S. H., and Reiter, R. J.,** Nocturnal elevation of plasma melatonin and urinary 5-hydroxy-indoleacetic acid in young men: attempts at modification by brief changes in environmental lighting and sleep and by autonomic drugs, *J. Clin. Endocrinol. Metab.,* 42, 752, 1976.

14. **Arendt, J. and Wilkinson, M.,** Melatonin radioimmunoassay, in *Methods of Hormone Radioimmunoassay,* Jaffe, B. M. and Behrman, M. R., Eds., Academic Press, New York, 1978, 101.

15. **Lynch, H. J., Ozaki, Y., and Wurtman, R. J.,** The measurement of melatonin in mammalian tissues and bodily fluids, *J. Neural Transm. Suppl.,* 13, 251, 1978.

16. **Waldhauser, F. and Wurtman, R. J.,** The secretion and action of melatonin, *Biochem. Action Horm.,* 10, 187, 1983.

17. **Wurtman, R. J., Axelrod, J., and Kelly, D. E.,** *The Pineal,* Academic Press, New York, 1968.

18. **Studnicka, F. K.,** Die parietalorgane, in *Lehrbuch der vergleichenden mikroskopischen Anatomie der Wir-beltiere,* Part 5, Opple, A., Ed., Gustav Fischer, Jena, 1905.

19. **Oksche, A.,** Survey of the development and comparative morphology of the pineal organ, in *Progress in Brain Research,* Vol. 10, Kappers, A. J. and Schade, J. P., Eds., Elsevier, Amsterdam, 1965, 3.

20. **DeGraaf, H. W.,** Zur Anatomie und Entwicklung der Epiphyse bei Amphibien und Reptilien, *Zool. Anz.,* 9, 191, 1886.

21. **VandeKamer, J. C.,** Histological structure and cytology of the pineal complex in fishes, amphibians and reptiles, *Prog. Brain Res.,* 10, 30, 1965.

22. **Kalsow, C. M. and Wacker, W. B.** Pineal reactivity of anti-retina sera, *Invest. Ophthalmol.,* 16, 181, 1977.

23. **Li., K. and Welsh, M. G.,** S-antigen and glial fibrillary acidic protein immunoreactivity in the *in situ* pineal gland of hamster and gerbil and in pineal grafts: developmental expression of pinealocyte and glial markers, *Am. J. Anat.,* 192, 510, 1991.

24. **Rodriguez, M., Gaskins, R., Wiggert, B., Redmond, M., and Chader, G.,** Immunocytochemical localization of interphotoreceptor retinoid-binding protein in the primate retina and pineal gland, *Invest. Ophthalmol. Vis. Sci. Suppl.,* 26, 340, 1985.

25. **Pepperberg, D. R., Okamjima, T. L., Wiggert, B., Ripps, H., Crouch, R. K., and Chader, G. J.,** Interphotoreceptor binding-protein (IRBP). Molecular biology and physiological role in the visual cycle of rhodopsin, *Mol. Neurobiol.,* 7, 61, 1993.

26. **Ostholm, T., Ekstrom, P., Bruun, A., and Van Veen, T.,** Temporal disparity in pineal and retinal ontogeny, *Brain Res.,* 470, 1, 1988.

27. **Craft, C. M., Lolley, R. N., Seldin, M. F., and Lee, R. H.,** Rat pineal phosducin: cDNA isolation, nucleotide sequence, and chromosomal assignment in the mouse, *Genomics,* 10, 400, 1991.

28. **Reig, J. A., Yu, L., and Klein, D. C.,** Pineal transduction. Adrenergic–cyclic AMP-dependent phosphorylation of cytoplasmic 33-kDa protein (MEKA) which binds beta gamma-complex of transducin, *J. Biol. Chem.,* 265, 5816, 1990.

29. **Lolly, R. N., Craft, C. M., and Lee, R. H.,** Photoreceptors of the retina and pinealocytes of the pineal gland share common components of signal transduction, *Neurochem. Res.,* 17, 81, 1992.

30. **Illum, N., Korf, H. W., Julian, K., Rasmussen, T., Herning, M., and Krabbe, S.,** Concurrent uveoretinitis and pineocytoma in a child suggests a causal relationship, *Br. J. Ophthalmol.,* 76, 574, 1992.

31. **Lopes, M. B., Gonzalez-Fernandez, F., Scheithauer, B. W., and Vandenberg, S. R.,** Differential expression of retinal proteins in a pineal parenchymal tumor, *J. Neuropathol. Exp. Neurol.,* 52, 516, 1993.

32. **Kazula, A., Nowak, J. Z., and Iuvone, P. M.,** Regulation of melatonin and dopamine biosynthesis in the chick retina: the role of GABA, *Vis. Neurosci.,* 10, 621, 1993.

33. **Best, S. A., Midgley, J. M., Huang, W., and Satson, D. G.,** The determination of 5-hydroxytryptamine, related indolealkylamines and 5-hydroxindoleacetic acid in the bovine eye by gas chromatography-negative ion chemical ionization mass spectrometry, *J. Pharm. Biomed. Anal.,* 11, 323, 1993.

34. **Bhatnagar, K. P.,** Comparative morphology of the pineal gland, in *Biological Rhythms, Mood Disorders, Light Therapy, and the Pineal Gland,* Shafii, M. and Shafii, S. L., Eds., American Psychiatric Press, Washington, D.C., 1990, 3.

35. **Rudeberg, C.,** Light and electron microscopic studies on the pineal organ of the dogfish *Scyliorhinus canicula* Linne., *Z. Zellforsch. Mikrosk. Anat.,* 85, 521, 1968.

36. **Ueck, M.,** Structure of the pineal organ of the sardine *Sardina polchardus sardina* (Risso), *Z. Zellforsch. Mikrosk. Anat.,* 92, 452, 1968.

37. **Collin, J. P.,** La capule sensorielle de l'organe pineal de la lamproie de planer. L'ultrastructure des cellules sensorielles et ses implications functionelles, *Arch. Anat. Microsc. Morphol. Exp.,* 58, 145, 1969.

38. **Petit, A.,** Ultrastructure, innervation et function de l'epiphyse et l'epiphyse de l'orvet (*Anguis fragilis* L.), *Z. Zellforsch. Mikrosk. Anat.,* 96, 437, 1969.

39. **Charlton, H. M.,** The pineal gland of *Xenopus laevis*. Daudin: a histological, histochemical, and electron microscopic study, *Gen. Comp. Endocrinol.,* 11, 465, 1968.

40. **Collin, J. P.,** Structure, nature secretoire, degenerescence partielle des photorecepteurs rudimentaires epiphysaire chez *Lacerta viridis* (Laurenti), *C. R. Acad. Sci. Ser. D,* 264, 647, 1967.

41. **Oksche, A. and Vaupel-VonHarnack, M.,** Electronen mikroskopische untersuchungen zur frage der sinneszellen im pinealorgan der vogel, *Z. Zellforsch. Mikrosk. Anat.,* 69, 41, 1966.

42. **Collin, J. P.,** Etude preliminaire de photorecepteurs rudimentaires de l'epiphyse de *Pica Pica* L. pendant la vie embryonnaire et post embryonnaire, *C. R. Acad. Sci. Ser. D,* 263, 660, 1966.

43. **Collin, J. P.,** Sur l'evolution des photorecepteurs rudimentaires chez la pie (*Pica pica* L.), *C. R. Seances Soc. Biol. Paris,* 160, 1876, 1966.

44. **Collin, J. P.,** Le photorecepteur rudimentaire de l'epiphyse d'oiseau: le prolongement basal chez le passereau *Pica Pica* L., *C. R. Acad. Sci. Ser. D,* 265, 48, 1967.

45. **Oksche, A. and Kirschstein, H.,** Electronenmikroskopische untersuchungen am pinealorgan von *Passer domesticus, Z. Zellforsch. Mikrosk. Anat.,* 102, 214, 1969.

46. **Bischoff, M. B.,** Photoreceptoral and secretory structures in the avian pineal organ, *J. Ultrastruct. Res.,* 28, 16, 1969.

47. **Collin, J. P.,** Rubans circonscrits par les vesicules dans les photorecepteurs rudimentaires epiphysaires de l'oiseau: *Vanellus vanellus* (L.) et nouvelles considerations phylogenetiques relatives aux pinealocytes (ou cellules principales) des mammiferes, *C. R. Acad. Sci. Ser. D,* 267, 758, 1968.

48. **Collin, J. P.,** Distinction et rapports entre les pedicules basaux des photorecepteurs rudimentaires secretoires et les afferences nerveuses monoaminergiques de l'epiphyse d'oiseau, *C. R. Seances Soc. Biol. Paris,* 163, 1137, 1969.

49. **Ueck, M.,** Weitere untersuchungen zur feinstruktur und innervation des pineal organs von *Passer domesticus* L., *Z. Zellforsch Mikrosk. Anat.,* 105, 276, 1970.

50. **Kappers, J. A.,** The sensory innervation of the pineal organ of the lizard, *Lacerta viridis,* with remarks on its position in the trend of pineal phylogenetic structural and functional evolution, *Z. Zellforsch.,* 81, 581, 1967.

51. **Hafeez, M. A. and Zerihun, L.,** Studies on central projections of the pineal nerve tract in rainbow trout, *Salmo gairdneri* Richardson, using cobalt chloride iontophoresis, *Cell Tissue Res.,* 154, 484, 1974.

52. **Zimmerman, P. and Paul, E.,** Reaktionsmuster verschiedener mittel- und zwischenhirnzentren von *Rana temporaria* L. Nach unterbrechung der nervenbahnen des pinealkomplexes, *Z. Zellforsch.,* 128, 512, 1972.

53. **Puzdrowski, R. L. and Northcutt, R. G.,** Central projections of the pineal complex in the silver lamprey Ichthyomyzon unicuspis, *Cell Tissue Res.,* 255, 269, 1989.

54. **Pevet, P. and Collin, J. P.,** Les pinealocytes de mammifere: diversite, homoligies, origin. Etude chez la taupe adulte (*Talpe europaea* L.), *J. Ultrastruct. Res.,* 57, 22, 1976.

55. **Anderson, E.,** The anatomy of bovine and ovine pineals: light and electron microscopic studies, *J. Ultrastruc. Res. Suppl.,* 8, 1, 1965.

56. **Arstila, A. V., Kalimo, H. O., and Hyyppa, M.,** Secretory organelles of the rat pineal gland: electron microscopic and histochemical studies *in vivo* and *in vitro*, in *The Pineal Gland, Ciba Found. Symp.,* Wolstenholme, G. E. W. and Knight, J., Eds., Churchill, London, 1971, 147.

57. **Upson, R. H., Benson, B., and Satterfield, V.,** Quantitation of ultrastructural changes in the mouse pineal in response to continuous illumination, *Anat. Rec.,* 184, 311, 1976.

58. **Upson, R. H., Benson, B., and Satterfield, V.,** Quantitation of ultrastructural changes in the mouse pineal in response to continuous illumination, *Anat. Rec.,* 184, 491, 1977.

59. **Karasek, M., Marek, K., and Pevet, P.,** Influence of a short light pulse at night on the ultrastructure of the rat pinealocyte: a quantitative study, *Cell Tissue Res.,* 254, 247, 1988.

60. **Vollrath, L.,** Comparative morphology of the vertebrate complex, *Prog. Brain Res.,* 52, 25, 1979.

61. **Vollrath, L., Diehl, B. J. M., and Boeckmann, D.,** The pineal complex in rats, *J. Neural Transm. Suppl.,* 13, 403, 1978.

62. **Elden, C. A., Keyes, M. C., and Marshall, C. E.,** Pineal body of the northern fur seal (*Callorhinus ursinus*). A model for studying the probable function of the mammalian pineal body, *Am. J. Vet. Res.,* 32, 639, 1971.

63. **Cuello, A. C. and Tramezzani, J. H.,** The epiphysis cerebri of the Weddell seal: its remarkable size and glandular pattern, *Gen. Comp. Endocrinol.,* 12, 153, 1969.

64. **Stammer, A.,** Studies on the pineal organ of the great horseshoe bat (Rhinolophus ferrum equinum), *Gen. Comp. Endocrinol.,* 18, 624, 1972.

65. **Ralph, C. L.,** The pineal gland and geographical distribution of animals, *Int. J. Biometeorol.,* 19, 189, 1975.

66. **Moller, M., Mollgard, K., and Kimble, J. E.,** Presence of a pineal nerve in sheep and rabbit fetuses, *Cell Tissue Res.,* 158, 451, 1975.

67. **Moller, M.,** Presence of a pineal nerve (nervus pinealis) in the human fetus: a light and electron microscopical study of the innervation of the pineal gland, *Brain Res.,* 154, 1, 1978.

68. **Hollmann, P.,** Uber herkunft und bedeutung der gliosen elemente inder epiphysis cerebri. Untersuchungen an Haussaugetieren, *Zbl. Vet. Med.,* 10, 203, 1963.

69. **Redecker, P. and Bargsten, G.,** Synaptophysin—a common constituent of presumptive secretory microvesicles in the mammalian pinealocyte: a study of rat and gerbil pineal glands, *J. Neurosci. Res.,* 34, 79, 1993.

70. **Wolfe, D. E.,** The epiphyseal cell: an electron microscopic study of its intercellualr relationships and intracellular morphology in the pineal body and other areas of brain tissue, *Progr. Brain Res.,* 10, 332, 1965.

71. **Wartenberg, H.,** The mammalian pineal organ: electron microscopic studies on the fine structure of pinealocytes, glial cells and on the perivascular compartment, *Z. Zellforsch.,* 86, 74, 1968.

72. **Karasek, M.,** Functional ultrastructure of the mammalian pinealocyte, in *Advances in Pineal Research, Vol. 2,* Reiter, R. J. and Fraschini, F., Eds., Libbey, London, 1987.

73. **Milofsky, A.,** The fine structure of the pineal in the rat, with special reference to parenchyma, *Anat. Rec.,* 127, 435, 1957.

74. **Gusek, W. and Santoro, A.,** Zur ultrastruktur der epiphysis cerebri der ratte, *Endokrinologie,* 41, 105, 1961.

75. **Bostelmann, W.,** Beitrag zur submikrosakopischen zytologie der epiphysis cerebri und zur experimentellen beeinflussung ihrer zellelemente, *Zentralbl. Allg. Pathol. Anat.,* 107, 430, 1965.

76. **Lin, H. S.,** Transformation of centrioles in pinealocytes of adult guinea pigs, *J. Neurocytol.,* 1, 61, 1972.

77. **Clabough, J. W.,** Cytological aspects of pineal developments in rats and hamsters, *Am. J. Anat.,* 127, 215, 1973.

78. **Lin, H. S.,** The fine structure and transformation of centrioles in the rat pinealocyte, *Anat. Rec.,* 163, 313, 1969.

79. **Vollrath, L. and Huss, H.,** The synaptic ribbons of the guinea pig pineal gland under normal and experimental conditions, *Z. Zellforsch.,* 139, 417, 1973.

80. **Vollrath, L.,** Synaptic ribbons of a mammalian pineal gland: Circadian changes, *Z. Zellforsch.,* 145, 171, 1973.

81. **Sjostrand, F. S.,** Ultrastructure of retinal rod synapses of the guinea pig eye as revealed by three dimensional reconstructions from serial sections, *J. Ultrastruct. Res.,* 2, 122, 1958.

82. **Arstila, A. U.,** Electron microscopic studies on the structure and histochemistry of the pineal gland of the rat, *Neuroendocrinology,* 2 (Suppl. 1), 7, 1967.

83. **Ito, T. and Matsushija, S.,** Electron microscopic observations on the mouse pineal, with particular emphasis on its secretory nature, *Arch. Histol., Jpn.,* 30, 1, 1968.

84. **Karasek, M. and Hansen, J. T.,** Presence of dense core vesicles in pinealocytes of the cat, *Cell Tissue Res.,* 222, 695, 1982.

85. **Karasek, M., King, T. S., Hansen, S. T., and Reiter, R. J.,** Quantitative changes in the numbers of dense core vesicles and synaptic ribbons in pinealocytes of the Djungarian hamster (phodopus sungorus) following sympathectomy, *Cytobios,* 35, 157, 1983.

86. **Sheridan, M. N. and Sladek, J. R.,** Histofluorescence and ultrastructural analysis of hamster and monkey pineal, *Cell Tissue Res.,* 164, 145, 1975.

87. **Romijn, H. J. and Gelsema, A. J.,** Electron microscopy of the rabbit pineal organ in vitro. Evidence of norepinephrine stimulated secretory activity of the Golgi apparatus, *Cell Tissue Res.,* 173, 365, 1976.

88. **Romijn, H. J., Mud, M. T., and Wolters, P. S.,** Diurnal variations in number of Golgi dense core vesicles in light pinealocytes of the rabbit, *J. Neural Transm.,* 38, 231, 1976.

89. **Benson, B. and Krasovich, M.,** Circadian rhythm in the number of granulated vesicles in the pinealocytes of mice. Effects of sympathectomy and melatonin treatment, *Cell Tissue Res.,* 184, 499, 1977.

90. **Karasek, M.,** Influence of TRH and TSH on the ultrastructure of the rat pineal gland, *Acta Med. Pol.,* 21, 347, 1981.

91. **Karasek, M., Marek, K., and Pevet, P.,** Influence of a short light pulse at night on the ultrastructure of the rat pinealocyte: a quantitative study, *Cell Tissue Res.,* 254, 247, 1988.

92. **Karasek, M.,** Some functional aspects of the ultrastructure of rat pinealocytes, *Endocrinol. Exp.,* 15, 17, 1981.

93. **Vaughan, M. K., Vaughan, G. M., Little, J. C., Buzzell, G. R., Chambers, J. P., and Reiter, R. J.,** Pineal lysosomal enzymes in the Syrian hamster: circadian rhythm and effects of castration or short photoperiod treatment, *Brain Res.,* 489, 318, 1989.

94. **Krstic, R.,** A combined scanning and transmission electron microscopic study and elctron probe microanalysis of human pineal acervuli, *Cell Tissue Res.,* 174, 129, 1976.

95. **Lubaszyk, A. and Reiter, R. J.,** Neurosecretion in the pineal gland of Macaca rheus, *Experientia,* 30, 654, 1974.

96. **Lewinski, A., Vaughan, M. K., Champney, T. H., Reiter, R. J., and Smither, N. K. R.,** Dark exposure increases the number of pineal concretions in male gerbils (Meriones ungui culatus), *IRCS Med. Sci., Biochem.,* 111, 977, 1983.

97. **Diehl, B. J. M.,** Occurrence and regional distribution of calcareous concretions in the rat pineal gland, *Cell Tissue Res.,* 195, 359, 1978.

98. **Vigh, B. and Vigh-Teichmann, I.,** Two components of the pineal organ of the mink (Mustela vison): their structural similarity to submammalian pineal complexes and calcification, *Arch. Histol. Cytol.,* 55, 477, 1992.

99. **Vigh, B. and Vigh-Teichmann, I.,** The pinealocyte forming receptor and effector endings: immunoelectron microscopy and calcium histochemistry, *Arch. Histol. Cytol. Suppl.,* 52, 433, 1989.

100. **Wallace, R. B., Altman, J., and Gas, G. D.,** An autoradiographic and morphological investigation of the postnatal development of the pineal body, *Am. J. Anat.,* 126, 175, 1969.

101. **Moller, M., Ingild, A., and Bock, E.,** Immunohistochemical demonstration of S-100 protein and GFA protein in interstitial cells of rat pineal gland, *Brain Res.,* 140, 1, 1978.

102. **Borregon, A., Boya, J., Calvo, J. L., and Lopez-Munoz, F.,** Immunohistochemical study of the pineal cells in the postnatal development of the rat pineal gland, *J. Pineal Res.,* 14, 78, 1993.

103. **Lopez-Munoz, F., Boya, J., Calvo, J. L., and Marin, F.,** Immunohistochemical localization of glial fibrillary acidic protein (GFAP) in rat pineal stalk astrocytes, *Histol. Histopathol.,* 7, 643, 1992.

104. **Le Gros Clark, W. E.,** The nervous and vascular relations of the pineal gland, *J. Anat.,* 74, 471, 1940.

105. **Von Bartheld, F. and Moll, J.,** The vascular system of the mouse epiphysis with remarks on the comparative anatomy of the venous trunks in the epiphyseal area, *Acta Anat.,* 22, 227, 1954.

106. **Ganti, S. R., Hilala, S. K., Stein, B. M., Silver, A. J., Mawad, M., and Sane, P.,** CT of pineal region tumors, *Am. J. Radiol.,* 146, 451, 1986.

107. **Kappers, J. A.,** The development, topographical relations and innervation of the epiphysis cerebri in the albino rat, *Z. Zellforsch.,* 52, 163, 1960.

108. **Kappers, J. A.,** Die innervation der epiphyse cerebri der albinoratte, *Acta Neuroveg.,* 23, 111, 1961.

109. **Kappers, J. A.,** Survey of the innervation of the pineal organ in vertebrates, *Am. Zool.,* 4, 47, 1964.

110. **Klein, D. C. and Weller, J.,** Pineal gland in culture: serotonin N-acetyltransferase activity is stimulated by norepinephrine and dibutyryl cyclic adenosine monophosphate, *Fed. Proc.,* 29, 615, 1970.

111. **Wurtman, R. J., Shein, H. M., and Larin, F.,** Mediation by β-adrenergic receptors of effect of norepineph-rine on pineal synthesis of ^{14}C-serotonin and ^{14}C-melatonins, *J. Neurochem.,* 18, 1683, 1971.

112. **Deguchi, T. and Axelrod, J.,** Induction and superinduction of serotonin N-acetyltransferase by adrenergic drugs and denervation in rat pineal organ, *Proc. Natl. Acad. Sci. U.S.A.,* 69, 2208, 1972.

113. **Zatz, M., Kebabian, J. W., Romero, J. A., Lefkowitz, R. J., and Axelrod, J.,** Pineal beta adrenergic receptor: correlation of binding of ^{3}H-1-alprenolol with stimulation of adenylate cyclase, *J. Pharmacol. Exp. Ther.,* 196, 714, 1966.

114. **Fontan, J. A. and Lovenberg, W.,** Pineal protein kinase: effect of enzyme phosphorylation on actinomycin D binding by, and template activity of, chromatin, *Proc. Natl. Acad. Sci. U.S.A.,* 70, 755, 1973.

115. **Moore, R. Y.,** The innervation of the mammalian pineal gland, *Prog. Reprod. Biol.,* 4, 1, 1978.

116. **Moore, R. Y.,** Neural control of pineal function in mammals and birds, *J. Neural Transm. Suppl.,* 13, 47, 1978.

117. **Moore, R. Y. and Traynor, M. E.,** Diurnal rhythms in pineal N-acetyltransferase and hippocampal norepi-nephrine: effects of water deprivation, blinding and hypothalamic lesions, *Neuroendocrinology,* 20, 250, 1976.

118. **Moore, R. Y.,** The enigma of the geniculohypothalamic tract—why 2 visual entraining pathways, *J. Inter-discip. Cycle Res.,* 23, 144, 1992.

119. **Moore, R. Y.,** The organization of the human circadian timing system, *Prog. Brain Res.,* 93, 99, 1992.

120. **Mikkelsen, J. D., Cozzi, B., and Muller, M.,** Efferent projections from the lateral geniculate nucleus to the pineal complex of the Mongolian gerbil (Meriones unguiculatus), *Cell Tissue Res.,* 264, 95, 1991.

121. **Mikkelsen, J. D.,** The organization of the crossed geniculogeniculate pathway of the rat: a Phaseolus vulgaris–leucoagglutinin study, *Neuroscience,* 48, 953, 1992.

122. **Kenny, G. C. T.,** The "nervus conarii" of the monkey, *J. Neuropathol. Exp. Neurol.,* 20, 563, 1961.

123. **Romijn, H. J.,** Parasympathetic innervation of the rabbit pineal gland, *Brain Res.,* 55, 431, 1973.

124. **Moller, M.,** Fine structure of the pinealopetal innervation of of mammalian pineal gland, *Microsc. Res. Tech.,* 21, 188, 1992.

125. **Laitinen, J. T., Torda, T., and Saavedra, J. M.,** Cholinergic stimulation of phosphoinositide hydrolysis in the rat pineal, *Eur. J. Pharmacol.,* 161, 237, 1989.

126. **Finocchiaro, M., Scheucher, A., Alvarez, A. L., Finkielman, S., Nahmod, V. E., and Pirola, C. J.,** Pineal hyperactivity in spontaneously hyperactive rats: muscarinic regulation of indole metabolism, *Clin. Sci. Colch.,* 79, 437,. 1990.

127. **Quay, W. B.,** Histological structure and cytology of the pineal organ in birds and mammals, *Prog. Brain Res.,* 10, 49, 1965.

128. **Romijn, H. J.,** Structure and innervation of the pineal gland of the rabbit, *Orycytolagus cuniculus* L. A light microscopic investigation, *Z. Zellforsch.,* 139, 473, 1973.

129. **David, G. F. X. and Herbert, J.,** Experimental evidence for a synaptic connection between habenula and pineal ganglion in the ferret, *Brain Res.,* 64, 327, 1973.

130. **David, G. F. X., Herbert, J., and Wright, G. D. S.,** The ultrastructure of the pineal ganglion in the ferret, *J. Anat.,* 115, 79, 1973.

131. **Kenny, G. C. T.,** The innervation of the mammalian pineal body, a comparative study, *Proc. Aust. Assoc. Neurol.,* 3, 133, 1965.

132. **Gardner, J. H.,** Innervation of pineal gland in the hooded rat, *J. Comp. Neurol.,* 99, 319, 1953.

133. **Moller, M. and Korf, H. W.,** Neural connections between the brain and the pineal gland of the golden hamster (*Mesocricetus auratus*). Tracer study by horseradish peroxidase, *Cell Tissue Res.,* 247, 145, 1987.

134. **Patrickson, J. W. and Smith, T. E.,** Innervation of the pineal gland of the rat: an HRP study, *Exp. Neurol.,* 95, 207, 1987.

135. **Ronnekleiv, O. K., Kelly, M. J., Moller, M., and Wuttke, W.,** Electrophysiological and morphological evidence for a direct central innervation of the pineal gland, *Pfluegers Arch. (Suppl.),* 373, 187, 1978.

136. **McClung, R. and Dafny, N.,** Neurophysiological properties of the pineal body. II. Single unit recording, *Life Sci.,* 16, 621, 1975.

137. **Miline, R., Devecerski, V., and Krstic, R.,** Influence d'excitations olfactives sur le systeme habenulo-epiphysaire, *Ann. Endocrinol.,* 24, 377, 1963.

138. **Reiter, R. J. and Ellison, N. M.,** Delayed puberty in blinded anosmic female rats: role of the pineal gland, *Biol. Reprod.,* 2, 216, 1970.

139. **Moller, M., Phansuwan-Pujito, P., Govitrapong, P., and Schmidt, P.,** Indications for a central innervation of the bovine pineal gland with substance P-immunoreactive nerve fibers, *Brain Res.,* 611, 347, 1993.

140. **Cozzi, B. and Moller, M.,** Indications for the presence of two populations of serotonin-containing pinealocytes in the pineal complex of the golden hamster (Mesocricetus auratus), *Cell Tissue Res.,* 252, 115, 1988.

141. **Korf, H. W., Sato, T., and Oksche, A.,** Complex relationships between the pineal organ and the medial habenular nucleus—pretectal region of the mouse as revealed by S antigen immunocytochemistry, *Cell Tissue Res.,* 261, 493, 1990.

142. **Zhang, E. T., Mikkelsen, J. D., and Moller, M.,** Tyrosine hydroxylase and neuropeptide Y-immunoreactive nerve fibers in the pineal complex of untreated rats following removal of the superior cervical ganglia, *Cell Tissue Res.,* 265, 63, 1991.

143. **Harada, Y., Okubo, M., Yaga, K., Kaneko, T., and Kaku, K.,** Neuropeptide Y inhibits beta adrenergic agonist- and vasoactive intestinal peptide-induced cyclic AMP accumulation in rat pinealocytes through pertussis toxin-sensitive G protein, *J. Neurochem.,* 59, 2178, 1992.

144. **Olcese, J.,** Neuropeptide Y: an endogenous inhibitor of norepinephrine-stimulated melatonin secretion in the rat pineal gland, *J. Neurochem.,* 57, 943, 1991.

145. **Moller, M.,** Fine structure of the pinealopetal innervation of the mammalian pineal gland, *Microsc. Res. Tech.,* 21, 188, 1992.

146. **Hartmann, F.,** Uber die innervation der epiphysis cerebri einiger saugetiere, *Z. Zellforsch.,* 46, 416, 429.

147. **Mikkelsen, J. D. and Moller, M.,** A direct neural projection from the intergeniculate leaflet of the lateral geniculate nucleus to the deep pineal gland of the rat, demonstrated with Phaseolus vulgaris leucoagglutinin, *Brain Res.,* 520, 342, 1990.

148. **Mikkelsen, J. D., Panula, P., and Moller, M.,** Histamine-immunoreactive nerve fibers in the rat pineal gland: evidence for a histaminergic central innervation, *Brain Res.,* 597, 200, 1992.

149. **Nurnberger, F. and Korf, H. W.,** Oxytocin and vasopressin immunoreactive nerve fibers in the pineal gland of the hedgehog, *Erinaceus europaeus* L., *Cell Tissue Res.,* 220, 87, 1981.

150. **Korf, H. W. and Wagner, U.,** Evidence for a nervous connection between the brain and the pineal organ in the guinea pig, *Cell Tissue Res.,* 209, 505, 1980.

151. **Dogterom, J., Snijdewint, F. G. M., Pevet, P., and Swaab, D. F.,** Studies on the presence of vasopressin, oxytocin and vasotocin in the pineal gland, subcommissural organ and fetal pituitary gland: failure to detect vasotocin in mammals, *J. Endocrinol.,* 84, 115, 1980.

152. **McCord, C. P. and Allen, F. P.,** Evidences associating pineal gland function with alterations in pigmentation, *J. Exp. Zool.,* 23, 207, 1917.

153. **Wurtman, R. J. and Axelrod, J.,** The pineal gland, *Sci. Am.,* 213, 50, 1965.

154. **Neacsu, C.,** The mechanism of antigonadotropic action of a polypeptide extracted from a bovine pineal gland, *Rev. Roum. Physiol.,* 9, 161, 1972.

155. **Rosenbloom, A. A. and Fisher, D. A.,** Radioimmunoassay of arginine vasotocin, *Endocrinology,* 95, 1726, 1975.

156. **Bowie, E. P. and Herbert, D. C.,** Immunocytochemical evidence for the presence or arginine vasotocin in the rat pineal gland, *Nature (London),* 261, 5555, 1976.

157. **Coculescu, M., Azoral, M., and Matulevicius, V.,** Tentative identification of arginine vasotocin in the bovine pineal extract prepared by the Milcu-Nanu method, *Rev. Roum. Med. Endocrinol.,* 15, 27, 1977.

158. **Sartin, J. L., Bruot, B. C., and Orts, R. J.,** Neurotransmitter regulation of arginine vasotocin release from rat pineal glands in vitro, *Acta Endocrinol.,* 91, 571, 1979.

159. **Reiter, R. J. and Vaughan, M. K.,** Pineal antigonadotrophic substances: polypeptides and indoles, *Life Sci.,* 21, 159, 1977.

160. **Pavel, S.,** The mechanism of action of vasotocin in the mammalian brain, *Prog. Brain Res.,* 52, 445, 1979.

161. **Negro-Vilar, A., Sanchez-Franco, F., Kwiatkowski, M., and Samson, W. K.,** Failure to detect radioimmunoassayable arginine vasotocin in mammalian pineals, *Brain Res. Bull.,* 4, 789, 1979.

162. **Pevet, P., Dogterom, J., Buijs, R. M., and Reinharz, A.,** Is it the vasotocin or a vasotocin-like peptide which is present in the mammalian pineal and subcommissural organ?, *J. Endocrinol.,* 80, 49P, 1978.

163. **Liu, B. and Burbach, J. P.,** Characterization of vasopressin and oxytocin immunoreactivity in the sheep and rat pineal gland: absence of vasotocin and detection of a vasopressin-like peptide, *Peptides,* 8, 7, 1987.

164. **Benson, B., Ebels, I., and Hruby, V. J.,** Isolation and structure elucidation of bovine pineal arginine vasopressin: arginine vasotocin not identified, *Int. J. Pept. Protein Res.,* 36, 109, 1990.

165. **Osland, R. B., Cheesman, D. W., and Forscham, P. H.,** Studies on the mechanism of the suppression of the preovulatory surge of luteinizing hormone in the rat by arginine vasotocin, *Endocrinology,* 101, 1203, 1977.

166. **Blask, D. E., Vaughan, M. K., Reiter, R. J., and Johnson, L. Y.,** Influence of arginine vasotocin on the estrogen-induced surge of LH and FSH in adult ovariectomized rats, *Life Sci.,* 23, 1033, 1978.

167. **Goldstein, R.,** Arginine-vasotocin (AVT)—a pineal hormone in mammals, *Rom. J. Endocrinol.,* 30, 21, 1992.

168. **Bianchini, P. and Osima, B.,** Studi su di un probabile ormone della pineale: l'Anestrina, *Boll. Soc. Ital. Biol. Sper.,* 36, 1674, 1960.

169. **Chazov, Y. I., Isachenkov, V. A., Krivosheyev, O. G., Veselova, S. N., and Zhivoderova, G. V.,** A factor from the pineal body inhibiting the ovulation induced by luteinizing hormone, *Dokl. Akad. Nauk SSSR,* 27, 246, 1972.

170. **Ianas, O., Csuma, A., and Badescu, I.,** Total and free amino acids in the "Crinofizin" pineal extract, *Rom. J. Endocrinol.,* 30, 103, 1992.

171. **Damian, E., Ianas, O., Badescu, I., and Oprescu, M.,** Anti-LH and FSH activity of melatonin extract of bovine pineal glands, *Life Sci.,* 12, 513, 1973.

172. **Orts, R. J. and Benson, B.,** Inhibitory effects on serum and pituitary LH by a melatonin-free extract of bovine pineal glands, *Life Sci.,* 12, 513, 1973.

173. **Orts, R. J., Poe, R. W., and Liao, T. H.,** Studies on the characteristics of a partially purified antigonadotrophin from bovine pineal gland, *Life Sci.,* 24, 985, 1979.

174. **Ebels, I., Moszkowska, A., and Scemama, A.,** Etude in vitro des extraits epiphysaires fractiones, resultats preliminaires, *C. R. Acad., Sci.,* 260, 5120, 1965.

175. **Moszkowska, A., Citharel, A., L'Heritier, A., Ebels, I., and LaPlante, E.,** Some new aspects of a sheep pineal gonadotropic inhibiting activity in in vitro experiments, *Experientia,* 30, 964, 1974.

176. **Benson, B., Matthews, M. J., and Rodin, A. E.,** Studies on a non-melatonin pineal antigonadotropin, *Acta Endocrinol.,* 69, 257, 1972.

177. **Ota, M., Horiuchi, S., and Obara, K.,** Inhibition of ovulation induced with PMSG and HCG by a melatonin-free extract of bovine pineal powder, *Neuroendocrinology,* 18, 311, 1975.

178. **Cheesman, D. W. and Forsham, P. H.,** Inhibition of induced ovulation by a highly purified extract of the bovine pineal gland, *Proc. Soc. Exp. Biol. Med.,* 146, 722, 1974.

179. **Demoulin, A., Hudson, B., Legros, J. J., and Franchimont, P.,** Influence d'un extrait de glandes pineales ovines sur la liberation de prolactine in vitro, *C. R. Seances Soc. Biol. Paris,* 171, 1134, 1977.

180. **Blask, D. E. and Reiter, R. J.,** The pineal gland of the blind-anosmic female rat: its influence on medial basal hypothalamic LRH, PIF and/or PRF activity in vivo, *Neuroendocrinology,* 17, 362, 1975.

181. **Vriend, J., Hinkle, P. M., and Knigge, K. M.,** Evidence for a thyrotropin-releasing hormone inhibitor in the pineal gland, *Endocrinology,* 107, 1791, 1980.

182. **Piekut, D. T. and Knigge, K. M.,** Immunocytochemical analysis of the rat pineal gland using antisera generated against analogs of luteinizing hormone-releasing hormone (LHRH), *J. Histochem. Cytochem.,* 30, 106, 1982.

183. **Benson, B. and Ebels, I.,** Structure of a pineal gland-derived antigonadotropic decapeptide, *Life Sci.,* 54, 437, 1994.

184. **Duraiswami, W., Franchimont, P., Boucher, D., and Thieblot, M.,** Immunoreactive luteinizing hormone releasing hormone (LHRH) in the bovine pineal gland, *Horm. Metab. Res.,* 8, 232, 1976.

185. **King, J. A. and Millar, R. P.,** Decapeptide luteinizing hormone releasing hormone in ovine pineal gland, *J. Endocrinol.,* 91, 405, 1981.

186. **Guansing, A. R. and Murk, L. M.,** Distribution of thyrotropin releasing hormone in human brain, *Horm. Metab. Res.,* 8, 493, 1976.

187. **Dogterom, J., Snijdewint, F. G. M., Pevet, P., and Buijs, R. M.,** On the presence of neuropeptides in the mammalian pineal gland and subcommissural organ, *Prog. Brain Res.,* 52, 465, 1979.

188. **Pevet, P., Reinharz, A. C., and Dogterom, J.,** Neurophysins, vasopressin and oxytocin in the bovine pineal gland, *Neurosci. Lett.,* 16, 301, 1980.

189. **Reinharz, A. C. and Vallotton, M. B.,** Presence of two neurophysins in the human pineal gland, *Endocrinology,* 100, 994, 1977.

190. **Geelen, G., Allevard-Burguburu, A. M., Gauquelin, G., Ziao, Y. Z., Frutoso, J., Charib, C., Sempore, B., Meunier, C., and Augoyard, G.,** Radioimmunoassay of arginine vasopressin, oxytocin and arginine vasotocin-like material in the human pineal gland, *Peptides,* 2, 459, 1981.

191. **Lepetit, P., Fevre-Montange, M., Gay, N., Belin, M. F., and Bobillier, P.,** Vasopressin mRNA in the cerebellum and circumventricular organs: a quantitative in situ hybridization study, *Neurosci. Lett.,* 159, 171, 1993.

192. **Legros, J. J., Louis, F., Grotyschel-Stewardt, U., and Franchimont, P.,** Presence of immunoreactive neurophysin-like material in human target organs and pineal gland: physiological meaning, *Ann. N.Y. Acad. Sci.,* 248, 157, 1975.

193. **Axelrod, J.,** O-methylation of epinephrine and other catechols in vitro and in vivo, *Science,* 126, 400, 1957.

194. **Axelrod, J. and Weissbach, H.,** Enzymatic O-methylation of N-acetylation to melatonin, *Science,* 138, 1312, 1960.

195. **Weissbach, H., Redfield, B. G., and Axelrod, J.,** Biosynthesis of melatonin to N-acetylserotonin, *Biochim. Biophys. Acta,* 43, 352, 1960.

196. **Axelrod, J. and Weissbach, H.,** Purification and properties of hydroxyindole O-methyl-transferase, *J. Biol. Chem.,* 236, 211, 1961.

197. **Bubenik, G. A., Brown, G. M., and Grota, L. R.,** Differential localization of N-acetylated indolealkylamines in CNS and the Harderian gland using immunohistology, *Brain Res.,* 118, 417, 1976.

198. **Koslow, S. H. and Green, R.,** Analysis of pineal and brain indolealkylamines by gas chromatography-mass spectrometry, *Adv. Biochem. Psychopharmacol.,* 7, 33, 1973.

199. **Axelrod, J., Maclean, P. D., Albers, R. W., and Weissbach, H. W.,** Regional distribution of methyltransferase enzymes in the nervous system and glandular tissues, in *Regional Neurochemistry,* Kety, S. S. and Elkes, J., Eds., Pergamon Press, Oxford, 1961, 307.

200. **Quay, W. B.,** Retinal and pineal hydroxyindole-O-methyl transferase activity in vertebrates, *Life Sci.,* 4, 983, 1965.

201. **Cardinali, D. P. and Wurtman, R. J.,** Hydroxyindole-O-methyltransferases in rat pineal, retina and Harderian gland, *Endocrinology,* 91, 247, 1972.

202. **Wiechmann, A. F. and Craft, C. M.,** Localization of mRNA encoding the indoleamine synthesizing enzyme, hydroxyindole-O-methyltransferase, in chicken pineal and retina by *in situ* hybridization, *Neurosci. Lett.,* 150, 207, 1993.

203. **Nowak, J. Z., Szymanska, B., Zawilska, J. B., and Bialek, B.,** Hydroxyindole-O-methyltransferase activity in ocular and brain structures of rabbit and hen, *J. Pineal Res.,* 15, 35, 1993.

204. **Weichmann, A. F. and Hollyfield, J. G.,** HIOMT immunoreactivity in the vertebrate retina: a species comparison, *Exp. Eye Res.,* 49, 1079, 1989.

205. **Synder, S. H. and Axelrod, J.,** Circadian rhythms in pineal serotonin: effect of monoamine oxidase inhibition and reserpine, *Science,* 149, 542, 1965.

206. **Giarman, N. J., Freedman, D. X., and Picard-Ami, L.,** Serotonin content of the pineal glands of man and monkey, *Nature (London),* 186, 480, 1960.

207. **McIsaac, W. M., Farrell, G., Taborsky, R. G., and Taylor, A. M.,** Indole compounds: isolation from pineal tissue, *Science,* 148, 102, 1965.

208. **Lynch, H. J.,** Diurnal oscillations in pineal melatonin content, *Life Sci.,* 10, 791, 1971.

209. **Panke, E. S., Rollag, M. D., and Reiter, R. J.,** Pineal melatonin concentrations in the Syrian hamster, *Endocrinology,* 104, 194, 1979.

210. **Reiter, R. J., Hurlbut, E. C., Esquifino, A. I., Champney, T. H., and Steger, R. W.,** Changes in serotonin levels, N-acetyltransferase activity, hydroxyindole-O-methyltransferase activity, and melatonin levels in the pineal gland of the Richardson's ground squirrel in relation to the light-dark cycle, *Neuroendocrinology,* 39, 356, 1984.

211. **Arendt, J., Symons, A. M., and Laud, C. A.,** Pineal function in sheep: evidence for a possible mechanism mediating seasonal reproductive activity, *Experientia,* 37, 584, 1981.

212. **Hedlund, L., Lischiko, M. M., Rollag, M. D., and Niswender, G. D.,** Melatonin: daily cycle in plasma and cerebrospinal fluid of calves, *Science,* 195, 686, 1977.

213. **Kennaway, D. J., Porter, K. J., and Seamark, R. F.,** Changes in plasma tryptophan and melatonin content in penned sheep, *Aust. J. Biol. Sci.,* 31, 49, 1978.

214. **Reppert, S. M., Perlow, M. J., Tamarkin, L., and Klein, D. C.,** A diurnal melatonin rhythm in primate cerebrospinal fluid, *Endocrinology,* 104, 295, 1979.

215. **Lewy, A. J. and Markey, S. P.,** Analysis of melatonin in human plasma by gas chromatrography negative chemical ionization mass spectrometry, *Science,* 201, 741, 1978.

216. **Ellison, N., Weller, J., and Klein, D.,** Development of a circadian rhythm in the activity of pineal serotonin N-acetyltransferase, *J. Neurochem.,* 19, 1335, 1972.

217. **Klein, D. and Weller, J.,** Rapid light-induced decrease in pineal serotonin N-acetyltransferase activity, *Science,* 177, 532, 1972.

218. **Hoffmann, K., Illnerova, H., and Vanecek, J.,** Effect of photoperiod and of one minute light at night-time on the pineal rhythm in N-acetyltransferase activity in the Djungarian hamster Phodopus sungorus, *Biol. Reprod.,* 24, 551, 1981.

219. **Axelrod, J., Shein, H. M., and Wurtman, R.J.,** Stimulation of C^{14}-melatonin synthesis from C^{14}-tryptophan by noradrenaline in rat pineal in organ culture, *Proc. Natl. Acad. Sci. U.S.A.,* 62, 544, 1969.

220. **Wurtman, R. J., Shein, H. M., Axelrod, J., and Larin, F.,** Incorporation of ^{14}C-tryptophan into ^{14}C-protein by cultured rat pineals: stimulation by L-norepinephrine, *Proc. Natl. Acad. Sci. U.S.A.,* 62, 749, 755.

221. **Vaughan, G. M., Pelham, R. W., Pang, S. F., Loughlin, L., Wilson, K. M., Sandock, K. L., Vaughan, M. K., Kowlow, S. H., and Reiter, R. J.,** Nocturnal elevation of plasma melatonin and urinary 5-hydroxy-indoleacetic acid in young men: attempts at modification by brief changes in environmental lighting and sleep and by autonomic drugs, *J. Clin. Endocrinol.,* 42, 752, 1976.

222. **Wetterberg, L.,** Clinical importance of melatonin, *Prog. Brain Res.,* 52, 539, 1979.

223. **Moore, D. C., Paunier, L., and Sizonenko, P. C.,** Effects of adrenergic stimulation and blockade on melatonin secretion in the human, *Prog. Brain Res.,* 52, 517, 1979.

224. **Fontana, J. A. and Lovenberg, W.,** A cyclic AMP-dependent protein kinase of the bovine pineal gland, *Proc. Natl. Acad. Sci. U.S.A.,* 68, 2787, 1971.

225. **Romero, J. A., Zatz, M., and Axelrod, J.,** Beta-adrenergic stimulation of pineal N-acetyltransferase: adenosine 3′,5′-cyclic monophosphate stimulates both RNA and protein synthesis, *Proc. Natl. Acad. Sci. U.S.A.,* 72, 2107, 1975.

226. **Deguchi, T. and Axelrod, J.,** Superinduction of serotonin N-acetyltransferase and supersensitivity of adenyl cyclase to catecholamines in denervated pineal gland, *Mol. Pharmacol.,* 9, 612, 1973.

227. **Klein, D. C., Sugden, D., and Weller, J. L.,** Postsynaptic α-adrenergic receptors potentiate the β-adrenergic stimulation of serotonin N-acetyltransferase, *Proc. Natl. Acad. Sci. U.S.A,* 80, 599, 1983.

228. **Klein, D. C., Chik, C. L., Weller, J., and Ho, A. K.,** Adrenergic regulation of pineal cAMP and cGMP: evidence for a gating mechanism, in *Progress in Catecholamine Research,* Dahlstrom, A., Baelmaker, R. H., and Sandler, M., Eds., Liss, New York, 1988, 415.

229. **Vanecek, J., Sugden, D., Weller, J., and Klein, D. C.,** Atypical synergistic α_1- and β-adrenergic regulation of adenosine 3′,5′-monophosphate and guanosine 3′,5′-monophosphate in rat pinealocytes, *Endocrinology,* 116, 2167, 1985.

230. **Sugden, D. and Klein, D. C.,** A cholera toxin substrate regulates cyclic GMP content of rat pinealocytes, *J. Biol. Chem.,* 262, 7447, 1987.

231. **Sugden, A. L., Sugden, D., and Klein, D. C.,** Essential role of calcium influx in the adrenergic regulation of cAMP and cGMP in rat pinealocytes, *J. Biol. Chem.,* 261, 11608, 1986.

232. **Ho, A. K., Chik, C. L., and Klein, D. C.,** Protein kinase C is involved in adrenergic stimulation of pineal cGMP accumulation, *J. Biol. Chem.,* 262, 10059, 1987.

233. **Reiter, R. J., Trakulrungsi, W. K., Trakulrungsi, C., Vriend, J., Morgan, W. W., Vaughan, M. K., and Johnson, L. Y.,** Pineal melatonin production: endocrine and age effects, in *Melatonin Rhythm Generating System,* Klein, D. C., Ed., S. Karger, Basel, 1983, 143.

234. **Reiter, R. J. and Richardson, B. A.,** Some perturbations that disturb the circadian melatonin rhythm, *Chronobiol. Int.,* 9, 313, 1992.

235. **Bauer, M. S., Poland, R. E., Whybrow, P. C., and Frazer, A.,** Pituitary adrenal and thyroid effects on melatonin content of the rat pineal gland, *Psychoneuroendocrinology,* 14, 165, 1989.

236. **Tannenbaum, M. G., Reiter, R. J., Vaughan, M. K., Troiani, M. E., and Gonzalez-Brito, A.,** Adrenalectomy prevents changes in rat pineal melatonin content and N-acetyltransferase activity induced by acute insulin stress, *J. Pineal Res.,* 4, 395, 1987.

237. **Johnson, L. Y., Vaughan, M. K., Richardson, B. A., Petterborg, L. J., and Reiter, R. J.,** Variation in pineal melatonin content during the estrous cycle of the rat, *Proc. Soc. Exp. Biol. Med.,* 169, 416, 1982.

238. **Daya, S. and Potgieter, B.,** The effect of castration, testosterone and estradiol on $^{[14]}$C-serotonin metabolism by organ cultures of male rat pineal glands, *Experientia,* 41, 275, 1985.

239. **Nir, I. and Hirschmann, N.,** The effect of thyroid hormones on rat pineal indoleamine metabolism in vitro, *J. Neural Transm.,* 42, 117, 1978.

240. **Parfitt, A. G. and Klein, D. C.,** Sympathetic nerve endings in pineal gland protect against acute stress-induced increase in N-acetyltransferase activity, *Endocrinology,* 99, 940, 1976.

241. **Gibbs, F. P. and Vriend, J.,** The half-life of melatonin elimination from plasma, *Endocrinology,* 109, 1796, 1981.

242. **Kopin, I. J., Pare, C. M. B., Axelrod, J., and Weissbach, H.,** The fate of melatonin in animals, *Biol. Chem.,* 236, 3072, 1971.

243. **Wurtman, R. J., Axelrod, J., and Kelly, D. E.,** *The Pineal,* Academic Press, New York, 1968.

244. **Rollag, M. D., Panke, E. S., Trakulrungsi, W. K., Trakulrungsi, C., and Reiter, R. J.,** Quantitation of daily melatonin synthesis in the hamster pineal gland, *Endocrinology,* 106, 231, 1980.

245. **Illnerova, H. and Vanecek, J.,** Response of rat pineal serotonin N-acetyltransferase to one minute light pulse at different times of the night, *Brain Res.,* 167, 431, 1979.

246. **Pardridge, W. M. and Mietus, L. J.,** Transport of albumin-bound melatonin through the blood-brain barrier, *J. Neurochem.,* 34, 1761, 1980.

247. **Kveder, S. and McIsaac, W. M.,** The metabolism of melatonin (N-acetyl-5-methoxytryptamine) and methoxytryptamine, *J. Biol. Chem.,* 236, 3214, 1961.

248. **Taborsky, R. G., Deloigs, P., and Page, I. H.,** 6-Hydroxyindole and the metabolism of melatonin, *J. Med. Chem.,* 8, 855, 1965.

249. **Kennaway, D. J.,** Urinary 6-hydroxymelatonin excretory rhythms in laboratory rats: effects of photoperiod and light, *Brain Res.,* 603, 338, 1993.

250. **Hirata, F., Hayaishi, O., Tokuyama, T., and Senoh, S.,** In vitro and in vivo formation of two new metabolites of melatonin, *J. Biol. Chem.,* 249, 1311, 1974.

251. **Lerner, A. B., Case, J. D., and Takahashi, Y.,** Isolation of melatonin and 5-methoxyindole-3-acetic acid from bovine pineal gland, *J. Biol. Chem.,* 235, 1992, 1960.

252. **Quay, W. B.,** Circadian rhythm in rat pineal serotonin and its modification by estrous cycle and photoperiod, *Gen. Comp. Endocrinol.,* 3, 473, 1963.

253. **Quay, W. B.,** Circadian and estrous rhythms in pineal melatonin and 5-hydroxyindole-3-acetic acid, *Proc. Soc. Exp. Biol. Med.,* 115, 710, 1964.

254. **Grota, L. J. and Brown, G. M.,** Antibodies to indolealkylamines: serotonin and melatonin, *Can. J. Biochem.,* 52, 196, 1974.

255. **Arendt, J., Paunier, L., and Sizonenko, P. C.,** Melatonin radioimmunoassay, *J. Clin. Endocrinol.,* 40, 347, 1975.

256. **Rollag, M. P. and Niswender, G. D.,** Radioimmunoassay of serum concentrations of melatonin in sheep exposed to different lighting regimens, *Endocrinology,* 98, 482, 1976.

257. **Kennaway, D. J., Frith, R. G., Phillipou, G., Matthews, C. D., and Seamark, R. F.,** A specific radioimmunoassay for melatonin in biological fluids and its validation by gas chromatography mass spectrometry, *Endocrinology,* 101, 119, 1977.

258. **Wetterberg, L., Eriksson, O., Friberg, Y., and Vangbo, B.,** A simplified radioimmunoassay for melatonin and its application to biological fluids. Preliminary observations on the half-life of plasma melatonin in man, *Clin. Chim. Acta,* 86, 169, 1978.

259. **Yu, H. S., Pang, S. F., Tang, P. L., and Brown, G. M.,** Persistence of circadian rhythms of melatonin and N-acetylserotonin in the serum of rats after pinealectomy, *Neuroendocrinology,* 32, 262, 1981.

260. **Lewy, A. J., Tetsuo, M., Markey, S. P., Goodwin, F. K., and Kopin, I. J.,** Pinealectomy abolishes plasma melatonin in the rat, *J. Clin. Endocrinol. Metab.,* 50, 204, 1980.

261. **Wetterberg, L.,** Melatonin in serum, *Nature (London),* 269, 646, 1977.

262. **Vaughan, G. M.,** New sensitive serum melatonin radioimmunoassay employing the Kennaway G280 antibody: Syrian hamster morning adrenergic responses, *J. Pineal Res.,* 15, 88, 1993.

263. **Kennaway, D. J.,** Urinary 6-hydroxymelatonin excretory rhythms in laboratory rats: effects of photoperiod and light, *Brain Res.,* 603, 338, 1993.

264. **Peniston-Bird, J. F., Di, W. L., Street, C. A., Kadva, A., Stalteri, M. A., and Silman, R. E.,** HPLC of melatonin in plasma with fluorescence detection, *Clin. Chem.,* 39, 2242, 1993.

265. **Vieira, R., Miquez, J., Lema, M., and Aldegunde, M.,** Pineal and plasma melatonin as determined by high-performance liquid chromatography with electrochemical detection, *Anal. Biochem.,* 205, 300, 1992.

266. **Smith, I., Mullen, P. E., Silman, R. E., Snedden, W., and Wilson, B. W.,** Absolute identification of melatonin in human plasma and cerebrospinal fluid, *Nature (London),* 260, 718, 1976.

267. **Wilson, B. W., Lynch, H. J., and Ozaki, Y.,** 5-Methoxytryptophol in rat serum and pineal: detection, quantitation, and evidence for daily rhythmicity, *Life Sci.,* 23, 1019, 1978.

268. **Lewy, A. J. and Markey, S. P.,** Analysis of melatonin in human plasma by gas chromatography negative chemical ionization mass spectrometry, *Science,* 201, 741, 1978.

269. **Lewy, A. J.,** Effects of light on human melatonin production and the human circadian system, *Prog. Neuro-Psych. Biol. Psych.,* 7, 551, 1983.

270. **Wurtman, R. J., Roth, W., Altschule, M. D., and Wurtman, J. J.,** Interactions of the pineal and exposure to continuous light on organ weights of female rats, *Acta Endocrinol.,* 36, 617, 1961.

271. **Wurtman, R. J., Axelrod, J., and Phillips, L.,** Melatonin, a pineal substance: effect on the rat ovary, *Science,* 141, 277, 1963.

272. **Reiter, R. J.,** The pineal and its control of hormones in the control of reproduction in mammals, *Endocr. Res.,* 1, 119, 1980.

273. **Karsch, F. J., Bittman, E. L., Foster, D. L., Goodman, R. L., Legan, S. J., and Robinson, J. E.,** Neuroendocrine basis of seasonal reproduction, *Recent Prog. Horm. Res.,* 40, 112, 1984.

274. **Hoffman, R. A. and Reiter, R. J.,** Pineal gland: influence on gonads of male hamsters, *Science,* 148, 1609, 1965.

275. **Gaston, S. and Menaker, M.,** Photoperiodic control of hamster testes, *Science,* 158, 925, 1967.

276. **Frehn, J. L. and Liu, C.,** Effects of temperature, photoperiod and hibernation on the testes of golden hamsters, *J. Exp. Zool.,* 174, 317, 1970.

277. **Berdtson, W. E. and Desjardins, C.,** Circulating LH and FSH levels and testicular function in hamsters during light deprivation and subsequent photoperiodic stimulation, *Endocrinology,* 95, 195, 1974.

278. **Reiter, R. J.,** Pineal function in long-term blinded male and female golden hamsters, *Gen. Comp. Endocrinol.,* 12, 460, 1969.

279. **Reiter, R. J.,** Surgical procedures involving the pineal gland which prevent gonadal degeneration in adult male hamsters, *Ann. Endocrinol.,* 33, 571, 1972.

280. **Reiter, R. J.,** Pineal gland: interface between the photoperiodic environment and the endocrine system, *Trend Endocrinol. Metab.,* 2, 14, 1991.

281. **Reiter, R. J. and Hester, R. J.,** Interrelationships of the pineal gland, the superior cervical ganglia and the photoperiod in the regulation of the endocrine systems of hamsters, *Endocrinology,* 79, 1168, 1966.

282. **Reiter, R. J.,** Morphological studies on the reproductive organs of blinded male hamsters and the effects of pinealectomy or superior cervical ganglionectomy, *Anat. Rec.,* 160, 13, 1968.

283. **Reiter, R. J.,** The effect of pinealectomy, pineal grafts and denervation of the pineal gland on the reproductive organs of male hamsters, *Neuroendocrinology,* 2, 138, 1967.

284. **Smale, L., Cassone, J. M., Moore, R. Y., and Morin, L. P.,** Paraventricular nucleus projections mediating pineal melatonin and gonadal responses to photoperiod in the hamster, *Brain Res. Bull.,* 22, 263, 1989.

285. **Bittman, E. L. and Lehman, M. N.,** Paraventricular neurons control hamster photoperiodism by a predominantly uncrossed descending pathway, *Brain Res. Bull.,* 19, 687, 1987.

286. **Reuss, S., Stehle, J., Schroder, H., and Vollrath, L.,** The role of the hypothalamic paraventricular nuclei for the regulation of pineal melatonin synthesis: new aspects derived from the vasopressin-deficient Brattleboro rat, *Neurosci. Lett.,* 109, 196, 1990.

287. **Reiter, R. J., Vaughan, M. K., Blask, D. E., and Johnson, L. Y.,** Melatonin: its inhibition of pineal antigonadotrophic activity in male hamsters, *Science,* 185, 1169, 1974.

288. **Reiter, R. J., Vaughan, M. K., Blask, D. E., and Johnson, L. Y.,** Pineal methoxyindoles: new evidence concerning their function in the control of pineal mediated changes in the reproductive physiology of male golden hamsters, *Endocrinology,* 96, 206, 1975.

289. **Donofrio, R. J., Reiter, R. J., Sorrentino, S., Blask, D. E., and Talbot, J. A.,** A method for measurement of prolactin in the hamster by means of radioimmunoassay, *Neuroendocrinology,* 13, 79, 1973.

290. **Reiter, R. J. and Johnson, L. Y.,** Depressed action of the pineal gland on pituitary luteinizing hormone and prolactin in male hamster, *Horm. Res.,* 5, 311, 1974.

291. **Jackson, F. L., Heindel, J. J., Preslock, J. P., and Berkowitz, A. S.,** Alterations in hypothalamic content of luteinizing hormone-releasing hormone associated with pineal-mediated testicular regression in the golden hamster, *Biol. Reprod.,* 31, 436, 1984.

292. **Vriend, J.,** Testing the TRH hypothesis of pineal function, *Med. Hypotheses,* 4, 376, 1978.

293. **Hoffman, R. A., Hester, R. J., and Towns, C.,** Effects of light and temperature on the endocrine system of the golden hamster, *Comp. Biochem. Physiol.,* 15, 525, 1965.

294. **Reiter, R. J.,** Evidence for refractoriness of the pituitary-gonadal axis to the pineal gland in golden hamsters and its possible implications in animal reproductive rhythms, *Anat. Rec.,* 173, 365, 1972.

295. **Reiter, R. J.,** Pineal control of seasonal reproductive rhythm in male golden hamsters exposed to natural daylight and temperature, *Endocrinology,* 92, 423, 1973.

296. **Tamarkin, L., Westrom, W. K., Hamill, A. I., and Goldman, B. D.,** Effects of melatonin on the reproductive systems of male and female Syrian hamsters. A diurnal rhythm in sensitivity to melatonin, *Endocrinology,* 99, 1534, 1976.

297. **Bridges, R., Tamarkin, L., and Goldman, B. D.,** Effects of photoperiod and melatonin on reproductive cycles in the hamster, *Ann. Biol. Anim. Biochem. Biophys.,* 16, 399, 1976.

298. **Reiter, R. J., Blask, D. E., Johnson, L. Y., Rudeen, P. K., Vaughan, M. K., and Waring, P. J.,** Melatonin inhibition of reproduction in the male hamster: its dependency on time of day of administration and on an intact and sympathetically innervated pineal gland, *Neuroendocrinology,* 22, 107, 1977.

299. **Li, K., Reiter, R. J., Vaughan, M. K., Oaknin, S., Troiani, M. E., and Esquifino, A. I.,** Elevated ambient temperature retards the atrophic response of the neuroendocrine-reproductive axis of male Syrian hamsters to either daily afternoon melatonin injections or to short photoperiod exposure, *Neuroendocrinology,* 45, 356, 1987.

300. **Reiter, R. J.,** The melatonin message: duration verus coincidence hypotheses, *Life Sci.,* 40, 2119, 1987.

301. **Grosse, J., Maywood, E. S., Ebling, F. J. P., and Hastings, M. H.,** Testicular regression in pinealectomized Syrian hamsters following infusions of melatonin delivered on non-circadian schedules, *Biol. Reprod.,* 49, 666, 1993.

302. **Bittman, E. L. and Karsch, F. J.,** Nightly duration of pineal melatonin secretion determines the reproductive response to inhibitory daylength in the ewe, *Biol. Reprod.,* 30, 585, 1984.

303. **Carter, D. S. and Goldman, B. D.,** Progonadal role of the pineal gland in the Djungarian hamster (Phodopus sungorus sungorus): mediation by melatonin, *Endocrinology,* 113, 1268, 1983.

304. **Hoffmann, K.,** Testicular involution in short photoperiods inhibited by melatonin, *Naturwissenschaften,* 61, 364, 1974.

305. **Gibbs, F. P. and Vriend, J.,** Counterantigonadotropic effect of melatonin administered via the drinking water, *Endocrinology,* 113, 1447, 1983.

306. **Hoffmann, K.,** The influence of photoperiod and melatonin on testis size, body weight and pelage color in the Djungarian hamster (Phodopus sungorus), *J. Comp. Physiol.,* 85, 267, 1973.

307. **Sisk, C. L. and Turek, F. W.,** Developmental time course of pubertal and photoperiodic changes in testosterone negative feedback on gonadotropin secretion in the golden hamster, *Endocrinology,* 112, 1208, 1983.

308. **Stankov, B., Vucini, V., Snochowski, M., Cozzi, B., Fumagalli, P., Maccarinelli, G., and Fraschini, F.,** Cytosolic androgen receptors in the neuroendocrine tissues of the golden hamster: influence of photoperiod and melatonin treatment, *Endocrinology,* 125, 1742, 1989.

309. **Anderson, R. A., Lincoln, G. A., and Wu, F. C.,** Melatonin potentiates testosterone-induced suppression of luteinizing hormone secretion in normal men, *Hum. Reprod.,* 8, 1819, 1993.

310. **Lindsay, D. R., Pelletier, J., Pisselet, C., and Courot, M.,** Changes in photoperiod and nutrition and their effect on testicular growth of rams, *J. Reprod. Fertil.,* 71, 351, 1984.

311. **Lincoln, G. A. and Almeida, O. F.,** Inhibition of reproduction in rams by long daylengths and the acute effect of superior cervical ganglionectomy, *J. Reprod. Fertil.,* 66, 417, 1982.

312. **Lincoln, G. A., Almedia, O. F., and Arendt, J.,** Role of melatonin and circadian rhythms in seasonal reproduction in rams, *J. Reprod. Fertil.,* 30, 23, 1981.

313. **Lincoln, G. A.,** Central effects of photoperiod on cyclicity and serum gonadotropins in the Syrian hamster, *Biol. Reprod.,* 12, 223, 1972.

314. **Seegal, R. F. and Goldman, B. D.,** Effects of photoperiod on cyclicity and serum gonadotropins in the Syrian hamster, *Biol. Reprod.,* 12, 223, 1975.

315. **Reiter, R. J. and Johnson, L. Y.,** Elevated pituitary LH and depressed pituitary prolactin levels in female hamsters with pineal-induced gonadal atrophy and the effects of chronic treatment with synthetic LRF, *Neuroendocrinology,* 14, 310, 1974.

316. **Reiter, R. J.,** Changes in the reproductive organs of cold-exposed and light-deprived female hamsters (Mesocricetus auratus), *J. Reprod. Fertil.,* 16, 217, 1968.

317. **Sorrentino, S. and Reiter, R. J.,** Pineal-induced alterations in estrous cycles in blinded hamsters, *Gen. Comp. Endocrinol.,* 15, 39, 1970.

318. **Hoffman, R. A. and Reiter, R. J.,** Response of some endocrine organs of female hamsters to pinealectomy and light, *Life Sci.,* 5, 1147, 1966.

319. **Reiter, R. J.,** Failure of the pineal gland to prevent gonadotrophin-induced ovarian stimulation in blinded hamsters, *J. Endocrinol.,* 38, 199, 1967.

320. **Reiter, R. J. and Fraschini, F.,** Endocrine aspects of the mammalian pineal gland: a review, *Neuroendocrinology,* 5, 219, 1969.

321. **Bittman, E. L.,** Photoperiodic influences on testicular regression in the golden hamster: termination of scotorefractoriness, *Biol. Reprod.,* 18, 871, 1971.

322. **Vaughan, M. K., Herbert, D. C., Brainard, G. C., Johnson, L. Y., Zeagler, J. W., and Reiter, R. J.,** A comparison of blinding and afternoon melatonin injections on the histology of the reproductive organs, pineal ultrastructure and gonadotrophin hormone levels in female Syrian hamsters, *Adv. Biosci.,* 29, 65, 1981.

323. **Stetson, M. H. and Hamilton, B.,** The anovulatory hamster: a comparison of the effects of short photoperiod and daily melatonin injections on the induction and termination of ovarian cyclicity, *J. Exp. Zool.,* 215, 173, 1981.

324. **Tamarkin, L., Lefebvre, N. G., Hollister, C. W., and Goldman, B. D.,** Effect of melatonin administered during the night on reproductive function in the Syrian hamster, *Endocrinology,* 101, 631, 1977.

325. **Reiter, R. J.,** Comparative physiology: pineal gland, *Annu. Rev. Physiol.,* 35, 305, 1973.

326. **Trakulrungsi, C., Reiter, R. J., Trakulrungsi, W. K., Vaughan, M. K., and Waring-Ellis, P. J.,** Interaction of daily injections and subcutaneous reservoirs of melatonin on the reproductive physiology of female Syrian hamsters, *Acta Endocrinol.,* 91, 59, 1979.

327. **Trakulrungsi, C., Reiter, R. J., Trakulrungsi, W. K., Vaughan, M. K., and Johnson, L. Y.,** Effects of injections and/or subcutaneous implants of melatonin in pituitary and plasma levels of LH, FSH, PRL, in ovariectomized Syrian hamsters, *Ann. Biol. Anim. Biochem. Biophys.,* 19, 1647, 1979.

328. **Bast, J. D. and Greenwald, G. S.,** Serum profiles of follicle-stimulating hormone, luteinizing hormone and prolactin during the estrous cycle of the hamster, *Endocrinology,* 94, 1295, 1974.

329. **Bex, F. J. and Goldman, B. D.,** Serum gonadotropins and follicular development in the Syrian hamster, *Endocrinology,* 96, 928, 1975.

330. **Bittman, E. L. and Goldman, B. D.,** Serum levels of gonadotrophins in hamsters exposed to short photoperiods: effects of adrenalectomy and ovariectomy, *J. Endocrinol.,* 83, 113, 1979.

331. **Goldman, B. and Brown, S.,** Sex differences in LH and FSH patterns in hamsters exposed to short photoperiod, *J. Steroid Biochem.,* 11, 531, 1979.

332. **Reiter, R. J. and Johnson, L. Y.,** Pineal regulation of immunoreactive luteinizing hormone and prolactin in light-deprived female hamsters, *Fertil. Steril.,* 25, 958, 1974.

333. **Bex, F. J. and Goldman, B. D.,** Serum gonadotropins associated with puberty in the female Syrian hamster, *Biol. Reprod.,* 16, 557, 1977.

334. **Stetson, M. H., Watson-Whitmyre, M., and Matt, K. S.,** Cyclic gonadotropin release in the presence and absence of estrogenic feedback in ovariectomized golden hamster, *Biol. Reprod.,* 19, 40, 1978.

335. **Reiter, R. J., Blask, D. E., and Johnson, L. Y.,** Influence of ovariectomy and estrogen and/or progesterone treatment on pituitary and plasma LH and prolactin levels in female hamsters, *Endocr. Res. Commun.,* 1, 181, 1974.

336. **Goldman, B. D., Mahesh, V. B., and Porter, J. C.,** The role of the ovary in the control of LH release in the hamster, *Mesocricetus auratus, Biol. Reprod.,* 4, 57, 1971.

337. **Goldman, B. D. and Porter, J. C.,** Serum LH levels in intact and castrated golden hamster, *Endocrinology,* 87, 676, 1970.

338. **Bridges, R. S. and Goldman, B. D.,** Diurnal rhythms in gonadotropins and progesterone in lactating and photoperiod induced acyclic hamsters, *Biol. Reprod.,* 13, 617, 1975.

339. **Legan, S. J. and Karsch, F. J.,** Photoperiodic control of seasonal breeding in ewes: modulation of the negative feedback action of estradiol, *Biol. Reprod.,* 23, 1061, 1980.

340. **Arendt, J., Symons, A. M., Laud, C. A., and Pryde, S. J.,** Melatonin can induce early onset of the breeding season in ewes, *J. Endocrinol.,* 97, 395, 1983.

341. **Malpaux, B., Daveau, A., Maurice, F., Gayrard, V., and Thiery, J.,** Short-day effects of melatonin on luteinizing hormone secretion in the ewe: evidence for central sites of action in the mediobasal hypothalamus, *Biol. Reprod.,* 48, 752, 1993.

342. **Okatani, Y., Okada, M., and Sagara, Y.,** Amplification of nocturnal melatonin secretion in women with nocturnal hyperprolactinemia, *Asia Oceania J. Obstet. Gynaecol.,* 18, 289, 1992.

343. **Terzolo, M., Revelli, A., Guidetti, D., Piovesan, A., Cassoni, P., Paccotti, P., Angeli, A., and Massobrio, M.,** Evening administration of melatonin enhances the pulsatile secretion of prolactin but not of LH and TSH in normally cycling women, *Clin. Endocrinol.,* 39, 185, 1993.

344. **Cagnacci, A., Elliott, J. A., and Yen, S. S.,** Amplification of pulsatile LH secretion by exogenous melatonin in women, *J. Clin. Endocrinol. Metab.,* 73, 210, 1991.

345. **Voordouw, B. C., Euser, R., Verdonk, R. E., Alberda, B. T., deFong, F. H., Drugendijk, A. C., Fauser, B. C., and Cohen, M.,** Melatonin and melatonin-progestin combinations alter pituitary-ovarian function in women and can inhibit ovulation, *J. Clin. Endocrinol. Metab.,* 74, 108, 1992.

346. **Wetterberg, L., Arendt, J., Paunier, L., Sizonenko, P. C., VanDonselaar, W., and Heyden, T.,** Human serum melatonin changes during the menstrual cycle, *J. Clin. Endocrinol. Metab.,* 42, 185, 1976.

347. **Laughlin, G. A., Loucks, A. B., and Yen, S. S.,** Marked augmentation of nocturnal melatonin secretion in amenorrheic athletes, but not in cycling athletes: unaltered by opioidergic or dopaminergic blockade, *J. Clin. Endocrinol. Metab.,* 73, 1321, 1991.

348. **Houssay, A. B., Pazo, J. H., and Epper, C. E.,** Effects of the pineal gland upon the hair cycles in mice, *J. Invest. Dermatol.,* 47, 230, 1966.

349. **Lombard Des Gouttes, M. N.,** Epiphysectomie a la naissance chez la souris male, *C. R. Acad. Sci.,* 264, 2141, 1967.

350. **DeFronzo, R. A. and Roth, W. D.,** Evidence for the existence of a pituitary-adrenal and a pituitary-thyroid axis, *Acta Endocrinol.,* 70, 31, 1972.

351. **Houssay, A. B. and Pazo, J. H.,** Role of the pituitary in the thyroid hypertrophy of pinealectomized rats, *Experientia,* 24, 813, 1968.

352. **Miline, R.,** La part du noyau paraventriculaire dans l'histophysiologie correlative de la glande thyroide et de la glande pineale, *Ann. Endocrinol.,* 24, 255, 1963.

353. **Scepovic, M.,** Contribution a l'etude histophysiologique de la glande thyroide chez les rats epiphysectomises, *Ann. Endocrinol.,* 24, 371, 1963.

354. **Losada, J.,** Effects of experimental pinealectomy, *Ann. Anat.,* 26, 133, 1977.

355. **Csaba, G., Kiss, J., and Bodoky, M.,** Uptake or radioactive iodine by the thyroid after pinealectomy, *Acta Biol. Acad. Sci. Hung.,* 19, 35, 1968.

356. **Ishibashi, T., Hahn, P. W., Srivastava, L., Kumaresan, P., and Turner, C. W.,** Effect of pinealectomy and melatonin on feed consumption and thyroid hormone secretion rate, *Proc. Soc. Exp. Biol. Med.,* 122, 644, 1966.

357. **Relkin, R.,** Effects of pinealectomy, constant light and darkness on thyrotropin levels in the pituitary and plasma of the rat, *Neuroendocrinology,* 10, 46, 1972.

358. **Relkin, R.,** Use of melatonin and synthetic TRH to determine site of pineal inhibition of TSH secretion, *Neuroendocrinology,* 25, 310, 1978.

359. **Niles, L. P., Brown, G., and Grota, L. J.,** Role of the pineal gland in diurnal endocrine secretion and rhythm regulation, *Neuroendocrinology,* 29, 14, 1979.

360. **Vriend, J., Reiter, R. J., and Anderson, G. R.,** Effects of the pineal and melatonin on thyroid activity of male golden hamsters, *Gen. Comp. Endocrinol.,* 38, 189, 1979.

361. **Vriend, J., Sackman, J. W., and Reiter, R. J.,** Effects of blinding, pinealectomy and superior cervical ganglionectomy on free thyroxin index of male golden hamsters, *Acta Endocrinol.,* 86, 758, 1977.

362. **Vriend, J. and Reiter, R. J.,** Effects of melatonin and the pineal gland on thyroid physiology of female hamsters, *Neurosci. Abstr.,* 7, 716, 1981.

363. **Vriend, J., Richardson, B., Vaughan, M. K., Johnson, L. Y., and Reiter, R. J.,** Effects of melatonin on thyroid physiology of female hamsters, *Neuroendocrinology,* 35, 79, 1982.

364. **Reiter, R. J., Hester, R. J., and Hassett, C. C.,** Thyroidal-pineal-gonadal interrelationships in dark-exposed female hamsters, *Fed. Proc.,* 25, 252, 1966.

365. **Vriend, J. and Wilber, J. F.,** Influence of the pineal gland on hypothalamic content of TRH in the Syrian hamster, *Horm. Res.,* 17, 108, 1983.

366. **Miline, R.,** Influence d'excitations olfactives sur le systeme habenulo-epiphysaire, *Ann. Endocrinol.,* 24, 377, 1963.

367. **Baschieri, L., DeLuca, F., Cramarosa, L., DeMartino, C., Oliverio, A., and Negri, M.,** Modification of thyroid activity by melatonin, *Experientia,* 19, 15, 1963.

368. **DeFronzo, R. A. and Roth, W. D.,** Evidence for the existence of a pineal-adrenal and a pineal-thyroid axis, *Acta Endocrinol.,* 70, 31, 1972.

369. **DeProspo, N. D., Demartino, L. J., and McGuinness, E. T.,** Melatonin's effect on ^{131}I uptake by the thyroid glands in normal and ovariectomized rats, *Life Sci.,* 7, 183, 1968.

370. **DeProspo, N. D. and Hurley, J. A.,** A comparison of intracerebral and intraperitoneal injections of melatonin and its precursors on ^{131}I uptake by the thyroid glands of rats, *Agents Actions,* 2, 14, 1971.

371. **Reiter, R. J., Hoffman, R. A., and Hester, R. J.,** Inhibiton of ^{131}I uptake by thyroid glands of male rats treated with melatonin and pineal extracts, *Am. Zool.,* 5, 727, 1965.

372. **DeProspo, N. D., Safinski, R. J., DeMartino, L. J., and McGuinness, E. T.,** Melatonin and its precursors' effects on ^{131}I uptake by the thyroid gland under different photoconditions, *Life Sci.,* 8, 837, 1969.

373. **Narang, G. D., Singh, D. V., and Turner, C. W.,** Effect of melatonin on thyroid hormone secretion rate and feed consumption of female rats, *Proc. Soc. Exp. Biol. Med.,* 125, 184, 1967.

374. **Singh, D. V. and Turner, D. V.,** Effect of melatonin upon thyroid hormone secretion rate in female hamsters and adult rats, *Acta Endocrinol.,* 69, 35, 1972.

375. **Vriend, J. and Reiter, R. J.,** Free thyroxin index in normal, melatonin-treated and blind hamsters, *Horm. Metab. Res.,* 9, 231, 1977.

376. **Vaughan, G. M., Vaughan, M. K., Seraile, L. G., and Reiter, R. J.,** Thyroid hormones in male hamsters with activated pineals or melatonin treatment, in *The Pineal and Its Hormones,* Reiter, R. J., Ed., Alan R. Liss, New York, 1982, 187.

377. **Vriend, J. and Wasserman, R. A.,** Effects of afternoon injections of melatonin in hypothyroid male Syrian hamsters, *Neuroendocrinology,* 42, 498, 1986.

378. **Vaughan, M. K., Richardson, B. A., Petterborg, L. J., Holtorf, A. P., Vaughan, G. M., Champney, T. H., and Reiter, R. J.,** Effects of injections and/or chronic implants of melatonin and 5-methoxytryptamine on plasma thyroid hormones in male and female Syrian hamsters, *Neuroendocrinology,* 39, 361, 1984.

379. **DeLean, A., Ferland, L., Drouin, J., Kelly, A., and Labrie, F.,** Modulation of pituitary thyrotropin releasing hormone receptor levels by estrogens and thyroid hormones, *Endocrinology,* 100, 1496, 1977.

380. **Gershengorn, M. C.,** Bihormonal regulation of the thyrotropin-releasing hormone receptor in mouse pituitary thyrotropic tumor cells in culture, *J. Clin. Invest.,* 62, 937, 1978.

381. **Perrone, M. H. and Hinkle, P. M.,** Regulation of pituitary receptors for thyrotropin releasing hormone by thyroid hormones, *J. Biol. Chem.,* 253, 5168, 1978.

382. **Hinkle, P. M. and Goh, K. B.,** Regulation of thyrotropin-releasing hormone receptors and responses to L-triiodothyronine in dispersed rat pituitary cell cultures, *Endocrinology,* 110, 1725, 1982.

383. **Tanaka, K., Murakami, M., and Greer, M. A.,** Type-II thyroxine 5'-deiodinase is present in the rat pineal gland, *Biochem. Biophys. Res. Commun.,* 137, 863, 1986.

384. **Tanaka, K., Murakami, M., and Greer, M. A.,** Rhythmicity of triiodothyronine generation by Type II thyroxine 5'-deiodinase in rat pineal is mediated by a β-adrenergic mechanism, *Endocrinology,* 121, 74, 1987.

385. **Murakami, M., Greer, M. A., Hjulstad, S., Greer, S. E., and Tanaka, K.,** The role of the superior cervical ganglia in the nocturnal rise of pineal type-II thyroxine 5'-deiodinase activity, *Brain Res.,* 438, 366, 1988.

386. **Osuna, C., Rubio, A., and Guerrero, J. M.,** Potentiating effect of phenylephrine on isoproterenol activation of thyroxine type II deiodinase in the pineal gland of adult rats, *Experientia,* 49, 329, 1993.

387. **Murakami, M., Greer, M. A., Greer, S. E., Hjulstand, S., and Tanaka, K.,** Comparison of the nocturnal temporal profiles of N-acetyl-transferase and thyroxine 5'-deiodinase in rat pineal, *Neuroendocrinology,* 50, 88, 1989.

388. **Kniazewski, B., Ostrowska, Z., Zwirska-Korczala, K., and Buntner, B.,** The influence of pinealectomy and single dose of melatonin administered at different times of day on serum T3 and T4 concentrations in rats, *Acta Physiol. Pol.,* 41, 117, 1990.

389. **Vriend, J.,** Evidence for pineal gland modulation of the neuroendocrine-thyroid axis, *Neuroendocrinology,* 36, 68, 1983.

390. **Moenter, S. M., Woodfill, C. J., and Karsch, F. J.,** Role of the thyroid gland in seasonal reproduction: thyroidectomy blocks seasonal suppression of reproductive neuroendocrine activity in ewes, *Endocrinology,* 128, 1337, 1991.

391. **Webster, J. R., Moenter, S. M., Barrell, G. K., Lehman, M. N., and Karsch, F. S.,** Role of the thyroid gland in seasonal reproduction. III. Thyroidectomy blocks seasonal suppression of gonadotropin-releasing hormone secretion in sheep, *Endocrinology,* 129, 1635, 1991.

392. **Reiter, R. J., Li, K., Gonzalez-Brito, A., Tannenbaum, M. G., Vaughan, M. K., Vaughan, G. M., and Villanua, M. A.,** Elevated environmental temperature alters the responses of the reproductive and thyroid axes of female hamsters to afternoon melatonin injections, *J. Pineal Res.,* 5, 301, 1988.

393. **Vriend, J.,** Effects of melatonin and thyroxine replacement on thyrotropin, luteinizing hormone, and prolactin in male hypothyroid hamsters, *Endocrinology,* 117, 2402, 1985.

394. **Ziegels, J., Devecerski, V., and Duchesne, P. Y.,** Etude histochimique de la cortico-surrenale du rat apres epiphysectomie, *C. R. Seances Soc. Biol.,* 170, 206, 1976.

395. **Wurtman, R. J., Altschule, M. D., and Holmgren, U.,** Effects of pinealectomy and of bovine extract in rats, *Am. J. Physiol.,* 197, 108, 1959.

396. **Trentini, G. P., Barbanti-Silva, G., Vassanelli, P., and Botticelli, A.,** Modificazioni isoenzimatiche del corticosurrene di ratto conseguenti ad epifisectomia (studio istochimico), *Boll. Soc. Ital. Biol. Sper.,* 41, 967, 1965.

397. **Dickson, K. L. and Hasty, D. L.,** Effects of the pineal gland in unilaterally adrenalectomized rats, *Acta Endocrinol.,* 70, 438, 1972.

398. **Wurtman, R. J., Roth, W., Altschule, M. D., and Wurtman, J. J.,** Interactions of the pineal and exposure to continuous light on organ weights of female rats, *Acta Endocrinol.,* 36, 617, 1961.

399. **Vaughan, M. K., Vaughan, G. M., Reiter, R. J., and Benson, B.,** Effect of melatonin and other pineal indoles on adrenal enlargement produced in male and female mice by pinealectomy, unilateral adrenalectomy, castration and cold stress, *Neuroendocrinology,* 10, 139, 1972.

400. **Ogle, T. F. and Kitay, J. I.,** Effects of pinealectomy on adrenal function in vivo and in vitro in female rats, *Endocrinology,* 98, 20, 1976.

401. **Henzl, M. R., Spaur, C. L., Magoun, R. E., and Kincl, F. A.,** A note on endocrine functions of neonatally pinealectomized rats, *Endocrinol. Exp.,* 4, 77, 1970.

402. **Nir, I., Schmidt, U., Hirschmann, N., and Sulman, F. G.,** The effect of pinealectomy on rat plasma corticosterone levels under various conditions of light, *Life Sci.,* 10, 317, 1971.

403. **Motta, M., Fraschini, F., Piva, F., and Martini, L.,** Hypothalamic and extra-hypothalamic mechanisms controlling adrenocorticotropin secretion, *Mem. Soc. Endocrinol.,* 17, 3, 1968.

404. **Golikov, P. P. and Fominykh, E. S.,** Melatonin action on the rate of aldosterone and corticosterone secretion in intact, pseudoepiphyse- and epiphysectomized rats, *Farmakol. Toksikol. (Moscow),* 37, 696, 1974.

405. **Yamada, K.,** Effects of melatonin on adrenal function in male rats, *Res. Commun. Chem. Pathol. Pharmacol.,* 69, 241, 1990.

406. **Kinson, G. A. and Singer, B.,** Effect of pinealectomy on adreno-cortical hormone secretion in normal rats and in rats with experimental renal hypertension, *J. Endocrinol.,* 37, XXXVII, 1967.

407. **Kinson, G. A., Wahid, A. K., and Singer, B.,** Effect of chronic pinealectomy on adreno-cortical hormone secretion rates in normal and hypertensive rats, *Gen. Comp. Endocrinol.,* 8, 445, 1967.

408. **Laakso, M. L., Porkka-Heiskanen, T., Leinonen, L., Joutsiniemi, S. L., and Mannisto, P. T.,** Hormonal and locomotor activity rhythms in rats under 90-min dark pulse conditions, *Am. J. Physiol.,* 264, R1058, 1993.

409. **Ng, T. B.,** Effects of pineal indoles on corticosterone and aldosterone production by isolated rat adrenal cells, *Biochem. Int.,* 14, 635, 1987.

410. **Vaughan, G. M., Allen, J. P., Vaughan, M. K., and Siler-Khodr, T. M.,** Influence of pinealectomy on corticotropin (ACTH), *Experientia,* 36, 364, 1980.

411. **Yasin, S. A., Costa, A., Besser, G. M., Hucks, D., Grossman, A., and Forsling, M. L.,** Melatonin and its analogs inhibit the basal and stimulated release of hypothalamic vasopressin and oxytocin in vitro, *Endocrinology,* 132, 1329, 1993.

412. **Petrescu, C. and Simionescu, N.,** Experimental studies on the relation between the pineal body and the adrenal medulla in the albino rat, *Stud. Cercet. Endocrinol.,* 21, 339, 1970.

413. **Banerji, T. K. and Quay, W. B.,** Role of the pineal gland in the nocturnal rise in plasma dopamine-hydroxylase activity, *Fed. Proc.,* 35, 691, 1967.

414. **Banerji, T. K. and Quay, W. B.,** Adrenal dopamine-B-hydroxylase activity: 24 hour rhythmicity as evidence for pineal control, *Experientia, 32,* 253, 1976.

415. **Lynch, H. J., Ho, M., and Wurtman, R. J.,** The adrenal medulla may mediate the increase in pineal melatonin synthesis induced by stress, but not that caused by exposure to darkness, *J. Neural Transm.,* 40, 87, 1977.

416. **Lynch, H. J., Eng, J. P., and Wurtman, R. J.,** Control of pineal indole biosynthesis by changes in sympathetic tone caused by factors other than environmental lighting, *Proc. Natl. Acad. Sci. U.S.A.,* 70, 1705, 1973.

417. **Enero, M. A., Langer, S. Z., Rothlin, R. P., and Stefano, F. J. E.,** Role of the α-adrenoceptor in regulating noradrenaline overflow by nerve stimulation, *Br. J. Pharmacol.,* 44, 672, 1972.

418. **Monteleone, P., Maj, M., Fusco, M., Orazzo, C., and Kemali, D.,** Physical exercise at night blunts the nocturnal increase of plasma melatonin in healthy subjects, *Life Sci.,* 47, 1989, 1990.

419. **Monteleone, P., Maj, M., Franza, M., Fusco, R., and Kemali, D.,** The human pineal gland responds to stress-induced sympathetic activation in the second half of the dark phase, *J. Neural Transm.,* 92, 25, 1993.

420. **Skrinar, G. J., Bullen, B. A., Reppert, S. M., Peachey, S. E., Turnbull, B. A., and McArthur, J. W.,** Melatonin response to exercise training in women, *J. Pineal Res.,* 7, 185, 1989.

421. **Relkin, R.,** Effects of pinealectomy, constant light and darkness on growth hormone in the pituitary and plasma of the rat, *J. Endocrinol.,* 53, 289, 1972.

422. **Sorrentino, S., Reiter, R. J., and Schalch, D. S.,** Pineal regulation of growth hormone synthesis and release in blinded and blinded-anosmic male rats, *Neuroendocrinology,* 7, 210, 1971.

423. **Sorrentino, S., Reiter, R. J., Schalch, D. S., and Donofrio, R. J.,** Role of the pineal gland in growth restraint of adult male rats by light and smell deprivation, *Neuroendocrinology,* 8, 116, 1971.

424. **Reiter, R. J., Vaughan, M. K., Vaughan, G. M., Sorrentino, S., and Donofrio, R. J.,** The pineal gland as an organ of internal secretion, in *Frontiers of Pineal Physiology,* Altschule, M. D., Ed., MIT Press, Cambridge, MA, 1975, 54.

425. **Ronnelkeiv, O. K. and McCann, S. M.,** Growth hormone release in conscious pinealectomized and sham-operated male rats, *Endocrinology,* 102, 1964, 1978.

426. **Klemcke, H. G., Bartke, A., and Borer, K. T.,** Testicular prolactin receptors and serum growth hormone in golden hamsters: effects of photoperiod and time of day, *Biol. Reprod.,* 29, 605, 1983.

427. **Borer, K. T., Kelch, R. P., and Hayashida, T.,** Hamster growth hormone—species specificity and physiological changes in blood and pituitary, *Neuroendocrinology,* 35, 349, 1982.

428. **Vriend, J., Sheppard, M. S., and Bala, R. M.,** Melatonin increases serum insulin-like growth factor-I in male Syrian hamsters, *Endocrinology,* 122, 2558, 1988.

429. **Vriend, J., Sheppard, M. S., and Borer, K. T.,** Melatonin increases serum growth hormone and insulin-like growth factor I (IGF-I) levels in male Syrian hamsters via hypothalamic neurotransmitters, *Growth Dev. Age.,* 54, 165, 1990.

430. **Vriend, J., Borer, K. T., and Thliveris, J. A.,** Melatonin: its antagonism of thyroxine's antisomatotrophic activity in male Syrian hamsters, *Growth,* 51, 35, 1987.

431. **Cramer, V. H., Bohme, W., Kendel, K., and Donnadieu, M.,** Freisetzung von wachstumshormon und von melanozyten stimulierendem hormon im durch melatonin gebahnten schalf bein menschen, *Arzneim. Forsch.,* 26, 1076, 1976.

432. **Valcavi, R., Zini, M., Maestroni, G. J., Conti, A., and Portioli, I.,** Melatonin stimulates growth hormone through pathways other than the growth hormone releasing hormone, *Clin. Endocrinol. (Oxford),* 39, 193, 1993.

433. **Ralph, C. L., Firth, B. T., Gern, W. A., and Owens, D. W.,** The pineal complex and thermoregulation, *Biol. Rev.,* 54, 41, 1979.

434. **Binkley, S. A.,** Pineal and melatonin: circadian rhythms and body temperature of sparrows, in *Chronobiology,* Scheving, L. E., Halberg, F., and Pauly, J. E., Eds., Igaku Shoin, Tokyo, 1974, 582.

435. **Hagelstein, K. A. and Folk, C. E.,** Effects of photoperiod, cold acclimation and melatonin on the white rat, *Comp. Biochem. Physiol.,* 62C, 225, 1979.

436. **Fitzgerald, J., Michel, F., and Butler, W. R.,** Growth and sexual maturation in ewes: the role of photoperiod, diet and temperature on growth rate and the control of prolactin, thyroxine and luteinizing hormone secretion, *J. Anim. Sci.,* 55, 1431, 1982.

437. **Sod-Moriah, U. A., Magal, E., Kaplanski, J., Hirschman, N., and Nir, I.,** The role of the pineal gland in thermoregulation in male hamsters, *Comp. Biochem. Physiol.,* 74A, 649, 1983.

438. **Kastin, A. J., Redding, T. W., and Schally, A. V.,** MSH activity in rat pituitaries after pinealectomy, *Proc. Soc. Exp. Biol. Med.,* 124, 1275, 1967.

439. **Rickards, D. A.,** The therapeutic effect of melatonin on canine melanosis, *J. Invest. Dermatol.,* 44, 13, 1965.

440. **Benson, B., Miller, C. W., and Sorrentino, S.,** Effects of blinding on blood glucose and serum insulin-like activity in rats, *Tex. Rep. Biol. Med.,* 29, 513, 1971.

441. **Csaba, G. and Barath, P.,** Are Langerhans' islets influenced by the pineal body?, *Experientia, 27,* 962, 1971.

442. **Milcou, S. M., Nanu-Ionescu, L., and Milcou, I.,** The effect of pinealectomy on plasma insulin in rats, in *The Pineal Gland,* Wolstenholme, G. E. W. and Knight, J., Eds., Churchill Livingstone, London, 1971, 345.

443. **Mori, N., Aoyama, H., Murase, T., and Mori, W.,** Anti-hypercholesterolemic effect of melatonin in rats, *Acta Pathol. Jpn.,* 39, 613, 1989.

444. **Chuang, J. I., Chen, S. S., and Lin, M. T.,** Melatonin decreases brain serotonin release, arterial pressure and heart rate in rats, *Pharmacology,* 47, 91, 1993.

445. **Benson, B., Matthews, M. J., and Rodin, A. E.,** A melatonin-free extract of bovine pineal with antigonadotrophic activity, *Life Sci.,* 10, 607, 1971.

446. **Damian, E., Ianas, O., Badescu, I., and Oprescu, M.,** Anti-LH and FSH activity of melatonin-free pineal extract, *Neuroendocrinology,* 26, 325, 1978.

447. **Pavel, S. and Petrescu, S.,** Inhibition of gonadotrophin by a highly purified pineal peptide and by synthetic arginine vasotocin, *Nature (London),* 212, 1054, 1966.

448. **Pang, S. F. and Ralph, C. L.,** Mode of secretion of pineal melatonin in the chicken, *Gen. Comp. Endocrinol.,* 27, 125, 1975.

449. **Rollag, M. D., Morgan, R. J., and Niswender, G. D.,** Route of melatonin secretion in sheep, *Biomed. Sci. Instrum.,* 13, 111, 1977.

450. **Anton-Tay, F. and Wurtman, R. J.,** Regional uptake of ^{3}H-melatonin from blood or cerebrospinal fluid by rat brain, *Nature (London),* 221, 474, 1965.

451. **Reiter, R. J., Dinh, D. T., De Los Santos, R., and Guerra, J. C.,** Hypothalamic cuts suggest a brain site for the antigonadotrophic actions of melatonin in the Syrian hamster, *Neurosci. Lett.,* 23, 315, 1981.

452. **Glass, J. D. and Lynch, G. R.,** Melatonin: identification of sites of antigonadal action in mouse brain, *Science,* 214, 821, 1981.

453. **Cardinali, D. P., Vacas, M. I., and Boyer, E. E.,** Specific binding of melatonin in bovine brain, *Endocrinology,* 105, 437, 1979.

454. **Niles, L. P., Wong, Y. W., Mishra, R. K., and Brown, G. M.,** Melatonin receptors in brain, *Eur. J. Pharmacol.,* 55, 219, 1979.

455. **Vakkuri, O., Lamsa, E., Rahkamaa, E., Ruotsalainen, H., and Leppaluoto, J.,** Iodinated melatonin: preparation and characterization of molecular structure by mass or ^{1}H NMR spectroscopy, *Anal. Biochem.,* 142, 284, 1984.

456. **Sugden, D.,** Effect of putative melatonin receptor antagonists on melatonin-induced pigment aggregation in isolated Xenopus laevis melanophores, *Eur. J. Pharmacol.,* 213, 405, 1992.

457. **Stankov, B., Fraschini, F., and Reiter, R. J.,** Melatonin binding sites in the central nervous system of mammals, *Brain Res. Rev.,* 16, 245, 1991.

458. **Krause, D. N. and Dubocovich, M. L.,** Regulatory sites in the melatonin system of mammals, *Trends Neurosci.,* 13, 464, 1990.

459. **Vanecek, J. and Jansky, L.,** Short days induce changes in specific melatonin binding in hamster median eminence and anterior pituitary, *Brain Res.,* 477, 387, 1989.

460. **Reppert, S. M., Weaver, D. R., Rivkees, S. A., and Stopa, E. G.,** Putative melatonin receptors in human biological clock, *Science,* 242, 78, 1988.

461. **Williams, L. M., Morgan, P. J., Hastings, M. H., Lawson, W., Davidson, G., and Howell, H. E.,** Melatonin receptor sites in the Syrian hamster brain and pituitary: localization and characterization using [^{125}I]iodomelatonin, *J. Neuroendocrinol.,* 1, 315, 1989.

462. **Duncan, M. J., Takahashi, J. S., and Dubocovich, M. L.,** Characteristics and autoradiographic localization of 2-^{125}I-iodomelatonin binding sites in Djungarian hamster brain, *Endocrinology,* 125, 1011, 1989.

463. **Weaver, D. R., Rivkees, S. A., and Reppert, S. M.,** Localization and characteristics of melatonin receptors in rodent brain by in vitro autoradiography, *J. Neurosci.,* 9, 2581, 1989.

464. **Vanecek, J., Pavlik, A., and Illnerova, H.,** Hypothalamic melatonin receptor sites revealed by autoradiography, *Brain Res.,* 435, 359, 1987.

465. **Morgan, P. J., Barrett, P., Davidson, G., and Lawson, W.,** Melatonin regulates the synthesis and secretion of several proteins by pars tuberalis cells of the ovine pituitary, *J. Neuroendocrinol.,* 4, 557, 1992.

466. **Morgan, P. J., Barrett, P., Howell, H. E., and Helliwell, R.,** Melatonin receptors: localization, molecular pharmacology and physiological significance, *Neurochem. Int.,* 24, 101, 1994.

467. **Arendt, J.,** Melatonin. A review, *Clin. Endocrinol.,* 29, 205, 1988.

468. **Cassone, V. M.,** Effects of melatonin on vertebrate circadian systems, *Trends Neurosci.,* 149, 457, 1990.

469. **Yu, H. S., Yuan, H., Lu, Y., and Pang, S. F.,** [^{125}I]-iodomelatonin binding sites in spleens of birds and mammals, *Life Sci.,* 125, 175, 1991.

470. **Martin-Cacao, A., Lopez-Gonzalez, M. A., Reiter, R. J., Calvo, J. R., and Guerrero, J. M.,** Binding of 2-[125] melatonin by rat thymus membranes during postnatal development, *Immunol. Lett.,* 36, 59, 1993.

471. **Song, Y., Poon, A. M., Lee, P. P., and Pang, S. F.,** Putative melatonin receptors in the male guinea pig kidney, *J. Pineal Res.,* 15, 153, 1993.

472. **Acuna-Castroviejo, D., Pablos, M. I., Menendez-Pelaez, A., and Reiter, R. J.,** Melatonin receptors in purified cell nuclei of liver, *Res. Commun. Chem. Pathol. Pharmacol.,* 82, 253, 1993.

473. **Van-Vuuren, R. J., Pitout, M. J., Van-Aswegen, C. H., and Theron, J. J.,** Putative melatonin receptors in human spermatozoa, *Clin. Biochem.,* 25, 125, 1992.

474. **Wiechmann, A. F. and Wirsig-Wiechmann, C. R.,** Distribution of melatonin receptors in the brain of the frog *Rana pipiens* as revealed by in vitro autoradiography, *Neuroscience,* 52, 469, 1993.

475. **Wiechmann, A. F. and Wirsig-Wiechmann, C. R.,** Melatonin receptor distribution in the brain and retina of a lizard, *Brain Behav. Evol.,* 43, 25, 1994.

476. **Brooks, D. S. and Cassone, V. M.,** Daily and circadian regulation of 2-[I-125]iodomelatonin binding in the chick brain, *Endocrinology,* 131, 1297, 1992.

477. **Martinoli, M. G., Williams, L. M., Kah, O., Titchener, L. T., and Pelletier, G.,** Distribution of central melatonin binding sites in the goldfish (*Carassius auratus*). *Mol. Cell. Neurosci.,* 2, 78, 1991.

478. **Laitinen, J. T. and Saavedra, J. M.,** The chick retinal melatonin receptor revisited: localization and modulation of agonist binding with guanine nucleotides, *Brain Res.,* 528, 349, 1990.

479. **Blazynski, C. and Dubocovich, M. L.,** Localization of 2-[125]iodomelatonin binding sites in mammalian retina, *J. Neurochem.,* 56, 1873, 1991.

480. **Dubocovich, M. L.,** Melatonin receptors in the central nervous system, *Adv. Exp. Med. Biol.,* 294, 255, 1991.

481. **Sugden, D.,** Melatonin: binding site characteristics and biochemical and cellular responses, *Neurochem. Int.,* 24, 147, 1994.

482. **Kennaway, D. J. and Hugel, H. M.,** Melatonin binding sites: are they receptors?, *Mol. Cell. Endocrinol.,* 88, C1, 1992.

483. **Menendez-Pelaez, A., Poeggeler, B., Reiter, R. J., Barlow-Walden, L., Pablos, M. I., and Tan, D.,** Nuclear localization of melatonin in different mammalian tissues: immunocytochemical and radioimmunoassay evidence, *J. Cell Biochem.,* 53, 373, 1993.

484. **Benitez-King, G., Huerto-Delgadilo, L., and Anton-Tay, F.,** Binding of ³H-melatonin to calmodulin, *Life Sci.,* 53, 201, 1993.

485. **Vanecek, J. and Vollrath, L.,** Developmental changes and daily rhythm in melatonin-induced inhibition of 3′,5′-cyclic AMP accumulation in the rat pituitary, *Endocrinology,* 126, 1509, 1990.

486. **Niles, L. P. and Hashemi, F.,** Picomolar-affinity binding and inhibition of adenylate cylase activity by melatonin in Syrian hamster hypothalamus, *Cell. Mol. Neurobiol.,* 10, 553, 1990.

487. **Daniolos, A., Lerner, A. B., and Lerner, M. R.,** Action of light on frog pigment cells in culture, *Pigment Cell Res.,* 3, 38, 1990.

488. **Carlson, L. L., Weaver, D. R., and Reppert, S. M.,** Melatonin signal transduction in hamster brain: inhibition of adenylyl cyclase by a pertussis toxin-sensitive G protein, *Endocrinology,* 125, 2670, 1989.

489. **Weaver, D. R., Carlson, L. L., and Reppert, S. M.,** Melatonin receptors and signal transduction in melatonin-sensitive and melatonin-insensitive populations of white-footed mice (*Peromyscus leucopus*), *Brain Res.,* 506, 353, 1990.

490. **Morgan, P. J., Lawson, W., Davidson, G., and Howell, H. E.,** Melatonin inhibits cyclic AMP production in cultured ovine pars tuberalis cells, *J. Mol. Endocrinol.,* 3, R5, 1989.

491. **Anton-Tay, F., Chou, C., Anton, S., and Wurtman, R. J.,** Brain serotonin concentration: elevation following intraperitoneal administration of melatonin, *Science,* 162, 177, 1968.

492. **Dahlstrom, A. and Fuxe, K.,** Evidence for the existence of monoamine containing neurons in the central nervous system, *Acta Physiol. Scand. Suppl.,* 232, 3, 1964.

493. **Ruzsas, C., DeGaetani, C., Criscuolo, M., Mess, B., and Trentini, G. P.,** Possible role of the midbrain seortonergic raphe nuclei in the regulation of ovulation exerted by melatonin in the rat, *Neuroendocrinol. Lett.,* 3, 331, 1981.

494. **Walker, R. F. and Wilson, C. A.,** Changes in hypothalamic serotonin associated with amplification of LH surges by progesterone in rats, *Neuroendocrinology,* 37, 200, 1983.

495. **Fuller, R. W.,** Serotonergic stimulation of pituitary-adrenocortical function in rats, *Neuroendocrinology,* 32, 118, 1981.

496. **Fuller, R. W.,** Role of serotonin in the hypothalamic regulation of pituitary function, *Adv. Exp. Biol. Med.,* 133, 431, 1981.

497. **Ferrari, C., Paracchi, A., Rondena, M., Beck-Peccoz, P., and Faglia, G.,** Effect of two serotonin antagonists on prolactin and thyrotropin in man, *Clin. Endocrinol.,* 5, 575, 1976.

498. **Egge, A. C., Rogol., A. D., Varma, M. M., and Blizzard, R. M.,** Effect of cyproheptadine on stimulated prolactin and TSH release in man, *J. Clin. Endocrinol. Metab.,* 44, 210, 1977.

499. **Vriend, J.,** Melatonin increases the ratio of 5-hydroxyindoleacetic acid to serotonin in the hypothalamus and brainstem concurrently with gonadal involution in male Syrian hamsters, *Can. J. Zool.,* 69, 1004, 1991.

500. **Vriend, J.,** Endocrine effects of blinding in male Syrian hamsters are associated with increased hypothalamic 5-hydroxyindoleacetic acid/serotonin ratios, *J. Pineal Res.,* 7, 401, 1989.

501. **Steger, R. W., Dennis, C., VanAbbema, A., and Gay-Primel, E.,** Alterations in hypothalamic serotonin metabolism in male hamsters with photoperiod-induced testicular regression, *Brain Res.,* 514, 11, 1990.

502. **Alexiuk, N. A. M. and Vriend, J. P.,** Extrahypothalamic effects of melatonin administration on serotonin and norepinephrine synthesis in female Syrian hamsters, *J. Neural Transm.,* 94, 43, 1993.

503. **Alexiuk, N. A. and Vriend, J.,** Effects of daily afternoon melatonin administration on monoamine accumulation in median eminence and striatum of ovariectomized hamsters receiving pargyline, *Neuroendocrinology,* 54, 55, 1991.

504. **Alexiuk, N. A. M. and Vriend, J. P.,** Melatonin reduces dopamine content in the neurointermediate lobe of male Syrian hamsters, *Brain Res. Bull.,* 32, 433, 1993.

505. **Steger, R. W., Bartke, A. and Goldman, B. D.,** Alterations in neuroendocrine function during photoperiod-induced testicular atrophy and recrudescence in the golden hamster, *Biol. Reprod.,* 26, 437, 1982.

506. **Steger, R. W., Bartke, A., Matt, K. S., Soares, M. J., and Talamantes, F.,** Neuroendocrine changes in male hamsters following photostimulation, *J. Exp. Zool.,* 229, 467, 1984.

507. **Steger, R. W., Matt, K. S., Klemcke, H. G., and Bartke, A.,** Interactions of photoperiod and ectopic pituitary grafts on hypothalamic and pituitary function in male hamsters, *Neuroendocrinology,* 41, 89, 1985.

508. **Benson, B.,** Temporal changes in medial basal hypothalamic catecholamines in male Syrian hamsters exposed to short photoperiod, *Exp. Brain Res.,* 65, 371, 1987.

509. **Steger, R. W. and Bartke, A.,** Temporal sequence of neuroendocrine events associated with the transfer of male golden hamsters from a stimulatory to a nonstimulatory photoperiod, *Biol. Reprod.,* 44, 76, 1991.

510. **Fang, J. M. and Dubocovich, M. L.,** Activation of melatonin receptor sites retarded the depletion of norepinephrine following inhibition of synthesis in the C3H/HeN mouse hypothalamus, *J. Neurochem.,* 55, 76, 1990.

511. **Anton-Tay, F.,** Pineal-brain relationships, in *The Pineal Gland,* Wolstenholme, G. E. W. and Knight, J., Eds., Churchill Livingstone, London, 1971, 213.

512. **Anton-Tay, F.,** Melatonin: effects on brain function, *Adv. Biochem. Psychopharmacol.,* 11, 315, 1974.

513. **Rosenstein, R. E. and Cardinali, D. P.,** Melatonin increases in vivo GABA accumulation in rat hypothalamus, cerebellum, cerebral cortex and pineal gland, *Brain Res.,* 398, 403, 1986.

514. **Rosenstein, R. E., Estevez, A. G., and Cardinali, D. P.,** Time-dependent effects of melatonin on glutamic acid decarboxylase and $^{36}Cl-$ ion influx in rat hypothalamus, *J. Neuroendocrinol.,* 1, 443, 1989.

515. **Rosenstein, R. E. and Cardinali, D. P.,** Central GABAergic mechanisms as targets for melatonin activity in brain, *Neurochem. Int.,* 17, 373, 1990.

516. **Coloma, F. M. and Niles, L. P.,** Melatonin enhancement of [^{3}]-gamma-aminobutyric acid and [^{3}]muscimol binding in rat brain, *Biochem. Pharmacol.,* 37, 1271, 1988.

517. **Niles, L. P., Pickering, D. S., and Arciszewski, M. A.,** Effects of chronic melatonin administration on GABA and diazepam binding in rat brain, *J. Neural Transm.,* 70, 117, 1987.

518. **Reiter, R. J.,** Melatonin: the chemical expression of darkness, *Mol. Cell. Endocrinol.,* 79, C153, 1991.

519. **Rusak, B. and Morin, L. P.,** Testicular responses to photoperiod are blocked by lesions of the suprachiasmatic nuclei in golden hamsters, *Biol. Reprod.,* 15, 1366, 1976.

520. **Stetson, M. H. and Watson-Whitmyre, M.,** Nucleus suprachiasmaticus: the biological clock in the hamster?, *Science,* 191, 197, 1976.

521. **Rusak, B.,** Suprachiasmatic lesions prevent an antigonadal effect of melatonin, *Biol. Reprod.,* 22, 148, 1980.

522. **Stetson, M. H. and Gibson, J. T.,** The estrous cycle in golden hamsters: a circadian pacemaker times preovulatory gonadotropin release, *J. Exp. Zool.,* 201, 289, 1977.

523. **Gallo, R. V.,** Pulsatile LH release during the ovulatory LH surge on proestrus in the rat, *Biol. Reprod.,* 24, 100, 1981.

524. **Levine, J. E. and Ramirez, V. D.,** Luteinizing hormone-releasing hormone release during the rat estrous cycle and after ovariectomy, as estimated with push-pull cannulae, *Endocrinology,* 111, 1439, 1982.

525. **Vriend, J.,** Influence of pineal gland and circadian rhythms in circulating levels of thyroid hormones in hamsters, *J. Pineal Res.,* 1, 15, 1984.

526. **Takahashi, J. S. and Menaker, M.,** Entrainment of the circadian system of the house sparrow: a population of oscillators in pinealectomized birds, *J. Comp. Physiol.,* 146, 245, 1982.

527. **Underwood, H.,** Circadian organization in the lizard *Sceloporus occidentalis*: the effects of pinealectomy, blinding, and melatonin, *J. Comp. Physiol., Pt. B,* 141, 537, 1981.

528. **Armstrong, S. M., Cassone, V. M., Chesworth, M. J., Redman, J., and Short, R. V.,** Synchronization of mammalian circadian rhythms by melatonin, *J. Neural Transm.,* S21, 373, 1986.

529. **Puchalski, W. and Lynch, G. R.,** Daily melatonin injections affect the expression of circadian rhythmicity in Djungarian hamsters kept under a long-day photoperiod, *Neuroendocrinology,* 48, 280, 1988.

530. **Cassone, V. M., Chesworth, M. J., and Armstrong, S. M.,** Dose dependent entrainment of rat circadian rhythm by daily injection of melatonin, *J. Biol. Rhythms,* 1, 219, 1986.

531. **Dahlitz, M., Alvarez, B., Vignau, J., English, J., Arendt, J., and Parkes, J. D.,** Delayed sleep phase syndrome response to melatonin, *Lancet,* 337, 1121, 1991.

532. **Wurtman, R. J. and Lieberman, H. S.,** Melatonin secretion as a mediator of circadian variations in sleep and sleepiness, *J. Pineal Res.,* 1, 301, 1985.

533. **Cassone, V. M.,** Effects of melatonin on vertebrate circadian systems, *Trends Neurosci.,* 149, 457, 1990.

534. **Niles, L. P., Pickering, D. S., and Arciszewski, M. A.,** Effects of chronic melatonin administration on GABA and diazepam binding in rat brain, *J. Neural Transm.,* 70, 117, 1987.

535. **Sugden, D.,** Psychopharmacological effects of melatonin in rat and mouse, *J. Pharmacol. Exp. Ther.,* 227, 587, 1983.

536. **Holmes, S. W. and Sugden, D.,** Effects of melatonin on sleep and neurochemistry in the rat, *Br. J. Pharmacol.,* 76, 95, 1982.

537. **Lieberman, H. R., Waldhauser, F., and Garfield, G.,** Effects of melatonin on human mood and performance, *Brain Res.,* 323, 201, 1984.

538. **MacFarlane, J. G., Cleghorn, J. M., Brown, G. M., and Streiner, D. L.,** The effects of exogenous melatonin on the total sleep time and daytime alertness of chronic insomniacs, *Biol. Psychiatry,* 30, 371, 1991.

539. **Guardiola Lemaitre, B., Lenegre, A., and Porsolt, R. D.,** Combined effects of diazepam and melatonin in two tests for anxiolytic activity in the mouse, *Pharmacol. Biochem. Behav.,* 41, 405, 1992.

540. **Golombek, D. A., Martini, M., and Cardinali, D. P.,** Melatonin as an anxiolytic in rats: time dependence and interaction with the central GABAergic system, *Eur. J. Pharmacol.,* 234, 231, 1993.

541. **Lewy, A., Singer, C., and Gabourey, C.,** Evidence for a phase advance reponse curve and a clock-gate model for the regulation of the timing of the human melatonin production, *J. Steroid Biochem.,* 20, 1457, 1984.

542. **Marczynski, T. J., Yamaguchi, N., Ling, G. M., and Grodzinska, L.,** Sleep induced by the administration of melatonin (5-methoxy-N-acetyltryptamine) to the hypothalamus in unrestrained cats, *Experientia,* 20, 435, 1964.

543. **Cramer, H., Rudolph, J., Consbruch, V., and Kendel, K.,** On the effects of melatonin on sleep and behavior in man, *Adv. Biochem. Psychopharmacol.,* 11, 187, 1974.

544. **Petterborg, L. J., Thalen, B. E., Kjellman, B. F., and Wetterberg, L.,** Effect of melatonin replacement on serum hormone rhythms in a patient lacking endogenous melatonin, *Brain Res. Bull.,* 27, 181, 1991.

545. **Folkard, S., Arendt, J., Aldous, M., and Kennett, H.,** Melatonin stabilizes sleep onset time in a blind man without entrainment of cortisol or temperature rhythms, *Neurosci. Lett.,* 113, 193, 1990.

546. **Claustrat, B., Brun, J., David, M., Sassolas, G., and Chazot, G.,** Melatonin and jet-lag: confirmatory result using a simplified protocol, *Biol. Psychiatry,* 32, 705, 1992.

547. **Petri, K., Dawson, A. G., Thompson, L., and Brook, R.,** A double blind trial of melatonin as a treatment for jet lag in international cabin crew, *Biol. Psychiatry,* 33, 526, 1993.

548. **Czeisler, C. A., Kronauer, R. E., and Mooney, J. J.,** Biologic rhythm disorders, depression and phototherapy: a new hypothesis, *Psychiatr. Clin. North Am.,* 10, 687, 1987.

549. **Lino, A., Siluy, S., Condorelli, L., and Rusconi, A. C.,** Melatonin and jet-lag: treatment schedule, *Biol. Psychiatry,* 34, 587, 1993.

550. **Samuel, A., Wegmann, H. M., Vejvoda, M., Maass, H., Gundel, A., and Schulz, M.,** Influence of melatonin treatment on human circadian rhythmicity before and after a simulated 9-hr time shift, *J. Biol. Rhythms,* 6, 235, 1991.

551. **Iguchi, H., Kato, K.-I., and Ibayashi, H.,** Age-dependent reduction in serum melatonin concentrations in healthy human subjects, *J. Clin. Endocrinol. Metab.,* 55, 27, 1982.

552. **Monteleone, P., Maj, M., Fuscu, M., Kemali, D., and Reiter, R. J.,** Depressed nocturnal plasma melatonin levels in drug-free paranoid schizophrenics, *Schizophrenia Res.,* 7, 77, 1992.

553. **Claustrat, B., Chazot, G., Brun, J., Jordan, D., and Sassolas, G.,** A chronobiological study of melatonin and cortisol secretion in depressed subjects: plasma melatonin, a biochemical marker of major depression, *Biol. Psychiatry,* 19, 1215, 1984.

554. **Wetterberg, L., Beck-Friis, J., and Kjellman, B. F.,** Melatonin as a marker of a subgroup of depression in adults, in *Biological Rhythms, Mood Disorders, Light Therapy, and the Pineal Gland,* Shafii, M. and Shafii, S. L., Eds., American Psychiatric Press, Washington, D.C., 1990, 69.

555. **Berga, S. L., Mortola, J. F., and Yen, S. S. C.,** Amplification of nocturnal melatonin secretion in women with functional hypothalamic amenorrhea, *J. Clin. Endocrinol.,* 68, 242, 1988.

556. **Brzezinski, A., Lynch, H. J., Seibel, M. M., Deng, M. H., Nader, T. M., and Wurtman, R. J.,** The circadian rhythm of plasma melatonin during the normal menstrual cycle and in amenorrheic women, *J. Clin. Endocrinol.,* 66, 891, 1988.

557. **Brambilla, F., Fraschini, F., Esposti, G., Bossolo, P. A., Marelli, G., and Ferrari, E.,** Melatonin circadian rhythm in anorexia nervosa and obesity, *Psychiatry Res.,* 23, 267, 1988.

558. **Tortosa, F., Puig-Domingo, M., Peinado, M. A., Oriola, J., Webb, S. M., and DeLieva, A.,** Enhanced circadian rhythm of melatonin in anorexia nervosa, *Acta Endocrinol.,* 120, 574, 1989.

559. **Manz, B., Alexander, H., Wagner, B., and Pollow, K.,** 24 hr pattern of serum melatonin in patients with anorexia nervosa determined by a novel ^{125}I-radioimmunoassay without extraction, in *Neuroendocrinology: New Frontiers,* Gupta, D., Wollmann, H. A., and Ranke, M. B., Eds., Brain Research Promotion, Tubingen, Germany, 1990, 255.

560. **Wirz-Justice, A., and Arendt, J.,** Diurnal menstrual cycle and seasonal indole rhythms in man and their modification in affective disorders, in *Biological Psychiatry Today,* Obiols, J., Ballus, C., and Gonzales Monclus, E., Eds., Elsevier/North-Holland, Amsterdam, 1979, 294.

561. **Puig-Domingo, M., Webb, S. M., Serrano, J., Peinado, M., Corcoy, R., Ruscalleda, J., Reiter, R. J., and DeLeiva, A.,** Brief report melatonin-related hypogonadotropic hypogonadism, *N. Engl. J. Med.,* 327, 1356, 1992.

562. **Lewy, A. J., Wehr, T. A., and Gold, P. W.,** Plasma melatonin in manic depressive illness, in *Catecholamines: Basic and Clinical Frontiers, Vol. 2,* Usdin, E., Kopin, I. J., and Barchas, J., Eds., Pergamon Press, New York, 1979, 1173.

563. **Rosenthal, N. E., Sack, D. A., Gillin, J. C., Lewy, A. J., Goodwin, F. K., Davenport, Y., Mueller, P. S., Newsome, D. A., and Wehr, T. A.,** Seasonal affective disorder, *Arch. Gen. Psychiatry,* 43. 870, 1986.

564. **Wehr, T. A.,** Seasonal vulnerability to depression implications for etiology and treatment, *Encephale,* 18, 479, 1992.

565. **Rosenthal, N. E., Sack, D. A., and Carpenter, C. D.,** Antidepressant effects of light in seasonal affective disorder, *Am. J. Psychiatry,* 142, 163, 1985.

566. **Terman, M., Terman, J. S., and Quitkin, F. M.,** Light therapy for seasonal affective disorder, *Neuropsychopharmacology,* 2, 1, 1989.

567. **Reiter, R. J. and Morgan, W. W.,** Attempts to characterize the convulsive response of parathyroidectomized rats to pineal gland removal, *Physiol. Behav.,* 9, 203, 1972.

568. **Reiter, R. J., Blask, D. E., Talbot, J. A., and Barnett, M. P.,** Nature and time course of seizures associated with surgical removal of the pineal gland from parathyroidectomized rats, *Exp. Neurol.,* 38, 386, 1973.

569. **Philo, R. and Reiter, R. J.,** Characterization of pinealectomy induced convulsions in the Mongolian gerbil, *Epilepsia,* 19, 485, 1978.

570. **Albertson, T. E., Peterson, S. L., Stark, L. G., Lakin, M., and Winters, W. D.,** The anticonvulsant properties of melatonin on kindled seizures in rats, *Neuropharmacology,* 20, 61, 1981.

571. **Brailowsky, S.,** Effects of melatonin on the photosensitive epilepsy of the baboons, *Papio papio, Electroencephalogr. Clin. Neurophysiol.,* 41, 314, 1976.

572. **Izumi, K. J., Donaldson, J., Minnich, J., and Barbeau, A.,** Oubain-induced seizures in rats: modification by melatonin and melanocyte-stimulating hormone, *Can. J. Physiol. Pharmacol.,* 51, 572, 1973.

573. **Golombek, D. A., Duque, D. F., DeBritoSanchez, M., Burin, L., and Cardinali, D. P.,** Time-dependent anticonvulsant activity of melatonin in hamsters, *Eur. J. Pharmacol.,* 210, 253, 1992.

574. **Champney, T. H. and Champney, J. C.,** Novel anticonvulsant action of chronic melatonin in gerbils, *NeuroReport,* 3, 1152, 1992.

575. **Herrera, H. H., Morgan, W. W., and Reiter, R. J.,** Brain norepinephrine levels in parathyroidectomized rats induced to convulse by pinealectomy, *Exp. Neurol.,* 48, 595, 1975.

576. **Philo, R. and Reiter, R. J.,** Brain amines and convulsions in four strains of parathyroidectomized, pinealectomized rats, *Epilepsia,* 19, 485, 1978.

577. **Jankovic, B. D., Isakovic, K., and Petrovic, S.,** Effect of pinealectomy on immune reactions in the rat, *Immunology,* 18, 1, 1970.

578. **Maestroni, G. J. M. and Conti, A.,** Action of melatonin on immune system, in *Role of Melatonin and Pineal Peptides in Neuroimmunomodulation,* Fraschini, F. and Reiter, R. J., Eds., Plenum Press, New York, 1991, 201.

579. **Maestroni, G. S. and Conti, A.,** The pineal neurohormone melatonin stimulates activated CD4+, Th-1+ cells to release opioid agonist(s) with immunoenhancing and anti-stress properties, *J. Neuroimmunol.,* 28, 167, 1990.

580. **Maestroni, G. J. M. and Conti, A.,** Role of the pineal gland in immunity. III. Melatonin antagonizes the immunosuppressive effect of acute stress via an opiatergic mechanism, *Immunology,* 63, 465, 1988.

581. **Lissoni, P., Barnes, S., Tancini, G., Rovelli, F., Ardizzoia, A., Conti, A., and Maestroni, G. J.,** A study of the mechanisms involved in the immunostimulatory action of the pineal hormone in cancer patients, *Oncology,* 50, 399, 1993.

582. **Giordano, M., Vermeulen, M., and Palmero, M. S.,** Seasonal variations in antibody-dependent cellular cytotoxicity regulation by melatonin, *FASEB J.,* 7, 1052, 1993.

583. **Yu, Z. H., Yuan, H., Lu, Y., and Pang, S. F.,** ^{125}Iodomelatonin binding sites in the spleens of birds and mammals, *Neurosci. Lett.,* 125, 175, 1991.

584. **Lissoni, P., Barni, S., Tancini, G., Ardizzoia, A., Ricci, G., Aldeghi, R., Brivio, F., Tisi, E., Rovelli, F., and Rescaldani, R.,** A randomised study with subcutaneous low-dose interleukin-2 alone vs interleukin plus the pineal neurohormone melatonin in advanced solid neoplasms other than renal cancer and melanoma, *Br. J. Cancer,* 69, 196, 1994.

585. **Hill, S. M., Spriggs, L. L., Simon, M. A., Muraoka, H., and Blask, D. E.,** The growth inhibitory action of melatonin on human breast cancer cells is linked to the estrogen response system, *Cancer Lett.,* 64, 249, 1992.

586. **Reiter, R. J.,** Interactions of the pineal hormone melatonin with oxygen-centered free radicals: a brief review, *Braz. J. Med. Biol. Res.,* 26, 1141, 1993.

587. **Tan, D., Reiter, R. J., Chen, L. D., Poeggeler, B., Manchester, L. C., and Barlow-Walden, L. R.,** Both physiological and pharmacological levels of melatonin reduce DNA adduct formation induced by the carcinogen safrole, *Carcinogenesis,* 15, 215, 1994.

588. **Schild, S. E., Scheithauer, B. W., Schomberg, P. J., Hook, C. C., Kelly, P. J., Frick, L., Robinbow, J. S., and Buskirk, S. J.,** Pineal parenchymal tumors, *Cancer,* 72, 870, 1993.

589. **Burger, P. C. and Fuller, G. N.,** Management of intracranial germ cell tumors, *Neurol. Clinics,* 9, 266, 1991.

590. **Russell, D. S. and Rubenstein, L. J.,** *Pathology of Tumours of the Nervous System,* 4th ed., Arnold, London, 1971.

591. **Borit, A., Blackwood, W., and Mair, W. G. P.,** The separation of pineocytoma from pineoblastoma, *Cancer,* 35, 408, 1980.

592. **Min, K. W., Scheithauer, B. W., and Bauserman, S. C.,** Pineal parenchymal tumors: an ultrastructural study with prognostic implications, *Ultrastruct. Pathol.,* 18, 69, 1994.

593. **Herrick, M. K.,** Pathology of pineal tumors, in *Diagnosis and Treatment of Pineal Region Tumors,* Neuwelt, E. A., Ed., Williams & Wilkins, Baltimore, 1984, 31.

594. **Stolovich, C., Loewenstein, A., Varssano, D., and Lazar, M.,** Trilateral retinoblastoma, *Metab. Pediatr. Syst. Ophthalmol.,* 15, 57, 1992.

595. **Kitay, J. I. and Altschule, M. D.,** *The Pineal Gland,* Harvard University Press, Cambridge, MA, 1954.

596. **DeGirolami, U. and Schmidek, H.,** Clinicopathological study of 53 tumors of the pineal region, *J. Neurosurg.,* 39, 455, 1973.

597. **Rubinstein, L. J. and Russell, D. S.,** Tumors and tumor-like lesions of maldevelopmental origin, in *Pathology of Tumors of the Nervous System,* 5th ed., Williams & Wilkins, Baltimore, 1989, 664.

598. **Min, K. W. and Scheithauer, B. W.,** Pineal germinomas and testicular seminoma. A comparative ultrastructural study with special references to early carcinomatous transformation, *Ultrastruct. Pathol.,* 14, 483, 1990.

599. **Gouliamos, A. D., Kalovidouris, A. E., Kotoulas, G. K., Athanasopoulou, A. K., Kouvaris, J. R., Trakadas, S. J., Vlahos, L. S., and Papavasiliou, C. G.,** CR and MR of pineal region tumors, *Magn. Reson. Imaging,* 12, 17, 1994.

600. **Sklar, C. A., Conte, F. A., Kaplan, S. L., and Grumbach, M. M.,** Human chorionic gonadotropin-secreting pineal tumor: relation to pathogenesis and sex limitation of sexual precocity, *J. Clin. Endocrinol. Metab.,* 53, 656, 1981.

601. **Takahashi, H., Tokuda, N., and Kariya, H.,** Precocious puberty in a seven-year-old body due to human chorionic gonadotropin producing pineal tumor detected by magnetic resonance computed tomographic scanning, *Acta Paediatr.,* 32, 88, 1990.

602. **Arita, N., Ushio, Y., Hayakawa, T., Uozumi, T., Watanabe, M., Mori, T., and Mogami, H.,** Serum levels of alpha-fetoprotein, human chorionic gonadotropin and carcinoembryonic antigen in patients with primary intracranial germ cell tumors, *Oncodev. Biol. Med.,* 1, 235, 1980.

603. **Walton, K.,** Teratomas of the pineal region and their relationship to pinealomas, *J. Pathol. Bacteriol.,* 61, 11, 1949.

604. **DeGirolami, U. and Armbrustmacher, V. W.,** Juvenile pilocytic astrocytoma of the pineal region, *Cancer,* 50, 1185, 1982.

Chapter 4

ENVIRONMENTAL MODULATION
OF NEUROENDOCRINE FUNCTION

Richard W. Steger and Andrzej Bartke

CONTENTS

SEASONAL VARIATIONS IN ENDOCRINE FUNCTION

The neuroendocrine system has a primary role in the transduction of information from the nervous system regarding changes in an animal's environment into signals that produce the proper endocrine responses to these challenges. The survival and successful reproduction of an animal are often predicated on its ability to predict seasonal changes in temperature and the availability of food and water and to make the proper metabolic alterations to meet these changing environmental factors. Natural selection favors adaptation to environmental fluctuations, and it seems that there is an almost endless variety of strategies to meet this end.

The controlling environmental factors that affect physiological functions can be broken down into two primary classifications: ultimate or proximate.[11,324] For example, in the case of reproductive performance, ultimate factors are those that are maximized in breeding strategies of adaptive species, such as food, climate, and lack of predation. Proximate factors in this case would be environmental factors that trigger or turn off the reproductive effort, such as day length, temperature, food, rain, and social input.

In this review, we will discuss mechanisms by which environmental information is transformed into endocrine responses. Particular emphasis will be placed on control of the reproductive axis, but many of the mechanisms discussed apply to regulation of other physiological systems. Space limitations prevent a complete description of comparative neuroendocrinology of seasonal reproductive activity, but we will try to emphasize some important species differences.

ENVIRONMENTAL FACTORS AFFECTING REPRODUCTIVE FUNCTION

Seasonal breeding is a phenomenon exhibited by a wide variety of species in their natural habitats, but is of particular importance in animals living in a temperate or a polar region. Reproductive processes can put tremendous energy demands on the organism, as does provision of nourishment to the offspring. Thus, it is essential to the survival of a species to ensure that offspring are born during the time of the year when these demands can best be satisfied while also minimizing the waste of parental energy and the effects of predation or other environmental hazards. A stimulating discussion of the advantages and disadvantages associated with the development of various seasonal reproductive patterns and the selection of various seasonal predictors has recently been published.[45]

PHOTOPERIOD

Animals have evolved a number of different reproductive strategies to ensure that offspring are born during a time of year that provides maximum survival potential, and photic information is often used as a primary means to predict these times. Although there are many gaps in our understanding of how environmental factors control reproductive and other endocrine processes, data from a number of different laboratories are now beginning to allow us to understand how photoperiodic information is perceived by the animal and how this information is transduced into a signal(s) that can modulate reproductive function.

Although data on photoperiodic control of reproductive function for a number of species have appeared in the literature and will subsequently be reviewed in this chapter, more is probably known about the effect of day length on reproductive function in the golden (Syrian) hamster *(Mesocricetus auratus)* than for any other species.[19]

Golden Hamster
Natural Conditions

The golden or Syrian hamster *(Mesocricetus auratus)* is a seasonal breeder that is very responsive to changes in day length.[15,249,312] Field data on hamster behavior are still incomplete, but from laboratory data and limited field observations, it is hypothesized that, under natural conditions, the short days of fall and winter induce gonadal regression. Hamsters remain in this state of reproductive quiescence throughout most of the winter while in their burrows, but sometime prior to the vernal equinox, and before emerging from their burrows, the reproductive axis is reactivated and the animals regain reproductive competence. At this time, the animals are not responsive to artificial reduction in day length and are said to be photorefractory. During the long days of spring and summer, reproductive function is maintained, but the photorefractory state is "broken" and the animals can again respond to the forthcoming short days of fall and winter.

Laboratory Conditions

Seasonal reproductive activity can be mimicked in the laboratory by exposing the animals to short days (<12.5 h of light per day).[15,32,96,296,317,335] Testicular or cyclic ovarian function is fully suppressed within 10 to 12 weeks of short-day exposure, but certain endocrine and neuroendocrine events clearly precede these changes. Spontaneous gonadal recrudescence begins after 15 to 20 weeks of short-day exposure but can be advanced by returning the animals to a photoperiod of greater than 12.5 h of light per day. The animals will not respond to short-photoperiod exposure at this time (photorefractory), but become photosensitive after 7 to 11 weeks of long-day exposure.[313]

It has been shown that a skeleton photoperiod consisting of brief pulses of light given during the proper time of the circadian rhythm of photoresponsivity can maintain reproductive activity.[84] Thus, a period of several hours of light (which is usually interpreted by the animal as a short day and leads to gonadal regression) followed several hours later by a brief pulse of light appears to be interpreted by the animal as a long day in that it maintains gonadal activity. Detailed studies of the various skeleton photoperiods, the diurnal patterns of animals' locomotor activity, and the endocrine responses indicate that the animals are sensitive to light some 14 h after the natural or artificial sunrise, and their gonadal function can be maintained or activated by as little as 1 min of light exposure during this period of sensitivity, even if they experienced darkness in the intervening hours.[203] This observation may explain how day length actually affects neuroendocrine function in this supposedly nocturnally active animal that spends most of its daylight hours in deep underground burrows.

Endocrine Events
Hormone Levels
Males

Decreases in circulating and pituitary levels of luteinizing hormone (LH) and follicle-stimulating hormone (FSH) generally precede testicular atrophy in male golden hamsters housed under short-day conditions.[32,37,296,312,335] Decreases in testicular weight in short-day animals have been reported to occur in the absence of detectable changes in peripheral gonadotropin levels,[34,249] but it is unclear whether these results are an artifact of sampling time or methodology or whether, for some unknown reason, the gonadotropin response to photoperiod is variable in nature. Serum and pituitary levels of prolactin (PRL) also decline after short-day exposure, and this response is much more uniform than is the gonadotropin response.[107,154,307,308] The suppression of serum PRL leads to a loss of testicular PRL and LH (human chorionic gonadotropin, hCG) receptors, which could help to explain the loss of testicular gametogenic and steroidogenic function, despite a lack of detectable changes in circulating gonadotropin levels in some experiments.[154] Spontaneous or long-day-induced testicular recrudescence is preceded by increases in serum and pituitary levels of LH, FSH, and PRL, with the increase in FSH generally preceding the increase of LH and PRL levels.[189,296]

Females

Although the endocrine consequences of short-day exposure have not been as extensively studied in the female as in the male golden hamster, it has been well documented that short-day exposure or blinding leads to an anestrous condition, as evidenced by a constant diestrous type of vaginal smear and a cessation of follicular growth and ovulation.[144,248,277] Distinct hormonal changes including an increase in progesterone is seen within one cycle after transfer to short day, and LH increases are seen after 7 cycles.[143,144] These hormonal changes are seen in afternoon but not morning blood samples, suggesting that photoperiod changes may involve changes in the response to a circadian oscillator or clock. The increase in LH was suggested to be secondary to a reduction in estrogen negative feedback, which, if supported by direct experimental evidence, would be markedly different from observations of male hamsters who become exceedingly sensitive to steroid feedback when housed under SD conditions.[18,305,333] Interestingly, FSH secretion does not change, which provides another physiologic example of differential regulation of LH and FSH release.

One of the most fascinating hormonal events seen in the photoperiod-induced anovulatory hamster is the existence of a daily LH and FSH surge similar in magnitude and timing to the proestrous LH and FSH surge seen in the normally cycling female hamster.[21,43,143,144,219,251,358] These LH surges occur in the presence of estradiol levels that are as low as or lower than basal levels during the estrous cycle and lower than those needed to stimulate uterine water retention.[143,144,248,358] A daily progesterone surge, most likely in response to increasing LH, is also seen in the anestrous hamster.[43,78] Ovariectomy eliminates this progesterone surge and undoubtedly lowers estrogen levels even further but surprisingly does not affect LH levels. These findings suggest that the regulation and timing of the LH surge may be fundamentally different in the rat and hamster because it has been demonstrated that estrogen is required for the LH surge in the rat. Alternatively, the daily LH surge in the SD hamster might be due to a mechanism unrelated to that causing the preovulatory LH surge in an intact long-day hamster.

Furthermore, based on studies in the rat, the progesterone surge would be expected to extinguish the response to a daily signal for an LH surge and perhaps abolish cyclicity completely. It may be that the SD hamster does not respond to high levels of progesterone due to reduced levels of hypothalamic progesterone receptors brought about by low estrogen levels. Estrogen has previously been shown to induce progesterone receptors in a number of species including the hamster,[62] and estrogen replacement blocks the daily LH surge in SD hamsters.[1] The ovaries of photoperiod-induced anovulatory hamsters are characterized by marked proliferation of interstitial tissue, a source of progesterone in the hamster, and the lack of antral follicles, which explains the altered steroid profile.[248,268,283] Ovarian changes may be secondary to the occurrence of daily LH surges because exogenous LH injections can induce a similar histological transformation of the ovary.[112] However, this mechanism was discounted by Jorgenson and Schwartz,[143] who demonstrated that daily LH or LH and FSH injections disrupted cycles but did not induce an endocrine state mimicking anestrus.

Despite the daily surge of LH seen in the anestrous hamster, pituitary and serum PRL levels are severely attenuated in SD female hamsters, and there is no evidence for any diurnal changes in SD PRL levels as seen in LD females.[251,358] Furthermore, chronic estradiol treatment caused a modest increase in SD PRL levels but not comparable to that seen in LD hamsters. The high levels of progesterone seen in anestrous animals could partially explain the low PRL levels because progesterone has been shown to decrease basal and estrogen-stimulated PRL release in the rat,[122] but this effect is minor and other mechanisms are likely to be involved. Furthermore, reports of studies in the rat have demonstrated that progesterone prolongs the preovulatory PRL surge by reducing dopaminergic activity in the median eminence.[5] It is plausible that the decrease in PRL might also contribute to altered ovarian function in the SD hamster because PRL is necessary for maintaining LH receptors and gonadotropin responsiveness.

Hormone Responses

Male hamsters housed in a short photoperiod are much more sensitive to the negative feedback effect of testosterone on gonadotropin synthesis and release than are long-photoperiod animals.[85,317,333,335,336] Testicular recrudescence is preceded by a reduced sensitivity of the hypothalamo-pituitary axis to testosterone-negative feedback.[85,189,336]

It is not certain whether the decrease in gonadotropin secretion associated with short-day exposure is due to the changing sensitivity of the negative feedback system, as proponents of the "steroid-dependent" model suggest, or whether primary changes in LH and FSH secretion cause a change in feedback sensitivity, as supporters of the "steroid-independent" model propose.[37,307,336] On the basis of available evidence, we feel that the regulation of gonadotropin secretion in hamsters is the result of the combined effects of steroid-independent and -dependent mechanisms.[307] Data from our laboratory suggest that changes in feedback sensitivity may occur through PRL-mediated changes in androgen receptors that are separate from but not necessarily independent of steroid-independent changes in LH and FSH secretion.[16,17,188] More recently, we have demonstrated that nuclear androgen receptors in the pituitaries of castrated hamsters with testosterone implants were increased after exposure to a short photoperiod.[240] Furthermore, these nuclear androgen receptors decreased after photostimulation.

Inhibin, a Sertoli cell product that selectively inhibits FSH release without causing any major change in LH levels, may also be involved in seasonal changes in reproductive function. The rapid reduction in FSH levels after transfer of male hamsters to SD conditions precedes the decrease in both LH and inhibin levels, suggesting that the negative feedback effects of inhibin on FSH are also enhanced.[153] Serum inhibin levels remain low for several weeks after photostimulation, which may partially account for the rapid and sustained rise of FSH above levels seen in hamsters maintained continuously under LD conditions.[153,298]

Neuroendocrine Events
Role of Luteinizing Hormone-Releasing Hormone (LHRH)
Pituitary Response to LHRH

Photoperiod-induced changes in gonadotropin secretion may not necessarily be associated with changes in the response of the pituitary to stimulation by LHRH. Several studies using a wide range of LHRH doses in both intact and castrated male hamsters showed no differences in LHRH response between LD and SD animals.[233,236,334] However, these studies all involved acute treatment with LHRH and it still must be resolved if photoperiod affects the long-term ability of the pituitary to respond to physiological levels of LHRH.

In vitro studies of LH release using either hemipituitaries or dispersed cell cultures derived from normal, regressed, and recrudescing male hamsters likewise showed no difference in response to LHRH due to photoperiod.[133,297] In contrast, basal and LHRH-stimulated FSH release, as measured *in vitro*, may actually be greater in animals undergoing spontaneous testicular recrudescence than in normal controls or in animals undergoing SD-induced testicular regression.[297] This FSH response parallels the rise in FSH levels preceding testicular weight gain and hypothalamic LHRH decline and may explain how FSH increases without changes in LH and apparently LHRH secretion.

LHRH Content and Release

Hypothalamic LHRH content is increased after transferring male hamsters from long to short days, and these high levels are maintained until shortly before spontaneous testicular recrudescence, when LHRH content decreases to levels seen in LD controls.[132,233,260,261,296] However, the increase in LHRH content coincident with the fall in gonadotropins and the decrease in LHRH content during the period of rising gonadotropin levels suggests that SD exposure inhibits the release of hypothalamic LHRH.

Castration of LD male hamsters results in an attenuation of hypothalamic LHRH content, presumably due to an increase in its release.[233] However, in gonadally regressed hamsters, castration does not attenuate hypothalamic LHRH content, despite its effect of causing an increase in LH release of a magnitude similar to that observed in gonadally active male hamsters. This apparent paradox may be explained by the ability of SD, but not LD, animals to respond to the low levels of circulating androgens that remain after castration. In the rat, certain regimens of steroid replacement have been shown to reduce LHRH content without affecting LH levels.[145] In support of this hypothesis, we have shown that testosterone replacement is more effective in increasing hypothalamic LHRH content in castrated SD than in castrated LD animals.[306] Direct measurements of hypothalamic LHRH synthesis, turnover, and/or release are technically difficult to carry out, but preliminary studies have suggested that *in vitro* LHRH release in response to norepinephrine (NE) does not differ between LD and SD hamsters (Steger and Bartke, unpublished observations).

LHRH Receptors

Further evidence supporting the hypothesis that photoperiod-induced changes in gona-dotropin secretion are due to changes in LHRH secretion has been derived from studies on pituitary LHRH receptor content. Studies in the rat suggest that LHRH up-regulates its own receptor[64] and, although castration may not increase LHRH receptor concentration in the hamster pituitary, the total number of receptors in the gland is increased.[236] Two recent studies have reported that LHRH receptor content is decreased in male hamsters housed under SD conditions and, although acute LHRH treatment did not reverse this effect, it could not be ascertained whether these changes were dependent or independent of long-term changes in endogenous LHRH secretion.[236, 307] Increases in pituitary LHRH receptor content accompany spontaneous or LD-induced testicular recrudescence coincide with the presumed stimulation of LHRH release, which is evidenced by decreases in hypothalamic LHRH content and increases in gonadotropin secretion.[296,307,308,310]

Neurotransmitter Changes

Although a number of laboratories are involved in studies of the endocrine events asso-ciated with seasonal changes in reproductive activity in the golden hamster, the neurochemical events accompanying photoperiod-induced changes in endocrine function have not been extensively studied. Data from several species, most notably from the rat, have documented that a number of recognized and putative hypothalamic neurotransmitters are involved in the control of hypothalamic hypophysiotropic hormone secretion, which, in turn, controls pitu-itary hormone synthesis and release.[145,197,309] Data from our laboratories suggest that there are many parallels between the neuroendocrine control of gonadotropin release in the hamster and in the much more extensively studied laboratory rat.[307]

Gonadotropin Regulation

Space limitations prevent us from detailing the neuroendocrine control of the gonadal axis, but there are a number of recent reviews describing the hypothalamic control of pituitary hormone secretion.[145,197,309] In general, data from the rat suggest that NE is the principal neurotransmitter controlling gonadotropin release in both the male and female, although there is accumulating evidence that excitatory amino acids and the opiate peptides are also of great importance. The role of dopamine (DA) is much less clear and appears to depend on the relative degree of DA stimulation and on the steroid background during the DA stimula-tion.[145,304] Serotonin seems to be principally inhibitory to LH release in the male rat but may have a role in the generation of the proestrous LH surge in the female. Acetylcholine (Ach), gamma-aminobutyric acid (GABA), and numerous other factors may also modulate LH release, but little is known about the physiology of these substances in the rat, let alone the hamster.

Prolactin Regulation

Unlike LH and FSH, PRL is mainly under the inhibitory control of the hypothalamus, although there is considerable evidence that stimulatory factors from the hypothalamus are also involved in the control of PRL synthesis and secretion.[26,27,93,197] The tuberoinfundibular system exerts the principal inhibitory influence over PRL through DA secretion into the portal vasculature.[27,115] DA binds to specific receptors on the lactotrophs and is inhibitory to both PRL synthesis and secretion. PRL secretion is also regulated by gonadal steroids. Estrogens stimulate basal PRL release by a direct effect on the pituitary and also by inhibiting the release and effect of DA from the tuberoinfundibular system.[27,57,116,245] Androgens may inhibit PRL release and potentiate the effect of DA.[27,93,102] Finally, serotonin can also stimulate PRL release, although it is not known for sure whether this effect is mediated through the release of a PRL releasing factor or by inhibition of hypothalamic DA release.[152,197]

Decreases in DA release explain some physiological increases in PRL secretion, but increases in PRL release due to mating, suckling, stress, and other stimuli are not accompanied by changes in DA sufficient to account for the PRL surge. A variety of compounds including thyrotropin-releasing hormone, vasoactive intestinal peptide (VIP), oxytocin, angiotensin, and other unidentified compounds have been demonstrated to release PRL but their physiological importance is still being debated. A discussion of the role of these compounds in PRL regulation is beyond the scope of this chapter, but this topic was recently reviewed.[26,27]

The neurointermediate lobe (NIL) of the pituitary may also participate in the regulation of PRL release most likely via a functional humoral link involving the short portal vessels.[26,27,94] The NIL can exert both stimulatory and inhibitory effects on PRL secretion. Thus removal of the posterior pituitary in the rat leads to a 2 to 3 fold elevation of basal plasma PRL levels,[210,231] whereas surgical ablation of the NIL abolishes both the proestrous PRL surge and the suckling-induced rise in PRL.[26,209,210] A role for NIL VIP and α-melanocyte-stimulating hormone (α-MSH) in stimulating PRL release has been proposed, but evidence also exists for the involvement of other putative PRL releasing factors.[27,83,94] The inhibitory effects of the NIL on PRL secretion appear to be mediated by DA. The NIL is innervated by tuberohypohyseal DA neurons whose cell bodies are found in the rostral arcuate nucleus and possibly in the rostral periventricular region.[179]

Male
Gonadal Regression

Norepinephrine—The transfer of male hamsters from a long photoperiod (14 h of light to 10 h of dark, i.e., 14L/10D) to a short photoperiod (5L/19D) was shown to result in a significant depression of hypothalamic NE and DA metabolism as well as the expected decrease in circulating LH, FSH, and PRL levels.[29,295b,296] In these and subsequent studies dealing with photoperiod effects on hamster neurotransmitter dynamics, hypothalamic NE and DA metabolism or "turnover" was estimated by blocking the rate-limiting enzyme in catecholamine synthesis, tyrosine hydroxylase, with a-methyl-tyrosine and measuring the rate of decline of NE and DA content in defined brain regions.[44,300] The turnover rate is calculated using the formula

$$K = k[CA]_0 \qquad\qquad [4.1]$$

where $[CA]_0$ is the amine concentration at zero time and k is the rate constant of NE or DA efflux (the slope of the line describing the decline in NE or DA content between zero time and 1 and/or 2 h after α-MPT treatment) calculated by the least-squares method after natural log transformation.[44] Subsequent studies confirmed and extended these original observations and demonstrated that there were regional changes in hypothalamic neurotransmitter metabolism, some of which appeared independent of changes in gonadotropin secretion.[29,295b,296,298,301,307,308,310] Thus, median eminence (ME) and medial basal hypothalamic (MBH) NE turnover is consistently reduced after short photoperiod exposure, but changes in the metabolism of NE in the anterior hypothalamus and medial preoptic area (MPOA) are somewhat more variable. The variability of changes in NE turnover in the MPOA region may relate to the variable effects of short photoperiods on serum gonadotropin levels in different experiments, but insufficient data exist to prove or disprove this hypothesis. More recent data have demonstrated that changes in NE metabolism precede changes in pituitary and gonadal hormone levels and the onset of testicular regression and are not simply due to changes in circulating steroid levels.[295b,306]

Dopamine—DA turnover in the ME and MBH is consistently reduced within 4 weeks or less of SD exposure, whereas the turnover of DA in the MPOA remains unaffected or significantly elevated.[29,295b,296,298] Testosterone treatment of regressed animals restores DA turnover in the MBH to levels not different from those seen in LD control animals but fails to correct the deficiency in ME DA turnover.[306] The elevated levels of DA turnover as seen in the MPOA of SD animals are further elevated by testosterone replacement. These data still need to be confirmed and reconciled with observations in the castrated rat that show testosterone to selectively depress MPOA DA turnover when implanted in the MPOA or when administered systemically.[284, 285] It was also determined that, in the rat, systemic testosterone administration or testosterone implants into the MBH did not affect MBH DA turnover, but had significant effects on serum LH levels.[284, 285] However, the comparison of testosterone effects in castrated rats with those in gonadally regressed hamsters may not be valid because of the vast differences in gonadotropin secretion rates (increased in castrated rats; reduced in gonadally regressed hamsters).

Pinealectomy blocks the effect of short days to decrease MBH and to increase MPOA DA turnover as well as preventing decreases in gonadotropin secretion and sex behavior.[310] The role of the pineal gland in mediating photoperiod-induced neuroendocrine alterations will be discussed more fully in a later section. These data strengthen the hypothesis that SD-induced changes in DA metabolism may be responsible for many of the consequent changes in hormone secretion. In the same regard, administration of the catecholamine precursor L-DOPA to gonadally regressed animals causes an increase in FSH secretion, which is one of the first events associated with testicular recrudescence.[298]

Changes in hypothalamic DA metabolism in gonadally regressed hamsters may also be secondary to changes in PRL secretion, because pituitary homografts under the kidney capsule increase PRL levels and elevate both MBH and ME DA turnover rates.[308] The pituitary grafts also promote increased FSH secretion by the *in situ* pituitary,[16,17] providing further evidence for a link between DA metabolism and gonadotropin secretion.

Serotonin—Although it is becoming increasingly apparent that hypothalamic serotoninergic neurons or 5-hydroxytryptamine (5-HT) terminals from neurons originating in the midbrain raphe nuclei have a major role in the control of anterior pituitary hormone secretion in the rat,[145,152,197,309,345] little is known about such a role in the hamster. Serotonin metabolism in the whole brain or hypothalamus shows a distinct diurnal rhythm, but manipulations of the photoperiod resulting in testicular atrophy do not affect this rhythm.[92] Transfer of adult male hamsters to a short photoperiod leads to a significant increase of 5-HT synthesis in the MBH but no change is seen in the ME, anterior hypothalamus, or olfactory bulbs.[299] It is not certain if this change in 5-HT metabolism is responsible for changes in pituitary hormone secretion, but studies in the rat have demonstrated that 5-HT can act within the MBH to inhibit LH release.[345] Alternatively, the increase in 5-HT synthesis might be secondary to the reduction in PRL levels because PRL replacement reverses the effects of hypophysectomy to increase MBH but not anterior hypothalamus (AH) 5-HT synthesis.[152]

Excitatory Amino Acids—Excitatory amino acids such as aspartate and glutamate have recently been shown to play an important role in the control of gonadotropin release[41] and may be involved in the photoperiodic response of the hamster's hypothalamic-pituitary axis. Activation of N-methyl-D-aspartate (NMDA) receptors leads to an increase of plasma LH levels in both LD and SD male hamsters and also prevents SD-induced decrease in LH and FSH levels and the accompanying testicular regression.[338] It has been further demonstrated that SD hamsters have an increased sensitivity and responsiveness to NMDA, suggesting that endogenous glutamatergic stimulation is decreased in this photoperiod.[128] The effects of NMDA receptor agonists on LH release in regressed hamsters are gonad-independent.[339]

Opiate Peptides—Opiate peptides have important inhibitory effects on LH release while stimulating PRL release.[145,197] Injections of an opiate antagonist, naloxone, delays but does not prevent gonadal regression presumably by increasing LH release.[58] Naloxone has little effect on LH release in fully regressed SD hamsters and does not appear capable of stimulating gonadal recrudescence.[88, 257] Hypothalamic ^{3}H-naloxone binding is not affected by SD exposure although amygdaloid binding is slightly decreased.[329,330] Changes in amygdaloid binding do not appear to be involved with changes in pituitary-gonadal function.

Acetylcholine—In the male rat, ACh appears to be associated with neural systems excitatory to LH release,[145] but its role in controlling gonadotropin release in the hamster has not been determined. It has been hypothesized that ACh may be important in the control of circadian rhythmicity, because the suprachiasmatic nucleus (SCN), a (or the) biological clock, is richly innervated with ACh fibers and because light or ACh agonists and antagonists affect the firing rate of SCN neurons.[202] The ACh agonist carbachol, when injected at the proper time, can prevent the inhibitory effects of short photoperiods on hamster testicular function, possibly by continually resetting the (a) biological clock.[82]

Neurotransmitters in Gonadal Recrudescence—The neurotransmitter events associated with testicular regression are reversed in the time period preceding spontaneous testicular growth.[296] Thus, hypothalamic NE and DA metabolism in male hamsters housed under a 5L/19D photoperiod were shown to be depressed at 10 weeks into the short photoperiod, but at 15 weeks and coincident with increasing gonadotropin levels, NE and DA metabolism were significantly elevated above these levels, although not yet to the same degree as seen in 14L/10D control animals.

The timing of spontaneous testicular recrudescence is extremely variable, but recrudescence can be induced in regressed animals by transferring them from SD to LD conditions (photostimulation). Transfer of gonadally regressed male hamsters from a short (5L/19D) to a long (14L/10D) photoperiod was shown to elicit, within 24 h, a significant change in hypothalamic DA, serotonin, and possibly NE metabolism,[298] Coincident with changes in neurotransmitter metabolism seen in these experiments were changes in LHRH content in the hypothalamus and FSH concentrations in serum. Changes in serum LH levels were also seen within 6 days of transfer. The role of increased catecholamine metabolism in the control of endocrine events associated with testicular recrudescence was further strengthened by the observation that inhibitors of catecholamine synthesis blocked, whereas catecholamine agonists mimicked, the endocrine effects of photostimulation.[298]

SD-induced increases in hypothalamic 5-HT metabolism are reversed within 2 days of transfer to LD conditions,[299] but it has not been determined whether pharmacological blockade of hypothalamic 5-HT will lead to gonadal recrudescence.

Excitatory amino acids may also be involved in activation of the reproductive axis, because NMDA administration promotes testicular recrudescence.[338] This effect of NMDA is blocked by the NMDA antagonist, MK-801, as is the stimulatory action of light pulses given during the dark phase.[65,338]

Prolactin Regulation during Gonadal Regression and Recrudescence—Plasma PRL levels are reduced within one to four weeks of SD exposure.[29,295b] The blockade of DA synthesis with aMPT leads to a marked increase in PRL secretion, which is not compromised in the SD hamster,[29,295b] indicating that PRL is still under inhibitory control of DA. Although we initially hypothesized that an increase in tuberoinfundibular-dopaminergic activity might be the cause of reduced PRL secretion in SD animals, this hypothesis was rejected when TIDA neuronal activity was clearly shown to be reduced under SD conditions.[295b,296] The pituitary response to the inhibitory effects of DA on PRL secretion was shown to increase in short photoperiods but probably not to a degree that would explain the marked reduction in PRL release.[297,308] More recently we have demonstrated that dopamine turnover in the NIL is increased within one week of SD exposure and may provide the mechanism accounting for the decline in plasma PRL levels after SD exposure.[303a] Recently, it has been demonstrated that the neurohypophysis has important regulatory effects on anterior pituitary PRL secretion. Thus removal of the posterior pituitary in the rat leads to a 2- to 3-fold elevation of plasma PRL levels that can be reversed by intracarotid injections of DA.[209,231] Furthermore, removal of the posterior pituitary reduces the amount of DA reaching the pituitary,[208] and pituitary stalk section induces a time-dependent increase in plasma PRL that parallels the decline in posterior pituitary DA content.[26]

Female

Even less is known about the neurochemical events associated with the seasonal control of gonadotropin release in the female hamster than is known about the male hamster. In one study, it was reported that female hamsters maintained in constant dark conditions became acyclic within 6 weeks and, after ovariectomy, had lower serum gonadotropin and higher medial basal hypothalamic LHRH levels than did control animals receiving 14 h of light per day.[156] Associated with these constant dark-induced changes was a suggestion of higher MBH DA activity, which the authors suggested was inhibitory to LHRH release. DA activity in the anterior hypothalamus was not affected by constant dark, and the activity of NE in either brain area was not tested.

Role of the Pineal Gland in Mediating Photoperiod Effects

The pineal gland is an essential component of the neuroendocrine axis, controlling the reproductive response of the hamster to photoperiodic information. Pinealectomy blocks the endocrine and gonadal response to SD exposure[249-251,316] and, as was already mentioned, also blocks many of the changes in neurotransmitter metabolism associated with nonstimulatory photoperiods.[310] Removal of the pineal from gonadally regressed male hamsters initiates testicular recrudescence.[316]

Mediators of Pineal Effects

Although the pineal produces a number of peptides and indoles, many of which can be demonstrated to have some effect on reproductive function, pineal melatonin is most widely regarded as the principal product mediating the control of the pineal over various physiological functions.[50,249,251,316] Pineal melatonin synthesis and content have long been known to show a dramatic diurnal pattern, with nighttime peaks and daytime nadirs observed in all mammalian species that have been studied.[316] It is assumed that this rhythm in melatonin secretion conveys a time signal, but the actual nature of this signal has been the subject of considerable debate, because, changes in day length have different effects on melatonin secretory profiles in different species. Day-length effects on the profile of melatonin secretion include changes in the absolute amount of melatonin secreted, changes in the duration of the nocturnal surge, and/or changes in the timing of the nocturnal surge in relation to the activity cycle of the animal. The majority of evidence now suggests that the duration of the nighttime melatonin rise is the most important signal of day length.[53,55,192,316]

Studies on the effects of melatonin injections on the reproductive function in the Syrian hamster were hampered by the existence of "windows" of melatonin sensitivity. Thus, morning melatonin injections have little effect on the reproductive axis of a hamster maintained in a stimulatory photoperiod, whereas injections in the afternoon mimic the effects of SD exposure.[250,318] Subcutaneous implants that continually release melatonin have no noticeable effect on the neuroendocrine axis of animals maintained in long days. However, identical implants block the effects of transfer to a short photoperiod and the effects of daily afternoon melatonin injection, and can induce testicular recrudescence when implanted into a hamster maintained under SD conditions. It has been hypothesized that these effects are due to loss or down-regulation of melatonin receptors by continued exposure to high levels of melatonin, but there is little experimental evidence either to support or to refute this explanation.[316]

Mechanism(s) of Melatonin Action

The site(s) of melatonin action have not been fully elucidated, but the recent availability of high-affinity, high specific activity melatonin ligand, 2-[^{125}I]iodomelatonin (^{125}I-melatonin) and the subsequent identification of specific G protein-coupled melatonin receptors should allow rapid progress to be made.[155] Earlier studies using ^{3}H-melatonin, demonstrated that melatonin is taken up and concentrated in the hypothalamus, and there are diurnal changes in melatonin binding sites in the hamster and rat brain.[50,51,340] Data from implant studies have also suggested that the AH and SCN are important sites of melatonin action on reproduction, nesting behavior and brown fat metabolism, at least in the white-footed mouse *(Peromyscus leucopus)*.[104,105] In the hamster, destruction of the SCN or total hypothalamic deafferentation blocks the antigonadotropic action of daily melatonin injections as well as the effects of short photoperiod on testicular function and sensitivity of the neuroendocrine axis to steroid-negative feedback.[89,252,263,264] However, this conclusion has been questioned by a contradictory report where it was shown that SCN lesions alter but do not block the ability of properly timed melatonin injections to induce gonadal regression.[36]

Studies with ^{125}I-melatonin show binding in tissue homogenates from the cerebral cortex, cerebellum, hypothalamus, brain stem, olfactory bulb, striatum, and pituitary, with binding sites being most abundant in the hypothalamus and brain stem.[80,235]. Autoradiographic analysis of ^{125}I-melatonin binding presents a more detailed localization of binding sites. The most intense binding is seen in the SCN, ME, paraventricular nuclei, pituitary and pineal.[359] Intense melatonin binding is consistently seen in the pars tuberalis, where it has been shown that melatonin implants affect gonadotropin and PRL secretion in the sheep.[172] Melatonin binding sites in the hamster hypothalamus are probably neuronal because neurotoxin treatment eliminates ^{125}I-melatonin binding.[359] Daily rhythms in the density of melatonin receptors have been described but the regulation of receptor differs according to location.[97,98] For example, pars tuberalis melatonin receptor density is directly controlled by plasma melatonin concentration, whereas SCN receptor levels are controlled by the light-dark cycle independent of the presence of the pineal.

It is becoming increasingly apparent that melatonin affects certain neurotransmitter systems in the hypothalamus, which may, in part, affect the release of the pituitary hormones. *In vitro* studies have shown that melatonin inhibits DA release from the preoptic area and the medial and posterior hypothalamus without affecting DA release from the cerebral cortex, cerebellum, dorsal hippocampus, or striatum.[365] Studies from our laboratories have shown that pinealectomy reverses many of the short-photoperiod-induced changes in hypothalamic dopamine metabolism *in vivo* and alters pituitary responses to DA, lending further support to the hypothesis that melatonin effects are mediated through a dopaminergic mechanism.[310] Pinealectomy of gonadally active male hamsters in a stimulatory photoperiod has no effect on reproductive function or hypothalamic DA metabolism. Melatonin has also been shown to affect other hypothalamic neurotransmitter systems, but the physiological significance of these effects is not understood.[50] The effects of melatonin on neuroendocrine function also may be modulated by changes in hypothalamic prostaglandin metabolism.[218]

It is of interest that the pineal function and, more specifically, melatonin secretion appear to mediate the effects of photoperiod also on hormonal function not directly related to reproduction. In the golden hamster, the activity of the adenohypophyseal-thyroid axis, much like that of the pituitary-gonadal system, is increased by long and suppressed by short photoperiod.[224,346,347] The amplitude of these "seasonal" photoperiod-dependent fluctuations in the thyroid function is relatively small, which is probably not surprising in view of the vital role of thyroid hormones in metabolic regulation. The physiological significance of these changes is presently not understood, but there is evidence that seasonal alterations of thyroid hormone secretion have a role in metabolic adaptations to hibernation in some species of mammals[254,306] and may regulate alternating cycles of photosensitivity and photorefractoriness in birds and mammals.[108,220]

Visual Pathways and Other Brain Regions

An understanding of the neural pathways involved in the control of seasonal changes in endocrine and reproductive activity can provide important insights into mechanisms by which an animal responds to environmental cues. Despite the inherent problems associated with the interpretation of data from experiments involving the use of brain lesions, we are now beginning to understand some of the neural circuitry involved in the transduction of environmental input into neural and endocrine output controlling sex behavior and gonadal function.

The importance of the SCN has already been discussed in regard to its involvement in the relay of photic information from the retina to the pineal gland, but the SCN also appears to be the most important, if not the only, circadian pacemaker controlling a variety of circadian rhythms.[84,114,202] Lesions of the periventricular nuclei also disrupt photoperiod-induced testicular regression, but do not affect circadian activity cycles, suggesting that this area is also involved in the processing or relay of information from the retina to the pineal.[234] Fibers from the SCN project down to the superior cervical ganglia, where they synapse with fibers projecting to the pineal. The actual pathways involved in the functional interaction of these regions are not completely understood, but there is a considerable amount of evidence that destruction of the superior cervical ganglia has many of the same effects as does pinealectomy.[249,251,316]

Environmental Influences on the Rate of Sexual Maturation

In addition to affecting endocrine and reproductive functions in the adult, photoperiod and other environmental influences can profoundly alter the rate of sexual development in many species (the golden hamster may be an exception in this regard). Thus, young Djungarian hamsters maintained in long photoperiods become sexually mature at the age of approximately six weeks, whereas exposure to short days delays sexual development by as much as three to four months.[124] These dramatic effects of photoperiod on sexual maturation are pineal mediated, with the duration of nocturnal elevation of blood melatonin levels acting as a signal for stimulation or delay of the pubertal development.[54] It has also been determined that in some species, such as the Siberian hamster, prenatal photoperiod has significant effects on pubertal development.[125,311,350] The maternal pineal and melatonin is instrumental in mediating this process. The biological significance of this type of environmental regulation of sexual development is undoubtedly related to season fluctuations in the chances of successful reproduction as determined by the availability and quality of food and by ambient temperature. Thus, rapid maturation of animals born during long days of the spring would give them optimal chances for breeding and producing litters before the environmental conditions begin to deteriorate, whereas suppression of pubertal development in animals born later in the season would serve to prevent the birth of litters during fall and winter and to optimize the chances of these animals to survive until the following spring.

Similar effects of photoperiod on the rate of sexual maturation have been described in several rodent species, including deer mice *(Peromyscus maniculatus)*[354,355] and white-footed mice *(Peromyscus leucopus)*,[138] cotton rats *(Sigmodon hispidus)*,[139] and different species of voles *(Microtus arvalis,*[129,160,161] *M. agrestis*[66,344]*)*. The effects of photoperiod on pubertal development in deer mice and white-footed mice are mediated by the pineal, almost certainly via changes in melatonin secretion.[138,232,355] In contrast, pubertal development in the golden hamsters appears to be independent of photoperiodic influences, with animals becoming responsive to changes in day length only after attaining sexual maturity.[72,286] Melatonin administration has been reported either to have no effect[332] or to inhibit[250] testicular growth in immature hamsters.

Comparative Physiology
Reproductive Neuroendocrinology in the Sheep

Earlier in this chapter, we discussed mechanisms by which changes in photoperiod regulate pituitary and gonadal functions in the golden hamster and other small rodents. Neuroendocrine responses to day length obviously represent evolutionary adaptation to seasonal changes in environmental conditions. Thus, in these species in which the period of gestation is very short (two to four weeks), confining the breeding season to long days of spring and summer ensures birth of litters at a time when chances for their survival are optimal. However, in many seasonally breeding species, gestation is much longer, and thus arrival of the offspring in the spring can be assured only by breeding in the fall. Species in this group are often referred to as "short-day breeders" and include many ruminants. Of these, domestic sheep have been studied in greatest detail.

In the ewe, the average length of gestation is 147 days, behavioral estrus and ovulations in temperate zones of the northern hemisphere occur generally between September and January (with some differences related to breed and geographical location, as discussed by Ammar-Kodja and Brudieux[3]) and the lambing season is in the spring. In rams, there are seasonal variations in testis size and sperm production[223] as well as in plasma levels of LH, FSH, and testosterone, including both the frequency and the height of testosterone peaks.[174,271] As in the ewe, the exact timing and amplitude of these variations depend on breed and geographical latitude,[69,228] but in the northern hemisphere, all measures of testicular function are generally maximal in the fall and minimal in the spring. Experiments involving exposure to artificially controlled photoperiod have provided strong evidence that the annual cycle of reproductive functions in the sheep is due primarily to stimulatory effects of short days and inhibitory effects of long days on gonadotropin release and, consequently, on gonadal activity.[77,178,229,362] More recent studies of these relationships indicate that sheep, similarly to other seasonally breeding species, respond to the presence or absence of light during a daily, photoperiod-entrained period of sensitivity rather than to the length of the day per se,[168] and that termination of reproductive activity in the winter may not be due to changes in day length but rather to animals becoming refractory to photoperiodic influences.[360] However, there is also evidence for spontaneous onset and termination of the breeding season under constant photoperiod conditions, with the ambient photoperiod acting primarily to synchronize the endogenous "biological clock" of the animal with the seasons of the year.

Seasonal and artificial photoperiod-induced changes in peripheral LH levels were originally described in intact animals. It was subsequently demonstrated that similar fluctuations in plasma LH also occur in gonadectomized ewes and rams treated with injections or slow-release implants of estradiol or testosterone; that is, in the absence of seasonal changes in sex hormone levels.[147,163,164,225,230] This indicates that photoperiod-related changes in LH release are associated with and perhaps due to changes in the sensitivity of the hypothalamic-pituitary system to inhibition by gonadal steroids. This clearly resembles neuroendocrine responses to photoperiod in the golden hamster, except that exposure to short photoperiods causes sheep to become less, rather than more, sensitive to steroid feedback. There is some evidence that photoperiod-induced changes in the sensitivity to steroid feedback may be related to alterations in hypothalamic content of steroid receptors.[62]

Measurements of LH levels in blood samples collected at frequent intervals have revealed seasonal differences in the frequency and amplitude of LH pulses.[173,364] Episodes of LH release occur approximately every 2 h during the breeding season and every 3.5 to 12 h during the nonbreeding season in ewes.[181] In rams, seasonal fluctuations in LH pulse frequency have been found in some studies but not others.[173,178,228,253,271] Seasonal fluctuations in the response of ovine pituitary to LHRH stimulation,[158,171] are not of sufficient magnitude to account for differences in plasma LH levels during the breeding vs. the nonbreeding season. Thus, the existence of seasonal differences in the pattern of LH secretion can be considered as evidence that endogenous LHRH is normally released in a pulsatile fashion in the ewe and that short photoperiod stimulates gonadal function by increasing the frequency of these pulses, or, in other words, accelerating the hypothalamic "LHRH pulse generator." The inability of some investigators to find seasonal-related changes in LH or LHRH pulse frequency in the ram[253] still needs to be resolved before firm conclusions can be made. However, it has been demonstrated that administration of LHRH every 2 h during the nonmating season can increase plasma LH, FSH, and testosterone levels and testicular size in the ram[174] and induce ovulatory cycles with normal luteal function in the ewe.[193,195,196]

The possible role of PRL in mediating this response is unclear and, indeed, controversial. Prolactin release in the sheep, as in other mammalian species, is stimulated by long and inhibited by short photoperiod.[177,227,243] Thus, plasma PRL levels gradually increase during the period of gonadal quiescence in the spring and maximal levels are observed during the summer, either coinciding with the onset of gonadal growth and activation or preceding it by as much as two to three months.[177,243] Thus, temporal relationships between changes in plasma PRL levels and gonadal activity can be interpreted as an indication of either stimulatory or inhibitory effects of this hormone on the ovary and the testis. However, suppression of endogenous PRL release by treatment with bromocriptine appears to have little, if any, effect on gonadal function in the sheep, except for a slight delay of testicular growth in rams injected with bromocriptine during the summer.[12]

There is a considerable amount of evidence that the effects of photoperiod on the hypothalamic control of pituitary function in the sheep, as in other species, are mediated by the pineal and its secretory product melatonin. Thus, removal of the pineal or interruption of its sympathetic innervation prevent photoperiod from altering plasma levels of gonadotropins, PRL, or testosterone.[13,169,173] Moreover, feeding of melatonin in the afternoon can accelerate the onset of breeding season in intact ewes,[6] whereas infusions of melatonin for 8 or 16 h/day can mimic the effects of long and short photoperiods, respectively, on plasma LH levels in pinealectomized, ovariectomized, estrogen-treated sheep.[38] These findings provide further evidence for the role of the pineal in the regulation of pituitary and gonadal function and suggest that the duration of nocturnal melatonin release serves as a "signal," transducing photoperiodic information to hypothalamic centers controlling adenohypophyseal hormone release. It is interesting to note that the critical role of the duration of nocturnal melatonin elevation in the control of pituitary and gonadal function by photoperiod was originally demonstrated in a LD breeder, the Djungarian hamster *(Phodopus sungorus)*.[53]

Pharmacological studies suggest that the inhibition of LH release in the anestrous ewe could result from enhanced catecholaminergic activity.[110] The locus of this change appears to be in the retrochiasmatic area based on electrophysiologic data,[186] measurement of amine metabolites,[100,101,321] and the observation that lesions in this area increase LH release during anestrus.[322]

From the foregoing discussion, it must be evident that, in the domestic sheep, photoperiod exerts powerful regulatory influences on neuroendocrine processes related to reproduction. However, circannual rhythms of reproductive and endocrine function can be demonstrated in sheep maintained in a constant photoperiod[127] or deprived of eyesight,[162] suggesting possible importance of endogenous rhythms and/or environmental cues unrelated to photoperiod.

Infrahuman Primates

Of the representatives of this taxonomic group, endocrine and reproductive functions have been studied in greatest detail in the rhesus monkey *(Macaca mulatta)*. Rhesus monkeys are seasonal breeders with conceptions taking place mainly in the fall and births in the spring. This pattern of reproduction is characteristic of wild populations in India[294] as well as of animals maintained and bred in captivity.[11] Although autumnal increases in plasma testosterone levels and various measures of copulatory and aggressive behavior in males[200] and in the incidence of ovulatory cycles in females[349] temporarily coincide with seasonal decreases in day length at locations where these studies were conducted, there is no evidence that these changes in endocrine function represent responses to photoperiod. Indeed, the existence of a cause-effect relationship between photoperiod and gonadal activity in this species is seriously questioned by reports of significant seasonal fluctuations in plasma androgen levels and in copulatory behavior of male rhesus monkeys housed in laboratories under constant, carefully controlled conditions of photoperiod and temperature.[25,198,199,238,357] Additional studies will be necessary to determine whether seasonal changes in gonadal activity and behavior in animals maintained under constant environmental conditions represent persistence of circannual cycles entrained by previous exposure of these animals to seasonal changes in photoperiod, temperature, etc., or should be regarded as an expression of truly endogenous rhythms ("biological clock"). In this context, it is interesting to note that a seasonal pattern of sexual activity persists in castrated rhesus males kept under constant conditions of light and temperature and injected daily with identical amounts of testosterone.[199] Evidently, circannual rhythms of copulatory behavior can continue in the absence of any identifiable environmental cues and without circannual fluctuations in the rate of testicular androgen production.

Although the existence of seasonal alterations in peripheral androgen levels in the male rhesus monkey is very well documented, much less is known about the underlying changes in the functions of the hypothalamic-pituitary-testicular axis. Beck and Wuttke[25] reported that seasonal changes in serum testosterone levels coincided with seasonal changes in serum PRL levels and were, in general, inversely related to seasonal fluctuations of serum LH. The levels of serum FSH remained relatively stable throughout the year. It is very difficult to conclude from the temporal association of changes in peripheral PRL and testosterone levels whether increases in PRL release might act as a stimulatory influence on testicular androgen production or rather represent a response to seasonally elevated output of gonadal steroids. Examination of changes in serum hormone levels in individual animals fails to provide support for either of these possibilities because seasonal increase in serum testosterone appears to precede the increase in serum PRL in some animals and follow it in others.

Wickings and colleagues[357] demonstrated that infusion of male rhesus monkeys during nonbreeding season with 100-ng pulses of LHRH spaced 96 min apart produced elevations in LH and testosterone that closely resembled the pulsatile pattern of release of these hormones observed in untreated males during the breeding season. This indicates that seasonal suppression of the pituitary-testicular axis in the male rhesus is due primarily to reduced pulsatile discharge of LHRH from the hypothalamus. However, other experiments performed by these investigators[357] have provided evidence that responsiveness of pituitary gonadotropes to LHRH, as well as responsiveness of Leydig cells to LH stimulation, also exhibit seasonal fluctuations, with gonadotropes being most sensitive during testicular redevelopment in August and September and testes being most sensitive during periods of reproductive quiescence in April and May. The response of the testis to alterations in hormonal, vascular, and/or neural activity induced by severe stress also exhibits seasonal fluctuations. During the breeding season, plasma testosterone levels in adult rhesus males decline in response to immobilization stress, whereas during the nonbreeding season, they increase in response to the same treatment.[109]

Seasonal changes in the endocrine function of the gonads have also been described in other species of infrahuman primates, including baboons (sacred baboon, *Papio hamadryas*,[157] and chacma baboon, *Papio ursinus*[35]) and a New World species, the squirrel monkey, *Saimiri sciureus*.[81,212] In squirrel monkeys, seasonal increase in testicular function and breeding activity coincides with a marked increase in body weight, which has been termed "the fatted-male phenomenon" and apparently represents increases in muscle mass and regional subcutaneous fat deposition in response to rising titers of testicular androgens.[212]

In contrast, there is little, if any, seasonal variation in reproductive functions of the bonnet monkey, *Macaca radiata*,[207] in the laboratory-housed cynomologus macaque, *Macaca fascicularis*,[184] and in the pigtail macaque, *Macaca nemestrina*.[33]

Human

Similar to the situation in other animal species, neuroendocrine and reproductive functions in the human can be altered by environmental influences, including malnutrition, stress, toxic substances, and extremes of ambient temperature. In addition, the human neuroendocrine system is often subjected to environmental factors unique to our own species, including occupational or accidental exposure to chemicals; use of alcohol, psychotropic drugs, prescription and over-the-counter medication; self-imposed dietary restrictions; and intensive physical training. Detailed discussion of the impact of these environmental variables and the role of cultural and social factors is outside the scope of this review but have been reviewed elsewhere.[258,259] We will limit ourselves to discussing the possible significance of natural, primarily seasonal, fluctuations of photoperiod, temperature, and diet in the regulation of human neuroendocrine systems.

In comparison to representatives of other taxonomic groups discussed earlier in this chapter, the human exhibits few, if any, major seasonal shifts in the function of the endocrine glands or in what is known about their neural control. Reproduction continues throughout the year and "normal ranges" of blood hormone levels and endocrine responses to functional tests do not exhibit sufficient seasonal fluctuations to be considered in diagnostic evaluation. This stability of neuroendocrine parameters across seasons probably stems from a combination of biological characteristics of our species and the extent to which we control our environment, including periods of illumination, ambient temperature, and availability and composition of diet.

In spite of the absence of grossly evident seasonal patterns of endocrine or reproductive functions, careful longitudinal and cross-sectional studies have revealed statistically significant seasonal variations in numerous hormonal and hormone-dependent parameters. Thus, urinary excretion of neutral 17-ketosteroids, studied in one adult male subject, exhibited a peak (acrophase) in September and a trough in May,[119] although plasma testosterone levels in normal young males are highest in summer and autumn in the northern hemisphere,[246,247,288] and, surprisingly, during the local spring in the southern hemisphere. Acrophase of plasma LH levels occurs in the spring, regardless of sex and age of the studied subjects,[247, 327] although acrophase of plasma FSH levels was reported in the spring[247] or in the fall.[327] Sperm count, mobility, and morphology also exhibit seasonal variations, with fluctuations in sperm production generally following those in plasma LH levels and out of phase with those in plasma testosterone.[68,126,181,204,237,326] Sexual activity exhibits acrophase coinciding with the seasonal increase in plasma testosterone levels in males.[247,337] Seasonal differences were reported to occur also in the ovulation rate,[141] incidence of chromosomal abnormalities in the offspring,[28,120,142] time of onset of the ovulatory LH surge,[320] and conception rate, which, in northern Finland, was reported to be maximal during the summer.[325]

Occurrence of detectable seasonal variations is not limited to gonadotropic hormones, gonadal steroids, and gametogenesis. Adrenal function also varies with season of the year, as demonstrated by measurements of plasma cortisol levels and daily production rates in young adult males[351] and plasma dehydroepiandrosterone sulfate levels and urinary androgen excretion in postmenopausal women.[75] In both studies, maximal values were recorded in fall and winter.[75,351] In contrast, no seasonal fluctuations were detected in plasma GH levels in adult males.[351]

The existence of discernible seasonal fluctuations in various parameters of neuroendocrine function in the human raises questions as to which of the seasonally variable environmental influences serve to entrain and/or sustain these changes and by what mechanism(s) they act. From studies conducted in various animal species (some of which were discussed earlier in this chapter), the photoperiod-dependent changes in daily rhythms of pineal function would appear to be the most obvious possibility. This possibility is consistent with the evidence that the human pineal exhibits light-dependent diurnal rhythm of secretory activity[166,226] and that gonadotropin secretion is inversely related to peripheral levels of a pineal secretory product, melatonin, during sexual maturation[8,282,348] and during the menstrual cycle.[352] However, the occurrence of seasonal fluctuations in the function of the human pineal and the possible relationship of these fluctuations to hypothalamic and pituitary function remain to be demonstrated.[7] The reports of normal fertility and blood hormone levels in blind individuals[91,165] are difficult to accept as evidence against the role of photoperiod clues in the regulation of human neuroendocrine function, because adequate gonadal function may well be possible in spite of desynchronization or absence of environment-dependent physiological rhythms; and, more importantly, blind individuals may rely on sensory inputs unrelated to light perception for information on seasonal changes in the environment.

SURVEY OF SEASONAL RHYTHMS IN REPRODUCTIVE ACTIVITY IN MALE MAMMALS

We have discussed the effects of seasonal changes in photoperiod on neuroendocrine and reproductive function in one species breeding in the spring (the golden hamster) and one species breeding in the fall (the sheep), as well as in infrahuman primates and in man. Other species were mentioned only in the context of discussing relations and mechanisms that are either absent or have not been studied in detail in golden hamsters, sheep, or primates. To provide a more complete coverage of the subject as well as a guide to literature, we include a survey of seasonal fluctuations in male endocrine and reproductive function in male mammals (Table 1). This list is not exhaustive in terms of either species or citations and emphasizes species for which there is some information on seasonal changes in plasma levels of hypophyseal and/or testicular hormones in relation to environmental variables.

FACTORS OTHER THAN PHOTOPERIOD INFLUENCING SEASONAL REPRODUCTIVE ACTIVITY

Temperature

Ambient temperature is of considerable importance in influencing reproductive strategies of animals, because it can greatly affect the amount of energy needed for thermoregulatory activity at the expense of energy needed for reproductive activities.[45] For example, in male deer mice *(Peromyscus maniculatus bairdii)* exposure to elevated ambient temperature (32°C) severely compromised testicular function, and low temperatures (0°C) augmented the inhibitory effects of short photoperiod.[74] Despite their influence on the energy balance, temperatures in most areas vary widely during any season and thus would not be as good predictors of season as would changes in day length.

Food Availability

Food availability is without doubt the most important overall factor controlling reproduction, because the animal must meet basic metabolic needs before energy can be allocated for reproductive activity. In this regard, both the energy or caloric component and the nutrient component of food must be considered. In general, it appears that environmental factors such as photoperiod are used as predictors of seasonality and the corresponding change in expected food availability, but plant cues are used by certain animals to predict food availability. Although our knowledge of plant cues is limited, their use might be of great advantage to certain species living in highly unpredictable climates.

One such species, the mountain vole *(Microtus montanus)*, which lives in the highly variable climate of the higher altitudes in the Rocky Mountains, uses a phenol compound, 6-methoxybenzoxalinone, found in emerging grasses to predict food availability.[215,269] Interestingly, it appears that the males of this species come into breeding season in response to the photoperiod and wait for fresh grass to stimulate reproductive function in the female. In California voles *(Microtus californicus)*, supplementation of standard laboratory chow with spinach counteracts the inhibitory effects of short day length on testes weight.[216]

Food availability is much more critical to the female than the male, because of the higher energy requirements during pregnancy and lactation particularly in these species that produce large, rapidly growing litters to overcome a high mortality rate and a very short growing season. In a laboratory population of deer mice, food restriction to 70% of the *ad libitum* consumption resulted in suppression of plasma LH and testosterone levels, testicular and seminal vesicle weights, and testicular sperm numbers.[39]

TABLE 1
Seasonal Changes in Endocrine Function in Male Mammals

Marsupials

Australian brush-tailed possum *(Trichosurus vulpecula)*—Increase in Leydig cell number, prostate weight, and other androgen-dependent characteristics in April (New Zealand fall) coinciding with end of seasonal anestrus in female and onset of breeding.[103]

Tammar wallaby *(Macropus eugenii)*—Plasma testosterone and weight of the prostate and Cowper's glands increase during breeding season (January, i.e., Australian summer), presumably representing a pheromone-mediated response to seasonal changes in female reproductive functions.[130]

Placental Mammals

Insectivores

Hedgehog *(Erinaceus europaeus)*—Plasma testosterone levels are maximal during spring (February to April), corresponding to increase in testicular volume and to mating season; plasma testosterone binding is maximal during hibernation (September to January).[266,267]

Bats[a]

Pallid bat *(Antrozous pallidus)*—Increases in androgen production and onset of breeding activity occur in the fall, "out-of-phase" with spermatogenesis and testicular size, which are maximal in late summer; gametogenic and hormonal functions of the testes are controlled primarily by photoperiod, but food and temperature are also involved.[24]

Little brown bat *(Myotis lucifugus)*—Increase in plasma testosterone after arousal from hibernation is accompanied by increase in sex-steroid binding protein (SBP), possibly explaining lack of stimulation of the accessory reproductive glands.[70]

Rodents[b]

Field vole *(Microtus arvalis)*—Long photoperiods stimulate sexual maturation and redevelopment of the testes in adult males in the spring; autumnal involution of the testes depends on changes in availability of food and in photoperiod.[129,160,161]

Field vole *(Microtus agrestis)*—Short photoperiod delays sexual development by inhibiting pubertal increases in hypothalamic LHRH content, pituitary and plasma LH, and plasma FSH levels;[66,344] these effects of photoperiod are pineal mediated;[56] in adult males short photoperiod produces testicular regression followed by spontaneous recrudescence after approximately 6 months (presumably corresponding to testicular growth occurring between December and March under field conditions).[113]

Montane vole *(Microtus montanus)*—Effect of diet on reproductive function in this species is discussed elsewhere in this chapter; photoperiodic regulation of endocrine and gametogenic functions of the testes involve responses to increases and decreases in the day length rather than to day length per se and an effect of prenatal photoperiod on responses to subsequent photoperiodic conditions.[125]

Bank vole *(Clethrionomys glareolus)*—Long photoperiod stimulates sexual development of juveniles with corresponding increases in the activity of steroidogenic enzymes in the testes and alterations in testicular steroid metabolism *in vitro*; steroid secretion by the adrenals appears to increase concomitantly.[314,315]

White-footed mouse *(Peromyscus leucopus)*—Effects of photoperiod, pinealectomy, melatonin, ambient temperature, and diet on sexual maturation and on endocrine and reproductive function in the adult in this species and in the related deer mouse *(Peromyscus maniculatus)* are discussed elsewhere in this chapter and by Johnston and Zucker;[140] in both species, responsiveness of the reproductive/endocrine function to photoperiod varies according to geographical origin of the animals, with those from more northern locations being most responsive;[71,180] in *P. leucopus,* seasonal changes in testicular growth and function are also influenced by an endogenous rhythm;[14] low ambient temperatures induce daily torpor and reduction in thyroid activity.[275]

Woodchuck *(Marmota monax)*—Reduction in body temperature during hibernation is accompanied by increased plasma binding of thyroid hormones with the corresponding reduction in free thyroxine and triiodothyronine in the plasma.[363]

Edible dormouse *(Glis glis)*—Plasma testosterone levels are maximal during May to July and plasma thyroxine levels are maximal in July.[135]

Sand rat *(Psammomys obesus)*—In this inhabitant of the Sahara desert, breeding season extends from October to May; testicular weight increases during summer; testicular levels of testosterone and androstenedione and metabolic clearance rate of testosterone are minimal in June and elevated between September and March;[151] cortisol production is maximal in the fall and subsequently declines, with minimum in June.[2]

TABLE 1 (continued)
Seasonal Changes in Endocrine Function in Male Mammals

Australian bush rat *(Rattus fuscipes)*—Plasma LH and FSH levels are maximal in September (Australian spring), with testosterone levels being maximal in December and January; the content of LH/hCG, FSH, and estradiol receptors is much greater in active than in regressed testes; depression of the testes can be induced experimentally by combining short photoperiod, low ambient temperature, and a low-protein diet.[131]

Cotton rat *(Sigmodon hispidus)*—Breeding is seasonal; short photoperiod, constant darkness of blinding delay pubertal development but do not affect adult testicular function.[139]

Grasshopper mouse *(Onychomys leucogaster)*—In this spring breeder, testicular regression can be induced by short photoperiod or by melatonin injections, and short photoperiod also delays sexual maturation.[95]

Pocket mouse *(Perognathus parvus)*—Gonadal function is initiated during hibernation and stimulated by long photoperiods after emergence, but seasonal changes in testicular weight occur also in animals exposed to invariant 12L/12D photoperiod.[149]

Golden-mantled ground squirrel *(Spermophilus lateralis)*—Seasonal increases in LH and testosterone levels (with maxima in April and May) appear to be due primarily to endogenous rhythm(s) because they persist in constant laboratory conditions;[167] LH response to castration is attenuated during the breeding season,[366] and melatonin content of the pineal is reduced during hibernation, especially close to arousal.[295]

Uinta ground squirrel *(Spermophilus armatus)*—Pineal melatonin synthesis (estimated from hydroxyindole-*O*-methyltransferase [HIOMT] activity) is lowest during the breeding season and maximal immediately before hibernation; testes size is maximal at emergence followed by maximal plasma testosterone levels and breeding season.[86]

Antelope ground squirrel *(Ammospermophilus leucurus)*—Seasonal differences in testes size (with maximum in winter and spring) were not altered by experimental exposure to short or long photoperiods, suggesting endogenous rhythm.[150]

American grey squirrel *(Sciurus carolinensis)*—Plasma testosterone and dihydrotestosterone are maximal in December at the start of the breeding season; during the breeding season, testicular conversion of pregnenolone to testosterone *in vitro* is increased, while output of 17a,20a-dihydroxyprogesterone is reduced and there are alterations in androgen metabolism in the prostate.[241,287]

Rock hyrax *(Procavia capensis)*—During the breeding season (March to May) there are increases in testicular and peripheral testosterone levels, and in the size but not the number of Leydig cells, with concomitant disappearance of lipid droplets and increases in smooth endoplasmic reticulum.[106,214]

Lagomorphs

Snowshoe hare *(Lepus americanus)*—Breeding season extends from January to August and coincides with increased pituitary content of LH and FSH (maximal levels in May and June); gonadotropin content of the pituitary is elevated in the spring also in castrated males.[73]

European hare *(Lepus europaeus)*—Seasonal increase in testicular size and in plasma testosterone levels is associated with reductions in pineal weight and in morphological indices of pineal activity.[170]

Armadillo *(Dasypus novemcinctus)*—Plasma testosterone levels are maximal in the summer.[67]

Carnivores

Ferret *(Mustela furo)*—Plasma testosterone and dihydrotestrone levels are much higher during the spring breeding season than in the sexually quiescent adult animal, but there is little seasonal difference in testicular response to LH stimulation;[87,213] photoperiod does not modify estradiol binding in the brain, pituitary, or reproductive tract, or behavioral responses to estradiol in the female;[22,23] in the adult, pineal and melatonin appear to have little direct inhibitory effect on reproductive function but appear to be involved in synchronizing reproductive cycle with seasonal changes in the environment,[55] while puberty can be readily induced by exposure of young females to long photoperiods.[265]

Mink *(Mustela vison)*—Breeding season is in the winter; plasma testosterone and androstenedione levels increase gradually between November and March and rapidly decline thereafter; short photoperiod stimulates and long photoperiod prevents autumnal testicular activation in juvenile males;[40, 217] short photoperiod or pharmacologically induced suppression of PRL release causes molt into winter pellage,[187] and in the female, spring-related stimulation of PRL release terminates embryonic diapause and causes implantation.[211]

Stone martin *(Martes foina)*—Plasma testosterone levels are lowest between July and February and maximal during sexual activity in May and June.[9]

Mongoose *(Herpestes auropunctatus)*—In Hawaii (where mongoose was introduced by man), breeding season extends from March to June and is accompanied by increases in plasma LH, FSH, and testosterone levels, in testicular LH/hCG binding, in testicular androgen responses to large doses of LH *in vitro*, and in LH responses to gonadotropin-releasing hormone (GnRH) *in vitro*; melatonin may mediate these changes because it is capable of suppressing the gonadotropin response to gonadectomy.[290-293]

TABLE 1 (continued)
Seasonal Changes in Endocrine Function in Male Mammals

European badger *(Meles meles)*—In these spring-breeding carnivores, plasma LH levels are maximal in January and February, and plasma testosterone and testes size are maximal in winter and spring, with prominent plasma testosterone peaks during the night; PRL reaches maximum levels in the summer and thyroxine reaches maximum levels in summer and fall.[10,190,191]

Red fox *(Vulpes vulpes)*—Plasma LH levels are maximal between November and February, coinciding with the winter increase in plasma testosterone levels and testes size; PRL and thyroxine levels are maximal in the spring and reduced in the fall;[190,191] similar to other seasonally breeding mammals, testicular capillary blood flow is maximal during the breeding season.[136]

Blue fox *(Alopex lagopus)*—Plasma testosterone levels are maximal during the breeding season in March and April.[4]

Domestic dog *(Canis familiaris)*—In a group of laboratory-housed mongrel dogs there was a sharp peak of plasma testosterone in August and September.[90]

Masked civet cat *(Paguma larvata)*—Testicular production of testosterone *in vitro* was increased before and during the breeding season, which in this species occurs in May and June, and coincided with depletion of interstitial lipid cells.[328]

Black bear *(Ursus americanus)*—Testosterone levels are lowest in August and September and highest in May and June after a gradual increase during hibernation.[194]

Ungulates

White-tailed deer *(Odocoileus virginianus)*—Increases in plasma levels of LH, FSH, and testosterone occur in late summer before the onset of breeding season; PRL levels are highest in May and June and lowest between November and January; pinealectomy prevents the spring increase in plasma PRL, advances the autumnal increase in plasma LH, and disrupts normal temporal relationships between cycle of plasma PRL, plasma testosterone, and antler growth.[201,239,276,289]

Red deer *(Cervus elaphus)*—Breeding season is in the fall and the pituitary-testicular axis becomes activated in the summer with highest plasma LH in August and testosterone in September through October; seasonal increase in pituitary responsiveness to LHRH precedes the increase in testicular response to LH; subcutaneous melatonin implants in the spring advanced antler development, increase in plasma testosterone, and onset of rutting.[175,176]

Reindeer *(Rangifer tarandus)*—Rutting season extends from August to October and is associated with increases in testosterone plasma levels and production rate; metabolic clearance rate of testosterone is reduced, presumably reflecting increased binding to plasma proteins.[353] The magnitude of seasonal increase in plasma testosterone and testes size increased with age, correlating with earlier onset of rutting behavior in older bulls and their higher position in the social hierarchy during rut.[159]

Roe deer *(Capreolus capreolus)*—In this small European deer, rutting season occurs in midsummer, i.e., earlier than in other cervids; plasma LH increases between April and July, plasma PRL between March and June, plasma FSH in March, and plasma testosterone between March and July with precipitous decline thereafter.[272,279]

Pigmy goat *(Capra hircus)*—Baseline levels of LH and testosterone and frequency of their peaks began to increase in late summer and highest serum LH and testosterone levels were recorded in October; highest levels of FSH were recorded in April, while changes in PRL paralleled changes in day length.[206]

Domestic cattle *(Bos taurus)*—In both sexes, serum PRL levels are increased by long photoperiods and suppressed by short photoperiods; PRL levels are influenced also by ambient temperature, with high temperatures being stimulatory and low temperatures inhibitory;[99,255,273,331] exposure of bulls to elevated temperatures (35.5°C) caused a transient suppression of plasma testosterone levels.

European wild boar *(Sus scrofa)*—Concentrations of testosterone, estrogens, and 5α-androst-16-en-3-one ("boar taint" steroid) in the seminal plasma are greatly elevated between October and December, i.e., during the rutting season;[275] serum PRL shows a clear seasonal rhythm, with maximal values in June.[244]

Domestic pig *(Sus scrofa domestica)*—Androgen and estrogen levels in peripheral blood plasma and in semen exhibit wide seasonal fluctuations, with highest values between October and December,[63] while serum PRL does not vary with season;[244] supplemental lighting accelerated development of sexual behavior in maturing boars.[31,123]

Domestic horse *(Equus caballus)*—Breeding season is in the summer and is accompanied by elevations in plasma LH and FSH levels, testicular weight, frequency, and amplitude of testosterone pulses and semen volume;[49,137] exposure to long photoperiod in the winter causes earlier increase in plasma LH and increased plasma testosterone levels and male libido.[323]

One-humped camel *(Camelus dromedarius)*—Plasma testosterone levels are maximal between January and April, corresponding to behavioral changes in males and occurrence of estrus in females.[361]

TABLE 1 (continued)
Seasonal Changes in Endocrine Function in Male Mammals

Asiatic elephant *(Elephas maximus)*—Impressive increases in plasma testosterone occur in adult males during "musth," a period of increased aggressiveness and sexual activity.[134]

[a] For extensive review of reproductive patterns in hibernating and nonhibernating bats, and seasonal changes in the function of pituitary gonadal function in these animals, the reader is referred to material from a symposium on comparative aspects of reproduction in Chiroptera.[117]

[b] Environmentally controlled seasonal changes in male neuroendocrine function in the golden hamster, the Djungarian hamster, the white-footed mouse, and the deer mouse are discussed in detail elsewhere in this chapter.

Rainfall

Rainfall is an important factor controlling food availability, and thus indirectly controls the reproductive activity of some species.[42] Thus, areas in which rainfall is seasonal are often associated with determinate breeding seasons which can sometimes be extended by unusually high or unseasonal rainfall. Some desert rodent species are capable of breeding throughout the year, which allows them to take advantage of irregular and sporadic periods of rainfall and food availability.

Humidity

Humidity may affect energy balance and, therefore, reproductive function by affecting thermoregulatory processes. There may also be a more direct effect of humidity on the neuroendocrine system. For example, ovulation induction procedures on caged squirrel monkeys are more successful in low-humidity conditions than in high-humidity conditions.[121] These results are similar to observations in the natural habitat, where mating is associated with the season of low humidity and births occur approximately 170 days later, during the season of high humidity and greater availability of food.

Social Factors

A regulatory mechanism that can adjust the onset or cessation of a breeding season can be a great advantage to a variety of species.[45] A variety of social factors are used to maximize reproductive performance in small short-lived mammals when this is energetically possible and such factors are also used by larger long-lived animals to shorten the reproductive period and to minimize the energetic expenses of reproductive activity.

Pheromones

Environmental stimuli affecting neuroendocrine function include various signals from parents, siblings, and other individuals within the population. These include pheromones, generally airborne chemosignals that exert a variety of powerful effects on behavior, hormone production, and reproductive processes. The chemical nature and physiological significance of pheromones have been studied extensively in insects and other invertebrates, but there is also a substantial amount of information on pheromonal communication in mammals. In the house mouse *(Mus musculus)*, adult males exert a variety of effects on female reproductive function, including acceleration of pubertal development,[343] induction of estrus in adult females (the "Whitten effect"[356]), and resorption of embryos in females recently inseminated by another male (the "Bruce effect"[48]). These effects do not require physical contact between the animals and can be produced by exposure of the females to cages or bedding soiled by the males or by placing them "downwind" from cages containing males.[46,79,356] There is also evidence that these diverse effects may have a common physiological mechanism; namely, stimulation of gonadotropin release from the female pituitary leading to development of ovarian follicles, increase in estrogen titers, estrus, and ovulation.[47] Female mice produce pheromones that delay puberty, suppress estrous cyclicity of other females, and accelerate pubertal development of males.[79,341] These effects were discovered in various laboratory strains of house mice, but occur also in wild *M. musculus* and their laboratory descendants, as well as in other rodent species.[30,79] Bronson[46] proposed an interesting hypothesis relating these pheromonal effects to ecology and behavior of small rodents in their natural habitat. In some rodent species, high population density stimulates migration in search of new habitats. Under these conditions, pubertal development of "resident" juvenile females would be suppressed by pheromones from adult females, and the young animals migrating from the densely populated area into another territory would be induced to mature and ovulate in response to pheromones from adult males. Clearly, pheromonal control of reproductive development and function can optimize the chances for successful reproduction in short-living animals.

Pheromonal communication is not limited to rodents, as exemplified by the ability of rams to hasten and synchronize the onset of ovulatory cycles in ewes at the beginning of the breeding season.[185,221,274]

Pheromones also play a role in mediating the acute effects of a female on the pituitary function in the male. Olfactory and visual stimuli originating from female conspecifics stimulate release of LH, and in some species also PRL, from the male's pituitary. These effects occur within minutes after exposure to a female and are followed by elevations in peripheral testosterone levels. Female-induced acute elevations of plasma LH and/or testosterone levels have been detected in numerous species, including mice,[182] rats,[117b,146,295c] hamsters,[183] rabbits,[118] cattle,[148] and monkeys.[262] The mechanism(s) for these acute endocrine responses to female conspecifics have not been fully elucidated, but Dluzen et al.[76] reported an increase in LHRH levels and a decrease in NE levels in the posterior olfactory lobes of male voles after exposure to female urine. We have demonstrated that ME NE turnover increases prior to a female-induced rise of LH in male rats.[117b,295c] Furthermore, there is no female-induced change in ME NE turnover in hyperprolactinemic or diabetic males, in which female exposure does not induce an increase in LH or testosterone levels.[117b,295c] It has also been demonstrated that exposure to sexually receptive females or cages soiled by these females significantly enhanced testicular recrudescence in male hamsters transferred from SD to LD conditions.[342]

The biological significance of female-induced surges of LH is unknown, but a role of the resulting increase of testosterone production in the control of male sexual behavior and pheromone secretion has been suggested.[183] We have indirect evidence that sexual arousal in the male increases release of hypothalamic LHRH leading to a surge of LH and perhaps also to stimulation of copulatory behavior via direct effects of this neuropeptide in the brain.[278,295c]

Stress

The stress response is the nonspecific reaction of the body to a "noxious" stimulus or demand.[280] As first put forth by Selye,[280] an animal reacts to a stressor with a generalized alarm reaction followed by a period of adaptation and a return to a normal physiologic state or to exhaustion and death if the stress is not relieved. The endocrine responses to stress have been extensively studied and, in general, include an increased release of catabolic hormones such as the glucocorticoids (stimulated by adrenocorticotropic hormone [ACTH] release), catecholamines, thyroid hormones (stimulated by thyroid-stimulating hormone [TSH] release), and growth hormone.[242] Anabolic hormones such as testosterone and insulin are generally suppressed by stress.

The reproductive system is often adversely affected by stress, but these effects vary greatly due to sex and age and can also be modified by various social factors.[242] Reproductive hormones such as LH, PRL, and testosterone are usually much more affected than FSH, and although changes in adrenal and thyroid function can affect the secretion of these reproductive hormones, there appear to be other mediators of the stress response. A detailed study of these responses can tell us a great deal about the control of the neuroendocrine axis, but a more complete discussion of the stress response is beyond the scope of this chapter and the interested reader is referred to several recent reviews on the subject.[61,242]

Population Density

There is a considerable amount of literature on the effects of stress of overcrowding on physiologic functions, including, most dramatically, the effect on reproduction. For example, as the population density of a large cage of house mice increases, there is a dramatic inhibition of sexual maturation in the young and a cessation of reproduction by many of the adults.[60] A similar phenomenon has also been described in deer mice, where, under conditions of high population density, a large proportion of a population may never achieve fertility.[319] These responses could be very important for the control of population numbers under natural conditions by preventing the increase in the number of animals beyond the carrying capacity of their environment. The mechanisms responsible for density-dependent modifications of the age of puberty; fertility; reproductive, parental, agonistic, and cannibalistic behavior; and survival of the young are not well understood, but a role for the ACTH-adrenal axis and for endogenous opiates has been suggested.[59]

ACKNOWLEDGMENTS

Work from the authors' labs has been supported by NIH (HD 20033) and NSF (DCB-8619702). We wish to thank many colleagues for valuable discussions and apologize to those whose work related to this subject has been inadvertently omitted or could not be discussed due to limitations of space.

REFERENCES

1. **Albers, H. E., Moline, M. L., and Moore-Ede, M. C.,** Sex differences in circadian control of LH secretion, *J. Endocrinol.,* 100, 101, 1984.
2. **Amirat, Z. and Brudieux, R.,** Seasonal changes in the metabolic clearance rate of cortisol in the adult male sand rat (Psammomys obesus), *Gen. Comp. Endocrinol.,* 53, 232, 1984.
3. **Ammar-Kodja, F. and Brudieux, R.,** Seasonal variations in the cyclic luteal ovarian activity in the Tadmit ewe in Algeria, *J. Reprod. Fertil.,* 65, 305, 1982.
4. **Andersen, K.,** Seasonal change in fine structure and function of Leydig cells in the blue fox (*Alopex lagopus*), *Int. J. Androl.,* 1, 424, 1978.
5. **Arbogast, L. A. and Ben-Jonathan, N.,** The preovulatory prolactin surge is prolonged by a progesterone-dependent dopaminergic mechanism, *Endocrinology,* 126, 246, 1990.
6. **Arendt, J., Symons, A. M., Laud, C. A., and Pryole, S. J.,** Melatonin can induce early onset of the breeding season in ewes, *J. Endocrinol.,* 97, 395, 1983.
7. **Arendt, J., Wirz-Justice, A., Brundtke, J., and Kornemark, M.,** Long-term studies on immunoreactive human melatonin, *Ann. Clin. Biochem.,* 16, 307, 1979.
8. **Attanasio, A., Borrelli, P., Marini, R., Cambiaso, P., Cappa, M., and Gupta, D.,** Serum melatonin in children with early and delayed puberty, *Neuroendocrinol. Lett.,* 5, 387, 1983.
9. **Audy, M. C.,** Endocrinologie—variations saisonnieres de la testosterone plasmatique chez la Fouine (Martes foina Erx.), *C.R. Acad. Sci. Paris Ser. D,* 287, 721, 1978.
10. **Audy, M. C.,** Physiologie animale—variations saisonnieres du rythme nycthemeral de la testosterone plasmatique chez le Blaireua europeen Meles meles L., *C.R. Acad. Sci. Paris Ser. D,* 291, 291, 1980.
11. **Baker, J. R.,** The evolution of breeding seasons, in *Evolution: Essays on Aspects of Evolutionary Biology,* de Beer, G. R., Ed., Oxford University Press, London, 1938, 161.
12. **Barenton, B. and Pelletier, J.,** Prolactin, testicular growth and LH receptors in the ram following light and 2-bromo-ergocryptine (CB-154) treatments, *Biol. Reprod.,* 22, 781, 1980.

13. **Barrell, G. K. and Lapwood, K. R.,** Effects of pinealectomy on the secretion of luteinizing hormone, testosterone and prolactin in rams exposed to various lighting regimes, *J. Endocrinol.*, 80, 397, 1979.

14. **Bartke, A. and Chang, M. C.,** Seasonal variation in male gonadal function in a laboratory population of Peromyscus leucopus, *Am. Midl. Nat.*, 89, 490, 1973.

15. **Bartke, A., Goldman, B. D., Klemcke, H. G., Bex, F. J., and Amador, A. G.,** Effects of photoperiod on pituitary and testicular function in seasonally breeding species, in *Functional Correlates of Hormone Receptors in Reproduction,* Mahesh, V., Muldoon, T, Saxena, B., and Sadler, W., Eds., Elsevier, New York, 1980, 171.

16. **Bartke, A., Siler-Khodr, T. M., Hogan, M. P., and Roychoudhury, P.,** Ectopic pituitary transplants stimulate synthesis and release of FSH in golden hamsters, *Endocrinology*, 108, 133, 1981.

17. **Bartke, A., Matt, K. S., Siler-Khodr, T. M., Soares, M. J., Talamantes, F., Goldman, B. D., Hogan, M. P., and Hebert, A.,** Does prolactin modify testosterone feedback in the hamster? Pituitary grafts alter the ability of testosterone to suppress luteinizing hormone and follicle-stimulating hormone release in castrated male hamsters, *Endocrinology*, 115, 1506, 1984.

18. **Bartke, A., Matt, K. S., Steger, R. W., Clayton, R. N., Chandrashekar, V., and Smith, M. S.,** Role of prolactin in the regulation of sensitivity of the hypothalamic-pituitary system to steroid feedback, in *Regulation of Ovarian and Testicular Function*, Mahesh, V. B., Dhindsa, D. S., Anderson, E., and Kalra, S. P., Eds., Plenum Press, New York, 1987, 153.

19. **Bartke, A. and Steger, R. W.,** Seasonal changes in the function of the hypothalamic-pituitary-testicular axis in the Syrian hamster, *Proc. Soc. Exp. Biol. Med.*, 199, 139, 1992.

21. **Bast, J. D. and Greenwald, G. S.,** Serum profiles of follicle-stimulating hormone, luteinizing hormone and prolactin during the estrous cycle of the hamster, *Endocrinology*, 94, 1295, 1974.

22. **Baum, M. J. and Schretlen, P. J. M.,** Cytoplasmic binding of oestradiol-17B in several brain regions, pituitary and uterus of ferrets ovariectomized while in or out of oestrus, *J. Reprod. Fertil.*, 55, 317, 1979.

23. **Baum, M. J. and Schretlen, P. J. M.,** Oestrogenic induction of sexual behavior in ovariectomized ferrets under short or long photoperiods, *J. Endocrinol.*, 78, 295, 1978.

24. **Beasleg, L. J. and Zucker, I.,** Photoperiod influences the annual reproductive cycle of the male pallid bat (Antrozous pallidus), *J. Reprod. Fertil.*, 70, 567, 1984.

25. **Beck, W. and Wuttke, W.,** Annual rhythms of luteinizing hormone, follicle-stimulating hormone, prolactin and testosterone in the serum of male rhesus monkeys, *J. Endocrinol.*, 83, 131, 1979.

26. **Ben-Jonathan, N., Arbogast, L. A., and Hyde, J. F.,** Neuroendocrine regulation of prolactin release, *Prog. Neurobiol.*, 33, 399, 1989.

27. **Ben-Jonathan, N. and Liu, J.-W.,** Pituitary lactotrophs: endocrine, paracrine, juxtacrine, and autocrine interactions, *Trends Endocrinol. Metab.*, 3, 254, 1992.

28. **Bennett, J. W. and Abroms, K. J.,** Gametogenesis and incidence of Down syndrome, *Lancet*, 2, 913, 1979.

29. **Benson, B.,** Temporal changes in medial basal hypothalamic catecholamines in male Syrian hamsters exposed to short photoperiod, *Exp. Brain Res.*, 65, 371, 1987.

30. **Berger, H. G., Baker, H. W. C., Hudson, B., and Pinkus-Tast, H.,** Gonadotrophic and gonadal function in the normal adult mouse, in *Gonadotropins*, Saxena, B. B., Berling, C. C., and Gandi, H. M., Eds., Interscience, New York, 1972, 569.

31. **Berger, T., Mahone, P., Svoboda, G. S., Metz, K. W., and Clegg, E. D.,** Sexual maturation of boars and growth of swine exposed to extended photoperiod during decreasing natural photoperiod, *J. Anim. Sci.,* 51, 672, 1980.

32. **Berndtson, W. E. and Desjardins, C.,** Circulating LH and FSH levels and testicular function in hamsters during light deprivation and subsequent photoperiodic stimulation, *Endocrinology*, 95, 195, 1974.

33. **Bernstein, I. S., Gordon, E. P., Rose, R. M., and Peterson, M. S.,** Influences of sexual and social stimuli upon circulating levels of testosterone in male pigtail macaques, *Behav. Biol.*, 24, 400, 1978.

34. **Bex, F. J., Bartke, A., Goldman, B. D., and Dalterio, S.,** Prolactin, growth hormone, luteinizing hormone receptors, and seasonal changes in testicular activity in the golden hamster, *Endocrinology*, 103, 2069, 1978.

35. **Bielert, C., Howard-Tripp, M. E., and Van der Walt, L. A.,** Environmental and social factors influencing seminal emission in chacma baboons (Papio ursinus), *Psychoneuroendocrinology*, 5, 287, 1980.

36. **Bittman, E. L., Goldman, B. D., and Zucker, I.,** Testicular responses to melatonin are altered by lesions of the suprachiasmatic nucleus in golden hamster, *Biol. Reprod.*, 21, 647, 1979.

37. **Bittman, E. L., Jonassen, J. A., and Hegarty, C. M.,** Photoperiodic regulation of pulsatile luteinizing hormone secretion and adenohypophyseal gene expression in female golden hamsters, *Biol. Reprod.*, 47, 66, 1992.

38. **Bittman, E. L. and Karsch, F. J.,** Nightly duration of pineal melatonin secretion determines the reproduction response to inhibitory day length in the ewe, *Biol. Reprod.,* 30, 585, 1984.

39. **Blank, J. L. and Desjardins, C.,** Differential effects of food restriction on pituitary-testicular function in mice, *Am. J. Physiol.*, 248, R181, 1985.

40. **Boissin-Agasse, L., Boissin, J., and Ortavant, R.,** Circadian photosensitive phase as photoperiodic control of testis activity in the mink (*Mustela vison*), a short-day mammal, *Biol. Reprod.*, 26, 110, 1982.

41. **Brann, D. W. and Mahesh, V. B.,** Excitatory amino acids: function and significance in reproduction and neuroendocrine regulation, *Front. Neuroendocrinol.*, 15, 1, 1994.

42. **Breed, W. G.,** Reproduction of the Australian hopping mouse *Notomys alexis* and other bipedal desert rodents, in *Environmental Factors in Mammal Reproduction*, Gilmore, D. and Cook, B., Eds., Macmillan, New York, 1981, 186.

43. **Bridges, R. S. and Goldman, B. D.,** Diurnal rhythms in gonadotropins and progesterone in lactating and photoperiod induced acyclic hamsters, *Biol. Reprod.*, 13, 616, 1975.

44. **Brodie, B. B., Costa, E., Dlabac, A., Nef, H., and Smooker, H. H.,** Application of steady state kinetics to the estimation and synthesis of rate and turnover time of tissue catecholamines, *J. Pharmacol. Exp. Ther.*, 154, 493, 1966.

45. **Bronson, F. H.,** Mammalian reproduction: an ecological perspective, *Biol. Reprod.*, 32, 1 1985.

46. **Bronson, F. H.,** The reproductive ecology of the house mouse, *Q. Rev. Biol.*, 54, 265, 1979.

47. **Bronson, F. H.,** Serum FSH, LH, and prolactin in adult ovariectomized mice bearing silastic implants of estradiol: responses to social cues, *Biol. Reprod.*, 15, 147, 1976.

48. **Bruce, H. M.,** Effect of castration on the reproductive pheromones of male mice, *J. Reprod. Fertil.*, 10, 141, 1965.

49. **Byers, S. W., Dorsett, K. F., and Abner, T. D.,** Seasonal and circadian changes of testosterone levels in the peripheral blood plasma of stallions and their relation to semen quality, *J. Endocrinol.*, 99, 141, 1983.

50. **Cardinali, D. P.,** Melatonin: a mammalian pineal hormone, *Endocr. Rev.*, 2, 327, 1981.

51. **Cardinali, D. P., Vacas, M. I., and Estevez Boyer, E.,** Specific binding of melatonin in bovine brain, *Endocrinology*, 103, 437, 1979.

52. **Carrillo, A. J., Goldman, B. D., and Bartke, A.,** Hypothalamic deafferentation inhibits the stimulatory influence of prolactin on follicle-stimulating hormone release in the golden hamster, *Endocrinology*, 114, 87, 1984.

53. **Carter, D. S. and Goldman, B. D.,** Antigonadal effects of timed melatonin infusion in pinealectomized male Djungarian hamsters (Phodopus sungorus sungorus): duration is the critical parameter, *Endocrinology*, 113, 1261, 1983.

54. **Carter, D. S. and Goldman, B. D.,** Progonadal role of the pineal in the Djungarian hamster (Phodopus sungorus sungorus): mediation by melatonin, *Endocrinology*, 113, 1268, 1983.

55. **Carter, D. S., Herbert, J., and Stacey, P. M.,** Modulation of gonadal activity by timed injections of melatonin in pinealectomized or intact ferrets kept under two photoperiods, *J. Endocrinol.*, 93, 211, 1982.

56. **Charlton, H. M., Grocock, C. A., and Ostberg, A.,** The effects of pinealectomy and superior cervical ganglionectomy on the testis of the vole, Microtus agrestis, *J. Reprod. Fertil.*, 48, 377, 1976.

57. **Chen, L. and Meites, J.,** Effects of estrogen and progesterone on serum and pituitary prolactin levels in ovariectomized rats, *J. Endocrinol.*, 86, 503, 1970.

58. **Chen, H. J., Targovnik, J., McMillan, L. and Randall, S.,** Age differences in endogenous opiate modulation of short photoperiod-induced testicular regression in golden hamsters, *J. Endocrinol.*, 101, 1, 1984.

59. **Christian, J. J.,** Social subordination, population density and mammalian evolution, *Science*, 168, 84, 1970.

60. **Christian, J. J. and Davis, D. E.,** Endocrines, behavior and population, *Science*, 145, 1550, 1964.

61. **Christian, J. J., Lloyd, J. A., and Davis, D. E.,** The role of endocrines in the self-regulation of mammalian populations, *Recent Prog. Horm. Res.*, 21, 501, 1965.

62. **Clarke, J., Burman, K., Funder, J. W., and Findlay, J. K.,** Estrogen receptors in the neuroendocrine tissues of the ewe in relation to breed, season, and stage of the estrous cycle, *Biol. Reprod.*, 24, 323, 1981.

63. **Claus, R., Schopper, D., and Wagner, H.-G.,** Seasonal effect on steroids in blood plasma and seminal plasma of boars, *J. Steroid Biochem.*, 19, 725, 1983.

64. **Clayton, R. N. and Catt, K. S.,** Gonadotropin-releasing hormone receptors: characterization, physiological regulation, and relationship to reproductive function, *Endocr. Rev.*, 2, 186, 1981.

65. **Colwell, C. S., Max, M., Hudson, D., and Menaker, M.,** Excitatory amino acid receptors may mediate the effects of light on the reproductive system of the golden hamster, *Biol. Reprod.*, 44, 604, 1991.

66. **Craven, R. P. and Clarke, J. R.,** Gonadotrophin levels in male voles (Microtus agrestis) reared in long and short photoperiods, *J. Reprod. Fertil.*, 66, 709, 1982.

67. **Czekala, N. M., Hodges, J. K., Gause, G. E., and Lasley, B. L.,** Annual circulating testosterone levels in captive and free-ranging male armadillos (Dasypus novemcinctus), *J. Reprod. Fertil.*, 59, 199, 1980.

68. **Czyba, J. C., Pinatel, M. C., and Souchier, C.,** Variations saisonnieres dans la composition cellulaire du sperme humain, *Sem. Hop.*, 55, 596, 1979.

69. **Dacheux, J. L., Pisselet, C., Blanc, M. R., Hocheresan-de-Reviers, M. T., and Canrot, M.,** Seasonal variations in rete testis fluid secretion and sperm production in different breeds of ram, *J. Reprod. Fertil.*, 61, 363, 1981.

70. **Damassa, D. S. and Gustafson, A. W.,** Control of plasma sex steroid-binding protein (SBP) in the little brown bat: effects of photoperiod and orchiectomy on the induction of SBP in immature males, *Endocrinology*, 115, 2355, 1984.

71. **Dark, J., Johnston, P. G., Healy, M., and Zucker, I.,** Latitude of origin influences photoperiodic control of reproduction of deer mice (Peromyscus maniculatus), *Biol. Reprod.*, 28, 213, 1983.

72. **Darrow, J. M., Davis, F. C., Elliott, J. A., Stetson, M. H., Turek, V. W., and Menaker, M.,** Influence of photoperiod on reproductive development in the golden hamster, *Biol. Reprod.*, 22, 443, 1980.

73. **Davis, G. J. and Meyer, R. K.,** Seasonal variation in LH and FSH of bilaterally castrated snowshoe hares, *Gen. Comp. Endocrinol.*, 20, 61, 1973.

74. **Desjardins, C. and Lopez, M. J.,** Environmental cues evoke differential responses in pituitary-testicular function in deer mice, *Endocrinology*, 112, 1398, 1983.

75. **Deslypere, J. P., DeBiscop, G., and Vermuelen, A.,** Seasonal variation of plasma dehydroepiandrosterone sulphate and urinary androgen excretion in post-menopausal women, *Clin. Endocrinol.*, 18, 25, 1983.

76. **Dluzen, D. E., Ramirez, V. D., Carter, C. S., and Getz, L. L.,** Male vole urine changes luteinizing hormone-releasing hormone and norepinephrine in female olfactory bulb, *Science*, 212, 573, 1981.

77. **D'Occhio, M. J., Schanbacher, B. D., and Kinder, J. E.,** Profiles of luteinizing hormone, follicle-stimulating hormone, testosterone and prolactin in rams of diverse breeds: effects of contrasting short (8L:16D) and long (16L:8D) photoperiods, *Biol. Reprod.*, 30, 1039, 1984.

78. **Donham, R. S., DiPinto, M. N., and Stetson, M. H.,** Twenty four-hour rhythm of gonadotropin release induces cyclic progesterone secretion by the ovary of prepubertal and adult golden hamsters, *Endocrinology*, 114, 821, 1984.

79. **Drickamer, L. C.,** Pheromones, social influences and population regulation in rodents, in *Environmental Factors in Mammal Reproduction*, Gilmore, D. and Cook, B., Eds., University Park Press, Baltimore, 1981, 100.

80. **Duncan, M. J., Takahashi, J. S., and Dubocovich, M. L.,** 2-[125-I]-iodomelatonin binding sites in hamster brain membranes: pharmacological characteristics and regional distribution, *Endocrinology*, 122, 1825, 1988.

81. **DuMond, F. and Hutchison, T. C.,** Squirrel monkey reproduction: the 'fatted' male phenomenon and seasonal spermatogenesis, *Science*, 158, 1067, 1967.

82. **Earnest, D. J. and Turek, F. W.,** Role for acetylcholine in mediating effects of light on reproduction, *Science*, 219, 77, 1983.

83. **Ellerkmann, E., Nagy, G. M., and Frawley, L. S.,** Rapid augmentation of prolactin cell number and secretory capacity by an estrogen-induced factor released from the neurointermediate lobe, *Endocrinology*, 129, 838, 1991.

84. **Elliott, J. A.,** Circadian rhythms and photoperiodic time measurement in mammals, *Fed. Proc.*, 35, 2339, 1976.

85. **Ellis, G. B. and Turek, F. W.,** Time course of the photoperiod-induced change in sensitivity of the hypothalamic-pituitary axis to testosterone feedback in castrated male hamsters, *Endocrinology*, 104, 625, 1979.

86. **Ellis, L. C. and Balph, D. F.,** Age and seasonal differences in the synthesis and metabolism of testosterone by testicular tissue and pineal HIOMT activity of uinta ground squirrels (Spermophilus armatus), *Gen. Comp. Endocrinol.*, 28, 42, 1976.

87. **Erskine, M. S. and Baum, M. J.,** Plasma concentrations of testosterone and dihydrotestosterone during prenatal development in male and female ferrets, *Endocrinology*, 111, 767, 1982.

88. **Eskes, G. A., Wilkinson, M., and Bhanot, R.,** Short day exposure eliminates the LH response to naloxone in golden hamsters, *Neuroendocrinology* 39, 281, 1984.

89. **Eskes, G. A., Wilkinson, M., Moger, W. H., and Rusak, B.,** Periventricular and suprachiasmatic lesion effects on photoperiodic responses of the hamster hypophyseal-gonadal axis, *Biol. Reprod.*, 30, 1073, 1984.

90. **Falvo, R. E., DePalatis, L. R., Moore, J., Kepic, T. A., and Miller, J.,** Annual variations in plasma levels of testosterone and luteinizing hormone in the laboratory male mongrel dog, *J. Endocrinol.*, 86, 425, 1980.

91. **Fatranska, M., Repcekova-Jezova, D., Jurcovicova, J., and Vigas, M.,** LH and testosterone response to LH-RH in blind men, *Horm. Metab. Res.*, 10, 82, 1978.

92. **Ferraro, J. S. and Steger, R. W.,** Diurnal variations in brain serotonin are driven by the photic cycle and are not circadian in nature, *Brain Res.*, 512, 121, 1990.

93. **Frantz, A. G.,** Prolactin, in *Endocrinology*, Vol. 1, DeGroot, L. J., Ed., Grune & Stratton, New York, 1979, 153.

94. **Frawley, L. S.,** Role of the hypophyseal neurointermediate lobe in the dynamic release of prolactin, *Trends Endocrinol. Metab.*, 5, 107, 1994.

95. **Frost, D. and Zucker, I.,** Photoperiod and melatonin influence seasonal gonadal cycles in the grasshopper mouse (Onychomys leucogaster), *J. Reprod. Fertil.*, 69, 237, 1983.

96. **Gaston, S. and Menaker, M.,** Photoperiodic control of hamster testis, *Science*, 158, 925, 1967.

97. **Gauer, F., Masson-Pevet, M., Stehle, J., and Pevet, P.,** Daily variations in melatonin receptor density of rat pars tuberalis and suprachiasmatic nuclei are distinctly regulated, *Brain Res.*, 641, 92, 1994.

98. **Gauer, F., Masson-Pévet, M., Skene, D. J., Vivien-Roels, B., and Pévet, P.,** Daily rhythms of melatonin binding sites in the rat pars tuberalis and suprachiasmatic nuclei: evidence for a regulation of melatonin receptors by melatonin itself, *Neuroendocrinology,* 57, 120, 1993.

99. **Gauthier, D. and Berbigier, P.,** The influence of nutritional levels and shade structure on testicular growth and hourly variations of plasma LH and testosterone levels in young Creole bulls in a tropical environment, *Reprod. Nutr. Dev.,* 22, 793, 1982.

100. **Gayrard, V., Malpaux, B., and Thiéry, J. C.,** Oestradiol increases the extracellular levels of amine metabolites in the ewe hypothalamus during anoestrus: a microdialysis study, *J. Endocrinol.,* 135, 421, 1992.

101. **Gayrard, V., Malpaux, B., Tillet, Y., and Thiéry, J. C.,** Estradiol increases tyrosine hydroxylase activity of the A15 nucleus dopaminergic neurons during long days in the ewe, *Biol. Reprod.,* 50, 1168, 1994.

102. **Giguere, V., Meunier, H., Veillieux, R., and Labrie, F.,** Direct effects of sex steroids on prolactin release at the anterior pituitary level: interactions with dopamine, thyrotropin-releasing hormone, and iso-butyl-methylxanthine, *Endocrinology,* 111, 857, 1982

103. **Gilmore, D. P.,** Seasonal reproductive periodicity in the male Australian brush-tailed possum (Trichosurus vulpecula), *J. Zool.,* 157, 75, 1969.

104. **Glass, J. D. and Lynch, G. R.,** Diurnal rhythm of response to chronic intrahypothalamic melatonin injections in the white-footed mouse, Peromyscus leucopus, *Neuroendocrinology,* 35, 117, 1982.

105. **Glass, J. D. and Lynch, G. R.,** Evidence for a brain site of melatonin action in the white-footed mouse, Peromyscus leucopus, *Neuroendocrinology,* 34, 1, 1982.

106. **Glover, T. D.,** The place of the seasonal breeder in research on male reproduction, *Adv. Biosci.,* 10, 235, 1972.

107. **Goldman, B. D., Matt, K. S., Rouchoudhury, P., and Stetson, M. H.,** Prolactin release in golden hamsters: photoperiod and gonadal influences, *Biol. Reprod.,* 24, 287, 1981.

108. **Goldsmith, A. R. and Nicholls, T. J.,** Prolactin is associated with the development of photorefractoriness in intact, castrated and testosterone-implanted starlings, *Cen. Comp. Endocrinol.,* 54, 247, 1984.

109. **Goncharov, N. P., Taradyan, D. S., Powell, J. E., and Stevens, V. C.,** Levels of adrenal and gonadal hormones in rhesus monkeys during chronic hypokinesia, *Endocrinology,* 111, 129, 1984.

110. **Goodman, R. L.,** Functional organization of the catecholaminergic neural system inhibiting luteinzing hormone secretion in the anestrous ewe, *Neuroendocrinology,* 50, 406, 1989.

111. **Gordon, T. P. and Bernstein, I. S.,** Seasonal variation in sexual behavior of all-male rhesus troops, *Am. J. Phys. Anthropol.,* 38, 221, 1973.

112. **Greenwald, G. S.,** Histological transformation of the ovary of the lactating hamster, *Endocrinology,* 77, 641, 1965.

113. **Grocock, C. A.,** Effects of age on photo-induced testicular regression, recrudescence, and refractiveness in the short-tailed field vole Microtus agrestis, *Biol. Reprod.,* 23, 15, 1980.

114. **Groos, G., Mason, R., and Meijer, J.,** Electrical and pharmacological properties of the suprachiasmatic nuclei, *Fed. Proc.,* 42, 2790, 1983.

115. **Gudelsky, G. A.,** Tuberoinfundibular dopamine neurons and the regulation of prolactin secretion, *Psycho-neuroendocrinology,* 6, 3, 1981.

116. **Gudelsky, G. A., Nansel, D. D., and Porter, J. C.,** Role of estrogen in the dopaminergic control of prolactin secretion, *Endocrinology,* 108, 440, 1981.

117. **Gustafson, A. W. and Weir, B. J.,** Comparative aspects of reproduction in Chiroptera, *J. Reprod. Fertil.,* 56, 317, 1979.

117b. **Hails, R., Fadden, C., and Steger, R. W.,** Diabetes disrupts copulatory behavior and neuroendocrine responses of male rats to female conspecifics, *Pharmacol. Biochem. Behav.,* 44, 837, 1993.

118. **Haltmeyer, G. C. and Eik-Nes, K. B.,** Plasma levels of testosterone in male rabbits following copulation, *J. Reprod. Fertil.,* 19, 273, 1969.

119. **Hamburger, C.,** Six years daily 17-ketosteroid determination in one subject: seasonal variation and independence of volume of urine, *Acta Endocrinol.,* 17, 116, 1954.

120. **Harlap, S.,** A time series analysis of the incidence of Down's syndrome in West Jerusalem, *Am. J. Epidemiol.,* 99, 210, 1974.

121. **Harrison, R. M. and Dukelow, W. R.,** Seasonal adaptation of laboratory-maintained monkeys (Saimiri sciureus), *J. Med. Primatol.,* 2, 277, 1973.

122. **Haug, E.,** Progesterone suppression of estrogen-stimulated prolactin secretion and estrogen receptor levels in the rat pituitary, *Endocrinology,* 104, 429, 1979.

123. **Hoagland, T. A. and Diekman, M. A.,** Influence of supplemental lighting during increasing daylength on libido and reproductive hormones in prepubertal boars, *J. Anim. Sci.,* 55, 1483, 1982.

124. **Hoffman, K.,** Effects of short photoperiods on puberty, growth and moult in the Djungarian hamster (Phodopus sungorus), *J. Reprod. Fertil.,* 54, 29, 1978.

125. **Horton, T. H.,** Growth and reproductive development of male Microtus montanus is affected by the prenatal photoperiod, *Biol. Reprod.,* 31, 499, 1984.

126. **Hotchkiss, R. S.,** Factors in stability and variability of semen observations on 640 successive samples from 23 men, *J. Urol.,* 45, 875, 1941.

127. **Howles, C. M., Craigon, J., and Haynes, N. B.,** Long-term rhythms of testicular volume and plasma prolactin concentrations in rams reared for 3 years in constant photoperiod, *J. Reprod. Fertil.,* 65, 439, 1982.

128. **Hui, Y., Hastings, M. H., Maywood, E. S. and Ebling, F. J. P.,** Photoperiodic regulation of glutamatergic stimulation of secretion of luteinizing hormone in male Syrian hamsters, *J. Reprod. Fertil.,* 95, 935, 1992.

129. **Huminski, S.,** Winter breeding in the field vole, Microtus arvalis (Pall.) in the light of an analysis of the effect of environmental factors on the condition of the male sexual apparatus, *Zool. Pol.,* 14, 157, 1963.

130. **Inns, R. W.,** Seasonal changes in the accessory reproductive system and plasma testosterone levels of the male tammar wallaby, Macropus eugenii in the wild, *J. Reprod. Fertil.,* 66, 675, 1982.

131. **Irby, D. C., Kerr, J. B., Risbridger, G. P., and deKretser, D. N.,** Seasonally and experimentally-induced changes in testicular function of the Australian bush rat (Rattus fuscipes), *J. Reprod. Fertil.,* 70, 657, 1984.

132. **Jackson, F. L., Heindel, J. J., Preslock, J. P., and Berkowitz, A. S.,** Alterations in hypothalamic content of luteinizing hormone-releasing hormone associated with pineal-mediated testicular regression in the golden hamster, *Biol. Reprod.,* 31, 436, 1984.

133. **Jackson, F. L., Philo, R. C., Berkowitz, A. S., and Preslock, J. P.,** Luteinizing hormone releasing hormone (LH-RH) response of primary monolayer cultures of pituitary cells from normal and regressed male hamsters, Proc and Abstr. 62nd Annu. Meet. Endocr. Soc., Washington, D.C., June 18 to 20, 1980, A#421, 180.

134. **Jainudeen, M. R., Katongole, C. B., and Short, R. V.,** Plasma testosterone levels in relation to musth and sexual activity in the male Asiatic elephant, Elephas maximus, *J. Reprod. Fertil.,* 29, 99, 1972.

135. **Jallageas, M. and Assenmacher, I.,** Annual plasma testosterone and thyroxine cycles in relation to hibernation in the edible dormouse, Glis glis, *Gen. Comp. Endocrinol.,* 50, 452, 1983.

136. **Joffre, J. and Joffre, M.,** Seasonal changes in the testicular blood flow of seasonally breeding mammals: dormouse, Glis glis, ferret, Mustelafuro, and fox, Vulpes vulpes, *J. Reprod. Fertil.,* 34, 227, 1973.

137. **Johnson, L. and Thompson, D. L., Jr.,** Age-related and seasonal variation in the Sertoli cell population, daily sperm production and serum concentrations of follicle-stimulating hormone, luteinizing hormone and testosterone in stallions, *Biol. Reprod.,* 29, 777, 1983.

138. **Johnston, P. G., Boskes, M., and Zucker, I.,** Photoperiodic inhibition of testicular development is mediated by the pineal gland in white-footed mice, *Biol. Reprod.,* 26, 597, 1982.

139. **Johnston, P. G. and Zucker, I.,** Photoperiodic influences on gonadal development and maintenance in the cotton rat, Sigmodon hispidus, *Biol. Reprod.,* 21, 1, 1979.

140. **Johnston, P. G. and Zucker, I.,** Photoperiodic regulation of the testes of adult white-footed mice (Peromyscus leucopus), *Biol. Reprod.,* 23, 859, 1980.

141. **Jongbloet, P. H.,** Month of birth and gametopathy. An investigation into patients with Down's, Klinefelter's and Turner's syndrome, *Clin. Genet.,* 2, 315, 1971.

142. **Jongbloet, P. H., Bezemer, P. D., Anneke, H. J., Erkelens-Zwets, V., and Theune, J. A.,** Seasonality of anencephalic births and pre-ovulatory overripeness ovopathy, *Chronobiologia,* 9, 273, 1982.

143. **Jorgenson, K. L. and Schwartz, N. B.,** Dynamic pituitary and ovarian changes occurring during the anestrus to estrus transition in the golden hamster, *Endocrinology,* 120, 34, 1987.

144. **Jorgenson, K. L. and Schwartz, N. B.,** Shifts in gonadtropin and steroid levels that precede anestrus in female golden hamsters exposed to short photoperiod, *Biol. Reprod.,* 32, 611, 1985.

145. **Kalra, S. P. and Kalra, P. S.,** Neural regulation of luteinizing hormone secretion in the rat, *Endocr. Rev.,* 4, 311, 1983

146. **Kamel, F., Wright, W. W., Mock, E. J., and Frankel, A. I.,** The influence of mating and related stimuli on plasma levels of luteinizing hormone, follicle stimulating hormone, prolactin and testosterone in the male rat, *Endocrinology,* 101, 421, 1977.

147. **Karsch, F. J., Dahl, G. E., Evans, N. P., et al.,** Seasonal changes in gonadotropin-releasing hormone secretion in the ewe: Alteration in response to the negative feedback action of estradiol, *Biol. Reprod.,* 49, 1377, 1993.

148. **Katongole, C. B., Naftolin, F., and Short, R. V.,** Relationship between blood levels of luteinizing hormone and testosterone in bulls, and the effects of sexual stimulation, *J. Endocrinol.,* 50, 457, 1971.

149. **Kenagy, G. J. and Barnes, B. M.,** Environmental and endogenous control of reproductive function in the Great Basin pocket mouse Perognathus parvus, *Biol. Reprod.,* 31, 637, 1984.

150. **Kenagy, G. J. and Bartholomew, G. A.,** Effects of day length and endogenous control on the annual reproductive cycle of the antelope ground squirrel, Ammospermophilus leucurus, *J. Comp. Physiol.,* 130 131, 1979.

151. **Khammar, F. and Brudieux, R.,** Seasonal changes in testicular contents of testosterone and androstenedione and in the metabolic clearance rate of testosterone in the sand rat (Psammomys obesus), *J. Reprod. Fertil.,* 71, 235, 1984.

152. **King, T. S., Steger, R. W., and Morgan, W. W.,** Effect of hypophysectomy and subsequent prolactin administration on hypothalamic 5-hydroxytryptamine synthesis in ovariectomized rats, *Endocrinology,* 116, 485, 1985.

153. **Kirby, J. D., Jetton, A. E., Ackland, J. F., Turek, F. W, and Schwartz, N. B.,** Changes in serum immunoreactive inhibin-α during photoperiod-induced testicular regression and recrudesence in the golden hamster, *Biol. Reprod.,* 49, 483, 1993.

154. **Klemcke, H. G., Bartke, A., and Borer, K. T.,** Regulation of testicular prolactin and luteinizing hormone receptors in golden hamsters, *Endocrinology,* 114, 594, 1984.

155. **Krause, D. N. and Dubocovich, M. L.,** Melatonin receptors, *Annu. Rev. Pharmacol. Toxicol.,* 31, 549, 568, 1991.

156. **Kumar, M. S. A., Chen, C. L., Besch, E. L., Simpkins, J. W., and Estes, K. S.,** Altered hypothalamic dopamine depletion rate and LHRH content in noncyclic hamsters, *Brain Res. Bull.,* 8, 33, 1982.

157. **Kummer, H.,** *Social Organization of Hamadryas Baboons,* University of Chicago Press, Chicago, 1968.

158. **Land, R. B., Carr, W. R., and Thompson, R.,** Genetic and environmental variation in the LH response of ovariectomized sheep to LH-RH, *J. Reprod. Fertil.,* 56, 243, 1979.

159. **Leader-Williams, N.,** Age-related changes in the testicular and antler cycles of reindeer, Rangifer tarandus, *J. Reprod. Fertil.,* 57, 117, 1979.

160. **Lecyk, M.,** The effect of the length of daylight on reproduction in the field vole (Microtus arvalis Pall.), *Zool. Pol.,* 12, 189, 1962.

161. **Lecyk, M.,** The effect of short daylight on sexual maturation in young individuals of the vole, Microtus arvalis Pall., *Zool. Pol.,* 13, 77, 1963.

162. **Legan, S. J. and Karsch, F. J.,** Importance of retinal photoreceptors to the photoperiodic control of seasonal breeding in the ewe, *Biol. Reprod.,* 29, 316, 1983.

163. **Legan, S. J. and Karsch, F. J.,** Photoperiodic control of seasonal breeding in ewes: modulation of the negative feedback action of estradiol, *Biol. Reprod.,* 23, 1061, 1980.

164. **Legan, S. J., Karsh, F. J., and Foster, D. L.,** The endocrine control of seasonal reproductive function in the ewe: a marked change in response to negative feedback action of estradiol on luteinizing hormone secretion, *Endocrinology,* 101, 818, 1977.

165. **Lehrer, S.,** Fertility of blind women, *Fertil. Steril.,* 38, 751, 1982.

166. **Lewy, A. J., Wehr, T. A., Goodwin, F. K., Newsome, D. A., and Markey, S. P.,** Light suppresses melatonin secretion in humans, *Science,* 210, 1267, 1980.

167. **Licht, P., Zucker, I., Hubbard, G., and Boshes, M.,** Circannual rhythms of plasma testosterone and luteinizing hormone levels in golden-mantled ground squirrels (Spermophilus lateralis), *Biol. Reprod.,* 27, 411, 1982.

168. **Lincoln, G. A.,** Induction of testicular growth and sexual activity in rams by a "skeleton" short-day photoperiod, *J. Reprod. Fertil.,* 52, 179, 1978.

169. **Lincoln, G. A.,** Photoperiodic control of seasonal breeding in the ram: participation of the cranial sympathetic nervous system, *J. Endocrinol.,* 82, 135, 1979.

170. **Lincoln, G. A.,** Seasonal changes in the pineal gland related to the reproductive cycle in the male hare, Lepus europaeus, *J. Reprod. Fertil.,* 46, 489, 1976.

171. **Lincoln, G. A.,** Use of a pulsed infusion of luteinizing hormone releasing hormone to mimic seasonally induced endocrine changes in the ram, *J. Endocrinol.,* 83, 251, 1979.

172. **Lincoln, G. A.,** Effect of placing micro-implants of melatonin in the pars tuberalis, pars distalis and the lateral septum of the forebrain on the secretion of FSH and prolactin, and testicular size in rams, *J. Endocrinol.,* 142, 267, 1994.

173. **Lincoln, G. A., Almeida, O. F. X., Klandorf, H., and Cunningham, R. A.,** Hourly fluctuations in the blood levels of melatonin, prolactin, luteinizing hormone, follicle-stimulating hormone, testosterone, triiodothyronine, thyroxine and cortisol in rams under artificial photoperiods, and the effects of cranial sympathectomy, *J. Endocrinol.,* 92, 237, 1982.

174. **Lincoln, G. A. and Davidson, W.,** The relationship between sexual and aggressive behaviour and pituitary and testicular activity during the seasonal sexual cycle of rams, and the influence of photoperiod, *J. Reprod. Fertil.,* 49, 267, 1977.

175. **Lincoln, G. A., Frasier, H. M., and Fletcher, T. J.,** Induction of early rutting in male red deer (Cervus elaphus) by melatonin and its dependence on LHRH, *J. Reprod. Fertil.,* 72, 339, 1984.

176. **Lincoln, G. A. and Kay, R. N. B.,** Effects of season on the secretion of LH and testosterone in intact and castrated red deer stags (Cervus elaphus), *J. Reprod. Fertil.,* 55, 75, 1979.

177. **Lincoln, G. A., McNeilly, A. S., and Cameron, C. L.,** The effects of a sudden decrease or increase in daylength on prolactin secretion in the ram, *J. Reprod. Fertil.,* 52, 305, 1978.

178. **Lincoln, G. A., Pett, M. J., and Cunningham, R. A.,** Seasonal and circadian changes in the episodic release of follicle-stimulating hormone, luteinizing hormone and testosterone in rams exposed to artificial photoperiods, *J. Endocrinol.,* 72, 337, 1977.

179. **Lindley, S. E., Lookingland, K. J. and Moore, K. E.,** Activation of tuberoinfundibular but not tuberohypophysial dopaminergic neurons following intracerebroventricular administration of alpha-melanocyte-stimulating hormone, *Neuroendocrinology,* 51, 394, 1990.

180. **Lynch, G. R., Heath, M. W., and Johnston, C. M.,** Effect of geographical origin on the photoperiodic control of reproduction in the white-footed mouse, Peromyscus leucopus, *Biol. Reprod.*, 25, 475, 1981.

181. **MacLeod, B. J. and Heim, L. M.,** Characteristics and variations in semen specimens in 100 normal young men, *J. Urol.*, 54, 474, 1945.

182. **Macrides, F., Bartke, A., and Dalterio, S.,** Strange females increase plasma testosterone levels in male mice, *Science*, 189, 1104, 1975.

183. **Macrides, F., Bartke, A., Fernandez, F., and D'Angelo, W.,** Effects of exposure to vaginal odor and receptive females on plasma testosterone in the male hamster, *Neuroendocrinology*, 15, 355, 1974.

184. **Mahone, J. P. and Dukelow, W. R.,** Seasonal variation of reproductive parameters in the laboratory-housed male cynomolgus macaque (Macaca fascicularis), *J. Med. Primatol.*, 8, 179, 1979.

185. **Martin, G. B., Scaramuzzi, R. J., and Lindsay, D. R.,** Effect of the introduction of rams during the anoestrous season on the pulsatile secretion of LH in ovariectomized ewes, *J. Reprod. Fertil.*, 67, 47, 1983.

186. **Martin, G. B. and Thiery, J. C.,** Hypothalamic multiunit activity and LH secretion in conscious sheep, *Exp. Brain Res.*, 67, 469, 1987.

187. **Martinet, L., Allain, D., and Weiner, C.,** Role of prolactin in the photoperiodic control of moulting in the mink (Mustela vison), *J. Endocrinol.*, 103, 9, 1984.

188. **Matt, K. S., Bartke, A., Soares, M. J., Talamantes, F., Hebert, A., and Hogan, M. P.,** Does prolactin modify testosterone feedback in the hamster? Suppression of plasma prolactin inhibits photoperiod-induced decreases in testosterone feedback sensitivity, *Endocrinology*, 115, 2098, 1984.

189. **Matt, K. S. and Stetson, M. H.,** Hypothalamic-pituitary-gonadal interactions during spontaneous testicular recrudescence in golden hamsters, *Biol. Reprod.*, 20, 739, 1979.

190. **Maurel, D. and Boissin, J.,** Comparative mechanisms of physiological metabolical and eco-ethological adaptation to the winter season in two wild European mammals: the European badger (Meles meles L.) and the red fox (Vulpes vulpes L.), in *Plant, Animal, and Microbial Adaptations to Terrestrial Environment*, Margaris, N. S., Arianoutsou-Faraggitalis, M., and Reiter, R. J., Eds., Plenum Press, New York, 1983, 219.

191. **Maurel, D., Lacroix, A., and Boissin, J.,** Seasonal reproductive endocrine profiles in two wild mammals, the red fox (Vulpes vulpes L.) and the European badger (Meles meles L.), considered as short-day mammals, *Acta Endocrinol.*, 105, 130, 1984.

192. **Maywood, E. S., Buttery, R. C., Vance, G. H. S., Herbert, J. and Hastings, M. H.,** Gonadal responses of the male Syrian hamster to programmed infusions of melatonin are sensitive to signal duration and frequency but not to signal phase nor to lesions of the suprachiasmatic nuclei, *Biol. Reprod.*, 43, 174, 1990.

193. **McLeod, B. J., Haresign, W., and Lemming, G. E.,** The induction of ovulation and luteal function in seasonally anoestrous ewes treated with small-dose multiple injections of Gn-RH, *J. Reprod. Fertil.*, 65, 215, 1982.

194. **McMillin, J. M., Seal, V. S., Rogers, L., and Ericson, A. W.,** Annual testosterone rhythm in the black bear (Ursus americanus), *Biol. Reprod.*, 15, 163, 1976.

195. **McNatty, K. P., Ball, K., Gibb, M., Hudson, N., and Thurley, D. C.,** Introduction of cyclic ovarian activity in seasonally anoestrous ewes with exogenous GnRH, *J. Reprod. Fertil.*, 64, 93, 1982.

196. **McNeilly, A. S., O'Connell, M., and Baird, D. T.,** Induction of ovulation and normal luteal function by pulsed injections of luteinizing hormone in anestrous ewes, *Endocrinology*, 110, 1292, 1982.

197. **Meites, J. and Sonntag, W. E.,** Hypothalamic hypophysiotropic hormones and neurotransmitter regulation: current views, *Annu. Rev. Pharmacol. Toxicol.*, 21, 295, 1981.

198. **Michael, R. P. and Keverne, E. B.,** An annual rhythm in the sexual activity of the male rhesus monkey, Macaca mulatta, in the laboratory, *J. Reprod. Fertil.*, 25, 95, 1971.

199. **Michael, R. P. and Wilson, M. I.,** Mating seasonality in castrated male rhesus monkeys, *J. Reprod. Fertil.*, 43, 325, 1975.

200. **Michael, R. P. and Zumpe, D.,** Relation between the seasonal changes in aggression, plasma testosterone and the photoperiod in male rhesus monkeys, *Psychoneuroendocrinology*, 6, 145, 1981.

201. **Mirarchi, R. E., Howland, B. E., Scanlon, P. F., Kirkpatrick, R. L., and Sanford, L. M.,** Seasonal variation in plasma LH, FSH, prolactin, and testosterone concentrations in adult male white-tailed deer, *Can. J. Zool.*, 56, 121, 1978.

202. **Moore, R. Y.,** Organization and function of a central nervous system circadian oscillator: the suprachiasmatic hypothalamic nucleus, *Fed. Proc.*, 42, 2783, 1983.

203. **Moore-Ede, M. C., Sulzman, F. M., and Fuller, C. A.,** *The Clocks That Time Us: Physiology of the Circadian Timing System*, Harvard University Press, Cambridge, MA, 1982.

204. **Mortimer, D., Templeton, A. A., Lenton, E. A., and Coleman, R. A.,** Annual patterns of human sperm production and semen quality, *Arch. Androl.*, 10, 1, 1983.

205. **Moss, R. L., Dudley, C. A., Foreman, M. M., and McCann, S. M.,** Synthetic LRF: a potentiator of sexual behavior in the rat, in *Hypothalamic Hormones*, Motta, M., Crosignani, P. G., and Martini, L., Eds., Academic Press, New York, 1975, 269.

206. **Muduuli, D. S., Sanford, L. M., Palmer, W. M., and Howland, B. E.,** Secretory patterns and circadian and seasonal changes in luteinizing hormone, follicle stimulating hormone, prolactin and testosterone in the male pygmy goat, *J. Anim. Sci.*, 49, 543, 1979.

207. **Mukku, V. R., Murty, G. S. R. C., Srinath, B. R., Ramsharma, K., Kotagi, S. G., and Moudgal, N. R.,** Regulation of testosterone rhythmicity by gonadotropins in bonnet monkeys (Macaca radiata), *Biol. Reprod.*, 24, 814, 1981.

208. **Mulchahey, J. J. and Neill J. D.,** Dopamine levels in the anterior pituitary gland monitored by in vivo electrochemistry, *Brain Res.*, 386, 322, 1986.

209. **Murai, I. and Ben-Jonathan, N.,** Posterior pituitary lobectomy abolishes the suckling-induced rise in prolactin: evidence for a prolactin releasing factor in posterior pituitary, *Endocrinology*, 121, 205, 1987.

210. **Murai, I. and Ben-Jonathan, N.,** Acute stimulation of prolactin release by estradiol: mediation by the posterior pituitary, *Endocrinology*, 126, 3179, 1990.

211. **Murphy, B. D., Mead, R. A., and McKibbin, P. E.,** Luteal contribution to the termination of preimplantation delay in the mink, *Biol. Reprod.*, 28, 497, 1983.

212. **Nadler, R. D. and Rosenblum, L. A.,** Hormonal regulation of the "fatted" phenomenon in squirrel monkeys, *Anat. Rec.*, 173, 181, 1972.

213. **Neal, J. and Murphy, B. D.,** Response of immature, mature non-breeding and mature breeding ferret testis to exogenous LH stimulation, *Biol. Reprod.*, 16, 244, 1977.

214. **Neaves, W. B.,** Changes in testicular Leydig cells and in plasma testosterone levels among seasonally breeding rock hyrax, *Biol. Reprod.*, 8, 451, 1973.

215. **Negus, N. C. and Berger, P. J.,** Experimental triggering of reproduction in a natural population of Microtus montanus, *Science*, 196, 1230, 1977.

216. **Nelson, R. J., Dark, J., and Zucker, I.,** Influence of photoperiod, nutrition and water availability on reproduction of male California voles (Microtus californicus), *J. Reprod. Fertil.*, 69, 473, 1983.

217. **Nieschlag, E. and Bieniek, H.,** Endocrine testicular function in mink during the first year of life, *Acta Endocrinol.*, 79, 375, 1975.

218. **Nir, I., Schmidt, U., and Zilber, N.,** The antigonadotrophic effect of melatonin in Syrian hamsters is modulated by prostaglandin, *J. Neural Transm.*, 95, 173, 1994.

219. **Norman, R. L. and Spies, H. G.,** Neural control of the estrogen-dependent twenty-four-hour periodicity of LH release in the golden hamster, *Endocrinology*, 95, 1367, 1974.

220. **O'Callaghan, D., Wendling, A., Karsch, F. J., and Roche, J. F.,** Effect of exogenous thyroxine on timing of seasonal reproductive transitions in ewes, *Biol. Reprod.*, 49, 311, 1993.

221. **Oldham, C. M., Martin, G. B., and Knight, T. W.,** Stimulation of seasonally anovular Merino ewes by rams. I. Time from introduction of rams to the preovulatory LH surge and ovulation, *Anim. Reprod. Sci.*, 1, 283, 1978.

223. **Ortavant, R.,** Le cycle Spermatogenetique chez les Belier, These Doc. Sci. No. 3990, University Paris VI, 1958.

224. **Panda, J. N. and Turner, C. W.,** The role of melatonin in the regulation of thyrotrophin secretion, *Acta Endocrinol.*, 57, 363, 1968.

225. **Parrott, R. F. and Davies, R. V.,** Serum gonadotrophin levels in prepubertally castrated male sheep treated for long periods with propionated testosterone, dihydrotestosterone, 19-hydroxytestosterone or oestradiol, *J. Reprod. Fertil.*, 56, 543, 1979.

226. **Pelham, R. W., Vaughan, G. M., Sandock, K. L., and Vaughan, M. K.,** Twenty-four-hour cycle of a melatonin-like substance in the plasma of human males, *J. Clin. Endocrinol. Metab.*, 37, 341, 1973.

227. **Pelletier, J.,** Evidence for photoperiodic control of prolactin release in rams, *J. Reprod. Fertil.*, 35, 143, 1973.

228. **Pelletier, J., Garnier, D. H., deReviers, M. M., Terqui, M., and Ortavant, R.,** Seasonal variation in LH and testosterone release in rams of two breeds, *J. Reprod. Fertil.*, 64, 341, 1982.

229. **Pelletier, J. and Ortavant, R.,** Photoperiodic control of LH release in the ram, I. Influence of increasing and decreasing light photoperiods, *Acta Endocrinol.*, 78, 435, 1975.

230. **Pelletier, J. and Ortavant, R.,** Photoperiodic control of LH release in the ram, II. Light-androgens interactions, *Acta Endocrinol.*, 78, 442, 1975.

231. **Peters, L. L., Hoefer, M. T., and Ben-Jonathan, N.,** The posterior pituitary: regulation of anterior pituitary secretion of prolactin, *Science*, 213, 659, 1981.

232. **Petterborg, L. J. and Reiter, R. J.,** Effect of photoperiod and melatonin on testicular development in the white-footed mouse, Peromyscus leucopus, *J. Reprod. Fertil.*, 60, 209, 1980.

233. **Pickard, G. E. and Silverman, A. J.,** Effects of photoperiod on hypothalamic luteinizing hormone releasing hormone in the male hamster, *J. Endocrinol.*, 83, 412, 1979.

234. **Pickard, G. E. and Turek, F. W.,** The hypothalamic paraventricular nucleus mediates the photoperiodic control of reproduction but not the effects of light on the circadian rhythm of activity, *Neurosci. Lett.*, 43, 67, 1983.

235. **Pickering, D. S. and Niles, L. P.,** Pharmacological characterization of melatonin binding sites in Syrian hamster hypothalamus, *Eur. J. Pharmacol.*, 175, 71, 1990.

236. **Pieper, D. R.,** Effects of photoperiod, castration, and gonadotropin-releasing hormone (GnRH) on the number of GnRH receptors in male golden hamsters, *Endocrinology*, 115, 1857, 1984.

237. **Pinatel, M. C., Souchier, C., Croze, J. P., and Czyha, J. C.,** Seasonal variation of necrospermia in man, *J. Interdiscip. Cycle Res.*, 12, 225, 1981.

238. **Plant, T. M., Zumpe, D., Sauls, M., and Michael, R. P.,** An annual rhythm in the plasma testosterone of adult male rhesus monkeys maintained in the laboratory, *J. Endocrinol.*, 62, 403, 1974.

239. **Plotka, E. D., Seal, U. S., Letellier, M. A., Verm, L. J., and Ozoga, J. J.,** Early effects of pinealectomy on LH and testosterone secretion in white-tailed deer, *J. Endocrinol.*, 103, 1, 1984.

240. **Prins, G. S., Bartke, A., and Steger, R. W.,** Influence of photoinhibition, photostimulation and prolactin on pituitary and hypothalamic nuclear androgen receptors in the male hamster, *Neuroendocrinology*, 52, 511, 1990.

241. **Pudney, J. and Lacy, D.,** Correlation between ultrastructure and biochemical changes in the testis of the American grey squirrel, Sciurus carolinensis during the reproductive cycle, *J. Reprod. Fertil.*, 49, 5, 1977.

242. **Ramaley, J. A.,** Stress and fertility, in *Environmental Factors in Mammal Reproduction*, Gilmore, D. and Cook, B., Eds., Macmillan, New York, 1981, 127.

243. **Ravault, J. P.,** Prolactin in the ram: seasonal variations in the concentration of blood plasma from birth until three years old, *Acta Endocrinol.*, 83, 720, 1976.

244. **Ravault, J. P., Martinot-Botte, F., Mauget, R., Martinot, N., Locatelli, A., and Bariteau, F.,** Influence of the duration of daylight on prolactin secretion in the pig: hourly rhythm in ovariectomized females, monthly variation in domestic (male and female) and wild strains during the year, *Biol. Reprod.*, 27, 1084, 1982.

245. **Raymond, V., Beaulieu, M., Labrie, F., and Boissier, J. R.,** Potent antidopaminergic activity of estradiol at the pituitary level on prolactin release, *Science*, 200, 1173, 1978.

246. **Reinberg, A., Lagoguey, M., Chauflournier, J.-M., and Cesselin, F.,** Circannual and circadian rhythms in plasma testosterone in five healthy young Parisian males, *Acta Endocrinol.*, 80, 732, 1975.

247. **Reinberg, A. and Lagoguey, M.,** Circadian and circannual rhythms in sexual activity and plasma hormones (FSH, LH, testosterone) of five human males, *Arch. Sex. Behav.*, 7, 13, 1978.

248. **Reiter, R. J.,** Changes in the reproductive organs of cold-exposed and light-deprived female hamsters (Mesocricetus auratus), *J. Reprod. Fertil.*, 16, 217, 1968.

249. **Reiter, R. J.,** Exogenous and endogenous control of the annual reproductive cycle in the male golden hamster participation of the pineal gland, *J. Exp. Zool.*, 191, 111, 1975.

250. **Reiter, R. J.,** Influence of pinealectomy on the breeding capability of hamsters maintained under natural photoperiodic and temperature conditions, *Neuroendocrinology*, 13, 366, 1973/74.

251. **Reiter, R. J.,** The pineal and its hormones in the control of reproduction in mammals, *Endocr. Rev.*, 1, 109, 1980.

252. **Reiter, R. J., Dinh, D. T., de los Santos, R., and Guerra, J. C.,** Hypothalamic cuts suggest a brain site for the antigonadotrophic action of melatonin in the Syrian hamster, *Neurosci. Lett.*, 23, 315, 1981.

253. **Rhim, T.-J, Kuehl, D., and Jackson, G. L.,** Seasonal changes in the relationship between secretion of gonadotropin-releasing hormone, luteinizing hormone, and testosterone in the ram, *Biol. Reprod.*, 48, 197, 1993.

254. **Rhodes, D. H.,** Effects of temperature, photoperiod, and daily torpor on thyroid function in the whitefooted mouse, Peromyscus leucopus, *Gen. Comp. Endocrinol.*, 42, 134, 1980.

255. **Rhynes, W. E. and Ewing, L. L.,** Testicular endocrine function in Hereford bulls exposed to high ambient temperature, *Endocrinology*, 92, 509, 1973.

256. **Rissman, E. F.,** Prepubertal sensitivity to melatonin in male hamsters, *Biol. Reprod.*, 22, 277, 1980.

257. **Roberts, A. C., Martensz, N. D., Hastings, M. H., and Herbert, J.,** The effect of castration, testosterone replacement and photoperiod on hypothalamic B-endorphin levels in the male Syrian hamster, *Neuroscience*, 23, 1075, 1987.

258. **Roenneberg, T. and Aschoff, J.,** Annual rhythm of human reproduction. I. Biology, sociology, or both?, *J. Biol. Rhythms*, 5, 195, 1990.

259. **Roenneberg, T. and Aschoff, J.,** Annual rhythm of human reproduction. II. Environmental correlations, *J. Biol. Rhythms*, 5, 217, 1990.

260. **Ronchi, E., Aoki, C., Krey, L. C., and Pfaff, D. W.,** Immunocytochemical study of GnRH and GnRH-associated peptide in male Syrian hamsters as a function of photoperiod and gonadal alterations, *Neuroendocrinology*, 55, 134, 1992.

261. **Ronchi, E., Krey, L. C., and Pfaff, D. W.,** Steady state analysis of hypothalamic GnRH mRNA levels in male Syrian hamsters: influences of photoperiod and androgen, *Neuroendocrinology*, 55, 146, 1992.

262. **Rose, R. M., Gordon, T. P., and Bernstein, I. S.,** Plasma testosterone levels in the male rhesus: influences of sexual and social stimuli, *Science*, 178, 643, 1972.

263. **Rusak, B. and Morin, L. P.,** Testicular responses to photoperiod are blocked by lesions of the suprachiasmatic nuclei in golden hamster, *Biol. Reprod.*, 15, 366, 1976.

264. **Rusak, B. and Zucker, I.,** Neural regulation of circadian rhythm, *Physiol. Rev.*, 59, 449, 1979.

265. **Ryan, K. D.,** Hormonal correlates of photoperiod-induced puberty in a reflex ovulator, the female ferret (Mustela furo), *Biol. Reprod.*, 31, 925, 1984.

266. **Saboureau, M. and Dutourne, B.,** The reproductive cycle in the male hedgehog (Erinaceus europaeus L.): a study of endocrine and exocrine testicular functions, *Reprod. Nutr. Dev.*, 21, 109, 1981.

267. **Saboureau, M., Laurent, A.-M., and Boissin, J.,** Plasma testosterone binding protein capacity in relation to the annual testicular cycle in a hibernating mammal, the hedgehog (Erinaceus europaeus L.), *Gen. Comp. Endocrinol.*, 47, 59, 1982.

268. **Saidapur, S. K. and Greenwald,G. S.,** Sites of steroid synthesis in the ovary of the cyclic hamster: a histochemical study, *Am. J. Anat.*, 151, 71, 1978.

269. **Sanders, E. H., Gardner, P. D., Berger, P. J., and Negus, N. C.,** 6-Methoxybenzoxazolinone: a plant derivative that stimulates reproduction in Microtus montanus, *Science*, 214, 67, 1981.

271. **Sanford, L. M., Winter, J. S. D., Palmer, W. M., and Howland, B. E.,** The profile of LH and testosterone secretion in the ram, *Endocrinology*, 95, 627, 1974.

272. **Schams, D. and Barth, D.,** Annual profiles of reproductive hormones on peripheral plasma of the male red deer (Capreolus capreolus), *J. Reprod. Fertil.*, 66, 463, 1982.

273. **Schams, D., Stephan, E., and Hooley, R. D.,** The effect of heat exposure on blood serum levels of anterior pituitary hormones in calves, heifers and bulls, *Acta Endocrinol.*, 94, 309, 1980.

274. **Schinckel, P. G.,** The effect of the presence of the ram on the ovarian activity of the ewe, *Aust. J. Agric. Res.*, 5, 465, 1954.

275. **Schopper, D., Gaus, J., Claus, R., and Bader, H.,** Seasonal changes of steroid concentrations in seminal plasma of a European wild boar, *Acta Endocrinol.*, 107, 425, 1984.

276. **Schutte, B. A., Seal, V. S., Plotka, E. D., Letellier, M. A., Verne, L. J., Ozoga, J. J., and Parsons, J. A.,** The effect of pinealectomy on seasonal changes in prolactin secretion in the white-tailed deer (Odocoileus virginianus borealis), *Endocrinology*, 108, 173, 1981.

277. **Seegal, R. F. and Goldman, B. D.,** Effects of photoperiod on cyclicity and serum gonadotropins in the Synan hamster, *Biol. Reprod.*, 12, 223, 1975.

278. **Sellers, K., Shrenker, P., and Bartke, A.,** unpublished data, 1985.

279. **Sempere, A. J. and Lacroix, A.,** Temporal and seasonal relationships between LH, testosterone and antlers in fawn and adult male roe deer (Capreolus capreolus L.): a longitudinal study from birth to four years of age, *Acta Endocrinol.*, 99, 295, 1982.

280. **Selye, H.,** A syndrome produced by diverse nocuous agents, *Nature (London)*, 138, 32, 1936.

281. **Shander, D. and Goldman, B.,** Ovarian steroid modulation of gonadotropin secretion and pituitary responsiveness to luteinizing hormone releasing hormone in the female hamster, *Endocrinology*, 103, 1383, 1978.

282. **Silman, R. E., Leone, R. M., Hooper, R. J., and Preece, M. A.,** Melatonin, the pineal gland and human puberty, *Nature (London)*, 282, 301, 1979.

283. **Silavin, S. L. and Greenwald, G. S.,** In vitro progesterone production by ovarian interstitial cells from hypophysectomized hamsters, *J. Reprod. Fertil.*, 66, 291, 1982.

284. **Simpkins, J. W., Kalra, P. S., and Kalra, S. P.,** Effects of testosterone on catecholamine turnover and LHRH content in the basal hypothalamus and preoptic area, *Neuroendocrinology*, 30, 94, 1980.

285. **Simpkins, J. W., Kalra, P. S., and Kalra, S. P.,** Inhibitory effects of androgens on preoptic area dopaminergic neurons in castrate rats, *Neuroendocrinology*, 31, 177, 1980.

286. **Sisk, C. L. and Turek, F. W.,** Gonadal growth and gonadal hormones do not participate in the development of responsiveness to photoperiod in the golden hamster, *Biol. Reprod.*, 29, 439, 1983.

287. **Siwela, A. A. and Tam, W. H.,** Metabolism of androgens by the active and inactive prostate gland, and the seasonal changes in systemic androgen levels in the grey squirrel (Sciurus carolinensis, Gmelin), *J. Endocrinol.*, 88, 381, 1981.

288. **Smals, N. H., Kloppenborg, P. W. C., and Benraad, T. J.,** Annual cycle in plasma testosterone levels in man, *J. Clin. Endocrinol. Metab.*, 42, 979, 1976.

289. **Snyder, D. L., Cowan, R. L., Hagen, D. R., and Schanbacher, B. D.,** Effect of pinealectomy on seasonal changes in antler growth and concentrations of testosterone and prolactin in white-tailed deer, *Biol. Reprod.*, 29, 63, 1983.

290. **Soares, M. and Hoffmann, J.,** Melatonin suppression of postcastration serum luteinizing hormone and follicle-stimulating hormone responses in the male mongoose, Herpestes auropunctatus, *Gen. Comp. Endocrinol.*, 48, 525, 1982.

291. **Soares, M. J. and Hoffman, J. C.,** Seasonal reproduction in the mongoose, Herpestes auropunctatus. I. Androgen, luteinizing hormone, and follicle-stimulating hormone in the male, *Gen. Comp. Endocrinol.*, 44, 350, 1981.

292. **Soares, M. J. and Hoffmann, J. C.,** Seasonal reproduction in the mongoose, Herpestes auropunctatus. II. Testicular responsiveness to luteinizing hormone, *Gen. Comp. Endocrinol.*, 47, 226, 1982.

293. **Soares, M. J. and Hoffmann, J. C.,** Seasonal reproduction in the mongoose, Herpestes auropunctatus. III. Regulation of gonadotropin secretion in the male, *Gen. Comp. Endocrinol.*, 47, 235, 1982.

294. **Southwick, C. H., Beg, M. A., and Siddiqi, M. R.,** Rhesus monkeys in North India, in *Primate Behavior*, DeVore, I., Ed., Holt, Rinehart & Winston, New York, 1965, 111.

295. **Stanton, T. L., Craft, C. M., and Reiter, R. J.,** Decreases in pineal melatonin content during the hibernation bout in the golden-mantled ground squirrel, Spermophilus lateralis, *Life Sci.*, 35, 1461, 1984.

295b. **Steger R. W. and Bartke, A.,** Temporal sequence of neuroendocrine events associated with the transfer of male golden hamsters from a stimulatory to a non-stimulatory photoperiod, *Biol. Reprod.*, 44, 76, 1991.

295c. **Steger, R. W., Bartke, A., Bain, P. A., and Chandrashekar, V.,** Hyperprolactinemia disrupts neuroendocrine responses of male rats to female conspecifics, *Neuroendocrinology*, 46, 499, 1987.

296. **Steger, R. W., Bartke, A., and Goldman, B. D.,** Alterations in neuroendocrine function during photoperiod induced testicular atrophy and recrudesence in the golden hamster, *Biol. Reprod.*, 26, 437, 1982.

297. **Steger, R. W., Bartke, A., Goldman, B. D., Soares, M. J., and Talamantes, F.,** Effects of short photoperiod on the ability of golden hamster pituitaries to secrete prolactin and gonadotropins in vitro, *Biol. Reprod.*, 29, 872, 1983.

298. **Steger, R. W., Bartke, A., Matt, K. S., Soares, M. J., and Talamantes, F.,** Neuroendocrine changes in hamsters following photostimulation, *J. Exp. Zool.*, 229, 467, 1984.

299. **Steger, R. W., Dennis, C., Van Abbema, A., and Gay-Primel, E.,** Alterations in hypothalamic serotonin metabolism in male hamsters with photoperiod-induced testicular regression, *Brain Res.*, 514, 11, 1990.

300. **Steger, R. W., DePaolo, L. V., Asch, R. H., and Silverman, A. Y.,** Interactions of delta 9-tetrahydrocannabinol (THC) with hypothalamic neurotransmitters controlling luteinizing hormone and prolactin release, *Neuroendocrinology*, 37, 361, 1983.

302. **Steger, R. W. and Gay-Primel, E.,** Effects of melatonin injections on the ability of golden hamster pituitaries to secrete prolactin and luteinizing hormone, *Biol. Reprod.*, 42, 217, 1990.

303. **Steger, R. W., Huang, H. H., Chamberlain, D., and Meites, J.,** Changes in the control of gonadotropin secretion in the transition period between regular cycles and constant estrus in the old female rat, *Biol. Reprod.*, 22, 595, 1980.

303a. **Steger, R. W., Juszczak, M., Fadden, C., and Bartke, A.,** Photoperiod effects on neurohypophyseal and tuberoinfundibular dopamine metabolism in the male hamster, *Endocrinology,* 136, 3000, 1995.

304. **Steger, R. W. and Johns, A., Eds.,** *Handbook of Pharmacological Methods for the Study of the Neuroendocrine System*, CRC Press, Boca Raton, FL, 1985.

305. **Steger, R. W. and Matt, K. S.,** Prolactin modifies the response of the hamster neuroendocrine system to testosterone negative feedback. Program for the 19th Annual Meeting of the Society for the Study of Reproduction. Ithaca, NY, July 14–17, 1986. Abstract # 268.

306. **Steger, R. W., Matt, K. S., and Bartke, A.,** Interactions of testosterone and short-photoperiod exposure on the neuroendocrine axis of the male Syrian hamster, *Neuroendocrinology*, 43, 69, 1986.

307. **Steger, R. W., Matt, K. S., and Bartke, A.,** Neuroendocrine regulation of seasonal reproductive activity in the male golden hamster, *Neurosci. Biobehav. Rev.*, 9, 191, 1985.

308. **Steger, R. W., Matt, K. S., Klemcke, H. G., and Bartke, A.,** Interactions of photoperiod and ectopic pituitary grafts on hypothalamic and pituitary function in male hamsters, *Neuroendocrinology*, 41, 89, 1985.

309. **Steger, R. W. and Peluso, J. J.,** The gonadotrope, in *Handbook of Endocrinology*, Gass, G. H. and Kaplan, H. M., Eds., CRC Press, Boca Raton, FL, 1982, 27.

310. **Steger, R. W., Reiter, R. J., and Siler-Khodr, T. M.,** Interactions of pinealectomy and short-photoperiod exposure on the neuroendocrine axis of the male Syrian hamster, *Neuroendocrinology*, 38, 158, 1984.

311. **Stetson, M. H., Elliot, J. A., and Goldman, B. D.,** Maternal transfer of photoperiodic information influences the photoperiodic response of prepubertal Djungarian hamsters, *Biol. Reprod.*, 34, 664, 1986.

312. **Stetson, M. H. and Tate-Ostroff, B.,** Hormonal regulation of the annual reproductive cycle of golden hamsters, *Gen. Comp. Endocrinol.*, 45, 329, 1981.

313. **Stetson, M. H., Watson-Whitmyre, M., and Matt, K. S.,** Termination of photorefractoriness in golden hamsters—photoperiodic requirements, *J. Exp. Zool.*, 202, 81, 1977.

314. **Tahka, K. M.,** A histochemical study on the effects of photoperiod on gonadal and adrenal function in the male bank vole (Clethrionomys glareolus), *J. Reprod. Fertil.*, 54, 57, 1978.

315. **Tahka, K. M., Teravainen, T., and Wallgren, H.,** Testicular steroid metabolism in juvenile bank voles (Clethrionomys glareolus Schreber) exposed to different photoperiods: an in vivo study, *Gen. Comp. Endocrinol.*, 51, 1, 1983.

316. **Tamarkin, L., Baird, C. J., and Almeida, O. F. X.,** Melatonin: a coordinating signal for mammalian reproduction, *Science*, 227, 714, 1985.

317. **Tamarkin, L., Hutchison, J. S., and Goldman, B. D.,** Regulation of serum gonadotropins by photoperiod and testicular hormones in the Syrian hamster, *Endocrinology*, 99, 1528, 1976.

318. **Tamarkin, L., Westrom, M. K., Hamill, A. I., and Goldman, B. D.,** Effect of melatonin on the reproductive system of male and female Syrian hamsters: a diurnal rhythm in sensitivity to melatonin, *Endocrinology*, 99, 1534, 1976.

319. **Terman, C. R.,** Reproductive inhibition in asymptotic populations of prairie deer mice, *J. Reprod. Fertil. Suppl.*, 19, 457, 1973.

320. **Testart, J., Frydman, R., and Roger, M.,** Seasonal influence of diurnal rhythms in the onset of the plasma luteinizing hormone surge in women, *J. Clin. Endocrinol. Metab.,* 55, 374, 1982.

321. **Thiery, J.-C.,** Monoamine content of the stalk-median eminence and hypothalamus in adult female sheep as affected by daylength, *J. Neuroendocrinol.,* 3, 407, 1991.

322. **Thiery, J. C., Martin, G. B., Tillet, Y., Caldani, M., Quentin, M., Jamain, C., and Ravault, J. P.,** Role of hypothalamic catecholamines in the regulation of catecholamines and prolactin secretion in the ewe during seasonal anestrous, *Neuroendocrinology,* 49, 80, 1989.

323. **Thompson, D. L., Jr., Pickett, B. W., Berndtson, W. E., Voss, J. L., and Nett, T. M.,** Reproductive physiology of the stallion. VIII. Artificial photoperiod, collection interval and seminal characteristics, sexual behavior and concentrations of LH and testosterone in serum, *J. Anim. Sci.,* 44, 656, 1977.

324. **Thomson, A. L.,** Factors determining the breeding seasons of birds: an introductory review, *Ibis,* 92, 173, 1950.

325. **Timonen, S., Franzar, B., and Wichmann, K.,** Photosensibility of the human pituitary, *Ann. Chir. Gynaecol.,* 53, 165, 1964.

326. **Tjoa, W. S., Smolensky, M. H., Hsi, B. P., Steinherger, E., and Smith, K. D.,** Circannual rhythm in human sperm count revealed by serially independent sampling, *Fertil. Steril.,* 38, 454, 1982.

327. **Touitou, Y., Lagogney, M., Bogdan, A., Reinherg, A., and Beck, H.,** Seasonal rhythms of plasma gonadotropins: their persistence in elderly men and women, *J. Endocrinol.,* 96, 15, 1983.

328. **Tsui, H. W., Tam, W. H., Lofts, B., and Phillips, J. G.,** The annual testicular cycle and androgen production in vitro in the masked civet cat, Paguma l. larvata, *J. Reprod. Fertil.,* 36, 283, 1974.

329. **Tubbiola, M. L. and Bittman, E. L.,** Steroidal and photoperiodic regulation of opiate binding in male golden hamsters, *J. Neuroendocrinol,* 6, 317, 1994.

330. **Tubbiola, M. L., Nock, B., and Bittman, E. L.,** Photoperiodic changes in opiate binding and their functional implications in golden hamsters, *Brain Res.,* 503, 91, 1989.

331. **Tucker, H. A. and Wettermann, R. P.,** Effects of ambient temperature and relative humidity on serum prolactin and growth hormone in heifers, *Proc. Soc. Exp. Biol. Med.,* 151, 623, 1976.

332. **Turek, F. W.,** Effect of melatonin on photic-independent and photic-dependent testicular growth in juvenile and adult male golden hamsters, *Biol. Reprod.,* 20, 1119, 1979.

333. **Turek, F. W.,** The interaction of the photoperiod and testosterone in regulating serum gonadotropin levels in castrated male hamsters, *Endocrinology,* 101, 1210, 1977.

334. **Turek, F. W., Alvis, J. D., and Menaker, M.,** Pituitary responsiveness to LRF in castrated male hamsters exposed to different photoperiodic conditions, *Neuroendocrinology,* 24, 140, 1977.

335. **Turek, F. W., Elliot, J. A., Alvis, J. D., and Menaker, M.,** Effect of prolonged exposure to nonstimulatory photopenods on the activity of the neuroendocrine-testicular axis of golden hamsters, *Biol. Reprod.,* 13, 475, 1975.

336. **Turek, F. W. and Ellis, G. B.,** Steroid-dependent and steroid-independent aspects of the photoperiodic control of seasonal reproductive cycles in male hamsters, in *Biological Clocks in Seasonal Reproductive Cycles,* Follett, B. K. and Follett, D. E., Eds., John Wright and Sons, Bristol, England, 1981, 251.

337. **Udry, J. R. and Morris, N. M.,** Seasonality of coitus and seasonality of birth, *Demography,* 4, 673, 1967.

338. **Urbanski, H. F.,** A role for N-methyl-D-aspartate receptors in the control of seasonal breeding, *Endocrinology,* 127, 2223, 1990.

339. **Urbanski, H. F.,** Photoperiodic modulation of luteinizing hormone secretion in orchidectomized Syrian hamsters and the influence of excitatory amino acids, *Endocrinology,* 131, 1665, 1992.

340. **Vacas, M. I. and Cardinali, D. P.,** Diurnal changes in melatonin binding sites of hamster and rat brains: correlation with neuroendocrine responsiveness to melatonin, *Neurosci. Lett.,* 15, 259, 1979.

341. **Vandenbergh, J. G.,** The influence of the social environment on sexual interaction in male mice, *J. Reprod. Fertil.,* 24, 383, 1971.

342. **Vandenbergh, J. G.,** Reproductive coordination in the golden hamster: female influences on the male, *Horm. Behav.,* 9, 264, 1977.

343. **Vandenbergh, J. G., Whitsett, J. M., and Lombardi, J. R.,** Partial isolation of a pheromone accelerating puberty in female mice, *J. Reprod. Fertil.,* 43, 515, 1975.

344. **Versi, E., Chiappa, S. A., Fink, G., and Charlton, H. M.,** Pineal influences hypothalamic GnRH content in the vole, Microrus agrestis., *J. Reprod. Fertil.,* 67, 365, 1983.

345. **Vitale, M. L. and Chiocchio, S. R.,** Serotonin, a neurotransmitter involved in the regulation of luteinizing hormone release, *Endocr. Rev.,* 14, 480, 1993.

346. **Vriend, J.,** Pineal-thyroid interactions, in *Pineal Research Reviews,* Vol. 1, Reiter, R. J., Ed., Alan R. Liss, New York, 1983, 183.

347. **Vriend, J. and Reiter, R. J.,** Free thyroxin index in normal, melatonin treated and blind hamsters, *Horm. Metab. Res.,* 9, 231, 1977.

348. **Waldhauser, F., Weiszenbacher, G., Frisch, H., Zeithuber, U., Waldhauser, M., and Wurtman, R. J.,** Fall in nocturnal serum melatonin during prepuberty and pubescence, Lancet, 1, 362, 1984.

349. **Walker, M. C., Gordon, T. P., and Wilson, M. E.,** Menstrual cycle characteristics of seasonally breeding rhesus monkeys, *Biol. Reprod.*, 29, 841, 1983.

350. **Weaver, D. R. and Reppert S. M.,** Maternal melatonin communicates day length to the fetus in Djungarian hamsters, *Endocrinology*, 119, 2861, 1986.

351. **Weitzman, E. D., deGraaf, A. S., Sassin, J. F., Hansen, T., Godtlibsen, O. B., Perlow, M., and Hellman, L.,** Seasonal patterns of sleep stages and secretion of cortisol and growth hormone during 24 hour periods in northern Norway, *Acta Endocrinol.*, 78, 65, 1975.

352. **Wetterberg, L., Arendt, J., Paunier, L., Sizonenko, P. C., van Donselaar, W., and Heyden, T.,** Human serum melatonin changes during the menstrual cycle, *J. Clin. Endocrinol. Metab.*, 42, 185, 1976.

353. **Whitehead, P. E. and West, N. O.,** Metabolic clearance and production rates of testosterone at different times of the year in male caribou and reindeer, *Can. J. Zool.*, 55, 1692, 1977.

354. **Whitsett, J. M., Noden, P. F., Cherry, J., and Lawton, A. D.,** Effect of transitional photoperiods on testicular development and puberty in male deer mice (Peromyscus maniculatus), *J. Reprod. Fertil.*, 72, 277, 1984.

355. **Whitsett, J. M., Underwood, H., and Cherry, J.,** Influence of melatonin on pubertal development in male deer mice (Peromyscus maniculatus), *J. Reprod. Fertil.*, 72, 287, 1984.

356. **Whitten, W. K., Bronson, F. H., and Greenstein, J. A.,** Estrus-inducing pheromone of male mice: transport by movement of air, *Science*, 161, 584, 1968.

357. **Wickings, E. J., Zaidi, P., Brabant, G., and Neischlag, E.,** Stimulation of pituitary and testicular functions with LH-RH agonist or pulsatile LH-RH treatment in the rhesus monkey during the non-breeding season, *J. Reprod. Fertil.*, 63, 129, 1981.

358. **Widmaier, E. P. and Campbell, C. S.,** The interaction of estradiol and daylength in modifying serum prolactin secretion in female hamsters, *Endocrinology*, 108, 371, 1981.

359. **Williams, L. M., Morgan, P. J., Hastings, M. H., Lawson, W., Davidson, G., and Howell, H. E.,** Melatonin receptor sites in the Syrian hamster brain and pituitary: localization and characterization using 125-I iodomelatonin, *J. Neuroendocrinol.*, 5, 315, 1989.

360. **Worthy, K. and Haresign, W.,** Evidence that the onset of seasonal anoestrus in the ewe may be independent of increasing prolactin concentrations and daylength, *J. Reprod. Fertil.*, 69, 41, 1983.

361. **Yagil, R. and Etzion, Z.,** Hormonal and behavioural patterns in the male camel (Camelus dromedarius), *J. Reprod. Fertil.*, 58, 61, 1980.

362. **Yeates, N. T. M.,** The breeding season of the sheep with particular reference to its modification by artificial means using light, *J. Agric. Sci.*, 39, 1, 1949.

363. **Young, R. A., Danforth, E., Jr., Vagenakis, A. G., Krupp, P. P., Frick, R., and Sims, E. A. M.,** Seasonal variation and the influence of body temperature on plasma concentrations and binding of thyrosine and triiodothyronine in the woodchuck, *Endocrinology*, 104, 996, 1979.

364. **Yuthasastrakosol, P., Palmer, W. M., and Howland, B. E.,** Release of LH in anoestrous and cyclic ewes, *J. Reprod. Fertil.*, 50, 319, 1977.

365. **Zisapel, N. Y., Egazi, V., and Laudon, M.,** Inhibition of dopamine release by melatonin: regional distribution in the rat brain, *Brain Res.*, 246, 161, 1982.

366. **Zucker, I. and Licht, P.,** Seasonal variations in plasma luteinizing hormone levels of gonadectomized male ground squirrels (*Spermophilus laferalis*), *Biol. Reprod.*, 29, 278, 1983.

Chapter 5

HYPOTHALAMIC NEUROENDOCRINE REGULATION

Warren E. Finn

CONTENTS

INTRODUCTION

The hypothalamus regulates many somatic and visceral functions and serves as one of the main homeostatic control centers in the body. These functions include such diverse activities as the regulation of temperature, water balance, feeding behavior, aggression, reproductive processes, and sleep-wake cyclic activity.[1] In regulating these activities, the hypothalamus participates in a complex interaction between the nervous system and the endocrine system.

Our knowledge of hypothalamic neuroendocrine control emerged with the development of the neurobiology of neurosecretion.[2] In the following years, the biochemical isolation and identfication of the hypothalamic neuropeptides enabled investigators to study the factors that participate in the regulation of the synthesis and release of the hypothalamic neuropeptides.

Recent developments in immunohistochemistry and molecular biology have greatly contributed to the advancement of our understanding of neuroendocrine regulation. Through the increased application of these methods on tissue sections and cell cultures of the hypothalamus,

0-8493-9429-5/96/$0.00+$.50
© 1996 by CRC Press, Inc.

157

it has been possible to begin constructing the complex patterns of interaction of hormones, neurohormones, and neurotransmitters involved in the control processes.

In the review that follows, three areas dealing with the advancing field of hypothalamic neuroendocrine regulation will be considered. First, some of the recent developments in the experimental methods being utilized to investigate this field will be discussed. Second, the functional anatomy of the hypothalamic nuclei and their associated membrane receptors will be outlined. And last, based on recent studies, the factors that regulate the synthesis and release of the hypothalamic neurohormones will be reviewed.

EXPERIMENTAL METHODS IN THE STUDY OF HYPOTHALAMIC AND PITUITARY REGULATION

The study of hypothalamic regulation had its beginning with the work of Scharrer, Scharrer, and Bargmann and their descriptions of neurosecretory neurons using the Gomori chrome alum hematoxylin stain methods.[3,4] In the 40 years since, the chemical neuroanatomical research of the hypothalamus has established a detailed description of the hypothalamic cell types and their processes. The distribution of peptidergic and monaminergic cells and their processes were studied first.[5] Until recently, the investigations concentrated on the posterior pituitary and the anterior hypophysiotropic pituitary hormones.

During the two last decades, many biochemical experimental methods have been applied to the study of hypothalamic neuroendocrine regulation, as shown in Table 1. With the biochemical identification of many of the chemical substances utilized in the signal integration at the hypothalamus and the pituitary levels, immunological techniques could be applied.[6] The classical hypothalamic hormones have been chemically characterized, primarily as peptides. In addition to the classical hypothalamic peptide hormones, including corticotropin-releasing hormone (CRH), growth hormone-releasing hormone (GHRH), thyrotropin-releasing hormone (TRH), and somatostatin, and several other peptides have been demonstrated within the hypothalamic neurons.[7] An important development was that of the high-affinity binding techniques using radiolabeled ligand. This led to the direct study of ligand receptor interaction and pharmacological characterization of receptor binding sites.[8] Receptor proteins that enabled probes to be derived and cloned were isolated and purified.[9,10] Eventually, by applying the methodologies of molecular biology, it was possible to isolate gene coding for many of the receptor proteins. Membrane receptors have been found to belong to at least four different classes of protein.[11] This increased understanding of receptor structure and function at the gene and protein levels made possible the development of probes for the protein itself. These protein probes could be produced by raising antibodies against synthetic peptides derived from the predicted amino acid sequence of a receptor or from a recombinantly produced receptor protein. It was then possible to estimate levels of mRNA for a given receptor protein.

The development of receptor ligand binding was also instrumental in facilitating the purification and isolation of the receptor proteins on the neuron membranes. The type and distribution of the membrane receptors for many of the hypothalamic chemical signals have been mapped within the hypothalamic nuclei (Table 2). Radioimmunological, immunohistochemical, and *in situ* hybridization techniques have been utilized to define the levels, location, and regulation of the various peptides.[12] Immunohistochemistry of receptors has demonstrated the association of specific receptor sites with different parts of the neuron. *In situ* hybridization has permitted the visualization of the perikarya, where receptor mRNAs are synthesized for the peptides, whereas receptor autoradiography has revealed the localization of the receptor polypeptides themselves.[13]

These techniques have been applied to study the maturation process of the brain's neurochemistry. Biochemical and immunohistochemical studies on rats and humans have revealed important differences in distribution of hypothalamic factors such as luteinizing hormone-

TABLE 1
Methods Applied in Hypothalamic Research

Method	Animal	Measurement	References
Microdialysis	Rat	Measure noradrenalin release in medial preoptic area	Barraclough[21]
	Rat	Measure extracellular serotonin release	Hernandez et al.[22]
In situ hybridization and immunocytochemistry	Rat	Map distribution of oxytocin-expressing neurons in nuclei	Chung et al.[23]
Immunocytochemistry	Human	Map distribution of LHRH prohormone product in hypothalamus	Bloch et al.[24]
	Human	Map distribution of vasopressin and oxytocin sites in separate neuronal types	Braak and Braak[25]
	Human	Map distribution of LHRH neurons	Najimi et al.[26]
	Human	Map location of opioid and vasopressin neurons in the paraventricular nucleus	Goldsmith and Dudek[27]
Retrograde tracers	Rat	Labeling spinal cord projections to hypothalamus	Burstein et al.[28]
Patch-clamp analysis	Rat	Analyzing spontaneous synaptic currents: IPSC and EPSC in supraoptic magnocellular neurons	Wuarin and Dudek[29]
Radioautography with highly selective ligands	Rat	Map distribution of μ, δ, and κ opioid receptors in the hypothalamus	Desjardins et al.[20]
	Rat	Map distribution of binding sites for vasopressin and oxytocin	Dreifuss et al.[30]
	Rat	Map distribution of somatostatin receptors	Epelbaum[31]

LHRH, luteinizing hormone-releasing hormone; IPSC, inhibitory postsynaptic current; EPSC, excitatory postsynaptic current.

releasing hormone (LHRH), somatostatin, and TRH between neonates and adults.[14] In addition, the opioid peptides have been shown to play a major role in hypothalamic regulation of a variety of autononic, behavioral, and neuroendocrine functions.[15,16] For example, intrahypothalamic administration of opioid analogues has been shown to decrease blood pressure,[17] stimulate eating,[18] and modulate the release of many hypothalamic hypophysiotropic factors.[19] The precise knowledge concerning the distribution of opioid receptor types within the hypothalamus is important to understanding their mode of action. A comprehensive study of μ, δ, and κ opioid binding sites in the rat has been completed.[20]

FUNCTIONAL ANATOMY OF THE HYPOTHALAMUS

OVERVIEW: THE HYPOTHALAMUS AND ITS NUCLEI

The hypothalamus is a complex part of the central nervous system (CNS), having rich interconnections with the forebrain, limbic, and brain stem structures.[41] Its outflow influences the endocrine system via the neurohypophyseal and adenohypophyseal neurosecretory systems.

The hypothalamus is the part of the diencephalon portion of the brain that extends from the region of the optic chiasma to the caudal border of the mamillary bodies.[42] It lies below the hypothalamic sulcus on the lateral wall of the third ventricle. The hypothalamus forms the floor and lower part of the lateral wall of the third ventricle.

Microscopically, the hypothalamus is composed of nerve cells arranged in groups or nuclei, many of which are not clearly segregated from one another (Figure 1). The principal nuclei and their connections can be divided into two major zones: the medial zone and the lateral zone.[41] In the medial zone, six groups are recognized: the paraventricular nuclei, the dorsomedial nucleus, the ventromedial nucleus, the infundibular (arcuate) nucleus, and the

TABLE 2
Receptors on Hypothalamic Cells

Receptor Type	Animal	Location	References
Opioid receptors			
μ	Rat	MPN, SCN, VMN	Desjardins et al.[20]
	Rat	ARC	Loose et al.[32]
	Guinea pig	PVN, SON	Wuarin and Dudek[29]
δ	Rat	SCN, VMN	Desjardins et al.[20]
κ	Rat	SCN	Desjardins et al.[20]
Adrenergic			
α₁	Duck	PVN, SON, POA	Gerstberger et al.[33]
α₂	Duck	PVN, POA	Gerstberger et al.[33]
β	Duck	PVN, POA	Gerstberger et al.[33]
Angiotensin-II	Duck	PVN, SON, POA	Gerstberger et al.[33]
Vasoactive intestinal peptide	Duck	PVN	Gerstberger et al.[33]
Antidiuretic hormone	Duck	PVN, SON, POA	Gerstberger et al.[33]
Vasopressin	Rat	SCN, ARC	Dreifuss et al.[30]
Oxytocin	Rat	VMN	Dreifuss et al.[30]
Melatonin	Rhesus monkey	SCN	Weaver et al.[34]
Corticosterone II	Rat	PVN, hippocampus, amygdala, septum	Jacobson and Sapolsky[35]
MSH and ACTH	Rat	ARC	Roselli-Rehfuss et al.[36]
Neuropeptide Y	Rat	ARC	Kalra and Crowley,[37] Pelletier[38]
Histamine	Human	Tuberomamillary	Panula et al.[39]
Muscarinic cholinergic	Human	VMN, tuberal nuclei, lateral area	Palacios et al.[40]
TRH	Human	POA, infundibular nucleus	Kopp et al.[14]
Somatostatin	Rat	Periventricular nucleus	Kopp et al.[14]
	Human	PVN	Kopp et al.[14]
	Human	Tuberal nuclei, lateral area, posterior nucleus	Palacios et al.[40]
	Rat	ARC	Epelbaum[31]

MPN, medial preoptic nucleus; SCN, suprachiasmatic nucleus; VMN, ventromedial nucleus; ARC, arcuate; PVN, paraventricular nucleus; SON, supraoptic nucleus; POA, preoptic area; ACTH, adrenocorticotropic hormone; MSH, melanocyte-stimulating hormone; TRH, thyrotropin-releasing hormone.

posterior nucleus. In the lateral zone, four major groupings are recognized: the supraoptic nucleus, the lateral nucleus, the tuberomamillary nucleus, and the lateral tuberal nucleus. The functions of many of these hypothalamic nuclei have been investigated (Table 3).

MORPHOLOGY OF THE HYPOPHYSIOTROPIC SYSTEM (ADENOHYPOPHYSEAL)

The hypophysiotropic system is less concisely organized. Only recently has its complexity been revealed by immunocytochemical techniques. The term describes the disparate system of neurons in the hypophysiotropic area projecting to the external layer of the median eminence where their terminals release their peptidergic, aminergic, and, probably, amino acid contents into the portal vessels to be transported to the adenohypophysis.[43] Many of these systems converge on the retrochiasmatic area during their projection to the median eminence and neurohypophysis. The hypothalamic hormones identified and visualized in these neurons are the following: gonadotropin-releasing hormone (GnRH), CRH, TRH,

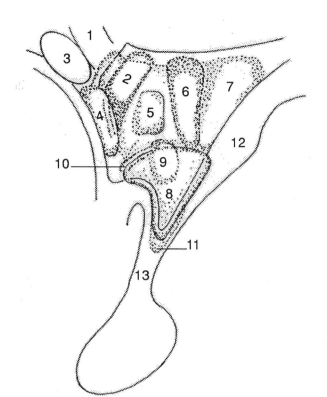

1. Fornix

2. Paraventricular nucleus

3. Anterior commissure

4. Preoptic area

5. Dorsomedial nucleus

6. Posterior nucleus

7. Lateral hypothalamus

8. Periventricular nucleus

9. Ventromedial nucleus

10. Supraoptic nucleus

11. Arcuate nucleus

12. Mammillary body

13. Infundibulum

FIGURE 1. Hypothalamic nucleus of the human brain.

somatostatin (growth hormone release inhibiting factor), GHRH, neurotensin, Met and Leu enkephalin, dynorphin, β-endorphin, adrenocorticotropic hormone (ACTH), galanin, vasoactive intestinal peptide (VIP), GABA, and dopamine.

MORPHOLOGY OF THE HYPOTHALAMIC NEUROHYPOPHYSEAL SYSTEM

The neurohypophyseal system is comprised of the projections of the large neurons of the paraventricular and supraoptic nuclei (and associated cell clusters in the anterior medial hypothalamus) to the neurohypophysis.[42] Axons of paraventricular neurons extend laterally over and around the fornix, and then ventrally to join axons of the supraoptic neurons as the supraoptico-hypothalamo, hypophyseal tract. The axons then turn caudally, to run in the internal layer of the median eminence to reach the neurohypophysis. Here, the terminals assume a close association with the capillary plexus of the posterior lobe. Approximately equal numbers of oxytocin- and vasopressin-containing neurons are present in both supraoptic and paraventricular nuclei of the rat.[43] Vasopressin neurons are largely retricted to ventral parts of the supraoptic nucleus and a spherical lateral zone in the posterior magnocellular paraventricular nucleus.[44]

THE MAGNOCELLULAR NEUROSECRETORY SYSTEM

The neurohypophysis contains neurosecretory nerve terminals that originate in the hypothalamus from magnocellular neurons.[57] Most of the magnocellular cells are concentrated in two paired structures, the supraopotic nuclei, located at the ventral surface of the brain near the optic chiasma, and the paraventricular nuclei, adjacent to the third ventricle. The neurosecretory terminals contain large amounts of oxytocin and vasopressin, which are synthesized in the cell somata and are transported down the axons into swellings in their nerve endings.

TABLE 3
Major Hypothalamic Nuclei

Hypothalamic Regions	Hypothalamic Nuclei	Comment	References
Chiasmatic and preoptic	Supraoptic, paraventricular	Vasopressin, oxytocin, and the hypothalamic-pituitary-adrenal system	Afifi,[45] Mohr,[46] Pittman[47]
	Supraoptic, paraventricular	Location of synthesis of CRF, vasopressin, and oxytocin	Jacobson and Sapolsky,[36] Kalsbeek,[48] Sawchenko[49]
	Paraventricular	Regulation of endocrine and modulation of autonomic function	Liposits et al.[50]
	Paraventricular	Regulation of ingestive behaviors	Grijalva[51]
	Paraventricular	Regulation of thyroid hormones via TRH, TSH	Kjos[52]
	Paraventricular	Role in control of thyroid function	Lechan and Jackson[53]
	Periventricular	1° source of CRH	Costa,[54] Delbende[55]
	Periventricular	Site for homeostasis: temperature, osmolality, appetite and behavioral drives	Bruce[56]
	Suprachiasmatic	Binding site of vasopressin	Dreifuss et al.[30]
	Suprachiasmatic	Principal component of the biological clock	Hofman,[57] Kalsbeek,[61] Bartke[58]
Tuberal	Arcuate	Site of highest concentration of neuropeptide Y-containing cell bodies	Pelletier[63]
	Arcuate	Site of cell bodies containing β-endorphin	Tang[59]
	Arcuate	Site for central signal generator of GnRH release	Cardenas,[60] Stuenkel[61]
	Ventromedial	Binding site of oxytocin	Dreifuss et al.[30]
	Ventromedial	Control site for satiety	Afifi and Bergman[45]
Mamillary	Lateral and medial	Medial nucleus is major component of mamillary body	Boshes[62]

CRF, corticotropin-releasing factor; TRH, thyrotropin-releasing hormone; TSH, thyroid-stimulating hormone; CRH, corticotropin-releasing hormone; GnRH, gonadotropin-releasing hormone.

The magnocellular neurosecretory system has served as a model for peptidergic neurons for many years. The mammalian magnocellular neurosecretory neurons secrete principally vasopression and oxytocin from the neurohypophyseal nerve terminals into the systemic circulation. The cells respond to a variety of stimuli: vasopressin release occurs in response to stimuli that change or threaten the water status in the body (plasma osmotic pressure and blood volume/blood pressure); oxytocin release is caused by parturition and suckling and also in some species by osmotic stimuli.

HYPOTHALAMIC NEUROENDOCRINE REGULATION OF ANTERIOR PITUITARY FUNCTION

HYPOPHYSIOTROPIC HORMONES

Growth Hormone-Releasing Hormone and Somatostatin and Their Regulation

The secretion of growth hormone (GH) is regulated by a complex neuroendocrine system that involves the CNS, hypothalamus, anterior pituitary, and various target tissues. Control of GH secretion occurs by an interplay between at least two hypothalamic hormones: the stimulatory GHRH and its inhibitory counterpart, somatostatin.[63] The hypothalamic GHRH is a 44-amino acid peptide that promotes an increased transcription of the GH gene. It also increases the translation of the mRNA encoding of GH and the release of the available GH from the cell.

The study of experimental animals and humans documents the key role of the two hypothalamic peptides, somatostatin and GHRH, in the regulation of GH secretion.[64] The inhibitory peptide is localized within the hypothalamic paraventricular nuclei and released by nerve terminals into the hypothalamic-pituitary portal microvasculature. Studies in conscious sheep and rat indicate that somatostatin is released into the portal venous blood.[65] After transport to the anterior pituitary gland, somatostatin is capable of inhibiting the stimulatory effects of the various hypothalamic releasing factors, including GHRH, GnRH, and TRH. Somatostatin suppresses the release of GHRH from the somatotroph cells but does not apppear to inhibit transcription of the GH gene or synthesis of GH protein.

In humans and experimental animals, there is an ultradian pattern of GH secretion from the anterior pituitary that is pulsatile.[66] In the male rat, pulses of GH secretions occur at regular 3–4-h intervals throughout the day with peak values greater than 100 ng/ml and with undetectable trough values.[67] In most mammalian species, the postpubertal growth and body size are sexually dimorphic. In the rat, there is a sexual difference in the pattern of GH secretion and the rate of somatic growth. Females show more frequent, lower amplitude GH pulses with elevated basal GH levels. Female rats show no clear rhythm or distinct trough phase. The mechanism underlying the generation of the rhythmic secretory patterns of somatostatin and GHRH is unknown.

In healthy adults, there is a physiologic correlation of GH secretion and slow-wave sleep (stages III and IV).[68] In contrast, sleep associated with rapid eye movement (REM) is accompanied by a suppression of GH secretion.[69] The mechanism involved is not known but it is suggested that it involves a somatostatin withdrawal during slow-wave sleep. In anorexia nervosa and malnutrition, and during fasting, a marked increase in mean serum GH levels has been observed.[70] When eating is resumed, there is a very rapid suppression of GH secretion.

There is evidence that in addition to exerting opposite actions on the anterior pituitary, somatostatin and GHRH may interact within the CNS to modulate hypophyseal GH secretion. Ultrastructural studies have indicated that the somatostatin-positive neuron terminals are in direct contact with GHRH-immunoreactive cells in the arcuate nucleus. In addition, findings suggest that somatostatin receptors may be directly associated with the perikarya of the GHRH-containing neurons. This implies a possible direct regulation of GHRH by somatostatin at the hypothalamic level. These morphological findings, together with physiological results, support the concept of a somatostatin-mediated central influence on GHRH-containing arcuate neuronal system.

Corticotropin-Releasing Hormone and Its Regulation

Baseline levels of glucocorticoids are necessary for the normal function of most tissues. Small deviation from normal levels of circulating glucocorticoids results in significant changes in a wide variety of physiological and biochemical variables in the body. Of the various regulatory mechanisms, the hypothalamic-pituitary-adrenal (HPA) axis plays a critical role in controlling the levels of the hypothalamic CRH. CRH-secreting neurons have been indentified by immunohistochemical techniques. Those neurons involved in anterior pituitary regulation arise in cells in the paraventricular nucleus and project to the median eminence.

In normal individuals, the HPA axis is regulated by a combination of circadian and stress-related excitatory inputs, inhibitory influences, and various negative feedback loops.[71] A variety of neurotransmitters appear to stimulate secretion of CRH. Cortisol and other corticosteriods are secreted by the adrenal cortex in response to stimulation with ACTH.[72] The secretion of ACTH by corticotroph cells in the anterior pituitary is principally influenced by CRH. However, vasopressin also releases ACTH and potentiates the ACTH response to CRH.[73] In fetal and neoplasic tissue, but not in healthy humans, VIP and cholecystokinin octapeptide also release ACTH.[74]

The effect of ACTH on cortisol is potentiated by *N*-proopiomelanocortin.[75] Acetylcholine directly stimulates CRH secretion. Central implants of atropine block the stress-induced HPA axis activation in rats.[76] This suggests that acetylcholine is a mediator of the stress response.[77]

Norepinephrine- and epinephrine-secreting neurons originating from the brain stem sympathetic nuclei also stimulates CRH secretion. This appears to be mediated by both α-1 and α-2 receptors.[78] In addition, the hypothalamic CRH neurons send projections to and stimulate these nuclei such as in the locus ceruleus. Studies indicate that local CRH administration at the locus ceruleus of awake, unrestrained rats increases its firing rate.[79] Therefore, it appears that the hypothalamic CRH neurons and the sympathetic nuclei are involved in a mutually reinforcing positive feedback loop.

Serotonin appears to activate the HPA axis via stimulation of both hypothalamic CRH and pituitary ACTH secretion. In addition, serotonin stimulates the release of hypothalamic AVP (arginine vasopressin), which also stimulates the corticotroph.[80] AVP and norepinephrine are synergistic with CRH in the regulation of the stress response.[80] CRH neurons co-contain AVP. CRH neurons receive regulatory signals from many parts of the brain. Important excitatory inputs are from the suprachiasmatic nucleus, the amygdala, and the raphe nuclei of the brain stem. The afferent control has been studied extensively.[81]

Inhibitory inputs on CRH secretion originate in the hippocampus and in the locus ceruleus of the midbrain. The excitatory influences are cholinergic, serotoninergic, or noradrenergic. The inhibitory influences are adrenergic also.

Glucocorticoids secreted by the adrenal gland exert negative feedback effects on the pituitary corticotroph cells, the hypothalamic CRH secreting neurons, and components of the limbic system. These studies indicate the presence of multiple regulatory negative feedback loops that act directly at the level of the CRH neurons.[82]

Endorphinergic pathways also play a role via ACTH regulation. Opioids have been shown to exert complex effects on the HPA axis.[83] Given acutely, morphine stimulates the secretion of β-endorphin, ACTH, and corticosteriods, whereas given chronically, it reduces the release of proopiomelanocortin-derived peptides.[84] It is reported that morphine and μ-agonists stimulate the secretion of CRH. Intrahypothalamic injections of CRH inhibit gonadotropin secretion and induce a characteristic pattern of behavior that suggests severe emotional distress.[86,87] There are several reviews dealing with the relationship between the HPA axis and various stress-induced clinical conditions.[88]

Gonadotropin-Releasing Hormone and Its Regulation

In the secretion of gonadotropins, the role of GnRH is well established.[89] The prevailing view was that only one GnRH, produced by the hypothalamic neurosecretory cells, was involved in the regulation of both LH and follicle-stimulating hormone (FSH) secretion. Recent work, however, provides evidence for a differential control of LH and FSH secretion.[90] Norepinephrine is the principal neurotransmitter promoting LH release, whereas serotonin inhibits LH release under most conditions. Opiates reduce hypothalamic norepinephrine activity and enhance serotonin activity, thus decreasing GnRH release. The gonadal steroids normally mimic these opiate effects by inhibiting norepinephrine activity and as a consequence reducing GnRH release.

Thyrotropin-Releasing Hormone and Its Regulation

TRH was characterized as a tripeptide amide[91] and shown to be present in high concentrations in the brain.[92] That brain region is now known as the paraventricular nucleus, located at the dorsal margin of the third ventricle. The paraventricular nucleus contains the hypophysiotropic neurons of the TRH-tuberoinfundibular system. These cells project to the median eminence mainly through the lateral retrochiasmatic area.

TRH was initially isolated from bovine and porcine hypothalamus and identified as the tripeptide amine pGlu-His-Pro-NH$_2$.[95] Its biological actions have been reported to be mediated by specific membrane receptors.[94] In the rat, the TRH binding sites are widely distributed in many brain regions. Radioimmunoassay studies on the human brain have indicated higher

TRH binding site levels in three structures: the ventromedial nucleus and the paraventricular and dorsal nuclei on the left side.

Prolactin and Its Regulation

Prolactin is an anterior pituitary hormone that acts directly on target tissue rather than as a tropic hormone. Although prolactin plays many physiologic roles in other animals, its known function in humans is postpartum stimulation of milk production. It is, however, present in males and nonpregnant females, where its function is unknown. In addition, bursts of prolactin release occur in sleep and during stress.[95] Unlike other pituitary hormones, prolactin is regulated mainly by tonic inhibition rather than by intermittent stimulation. The neurotransmitter dopamine appears to fit the criteria of a prolactin releasing inhibitory factor. Hence, prolactin's principal inhibitor is dopamine. Prolactin enhances dopamine secretion and thus inhibits its own secretion. Other known physiologic inhibitors are somatostatin and triiodothyronine. Prolactin release is stimulated by serotonin, acetylcholine, opiates, estrogens, TRH, and angiotensin-II. Which of these is physiologically important is not known.

Prolactin secretion rises during pregnancy. When estrogen levels begin to fall, lactation becomes possible. As lactation starts and the mother nurses the baby, prolactin levels begin to move toward nonpregnant levels. Lactation can continue at normal resting levels of prolactin. Prolactin is processed in the lactotrophic cell by undergoing a transformation into a releaseable form before exocytotic release.[97] Studies indicate that the dopamine prolactin inhibitory mechanism occurs during the transformation of prolactin within the lactotrophic cell of the anterior pituitary. In the suckling rat, the dopamine is transiently suppressed, enhancing the essential prolactin transformation process.

HYPOTHALAMIC NEUROENDOCRINE REGULATION OF POSTERIOR PITUITARY FUNCTION

NEUROHYPOPHYSEAL HORMONES: OXYTOCIN AND VASOPRESSIN AND THEIR REGULATION

When release of neurohypophyseal hormones is required, the magnocellular neurons develop specific firing patterns.[98] Oxytocin neurons can be characterized electrophysiologically by their synchronous high-frequency discharge during suckling, and vasopressin neurons by their asynchronous phasic activity.[99] The release of oxytocin and vasopressin is triggered by central inputs to the supraoptic and paraventricular nuclei or directly by osmotic stimuli at cells of the supraoptic nucleus.[100] At the level of the neurohypophysis, hormone release can be modulated by various neurotransmitters and neuropeptides. The modulatory factors are either colocalized and co-released with the vasopressin or oxytocin, or contained within separate transmitter endings.[101] It is clear that magnocellular neurons contain numerous peptides. They are present in smaller amounts than vasopressin and oxytocin. The peptides include dynorphin, enkephalins, galanin, cholecystokinin, TRH, CRH, neuropeptide Y, and other uncharacterized proteins.[102] The relative amounts of these co-packaged peptides vary under different physiological conditions.

SUMMARY

It is said that the advances in understanding of the physiological problems parallel the advances in understanding of the morphology of the system under investigation. This is certainly the case for the hypothalamic neuroendocrine system, in which the visualization of the location of the hormones, neurohormones, and neurotransmitters has so greatly increased in detail recently, with the development of immunohistochemical and related methods. Specific ligand receptor binding studies have now revealed that a large number of potential chemical signal interactions are comon on the neurons of the hypothalamus. Also, the discovery of the typical occurrence of the co-packaging of different neuropeptides within the same hypothalamic neuron suggests a level of complexity not yet understood. The last 40 years of studies in the field of neuroendocrine regulation has been a time of active neuro-chemical mapping of the various hypothalamic nuclei and their afferent and efferent connections. These extensive details concerning the morphology of the hypothalamus are beginning to generate new insights into this complex regulatory system.

REFERENCES

1. **Swanson, L. W.,** The hypothalamus, in *Handbook of Chemical Neuroanatomy: Integrated Systems of the CNS, Part 1, 5,* Björklund, A., Hökfelt, T., and Swanson, L. W., Eds., Elsevier, Amsterdam, 1987, 1.
2. **Harris, G. W.,** Humors and hormones, *J. Endocrinol.,* 53, 2, 1972.
3. **Scharrer, E. and Scharrer, B.,** Hormones produced by neurosecretory cells, *Recent Prog. Horm. Res.,* 10, 183, 1954.
4. **Bargmann, W. and Scharrer, E.,** The site of origin of the hormones of the posterior pituitary, *Am. Sci.,* 39, 255, 1951.
5. **Silverman, A. and Pickard, G. E.,** The hypothalamus, in *Chemical Neuroanatomy,* Emson, P. C., Ed., Raven Press, New York, 1983, 295.
6. **Kuhar, M. J., DeSouza, E. D., and Unnerstall, J. R.,** Neurotransmitter receptor mapping by autoradiography and other methods, *Annu. Rev. Neurosci.,* 9, 27, 1986.
7. **Yamamura, H. I., Enna, S. J., and Kuhar, M. J.,** *Methods in Neurotransmitter Receptor Analysis,* Raven Press, New York, 1990.
8. **Seifert, G., Ed.,** *Cell Receptors, Morphological Characterization and Pathological Aspects,* Springer, Berlin, 1991.
9. **Barnard, E. A., Darlison, M. G., and Seeburg, P.,** Molecular biology of the GABA: the receptatory channel superfamily, *Trends Neurosci.,* 10, 502, 1987.
10. **Hall, Z. W.,** Three of a kind: the β-adrenergic receptor, the muscarinic acetylcholine receptor, and rhodopsin, *Trends Neurosci.,* 10, 99, 1987.
11. **Valentino, K. L., Eberwine, J. H., and Barchas, J. D., Eds.,** *In situ* hybridization, in *Applications to Neurobiology,* Oxford University Press, Oxford, 1987.
12. **Diericks, K. and Vandesande, F.,** Immunocytochemical localization of the vasopressinergic and the oxytocinergic neurons in the human hypothalamus, *Cell Tissue Res.,* 184, 15, 1977.
13. **Meister, B.,** Gene expression and chemical diversity in hypothalamic neurosecretory neurons, *Mol. Neurobiol.,* 7, 87, 1993.
14. **Kopp, N., Najimi, M., Champier, J., Chigr, F., Charnay, Y., Epelbaum, J., and Jordan, D.,** Ontogeny of peptides in human hypothalamus in relation to sudden infant death syndrome (SIDS), in *Progress in Brain Research,* 93, Swaab, D. F., Hofman, M. A., Mirmiran, M., Ravid, R., and van Leeuwen, F. W., Eds., Elsevier, London, 1992, 167.
15. **Olson, G. A., Olson, R. D., and Kastin, A. J.,** Endogenous opiates: 1986, *Peptides,* 8, 1135, 1987.
16. **Olson, G. A., Olson, R. D., and Kastin, A. J.,** Endogenous opiates: 1987, *Peptides,* 10, 205, 1989.
17. **Kregel, K. C., Reynolds, D. G., Guril, N. J., and Gisolfi, C. V.,** Effects of opiate receptor drugs injected intracerebrally into normovolemic and hypervolemic monkey, *Peptides,* 6, 1161, 1985.
18. **Gosnell, B. A., Grace, M., and Levine, A. S.,** Effects of beta-chlornaltrexamine on food intake, body weight, and opioid-induced feeding, *Life Sci.,* 40, 1459, 1987.
19. **Kalra, S. P., Kalra, P. S., Sahu, A., Allen, L. G., and Crowley, W. R.,** The steroid-neuropeptide connection in the control of LHRH secretion, *Adv. Exp. Med. Biol.,* 219, 65, 1987.
20. **Desjardins, G. C., Brawer, J. R., and Beaudet, A.,** Distribution of mu, delta, and kappa opioid receptors in the hypothalamus of the rat, *Brain Res.,* 536, 114, 1990.
21. **Barraclough, C. A.,** Neural control of the synthesis and release of luteinizing hormone-releasing hormone, in *Functional Anatomy of the Neuroendocrine Hypothalamus,* 168, Ciba Foundation Symposium, John Wiley & Sons, Chichester, 1992, 233.
22. **Hernandez, L., Parada, M., Baptista, T., Schwartz, D., West, H. L., Mark, G. P., and Hoebel, B. G.,** Hypothalamic serotonin in treatments for feeding disorders and depression as studied by brain microdialysis, *J. Clin. Psychiatry,* 52 (Suppl. 12), 32, 1991.
23. **Chung, S. K., McCabe, J. T., and Pfaff, D. W.,** Estrogen influences on oxytocin mRNA expression in preoptic and anterior hypothalamic regions studied by *in situ* hybridizations, *J. Comp. Neurol.,* 307, 281, 1991.

24. **Bloch, B., Gaillard, R. C., Culler, M. D., and Negro-Vilar, A.,** Immunohistochemical detection of proluteinizing hormone-releasing hormone peptides in neurons in the human hypothalamus, *J. Clin. Endocrinol. Metab.,* 74, 135, 1992.

25. **Braak, H. and Braak, E.,** Anatomy of the human hypothalamus (chiasmatic and tuberal region), in *Progress in Brain Research,* 93, Swaab, D. F., Hofman, M. A., Mirmiran, M., Ravid, R., and van Leeuwen, F. W., Eds., Elsevier, London, 1992, 3.

26. **Najimi, M., Chigr, F., Jordan, D., Leduque, P., Bloch, B., Tommasi, M., Rebaud, P., and Kopp, N.,** Anatomical distribution of LHRH-immunoreactive neurons in the human infant hypothalamus and extrahypothalamic regions, *Brain Res.,* 516, 280, 1990.

27. **Goldsmith P. C. and Dudek F. E.,** Patch-clamp analysis of spontaneous synaptic currents in supraoptic neuroendocrine cells of the rat hypothalamus, *J. Neurosci.,* 13, 2323, 1993.

28. **Burstein, R., Cliffer, K. D., and Giesler, G. J.,** Cells of origin of the spinohypothalamic tract in the rat, *J. Comp. Neurol.,* 291, 329, 1990.

29. **Wuarin, J. P. and Dudek, F. E.,** Patch-clamp analysis of spontaneous synaptic currents in supraoptic neuroendocrine cells of the rat hypothalamus, *J. Neurosci.,* 13, 2323, 1993.

30. **Dreifuss, J. J., Tribollet, E., Dubois-Dauphin, M., and Raggenbass, M.,** Receptors and neural effects of oxytocin in the rodent hypothalamus and preoptic region, in *Functional Anatomy of the Neuroendocrine Hypothalamus,* 168, Ciba Foundation, John Wiley & Sons, Chicester, 1992, 187.

31. **Epelbaum, J.,** Intrahypothalamic neurohormonal interactions in the control of growth hormone secretion, in *Functional Anatomy of the Neuroendocrine Hypothalamus,* 168, Ciba Foundation Symposium, John Wiley & Sons, Chichester, 1992, 54.

32. **Loose, M. D., Ronnekleiv, O. K., and Kelly, M. J.,** Neurons in the rat arcuate nucleus are hyperpolarized by GABA and mu-opioid receptors agonists: evidence for convergence at a ligand-gated potassium conductance, *Neuroendocrinology,* 54, 537, 1991.

33. **Gerstberger, R., Muller, A. R., and Simon-Oppermann, C.,** Functional Hypothalamic angiotensin II and catecholamine receptor systems inside and outside the blood-brain barrier, in *Progress in Brain Research,* 91, Ermisch, A., Landgraf, R., and Rühle, H. J., Eds., Elsevier, London, 1992, 423.

34. **Weaver, D. R., Stehle, J. H., Stopa, E. G., and Reppert, S. M.,** Melatonin receptors in human hypothalamus and pituitary: implications for circadian and reproductive responses to melatonin, *J. Clin. Endocrinol. Metab.,* 76, 295, 1993.

35. **Jacobson, L. and Sapolsky, R.,** The role of the hippocampus in feedback regulation of the hypothalamic-pituitary-adrenocortical axis, *Endocr. Rev.,* 12, 118, 1991.

36. **Roselli-Rehfuss, L., Mountjoy, K. G., Robbins, L. S., Mortrud, M. T., Low, M. J., Tatro, J. B., Entwistle, M. L., Simerly, R. B., and Cone, R. D.,** Identification of a receptor for gamma-melanotropin and other proopiomelanocortin peptides in the hypothalamus and limbic system, *Proc. Natl. Acad. Sci. U.S.A.,* 90, 8856, 1993.

37. **Kalra, S. P. and Crowley, W. R.,** Neuropeptide Y: a novel neuroendocrine peptide in the control of pituitary hormone secretion, and its relation to luteinizing hormone, *Front. Neuroendocrinol.,* 13, 1, 1992.

38. **Pelletier, G.,** Ultrastructural localization of neuropeptide Y in the hypothalamus, *Ann. N.Y. Acad. Sci.,* 611, 232, 1990.

39. **Panula, P., Airaksinen, M. S., Pirvola, U., and Kotilainen, E.,** A histamine-containing neuronal system in human brain, *Neuroscience,* 34, 127, 1990.

40. **Palacios, J. M., Probst, A., and Mengod, G.,** Receptor localization in the human hypothalamus, in *Progress in Brain Research,* 93, Swaab, D. F., Hofman, M. A., Mirmiran, M., Ravid, R., and van Leeuwen, F. W., Eds., Elsevier, London, 1992, 57.

41. **Everitt, B. J. and Hökfelt, T.,** Neuroendocrine anatomy of the hypothalamus, *Acta Neurochir. Suppl.,* 47, 1, 1990.

42. **Sofroniew, M. V.,** Vasopressin, oxytocin and their related neurophysins, in *Gaba and Neuropeptides in the CNS, Handbook of Chemical Neuroanatomy,* Björklund, A. and Hökfelt, T., Eds., Elsevier, Amsterdam, 1985, 93.

43. **Sawchenko, P. E. and Swanson, L. W.,** The organization of noradrenergic pathways from the brainstem to the paraventricular and supraoptic nuclei in the rat, *Brain Res. Rev.,* 4, 275, 1982.

44. **Hatton, G.I.,** Emerging concepts of structure-function dynamics in adult brain: the hypothalamo-neurohypophysial system, *Prog. Neurobiol.,* 34, 437, 1990.

45. **Afifi, A. and Bergman, R. A.,** *Basic Neuroscience,* 2, Urban & Schwarzenberg, Baltimore, 1986.

46. **Mohr, E. and Richter, D.,** Hypothalamic neuropeptide genes. Aspects of evolution, expression, and subcellular mRNA distribution, *Ann. N.Y. Acad. Sci.,* 689, 50, 1993.

47. **Pittman, Q. J. and Bagdan, B.,** Vasopressin involvement in central control of blood pressure, in *Progress in Brain Research,* 91, Ermisch, A., Landgraf, R., and Rühle, H. J., Eds., Elsevier, London, 1992, 69.

48. **Kalsbeek, A. and Buijs, R. M.,** Peptidergic transmitters of the suprachiasmatic nuclei and the control of circadian rhythmicity, in *Progress in Brain Research,* 92, Joosse, J., Buijs, R. M., and Tilders, F. J. H., Eds., Elsevier, London, 1992, 321.

49. **Sawchenko, P. E., Imaki, T., and Vale, W.,** Co-localization of neuroactive substances in the endocrine hypothalamus, in *Functional Anatomy of the Neuroendocrine Hypothalamus,* 168, Ciba Foundation Symposium, John Wiley & Sons, Chicester, 1992, 16.

50. **Liposits, Z.,** Ultrastructure of hypothalamic paraventricular neurons, *Crit. Rev. Neurobiol.,* 7, 89, 1993.

51. **Grijalva, C. V. and Novin, D.,** The role of the hypothalamus and dorsal vagal complex in gastrointestinal function and pathophysiology, *Ann. N.Y. Acad. Sci.,* 597, 207, 1990.

52. **Kjos, T., Gotoh, E., Tkacs, N., Shackelford, R., and Ganong, W. F.,** Neuroendocrine regulation of plasma angiotensinogen, *Endocrinology,* 129, 901, 1991.

53. **Lechan, R. M. and Jackson, I. M. D.,** Immunohistochemical localization of thyrotropin-releasing hormone in the rat hypothalamus and pituitary, *Endocrinology,* 111, 55, 1982.

54. **Costa, A., Trainer, P., Besser, M., and Grossman, A.,** Nitric oxide modulates the release of corticotrophin-releasing hormone from the rat hypothalamus *in vitro, Brain Res.,* 605, 187, 1993.

55. **Delbende, C., Delarue, C., Lefebve, H., Bunel, D. T., Szafarczyk, A., Mocaer, E., Kamoun, A., Jegou, S., and Vaudry, H.,** Glucocorticoids, transmitters and stress, *Br. J. Psychiatry,* 15 (Suppl.), 24, 1992.

56. **Bruce, D. A.,** Complications of third ventricle surgery, *Pediatr. Neurosurg.,* 17, 325, 1991.

57. **Hofman, M. A. and Swaab, D. F.,** Seasonal changes in the suprachiasmatic nucleus of man, *Neurosci. Lett.,* 139, 257, 1992.

58. **Bartke, A. and Steger, R. W.,** Seasonal changes in the function of the hypothalamic-pituitary-testicular axis in the Syrian hamster, *Soc. Exp. Biol. Med.,* 92, 139, 1992.

59. **Tang, F.,** Endocrine control of hypothalamic and pituitary met-enkephalin and beta-endorphin contents, *Neuroendocrinology,* 53 (Suppl. 1), 68, 1991.

60. **Cardenas, H., Ordog, T., O'Byrne, K. T., and Knobil, E.,** Single unit components of the hypothalamic multiunit electrical activity associated with the central signal generator that directs the pulsatile secretion of gonadotrophic hormones, *Proc. Natl. Acad. Sci. U.S.A.,* 90, 9630, 1993.

61. **Stuenkel, C. A.,** Neural regulation of pituitary function, *Epilepsia,* 32 (Suppl. 6), S2, 1991.

62. **Boshes, B.,** Syndromes of the diencephalon, in *Localization in Clinical Neurology,* Vinken, P. J. and Bruyn, G. W., Eds., North-Holland, Amsterdam, 1969, 432.

63. **Tannenbaum, G. S.,** Neuroendocrine control of growth hormone secretion, *Acta Paediatr. Scand.,* 372 (Suppl.), 5, 1991.

64. **Iranmanesh, A. and Veldhuis, J. D.,** Clinical pathophysiology of the somatotropic (GH) axis in adults, *Endocrinol. Metab. Clin. N. Am.,* 21, 783, 1992, Veldhuis J. D., Ed., W. B. Saunders, London.

65. **Frohman, L. A., Downs, T. R., and Clark, I. J.,** Measurement of growth hormone-releasing hormone and somatostatin in hypothalamic-portal plasma of unanesthetized sheep: spontaneous secretion and response to insulin-induced hypoglycemia, *J. Clin. Invest.,* 86, 17, 1990.

66. **Martin, J. B.,** Brain regulation of growth hormone secretion, *Frontiers Neuroendocrinol.,* 4, 129, 1976, Martini L. and Ganong W. F., Eds., Raven Press, New York.

67. **Tannenbaum, G. S. and Martin, J. B.,** Evidence for an endogenous ultradian rhythm governing growth hormone secretion in the rat, *Endocrinology,* 98, 562, 1976.

68. **Holl, R. W., Hartman, M. L., and Veldhaus, J. D.,** Thirty-second sampling of plasma growth hormone (GH) in man: correlation with sleep stages, *J. Clin. Endocrinol. Metab.,* 72, 854, 1991.

69. **Hartman, M. L., Veldhuis, J. D., and Johnson, M. L.,** Augmented growth hormone (GH) secretory burst frequency and amplitude mediate enhanced GH secretion during a two day fast in normal men, *J. Clin. Endocrinol. Metab.,* 74, 757, 1992.

70. **Ho, K. Y., Veldhuis, J. D., and Johnson, M. L.,** Fasting enhances growth hormone secretion and amplifies the complex rhythms of growth hormone secretion in man, *J. Clin. Invest.,* 81, 968, 1988.

71. **Keller-Wood, M. E. and Dallman, M. F.,** Corticosteroid inhibition of ACTH secretion, *Endocr. Rev.,* 5, 1, 1984.

72. **Checkley, S.,** Neuroendocrine mechanisms and the precipitation of depression by life events, *Br. J. Psychiatry Suppl.,* 15, 7, 1992.

73. **Gillies, G. E., Linton, E. A., and Lowry, P. J.,** Corticotropin releasing activity of the new CRF is potentiated several times by vasopressin, *Nature,* 299, 355, 1982.

74. **Jones, M. T. and Gillham, B.,** Factors involved in the regulation of adrenocorticotropic hormone/beta lipotropic hormone, *Physiol. Rev.,* 68, 743, 1988.

75. **Al-Dujaili, E. A. S., Hope J., Estivariz, F. E., et al.,** Circulating human pituitary pro-γ-melanotropin enhances the adrenal response to ACTH, *Nature,* 291, 156, 1981.

76. **Hedge, G. A. and Smelik, P. G.,** Corticotropin release: inhibition by intrahypothalamic implantation of atropine, *Science,* 159, 891, 1968.

77. **Hedge, G. A. and de Wied, D.,** Corticotropin and vasopressin secretion after hypothalamic implantation of atropine, *Endocrinology,* 88, 1257, 1971.

78. **Galogero, A. E., Gallucci, W. T., and Gold, P. W.,** Multiple feedback regulatory loops upon rat hypothalamic corticotropin-releasing hormone secretion: potential clinical implications, *J. Clin. Invest.,* 82, 767, 1988.

79. **Valentino, R. J., Foote, S. L., and Aston-Jones, G.**, Corticotropin-releasing factor activates noradrenergic neurons of the locus ceruleus, *Brain Res.*, 270, 363, 1983.

80. **Gibbs, D. M. and Vale, W.**, Effect of the serotonin reuptake inhibitor fluoxetine on corticotropin-releasing factor and vasopressin secretion into the hypophyseal protal blood, *Brain Res.*, 280, 176, 1983.

81. **Whitnall, M. H.**, Regulation of the hypothalamic corticotropin-releasing hormone neurosecretory system, *Prog. Neurobiol.*, 40, 573, 1993.

82. **Chrousos, G. P.**, Regulation and dysregulation of the hypothalamic-pituitary-adrenal axis, in *Endocrinology and Metabolism Clinics of North America*, 21, Veldhuis, J. D., Ed., W. B. Saunders, London, 1992, 833.

83. **Gonzalvez, M. L., Milanes, M. V., and Vargas, M. L.**, Effects of acute and chronic administration of mu- and delta-opioid agonists on the hypothalamic-pituitary-adrenocortical (HPA) axis in the rat, *Eur. J. Pharmacol.*, 200, 155, 1991.

84. **Buckingham, J. C. and Cooper, T. A.**, Differences in hypothalamo-pituitary-adrennocortical activity in the rat after acute and prolonged treatment with morphine, *Neuroendocrinology*, 38, 411, 1984.

85. **Pfeiffer, A., Herz, A., Loriaux, D. L., and Pfeiffer, D. G.**, Central kappa- and mu-opiate receptors mediate ACTH-release in rats, *Endocrinology*, 116, 2688, 1985.

86. **Cameron, O. G., Lee, M. A., Curtis, G. C., and McCann, D. S.**, Endocrine and physiological changes during 'spontaneous' panic attacks, *Psychoneuroendocrinology*, 12, 321, 1987.

87. **Gold, P. W., Goodwin, F. K., and Chrousos, G. P.**, Clinical and biochemical manifestations of depression, *N. Engl. J. Med.*, 319, 348, 1988.

88. **Rose, R. M. and Sachar, E.**, Psychoneuroendocrinology, in *Textbook of Endocrinology*, Williams, R., Ed., W. B. Saunders, Philadelphia, 1980, 646.

89. **Kalra, S. P. and Kalra, P. S.**, Neural regulation of luteinizing hormone secretion in the rat, *Endocr. Rev.*, 4, 311, 1983.

90. **Hall, J. E., Brodie, T. D., Badger, T. M., Rivier, J., Vale, W., Conn, M., Schoenfeld, D., and Crowley, W. F.**, Evidence of differential control of FSH and LH secretion by gonadotropin-releasing hormone (GnRH) form the use of a GnRH antagonist, *J. Clin. Endocrinol. Metab.*, 67, 524, 1988.

91. **Burgus, R., Dunn, T. F., DeSiderio, D., Ward, D. W., Vale, W., and Guillemin, R.**, Characterization of ovine hypothalamic hypophysiotrophic TSH-releasing factor, *Nature (London)*, 226, 321, 1970.

92. **Nair, R. M. G., Barrett, J. F., Bowers, C. Y., and Schally, A. V.**, Structure of porcine thyrotropin releasing hormone, *Biochemistry*, 9, 1103, 1970.

93. **Boler, R. M., Enzman, F., Folkers, K., Bowers, C. Y., and Schally, A. V.**, The identity of chemical and hormonal properties of the thyrotropin-releasing hormone and pyroglutamyl-histidyl-proline amide, *Biochem. Biophys. Res. Commun.*, 37, 705, 1969.

94. **Makara, G. B.**, The relative importance of hypothalamic neurons containing corticotrophin-releasing factor or vasopressin in the regulation of adrenocorticotropic hormone secretion, in *Functional Anatomy of the Neuroendocrine Hypothalamus*, 168, Ciba Foundation Symposium, John Wiley & Sons, Chichester, 1992, 43.

95. **Archer, D. F.**, Current concepts and treatment of hyperprolactinemia, *Obstet. Gynecol. Clin. North Am.*, 14, 979, 1978.

96. **Van de Kar, L. D., Richardson-Morton, K. D., and Rittenhouse, P. A.**, Stress: Neuroendocrine and pharmacological mechanisms, *Methods Achiev. Exp. Pathol.*, 14, 133, 1991.

97. **Grosvenor, C. E. and Mena, F.**, Regulation of prolactin transformation in the rat pituitary, in *Functional Anatomy of the Hypothalamus*, 168, Ciba Foundation, John Wiley & Sons, Chicester, 1992, 69.

98. **Renaud, L. P., Allen, A. M., Cunningham, J. T., Jarvis, C. R., Johnson, S. A., Nissen, R., Sullivan, M. J., van Vulpen, E., and Yang, C. R.**, Synaptic and neurotransmitter regulation of activity in mammalian hypothalamic magnocellular neurosecretory cells, in *Progress in Brain Research*, 92, Joosse, J., Buijs, R. M., and Tilders, F. J. H., Eds., Elsevier, London, 1992, 277.

99. **Poulain, D. A. and Wakerley, J. B.**, Electrophysiology of hypothalamic magnocellular neurons secreting oxytocin and vasopressin, *Neuroscience*, 7, 773, 1982.

100. **Mason, W. T.**, Supraoptic neurons of rat hypothalamus are osmosensitive, *Nature*, 287, 154, 1980.

101. **Falke, N.**, Modulation of oxytocin and vasopressin release at the level of the neurohypophysis, *Prog. Neurobiol.*, 36, 465, 1991.

102. **Meister, B., Villar, M. J., Ceccatelli, S., and Hökfelt, T.**, Localization of chemical messengers in magnocellular neurons of the hypothalamic supraoptic and paraventricular nuclei: an immunohistochemical study using experimental manipulations, *Neuroscience*, 37, 603, 1990.

103. **Renaud, L. P. and Bourque, C. W.**, Neurophysiology and neuropharmacology of hypothalamic magnocellular neurons secreting vasopressin and oxytocin, *Prog. Neurobiol.*, 36, 131, 1991.

Chapter 6

AN OVERVIEW OF THE BIOLOGICAL ACTIONS AND NEUROENDOCRINE REGULATION OF GROWTH HORMONE

William E. Sonntag

CONTENTS

INTRODUCTION

In the past 25 years, there have been tremendous strides in our understanding of the biological actions and neuroendocrine regulation of growth hormone. Although the existence of this hormone was originally proposed in the early part of this century and its structure determined in the 1940s, investigations of the mechanism of action and regulation of this hormone were impeded because of the difficulty in obtaining adequate amounts of purified hormone and the lack of a sensitive assay to detect changes in blood concentrations. With the development of radioimmunoassay (RIA) by Berson and Yalow in the 1960s and the first growth hormone RIA in 1968, scientific investigations into the regulation of growth hormone proceeded rapidly. The discovery of the structures for somatostatin and growth hormone-releasing hormone (GHRH), development of quantitative scientific techniques, new pharmaceutical agents, as well as modern techniques in molecular biology provided the impetus for further studies. Since the initial discovery of growth hormone, literally tens of thousands of papers have been published related to this topic. In this chapter, an overview of the biological actions of growth hormone and its neuroendocrine regulation are presented. Because it is not feasible to present an exhaustive review of this topic in the space provided, the focus of this chapter will be to provide an introduction into the history of, and current topics related to, the actions and regulation of growth hormone.

HISTORY AND BASIC ASPECTS OF GROWTH HORMONE

HISTORY

Since the early part of this century, it has been known that a substance present in blood promotes body growth, but it was only after Li et al.[1] isolated pure bovine growth hormone from the pituitary gland in 1945 that the specific biological effects of growth hormone became evident. This hormone was subsequently shown to stimulate amino acid uptake into tissues, promote DNA, RNA, and protein synthesis, have a role in cell division and hypertrophy, and increase bone growth and lean body mass. Soon after the discovery of growth hormone, highly purified pituitary extracts were used to stimulate growth in growth hormone-deficient children. An assay for determining circulating concentrations of growth hormone was developed by Utiger et al.[2] and the amino acid sequence was determined by Li et al.[3] and revised by Niall.[4] Early studies of plasma concentrations of growth hormone demonstrated marked variability, but in the late 1970s, it was recognized that this variability resulted in large part from discrete growth hormone pulses that increase after the onset of sleep.[5] Although the precise function of this ultradian pattern remains unknown, the pulsatile release of growth hormone has been confirmed in every species examined to date and has been demonstrated to be necessary for the biological actions of the hormone.

STRUCTURE OF GROWTH HORMONE

Growth hormone is a single-chain polypeptide composed solely of amino acids. The amino acid composition is similar among mammalian species as are the total number of amino acid residues.[10] It is generally accepted that these hormones are fairly uniform in molecular weight, ranging from 20,500 Da for human growth hormone to 26,000 Da for bovine growth hormone.[11] Growth hormone has two disulfide bridges formed from four cysteine residues which contribute to the secondary structure of the molecule. For porcine growth hormone, four alpha helices are present and helix 3 has an especially important role in function because substitution of amino acids in this region (e.g., Glu 117, Gly 119, and Ala 122) produces a molecule that binds to the growth hormone receptor but the biological activity is suppressed.[12] In transgenic mice expressing this mutation, growth rates are decreased, suggesting that endogenous growth hormone activity is inhibited.[13]

In humans, there appears to be alternative splicing of growth hormone mRNA leading to a 20-kDa variant of growth hormone.[14-16] Although, this variant represents 5–10% of growth hormone in the pituitary gland, specific regulation of this variant has not been demonstrated.[17] The 20-kDa variant retains activity in the rat tibia test for growth hormone biological activity but is not as efficient in inducing ^{14}C-glucose oxidation by adipose tissue, suggesting that the insulin-like activities of growth hormone can be separated from growth-promoting activities. Several other posttranslational modifications of growth hormone appear to be possible, although there are few data to suggest that these modifications impact the biological activity of the molecule. Phosphorylated, acetylated, glycosylated, and deaminated forms have been reported in the pituitary gland[17-21] but there is controversy concerning prevalence in serum. The multiple forms of growth hormone demonstrate that this is not a single protein but a family of related proteins which may have subtle variations in biological actions.

GROWTH HORMONE SECRETION

Studies of serum levels of growth hormone have revealed discrete pulses with amplitude and frequencies that vary between species and within males and females of the same species.[21-27] Although the biological basis for the pulsatile release of growth hormone is not entirely clear, the biological effects have been established. The response to growth hormone is increased when administered in discrete pulses compared to continuous infusions of the hormone. In children, growth hormone levels in serum are characterized by low-amplitude, low-frequency pulses, and, as puberty approaches, both the amplitude and the frequency increase, reaching a maximum at 12–15 years of age.[28-30] Trough levels of growth hormone are low or nondetectable. With increasing age, the amplitude of the pulses declines and in young adults the majority of growth hormone secretion is associated with the onset of slow-wave sleep although low amplitude pulses continue to occur throughout the day.[21] In mid-age and older adults, the amplitude of growth hormone pulses continues to decline, resulting in the characteristic reduction in IGF-I (insulin-like growth factor I) levels with age.[31,32] Similar changes in growth hormone are evident throughout the life cycle of rodents[33] and nonhuman primates except that the period of growth hormone secretion appears to be species specific[34,35] and sexually dimorphic. For example, in male rats the ultradian rhythm is characterized by high-amplitude secretory pulses every 3.5 h whereas in the female, these pulses occur approximately every hour.[36]

GROWTH HORMONE RECEPTORS

Recent studies using x-ray crystallography indicate that a single molecule of growth hormone binds to two membrane-bound receptors.[37] Site 1 binds to helix 4 and site 2 binds to helices 1 and 3 of growth hormone. The current model suggests that growth hormone binds to both receptors, which results in dimerization of the molecules and initiation of biological actions of growth hormone.[38] Dimerization results in activation of an independent tyrosine kinase, JAK 2 kinase, which phosphorylates the growth hormone receptor as well as other intracellular proteins (including MAP kinase) and appears to be necessary for the biological actions of the molecule.[39-43]

BIOLOGICAL ACTIONS OF GROWTH HORMONE

CARBOHYDRATE METABOLISM

Growth hormone is a potent diabetogenic agent, producing hyperglycemia and an insensitivity to elevated levels of insulin, which results from decreased uptake and utilization of carbohydrate. These changes have been observed after administration of growth hormone or after endogenous secretion of growth hormone. Early studies by Weil[44] described the response of organisms to exogenous growth hormone as triphasic. Initially, there is a transient hypoglycemia which may be attributed to an increase in fatty acid metabolism. In the second phase, glycolysis and glycogenesis are inhibited due to feedback by the degradation products of fatty acid metabolism and therefore the concentration of glucose in the circulation begins to rise. In the third phase, the increased concentrations of glucose are magnified due to decreased uptake, resulting in a marked release of insulin.

Similar findings were reported by Rabinowitz et al.[45,46] using a post-pyrandial model. In response to feeding, insulin secretion is increased whereas the level of growth hormone is reduced. The inverse relationship between insulin and growth hormone promotes glucose uptake and the formation of glycogen and triglycerides. Subsequently, insulin levels decline and growth hormone increases. In this phase, protein synthesis is promoted and excess storage of glucose is prevented. In the final phase, the secretion of growth hormone increases whereas insulin drops to basal levels. Growth hormone in this case attenuates tissue utilization of glucose and induces mobilization of fatty acids. The diabetogenic nature of endogenously secreted growth hormone has been shown by Schnure and Lipman.[47] These investigators reported a marked decline in glucose tolerance 90 min after the onset of sleep when growth hormone levels are elevated. From these studies, it is clear that growth hormone plays an important role in carbohydrate metabolism, but the actions of growth hormone are intimately related to effects on both lipid and protein metabolism.

LIPID METABOLISM

Recent studies have clearly indicated an important role for growth hormone in the regulation of adipose tissue. Studies indicated that growth hormone reduces adipose tissue mass in several species,[48,49] and studies by Rudman et al.[50] demonstrated that growth hormone decreases adipose tissue in older men. The primary effects of growth hormone are to retard lipogenesis by decreasing enzyme activity. Hypophysectomized rats treated with ovine growth hormone for four days demonstrate a reduction in the lipid content of epididymal and omental adipose tissue as compared to nontreated hypophysectomized rats.[51] Chronic administration of growth hormone results in inhibition of glyceride synthesis and decreased body fat content.[52] In addition, acute growth hormone treatment of fed, intact or hypophysectomized rats decreases fatty acid synthesis in both carcass and liver. A similar effect is not observed in starved rats, because lipogenesis is inhibited in these animals.

Growth hormone also facilitates mobilization of fatty acids when administered to fasted intact or hypophysectomized animals.[53] Treatment of hypophysectomized rats with growth hormone produces a significant release of free fatty acids by epididymal adipose tissue, and feeding reduces the magnitude of this response but does not abolish it completely.[53-55] The ability of growth hormone to promote mobilization of free fatty acids when administered *in vitro* is not nearly as pronounced as its *in vivo* effect. The release of fatty acids *in vitro* requires higher concentrations of growth hormone, suggesting that (a) growth hormone does not stimulate fatty acid mobilization by a direct action on adipose tissue or (b) other factors interact with growth hormone to regulate this effect.[53,56]

Early experiments suggested that growth hormone stimulated fatty acid oxidation, as indicated by a decrease in the respiratory quotient, an increase in ketogenesis, and subsequently a decrease in body fat. However, studies measuring respiratory $^{14}CO_2$ after injection of ^{14}C-palmitate failed to detect effects of growth hormone in fasted or fed hypophysectomized rats,[53,57] unanesthetized dogs,[58] or human diabetic subjects.[59] *In vivo* or *in vitro* administration of growth hormone also does not stimulate the oxidation of palmitate or acetate by rat liver slices or kidney homogenates.[60-62] Furthermore, neither hypophysectomy nor hypophysectomy with growth hormone replacement produced changes in the oxidation of ^{14}C-palmitate by isolated rat diaphragm.

PROTEIN METABOLISM

Growth hormone promotes protein synthesis, as indicated by decreased excretion of nitrogen subsequent to growth hormone administration. More specifically, early studies by Noall et al.[63] were able to show that growth hormone can stimulate amino acid transfer from the extracellular to the intracellular compartment utilizing the nonmetabolizable amino acid, ^{14}C-α-aminoisobutyric acid (^{14}C-AIB). Extending this observation, Riggs and Walker[64] reported that hypophysectomy diminishes the incorporation of ^{14}C-AIB into muscle, and this effect can be reversed by the administration of bovine growth hormone.

Employing *in vitro* experiments, Kostyo et al.[65] found that excised diaphragm from hypophysectomized rats accumulates less ^{14}C-AIB against a concentration gradient than does tissue from intact rats. Addition of either bovine or simian growth hormone to the preparations increased the transport of ^{14}C-AIB into the intracellular compartment. The transport induced by growth hormone is equivalent to that observed in diaphragms of intact rats. Similarly, diaphragms from hypophysectomized rats pretreated with growth hormone prior to sacrifice show higher intracellular levels of ^{14}C-AIB after *in vitro* incubation in ^{14}C-AIB than diaphragms of hypophysectomized rats that are not pretreated with growth hormone.[66]

In addition to an increase in AIB uptake, growth hormone can increase the intracellular transport of naturally occurring amino acids, such as glycine, alanine, serine, threonine, proline, histidine, tryptophan, glutamine, and asparagine.[67] The diminished total amino acid content of cartilage observed in hypophysectomized rats is replenished in hypophysectomized rats treated with growth hormone. Growth hormone stimulates the *in vitro* incorporation of labeled leucine and glycine into protein in diaphragms removed from hypophysectomized rats. A similar response is observed in preparations of the levator ani muscle.

Growth hormone also stimulates ^3H-leucine incorporation into protein.[68-70] This latter effect of growth hormone may be secondary to an increase in IGF-I because growth hormone increases IGF-I gene expression in a number of tissues. In addition, growth hormone has been reported to increase protein synthesis in the tibia,[71] collagen content of rat skin,[72] wound healing,[73,74] and erythropoiesis.[75]

INSULIN-LIKE GROWTH FACTORS

In 1957, Salmon and Daughaday[76] discovered a factor that was regulated by growth hormone and promoted the incorporation of sulfate into cartilage. These initial studies led to the identification and purification of the somatomedin family of hormones,[77] which are peptides of small molecular mass (about 7.5-kDA) that circulate in blood at high concentrations. These hormones have been shown to induce mitogenic activity in cultured fibroblasts and fetal cell lines, stimulate anabolic activity in many cell and tissue types, and induce DNA and protein synthesis.[78] Somatomedin C, which is also termed IGF-I, has been shown to be structurally related to insulin[79] and exerts similar though less potent effects on glucose regulation compared with insulin. IGF-I binds with high affinity to the type 1 IGF receptor through which it exerts its actions,[80] and receptors for these molecules are found in tissues throughout the body. It has been demonstrated that the type 1 IGF receptor shares 50% amino acid sequence similarity with insulin, and competitive binding and affinity cross-linking studies have demonstrated that IGF-I binds to the insulin receptor with 100 times lower affinity than to the IGF receptor.[80] IGF-I is synthesized mainly in the liver under regulation of growth hormone but is also synthesized in smaller quantities in almost all tissues.[81] Although the regulation of the paracrine activity of IGF-I is poorly understood, alterations in the activity of this hormone or its receptors at the tissue level have a significant effect on many intracellular processes.

IGF-I circulates in blood either free (with a half-life of 15–20 min) or bound to specific IGF-I binding proteins that prolong the half-life of the peptide. At present, six binding proteins have been identified[82] and constitute an intricate regulatory system that controls the availability of IGF-I to specific tissues. It is now clear that the binding proteins are important regulators of IGF-I activity and may also prevent hypoglycemic conditions that can be induced by IGF-I.

Over the past decade, there has been increasing interest in determining whether growth hormone acts directly on tissues or whether the effects of this hormone are mediated through IGF-I. Although investigators initially proposed that all the actions of growth hormone were mediated via IGF-I, other studies provided relatively convincing data that growth hormone could have direct anabolic effects on specific tissues.[83,84] However, subsequent studies demonstrated that IGF-I is present in most tissues of the body and that the "local" actions of growth hormone discovered by others were actually mediated via paracrine secretion of IGF-I. These studies have led to the concept that growth hormone has at least three actions: (1) stimulating IGF-I secretion from hepatic tissue, thereby increasing the concentration of IGF-I in plasma; (2) regulating IGF-I expression in tissues locally, thereby influencing the paracrine activity of IGF-I; and (3) acting directly on tissues to influence expression of specific proteins. With the technology available, it has been difficult to investigate the direct, independent actions of growth hormone because a large majority of tissues secrete IGF-I.

OTHER EFFECTS OF GROWTH HORMONE

As implied by its name, growth hormone has potent effects on growth including an increase in nitrogen retention, lean body mass, body length, body weight, and width of the epiphyseal cartilage plate. Classically, the tibia test is used as a bioassay for the effects of growth hormone.[85,86] This test compares the width of the epiphyseal plate after hypophysectomy and treatment with or without growth hormone. Comparisons are subsequently made in the width of the plate. The effects of growth hormone on body growth are supported by studies demonstrating that genetic dwarfs grow in response to growth hormone,[87,88] passive immunization with growth hormone antiserum decreases growth,[89-91] and transgenic animals expressing high levels of growth hormone exhibit increased body growth.[92,93]

While growth hormone administration results in the retention of minerals, such as sodium, potassium, and phosphorus, it produces an increased excretion of calcium as well as increased calcium absorption from the intestine.[94-99] This hypercalciuria may be mediated indirectly, through an effect of growth hormone on the parathyroid gland or by a rise in plasma phosphate also produced by growth hormone administration.[100,101] The elevation of plasma phosphate levels has been shown to be the result of an increase in kidney tubular phosphate reabsorption. In addition to effects on tubular function, renal plasma flow and glomerular filtration rate are increased by growth hormone administration; however, many of these effects can be mimicked by IGF-I, suggesting that the effects may not be direct. Growth hormone also promotes compensatory renal hypertrophy, which is absent in hypophysectomized rats.

Growth hormone has an important role as a "permissive factor" in a number of other endocrine systems. For example, growth hormone increases insulin secretion,[102-104] enhances the effects of adrenocorticotropic hormone (ACTH) on glucocorticoid release,[105,106] increases conversion of T_4 to T_3 in rats and humans,[107,108] augments effects of LH on steroid production by the ovary and testis,[109,110] and facilitates sexual maturation and puberty.[111]

In addition to a role in endocrine function, growth hormone is known to directly regulate the activity of specific proteins in liver. Estrogen receptors are increased by growth hormone[112] and growth hormone increases 5α-reductase and decreases 3α-hydroxysteroid dehydrogenase.[113] More recently, investigators have found that several hepatic enzymes are sexually dimorphic and are regulated by the pattern of growth hormone release (see review by Leakey et al.[114]). In male rats, growth hormone exhibits high-amplitude pulses with an interpulse interval of approximately 3.3 h whereas in the female both the amplitude of the pulses and the interpulse interval are reduced. Expression of the P450 enzymes 2C11 and 2C13 are influenced by the male pattern of growth hormone expression, whereas 2C12, steroid sulfotransferases, and testosterone 5α-reductase are stimulated by the female pattern. Other drug metabolizing enzymes are regulated by growth hormone and a combination of a number of other hormones such as glucocorticoids, thyroid hormones, and sex steroids.

REGULATION OF GROWTH HORMONE SECRETION BY HYPOTHALAMIC NEUROPEPTIDES

OVERVIEW

Growth hormone secretory dynamics result from an intricate interchange between somatostatin and growth hormone-releasing hormone (GHRH) secretion from the hypothalamus. GHRH increases growth hormone release,[115,116] and somatostatin inhibits its release.[117] The results of several studies suggest that both hormones are secreted in a phasic manner, with GHRH contributing to high-amplitude growth hormone pulses and somatostatin being secreted during trough periods.[118] The dynamic interrelationship between these hypothalamic hormones is responsible for pulsatile growth hormone secretion. Although somatostatin and GHRH have a critical role in the regulation of growth hormone, other factors contribute to growth hormone release by acting directly on the pituitary gland, by regulating hypothalamic GHRH or somatostatin secretion, or by influencing neurotransmitters that regulate somatostatin and GHRH release.

SOMATOSTATIN

Early evidence suggested the existence of a hypothalamic substance that can inhibit growth hormone release by rat pituitary cells *in vitro*.[119] A tetradecapeptide that inhibits growth hormone release was subsequently isolated by Vale et al.[120] and named GHRH or somatostatin. Both synthetic and ovine somatostatin inhibit the release of growth hormone by rat pituitary cells *in vitro* and inhibit the rise in growth hormone after the injection of sodium pentobarbital *in vivo*.[121]

Somatostatin inhibits the release of growth hormone and thyroid-stimulating hormone (TSH) in response to several pharmacological and physiological stimuli,[122] and chronic administration of somatostatin decreases pituitary and plasma growth hormone.[123] Passive immunization with antiserum against somatostatin increases basal levels of growth hormone, reverses the inhibition of growth hormone release by starvation or electric shock, and enhances thyrotropin-releasing hormone (TRH)-mediated TSH secretion.[124-129] Analysis of serial samples of blood revealed that somatostatin antiserum increases trough growth hormone levels, but the pulsatile nature of growth hormone release remained, providing convincing evidence for the existence of a GHRH which also controls the release of growth hormone.[36]

Somatostatin has been localized in the median eminence, arcuate nucleus, medial preoptic area, and periventricular nucleus of the rat hypothalamus.[130] Somatostatin immunoreactivity is also found in the ventromedial nucleus (VMN), amygdala, mamillary bodies, and olfactory tubercle.[131-134] Using immunocytochemical methods, somatostatin-containing fibers have been localized in the external zone of the median eminence and VMN of guinea pigs.[135] Somatostatin nerve fibers appear in the median eminence, forming part of the tuberoinfundibular tract.[136,137] Although perikarya for somatostatin were not localized in the same study, somatostatin fibers were generally localized in the arcuate, VMN, medial basal areas of the hypothalamus, and in the nerve endings of the organum vasculosum of the lamina terminalis of the rat in close proximity to the capillary network.[138] Somatostatin perikarya have been localized in the periventricular, VMN, and preoptic regions of the rat hypothalamus.[139-141] Studies on the anatomical localization of somatostatin cell bodies are supported by physiological evidence indicating that lesions of the preoptic-anterior hypothalamic area increase plasma growth hormone whereas stimulation of the VMN and periventricular regions increase somatostatin concentrations in portal blood and decrease plasma growth hormone concentrations.[142-144]

Somatostatin is synthesized as a prohormone and is enzymatically cleaved to the mature peptide during axonal transport to the median eminence. Two higher molecular weight forms of the hormone have been reported in hypothalamic extracts and there is evidence that higher molecular weight forms are released into portal blood.[145] Somatostatin-28 is a precursor to somatostatin-14 and has greater biological activity on a molar basis for inhibition of growth hormone release.[118] Although few data are available supporting an independent role for these molecules, somatostatin-28 release increases with age and appears to contribute to the age-related decline in growth hormone secretion.[146]

GROWTH HORMONE-RELEASING HORMONE

The existence of a GHRH was proposed in 1964 when it was found that hypothalamic extracts increase the release of growth hormone from incubated rat pituitaries in a dose-related manner.[147] GHRH was subsequently purified from a pancreatic tumor that induced acromegaly and was found to exhibit high homology to brain GHRH. GHRH is synthesized as a prohormone and subsequently processed to GHRH $(1-44)NH_2$ or GHRH $(1-40)OH$. Both forms of GHRH are released into hypophyseal portal blood and stimulate growth hormone release. Early studies demonstrated that GHRH is present in the VMN, because it has been shown that electrical stimulation of this area increases growth hormone release whereas lesions of this area decrease growth hormone release and result in growth retardation.[148,149] These studies were recently supported by immunocytochemical data showing immunoreactive GHRH material in the arcuate and VMN.[150-154] GHRH is transported to the median eminence and release into portal blood is enhanced by hypophysectomy,[155] opiates,[156] several neurotransmitters[157,158] including dopamine[159] and 5-HT (5-hydroxytryptamine)[160] and inhibited by IGF-I and somatostatin.[162-164] Passive immunization with antiserum against GHRH blocks growth hormone pulses[165,166] as well as the response to a number of physiological and pharmacological stimuli.[156,167]

Although mRNA and protein levels in the hypothalamus are not always an accurate indicator of GHRH activity and secretion, levels are greatest during trough periods and decline during growth hormone secretory episodes.[168] These results are consistent with the hypothesis that GHRH release into the portal circulation is necessary for high-amplitude growth hormone pulses.

INTEGRATION BETWEEN SOMATOSTATIN AND GHRH

The generally accepted model for regulation of growth hormone secretion proposes a dynamic interrelationship between somatostatin and GHRH. During trough periods, somatostatin secretion is high and GHRH secretion is low. Somatostatin secretion decreases and GHRH secretion subsequently increases resulting in high-amplitude growth hormone secretory episodes. However, several studies suggest that somatostatin can alter pituitary response to GHRH, and it is well known that withdrawal of the inhibitory effect of somatostatin alone results in a growth hormone surge. The amplitude of this latter surge is dependent on the levels of GHRH. Thus, phasic release of GHRH may not be a necessary precondition for high-amplitude growth hormone pulses.[169]

OPIOID PEPTIDES

The existence of opioid receptors in the brain had been suggested for many years by the profound analgesic and behavioral effects of plant opioid alkaloids on the mammalian central nervous system. Endocrine effects of morphine also had been suspected, based on observations of high infertility among narcotic addicts[170-172] and evidence that morphine initiated lactation in estrogen-primed rats.[173] Early work with morphine showed that it was a potent stimulator of growth hormone release in many species. The subsequent discovery of endogenous opioid peptides and opioid receptors in the brain strongly suggested a role in the neuroendocrine control of anterior pituitary hormones, including growth hormone.

Intraventricular or systemic administration of morphine or opioid peptides, such as β-endorphin and met^5-enkephalin, were shown to induce rapid increases in plasma growth hormone in rats.[174-177] β-endorphin was reported to be 500 to 2000 times more potent than met^5-enkephalin.[178] The stimulating activities of the opioid peptides were blocked by concomitant injection of naloxone, a specific opioid receptor antagonist.[176,177,179] The first evidence that endogenous opioid peptides had a physiologic role in the regulation of anterior pituitary hormone release was provided by the reports that naloxone alone can reduce basal serum growth hormone and prolactin and elevate serum luteinizing hormone (LH) and follicle-stimulating hormone (FSH) levels.[177-179]

The results on opioid regulation of anterior pituitary hormones have been confirmed and extended by a number of investigators, although data on growth hormone are controversial. Both naloxone and naltrexone are reported to decrease basal serum growth hormone levels.[177,179,180] However, early studies suggested that these drugs did not affect pulsatile growth hormone secretion in unanesthetized, unrestrained male rats.[181-183] More recent data demonstrate that naloxone can inhibit the growth hormone surge induced by suckling in postpartum lactating rats, suggesting that, at least under some circumstances, endogenous opioid peptides participate in the physiologic regulation of growth hormone. Similarly, naloxone can lower trough levels of growth hormone in female rats and pulse amplitude in male rats.[184]

In human subjects, enkephalin analogues have been found to stimulate growth hormone release, whereas naloxone can inhibit growth hormone release induced by arginine infusion or exercise stress, but does not influence basal growth hormone or growth hormone release induced by apomorphine, L-DOPA, insulin, hypoglycemia, or sleep.[186-189] These findings suggest that the endogenous opioid peptides have only a minor role in growth hormone secretion in humans. However, the doses of naloxone used in human studies usually have been low compared to those used in animal studies, and the timing of naloxone injections has been variable. Therefore, it is possible that higher doses of naloxone may have different effects on growth hormone release than those previously reported.

Opioid peptides do not appear to act directly on the anterior pituitary because they do not influence *in vitro* release of growth hormone or modulate response to somatostatin or GHRH.[178,179] The opiate-induced increase in growth hormone release also does not appear to be mediated exclusively through inhibition of hypothalamic somatostatin, because opiates can stimulate growth hormone release in rats passively immunized with antiserum to this peptide.[175,190]

There is evidence that the effects of opiates are mediated via hypothalamic neurotransmitters, which in turn can regulate the release of hypothalamic hormones into the portal vessels. Met^5-enkephalin and β-endorphin decrease dopamine and norepinephrine turnover in the median eminence,[191-193] whereas serotonin turnover is increased by acute administration of morphine or β-endorphin.[194-196] Because both dopamine and norepinephrine stimulate growth hormone release, it is unlikely that the opiate-induced increase in growth hormone is mediated through these neurotransmitters.

Although serotonin (5-HT) turnover is increased by β-endorphin, neither the 5-HT synthesis inhibitor, parachlorophenylalanine (PCPA), nor the 5-HT receptor blocker, metergoline, blocks growth hormone release induced by morphine[197] or enkephalin analogs.[198] The growth hormone releasing effect of an enkephalin analog is inhibited by the α-adrenergic receptor blocker, phenoxybenzamine, and by the norepinephrine synthesis inhibitor, diethyldithiocarbamate.[199] Stimulation of growth hormone by morphine is not affected by the α-adrenergic receptor blocker, prazosin, or the catecholamine synthesis inhibitor, α-methyl-paratyrosine in rats.[180,197] Thus, the precise mechanism through which opioid peptides increase growth hormone release remains unclear.

GALANIN

Galanin is found in the arcuate, periventricular, and supraoptic regions of the hypothalamus[200] and in several extrahypothalamic sites including the pituitary gland.[201] Galanin mRNA has been colocalized in GHRH neurons, and this, together with the distribution of galanin receptors throughout the hypothalamus and pituitary, suggests that the peptide may have an important paracrine role in regulation of growth hormone release. Both intraventricular and systemic injections of galanin have been reported to increase growth hormone secretion and to potentiate the actions of GHRH.[183,201-205] In addition, passive immunization with galanin antiserum decreases growth hormone pulse amplitude and increases pulse frequency.[206,207] Current studies suggest that galanin acts by increasing the secretion of GHRH, because its effects can be blocked by GHRH antiserum.[208] However, other investigators have proposed that galanin increases somatostatin secretion, which subsequently increases GHRH activity in a paracrine relationship.[209] This latter hypothesis is supported by several lines of evidence including data that suggest that somatostatin antiserum and other regimens that result in diminished somatostatin secretion decrease the galanin-induced rise in growth hormone. Many of the effects of galanin on growth hormone secretion appear to be estrogen dependent because they are greater in females and augmented by estrogen administration.[209]

SUBSTANCE P

Substance P is a decapeptide widely distributed in the brain and spinal cord. Previous studies indicate that this peptide is important both in the perception of pain and in the regulation of neuroendocrine functions.[210] The effect of substance P on growth hormone release is unclear but the majority of the evidence suggests an inhibitory role. Injection of substance P into the lateral ventricle of urethane-anesthetized rats decreases serum growth hormone levels. Because this effect can be abolished by systemic injection of somatostatin antiserum, it was concluded that substance P stimulates the secretion of somatostatin.[190] The same study indicated that substance P can potentiate the increase in growth hormone resulting from intraventricular injection of β-endorphin. Administration of the opioid antagonist, naloxone, prevented the rise in growth hormone produced by β-endorphin and substance P. These results support the conclusion that substance P modulates the opiate-induced release of growth hormone, possibly at a central level, because systemic injections of antiserum to substance P or somatostatin cannot antagonize the synergistic effect of substance P on the morphine-induced release of growth hormone. More recent studies suggest that intracerebroventricular and intravenous administration of substance P inhibit growth hormone secretion, and passive immunization with antiserum against substance P increases growth hormone release.[211,212] Thus, the current data support an inhibitory role for substance P on growth hormone release.

THYROTROPIN-RELEASING HORMONE

The tripeptide TRH can release growth hormone in cows and sheep,[213,214] although in other species the action of TRH is controversial. In intact rats and man, TRH does not increase growth hormone consistently, and it has been proposed that TRH can only increase growth hormone under specific pathologic conditions in these species. If the pituitary is transplanted beneath the kidney capsule, intravenous administration of TRH can stimulate both the biosynthesis and release of growth hormone.[215] Although studies supporting a physiological role for TRH are limited, passive immunization with TRH antiserum (intracerebroventricularly) has been shown to decrease growth hormone secretion.[216] These results have led to the hypothesis that TRH has the capacity to increase growth hormone, but the response may be tonically suppressed by hypothalamic hormones.

NEUROPEPTIDE Y

Neuropeptide Y is a peptide that is ubiquitously distributed throughout the hypothalamus.[217,218] Although this peptide increases growth hormone secretion from rat pituitary cell cultures,[219] inhibitory effects are observed after intravenous administration to male rats. In addition, intracerebroventricular administration to female rats has been shown to inhibit growth hormone secretion.[219,220] Antiserum to neuropeptide Y administered into the lateral ventricle increases growth hormone, although administation of neuropeptide Y (at low concentrations) has been shown to increase somatostatin secretion.[221] Thus, the importance of neuropeptide Y for growth hormone secretion is unclear but the peptide may regulate paracrine relationships between somatostatin and GHRH.

BOMBESIN

Bombesin was initially isolated from amphibian skin[222] and later reported to be present in mammalian brain.[223] Bombesin is a tetradecapeptide, and its role as a central nervous system neurotransmitter is currently under investigation. Early studies indicated that both intravenous and intracisternal administration of bombesin to steroid-primed male rats produced a considerable rise in plasma growth hormone, although intravenous injection was more effective. However, more recent studies suggest that intracerebroventricular administration of the peptide inhibits both growth hormone secretion and the response to opioid stimulation, possibly as a result of increased somatostatin secretion.[224] A possible confounding factor in several studies of the effects of bombesin (as well as other compounds) is that bombesin can increase growth hormone secretion from pituitary cells.[225,226]

NEUROTENSIN

Neurotensin is a tridecapeptide found in the hypothalamus[227] and intravenous injection of this peptide stimulates the release of growth hormone in normal and estrogen-progesterone primed male rats.[211] The increase in growth hormone is antagonized by the antihistaminergic drug, diphenhydramine.[228] Because the addition of neurotensin to rat pituitaries cultured *in vitro* does not stimulate the release of growth hormone, it was suggested that the neurotensin-induced release of growth hormone may be mediated by histamine, at a central level.[229]

VASOPRESSIN/OXYTOCIN

Vasopressin elicits the release of growth hormone in rats[230] and humans,[231] however, the mechanism for this effect appears to vary in each of these species. In the rat, the β-adrenergic antagonist, propranolol, blocks the effect of vasopressin on growth hormone secretion whereas, in humans, the α-adrenergic antagonist, phentolamine, suppresses the vasopressin-induced release of growth hormone. Vasopressin can directly stimulate growth hormone release from the pituitary.[232] However, rats with hereditary vasopressin deficiency appear to have normal plasma growth hormone levels and administration of antibodies to vasopressin has no effect on basal growth hormone secretion.[233] In summary, vasopressin increases circulating levels of growth hormone via a central adrenergic mechanism, which may be species dependent, but may have only a limited role in episodic growth hormone release.

Athough there is limited information of the effects of oxytocin on growth hormone release, a recent study demonstrated that passive immunization with oxytocin antiserum increased growth hormone secretion, suggesting that oxytocin may regulate GHRH or somatostatin secretion through a paracrine relationship.[233]

VASOACTIVE INTESTINAL POLYPEPTIDE

Vasoactive intestinal polypeptide (VIP) is present in the hypothalamus and brain in relatively high concentrations. The peptide is present in hypophyseal portal blood, suggesting that it may have a role in the control of anterior pituitary function.[234,235] Intraventricular injection of VIP, at concentrations ranging from 4 to 500 ng, stimulates the release of growth hormone from the pituitary.[236,237] This effect may be centrally mediated but direct effects on the pituitary cannot be discounted because there are some reports that VIP can stimulate growth hormone release from the pituitary.[238,239]

CALCITONIN

Calcitonin immunoreactivity is present in the hypothalamus, median eminence, and pituitary gland and recent studies suggest that this peptide can inhibit pulsatile release of growth hormone and growth hormone release induced by arginine or GHRH.[240-244] The effects of calcitonin appear not to be mediated through increased somatostatin secretion.

PITUITARY ADENYLATE CYCLASE ACTIVATING PEPTIDE

Pituitary adenylate cyclase activating peptide (PACAP) is found in the hypothalamus and median eminence of rodents and two molecular weight variants have been reported (27 and 38 amino acids).[245] Although there is limited information on possible paracrine interrelationships, both peptides are capable of increasing the release of growth hormone and other pituitary hormones directly from the pituitary gland.

NEUROTRANSMITTERS THAT INFLUENCE GROWTH HORMONE SECRETION

OVERVIEW

In addition to opioid and neuroactive peptides, various neurotransmitters also influence the release of somatostatin and GHRH and subsequently the release of growth hormone from the pituitary gland. The high concentrations of biogenic amines in the hypothalamus have led to extensive studies on their role in growth hormone secretion. Dopamine, norepinephrine, and serotonin (5-HT) have an important role in the neural regulation of growth hormone secretion in both animals and man.[246,247] These monoamines appear to act at the hypothalamic level to alter the release of somatostatin and/or GHRH, or possibly acting directly on the pituitary gland, thereby influencing growth hormone release. A number of other neurotransmitters have also been shown to influence growth hormone secretion including γ-aminobutyric acid (GABA), acetylcholine (ACh), histamine, and glutamate.

DOPAMINE AND NOREPINEPHRINE

Both dopamine and norepinephrine promote the release of growth hormone. L-DOPA, for example, increases basal growth hormone levels[248] and enhances growth hormone release induced by suckling in postpartum lactating rats.[249] The effects are abolished by pretreatment with the catecholamine synthesis inhibitor, α-methyl-para-tyrosine (αmpt).[250] Because dopamine can be converted into norepinephrine, it was unclear if the major effects of dopamine were mediated by activation of dopamine receptors or by conversion to norepinephrine. Dopamine receptor agonists, such as apomorphine and piribedil, were shown to increase plasma growth hormone levels in male rats.[251] Apomorphine also reversed the inhibition of growth hormone induced by haloperidol, a dopamine receptor blocker. Moreover, plasma growth hormone release was stimulated by intraventricular injections of either dopamine or piribedil, or by systemic administration of dopamine or apomorphine in ovariectomized or ovariectomized estrogen-progesterone-primed rats.[252]

There are other reports implicating dopamine as an important neurotransmitter in the regulation of growth hormone secretion.[253-255] Pulsatile growth hormone secretion is still evident with an increased number of secretory bursts in rats with a complete hypothalamic island produced by sectioning with a Halasz knife.[256] This technique depletes hypothalamic norepinephrine content without affecting hypothalamic dopamine content.[257] Furthermore, neonatal treatment with monosodium glutamate, which does not affect hypothalamic norepinephrine or somatostatin content, results in diminished hypothalamic dopamine content and reduced plasma growth hormone.[258] More recently, specific D_2 agonists have been shown to stimulate growth hormone secretion. Although these studies are not conclusive, they reinforce the importance of dopamine in the regulation of growth hormone secretion.

Because growth hormone secretion is under the dual control of somatostatin and GHRH, several studies have attempted to determine the role of monoamines in the regulation of these hypothalamic hormones. Dopamine and norepinephrine are reported to stimulate the release of somatostatin from rat hypothalamic synaptosomes or fragments.[259,260] The release can be blocked by addition of pimozide or phentolamine into the incubation media.[260] However, *in vivo*, dopamine can increase the growth hormone response to GHRH as well as other stimuli that increase growth hormone secretion, suggesting that dopamine may also decrease somatostatin release.

Clonidine, an α-adrenergic receptor agonist, also stimulates growth hormone release when injected intraventricularly. This increase is blocked by pretreatment with phenoxybenzamine, an α-adrenergic receptor blocker.[253] Serial sampling of blood in unanesthetized, unrestrained rats provided strong evidence that growth hormone secretory bursts are regulated by an α-adrenergic mechanism.[253,255] The drugs, αmpt and phenoxybenzamine, abolish the spontaneous bursts of growth hormone whereas dopamine receptor blockers have a minimal inhibitory effect. The α-adrenergic effects appear to be mediated by both decreased somatostatin and increased GHRH.

β-Adrenergic receptors appear to inhibit growth hormone secretion in the rat. Early studies suggested that propranolol, a β-adrenergic blocker, had no effect on pulsatile growth hormone secretion,[261] but growth hormone release induced by γ-hydroxybutyric acid (GHB), a derivative of GABA acid, was reported to be transiently augmented by propranolol and completely inhibited by the β-adrenergic agonist, isoproterenol.[262] More recent studies indicate that β-agonists inhibit growth hormone and these effects are mediated through increases in somatostatin because effects can be blocked by passive immunization to this peptide.

There appear to be species differences in growth hormone responses to catecholaminergic agents. Although data are not consistent, both dopamine and norepinephrine are involved in the release of growth hormone in conscious dogs. L-DOPA elicits an increase in plasma growth hormone in this species, but this can be prevented by the α-adrenergic blocker, phentolamine,[263,264] whereas the dopamine receptor blocker, pimozide,[265] has no effect. Clonidine stimulates growth hormone release whereas subemetic doses of apomorphine fail to increase growth hormone.[265] Although the data suggest that norepinephrine alone is important for growth hormone release, dopamine may play an independent role in growth hormone regulation, because the growth hormone-releasing activity of L-DOPA is not influenced by treatment with fusaric acid, a potent inhibitor of dopamine-β-hydroxylase.[264]

In nonhuman primates, growth hormone secretion appears to be regulated primarily by an α-adrenergic mechanism. Intravenous infusion of dopamine and norepinephrine stimulates growth hormone release, but the growth hormone-stimulating effect of dopamine can be blocked by either phentolamine or FLA63, an inhibitor of dopamine-β-hydroxylase. Norepinephrine microinjected into the hypothalamus stimulates growth hormone release whereas both phentolamine and dopamine suppress growth hormone.[266-268] In monkeys, growth hormone release is also stimulated by clonidine and dihydroxyphenylserine, a norepinephrine precursor, but apomorphine is effective only in emetic doses, which may act as a nonspecific stress.[269] Phentolamine, but not pimozide, blocks growth hormone secretion induced by amphetamine,[270] which stimulates both dopamine and norepinephrine release from nerve terminals. These data suggest that dopamine may only increase growth hormone after conversion to norepinephrine.

In humans, data indicate that dopaminergic and noradrenergic α-receptors are stimulatory and noradrenergic β-receptors are inhibitory to growth hormone release. Intravenous injection of epinephrine or norepinephrine has no effect on plasma growth hormone in man, possibly because they penetrate the blood-brain barrier poorly, but oral administration of L-DOPA, the precursor of both dopamine and norepinephrine, stimulates growth hormone release.[271] Norepinephrine is involved in growth hormone responses to various physiologic and pharmacologic stimuli in man. Phentolamine, an α-receptor blocker, blocks growth hormone release induced by insulin hypoglycemia, arginine, vasopressin, L-DOPA, exercise, and stresses such as surgery and electric shock. Propranolol, a β-receptor blocker, enhances growth hormone responses to insulin hypoglycemia, glucagon, L-DOPA, and exercise. The roles of noradrenergic α- and β-receptors are further supported by reports that clonidine, an α-receptor agonist, increases plasma growth hormone and isoproterenol inhibits the vasopressin-induced increase in growth hormone.

Dopamine also may have a distinct facilitatory role on growth hormone secretion in man.[272,273] Both apomorphine and bromoergocryptine produce a rise of plasma growth hormone, whereas pimozide, a dopamine receptor blocker, decreases growth hormone response to arginine and exercise.

SEROTONIN

Serotonin appears to have an important role in the regulation of growth hormone secretion in the rat. When intraventricular injections of serotonin (5-HT) are administered, plasma levels of growth hormone increase.[274] The stimulatory effect of the serotonin precursor, 5-hydroxytryptophan (5-HTP), on growth hormone secretion can be reversed by the structurally similar pineal hormone, melatonin, or the serotonin receptor antagonist, cyproheptadine.[275,276] Conversely, the severe depletion of brain serotonin by concomitant administration of the tyrosine hydroxylase inhibitor, or the neurotoxin, 5,6-dihydrotryptamine, produces a marked reduction in circulating levels of growth hormone in unanesthetized male rats.[277]

Participation of serotonin in the physiologic regulation of growth hormone secretion in the rat is suggested by the observation that the pulsatile release of growth hormone in unanesthetized male rats is inhibited by PCPA or the antiserotonergic drug, methysergide.[261] Moreover, the characteristic growth hormone pulse that occurs at the onset of the dark period is abolished by the serotonin-receptor antagonist, metergoline.[278] Studies suggest that the effects of serotonin are mediated both by inhibition of somatostatin secretion and an increase in GHRH release.[279]

Findings similar to those observed in the rat have not been obtained in studies on the effects of serotonin on growth hormone release in the dog. Mueller et al.[280] reported that infusion of tryptophan, the amino acid precursor of serotonin, produces only a slight elevation in growth hormone levels in the unanesthetized beagle. Administration of 5-HTP produces an elevated serum growth hormone but the dramatic side effects suggest that these responses may be associated with stress. PCPA has no effect on basal growth hormone secretion and potentiates rather than diminishes the rise in growth hormone induced by insulin hypoglycemia. The drug 5-HTP reduces the rise in serum growth hormone during insulin-induced hypoglycemia. Dogs maintained on a tryptophan-deficient diet show no change in basal growth hormone levels. When tryptophan is administered to these animals, it blunts rather than potentiates the insulin-induced rise in growth hormone. Thus, in the dog, serotonin appears to be of minor importance in the regulation of growth hormone secretion and may suppress rather than stimulate growth hormone release.

Generally, serotonin increases growth hormone release in humans. Administration of 5-HTP to normal human subjects has been reported to increase[281-283] or to have no effect[284,285] on circulating levels of growth hormone. However, cyproheptadine decreases or abolishes sleep-related growth hormone release[286] and diminishes the rise in serum growth hormone associated with exercise,[275] arginine infusion,[283] and insulin-induced hypoglycemia.[275,281] Administration of methysergide produces a 40% decrease in peak growth hormone values and a 35% decrease in overall mean growth hormone concentrations.[281] Mueller et al[285] reported that L-tryptophan produces only a slight increase in plasma growth hormone in female subjects and none in male subjects. They also found that L-tryptophan does not amplify the increase in serum growth hormone produced by insulin-induced hypoglycemia. Thus, the physiological regulation of growth hormone secretion by serotonin remains unclear.

Liuzzi et al.[287] cautioned that the data on the regulation of growth hormone secretion must be viewed with reservations. Systemic administration of serotonin precursors may lead to accumulation of serotonin in cells that do not usually contain this indoleamine and may also interfere with the storage or metabolism of catecholamines. There is some debate over the specificity of action of cyproheptadine, methysergide, and PCPA on the serotoninergic system, and these substances may indirectly affect the catecholaminergic systems as well. The majority of evidence leads to the conclusion that serotonin participates in the regulation of growth hormone secretion in the rat and human.

MELATONIN

Melatonin is synthesized and secreted by the pineal gland and appears to decrease the secretion of growth hormone in the rat. Conditions that favor the secretion of melatonin correlate well with states in which somatic growth is retarded. Sorrentino et al.[288] found that rats that are blinded or exposed to constant darkness, which increases melatonin synthesis, demonstrate a reduction in body weight, tibial length, and pituitary growth hormone content. These effects are abolished by pinealectomy. Smythe and Lazarus[289] reported that the increase in serum growth hormone after 5-HTP is antagonized by concomitant administration of melatonin. It is hypothesized that melatonin may antagonize the binding of serotonin to its receptor sites in the hypothalamus. Alternatively, melatonin may stimulate the metabolism of, or inhibit the release of, serotonin from its respective neurons.[290]

In the rat, the effect of melatonin on the pulsatile release of growth hormone is contradictory. Ronnelkeiv and McCann[291] found that pinealectomy decreases the duration, frequency, and amplitude of growth hormone pulses as compared to sham-operated controls. The result is a reduction in mean total growth hormone concentration. However, Willoughby[292] reported that pinealectomy had no effect on the pulsatile release of growth hormone. Therefore, it is difficult to discern the role of melatonin, if any, on the pulsatile release of growth hormone from these studies.

In humans, the effect of melatonin on growth hormone secretion is paradoxical. When administered to normal healthy male subjects, melatonin elevates circulating levels of growth hormone.[293] By contrast, melatonin antagonizes the rise in growth hormone produced by exercise or insulin hypoglycemia.[280] In humans, the effect of melatonin may be dependent on the physiologic status of the individual.

γ-AMINOBUTYRIC ACID

GABA is found in the hypothalamus, as well as other areas of the brain.[294] Administration of GABA or its metabolites to rats or humans has produced conflicting reports in regard to growth hormone secretion. In the urethane-anesthetized male rat, injection of GABA into the lateral ventricles produces a significant rise in growth hormone levels.[298,299] Similar results are obtained after intraventricular or intraperitoneal administration of the GABA metabolite γ-amino-O-hydroxybutyric acid.[298,299] Intraperitoneal injection of amino-oxyacetic acid, an agent that blocks the degradation of GABA, also produces a marked rise in serum growth hormone.[299] Intravenous administration of the potent GABA antagonist, picrotoxin, reduces plasma growth hormone.[277] However, others report that GABA and GABAergic drugs decrease serum growth hormone levels in rats.[298] The role of GABA on growth hormone secretion must therefore await further study. Little evidence is available to clarify the mechanism(s) by which GABA stimulates or inhibits the secretion of growth hormone. Takahara et al.[299] found that both GABA and amino-oxyacetic acid induce an increase in hypothalamic somatostatin content, suggesting that GABA promotes growth hormone secretion in the rat by inhibiting the release of somatostatin by the hypothalamus. It is also possible that the effect of GABA is mediated through other neurotransmitters, GHRH, or a combination of both. GABA does not appear to have a direct effect on the pituitary because it does not stimulate the release of growth hormone when added to *in vitro* pituitary cultures.[300]

ACETYLCHOLINE

ACh is present in high concentrations in the hypothalamus, and ACh receptors are found in the hypothalamus and pituitary gland. Several studies have been conducted to investigate the ability of ACh to facilitate the release of growth hormone by the pituitary. Casanueva et al.[301] reported that the cholinergic system stimulates the release of growth hormone in the dog. Similarly, ACh, pilocarpine (a cholinergic receptor agonist), and the cholinesterase inhibitor, physostigmine, all promote release of growth hormone in the rat.[302] Collu et al.[277] and Martin et al.[261] have shown that the cholinergic receptor blocker, atropine sulfate, decreases basal growth hormone levels in the rat. More recently, ACh and muscarinic agonists have been reported to increase growth hormone release in several species whereas muscarinic blockade decreases growth hormone release in response to a number of physiological stimuli.[303-316] These effects appear to be mediated by inhibition of somatostatin secretion because the effects of atropine are abolished after passive immunization with somatostatin antiserum.[303]

HISTAMINE

Histamine has not been established as a physiologic mediator of growth hormone release. Rudolph et al.[317] reported that neither H_1 nor H_1 agonists affects growth hormone levels in the dog, whereas the H_1 receptor antagonist, dexchlorpheniramine, significantly elevates baseline growth hormone levels in the rat. There is evidence that histamine may mediate the neurotensin and substance P-induced increase in growth hormone.[211] However, further studies are necessary to establish a relationship between the histaminergic system and growth hormone secretion.

NMDA AND EXCITATORY AMINO ACIDS

The presence of *N*-methyl-D-aspartate (NMDA) in the hypothalamus and brain has been recognized for several years.[318,319] However, only recently have studies been conducted to investigate a potential role for NMDA in growth hormone release. Stimulation of NMDA receptors with agonists consistently increases growth hormone release in several species.[320-322] Early studies concluded that these effects were mediated through interactions within the hypothalamus because NMDA had no effect on growth hormone release from the pituitary and the increase could be inhibited by GHRH antiserum.[323] However, more recent studies suggest that part of the actions of NMDA are mediated by direct effects on the pituitary to release growth hormone.[324]

It is well known that several other amino acids stimulate growth hormone secretion including, but not limited to, arginine, leucine, and isoleucine. These amino acids appear to decrease somatostatin secretion from the hypothalamus although specific mechanisms and interactions with other hypothalamic neuropeptides/transmitters are unknown.[325,326]

HORMONAL CONTROL OF GROWTH HORMONE SECRETION

THYROID HORMONES

The thyroid hormones, T_3 and T_4, influence the synthesis and release of growth hormone. In the rat, thyroidectomy results in a marked reduction of both serum and pituitary growth hormone[327-329] and abolishes the pulsatile release of growth hormone.[330] Administration of thyroid hormone to rats increases plasma and pituitary growth hormone within 24 h[329,331] and this effect may be mediated directly on the pituitary gland.[332,333] Growth hormone synthesis is decreased by prior thyroidectomy and stimulated by thyroid hormone. Similarly, in humans, it is well known that hypothyroidism in children is associated with growth failure. The growth hormone response to insulin-induced hypoglycemia or arginine infusion is impaired in many hypothyroid patients[334-336] and administration of thyroid hormone rapidly restores growth rate and normalizes growth hormone response to many stimuli.

Although it appears that thyroid hormones can potentiate growth hormone release at the level of the pituitary, it has not been determined if thyroid hormones also influence the synthesis and/or release of hypothalamic somatostatin or GHRH, or affect the function of neurotransmitters which regulate the secretion of these hypophysiotropic hormones into the portal vessels. A recent report indicates that thyroid hormones may affect the activity of hypothalamic enzymes that metabolize somatostatin,[337] but whether this alters the concentrations of somatostatin in portal blood remains to be determined.

ESTROGEN AND TESTOSTERONE

Estrogen and testosterone appear to have a potentiating effect on growth hormone secretion. Growth hormone levels are increased on the day of estrus and in ovariectomized rats treated with estradiol benzoate.[338] Estrogen causes a marked increase in pituitary sensitivity to GHRH, suggesting that estrogen acts at the level of the pituitary to sensitize the somatotroph.[339] The growth hormone response to arginine infusion in women is highest at midcycle when concentrations of estrogens are elevated compared to concentrations in other phases of the menstrual cycle.[340] Estrogen administration enhances the growth hormone response to arginine and exercise in children and adult men.[341] In prepubertal children, who have low circulating gonadal steroids, the growth hormone response to insulin-induced hypoglycemia and arginine infusion is lower than that of adults.[342] Finally, the pulsatile release of growth hormone becomes evident around puberty, when levels of estrogen and testosterone increase.[343]

PROGESTERONE

Unlike estrogens, progesterone appears to have an inhibitory effect on growth hormone secretion. Medroxyprogesterone acetate decreases the growth hormone response to insulin hypoglycemia or arginine infusion[344] and inhibits the sleep-related growth hormone release in humans.[345] The elevated plasma growth hormone levels in acromegalic patients may be reduced by medroxyprogesterone[346] but this has not been confirmed. The mechanism by which progesterone inhibits growth hormone secretion is unknown.

GLUCOCORTICOIDS

Decreased growth in children receiving glucocorticoid therapy or suffering from chronic hypercortisolemia (Cushing's syndrome) suggests that glucocorticoids inhibit growth hormone secretion. The growth hormone response to insulin hypoglycemia is impaired in patients with elevated glucocorticoids.[347-349] Although it is known that glucocorticoids are necessary for growth hormone synthesis, little is known about the mechanism by which glucocorticoids influence growth hormone release.

SLEEP, STRESS, AND EXERCISE EFFECTS ON GROWTH HORMONE

As noted previously, the major burst of growth hormone release occurs within 2 h after sleep onset in adult humans. About 70 to 90% of the total 24 h secretion of growth hormone may take place during this period.[350-352] The nocturnal rise of growth hormone is entrained to the onset of sleep and is not related to an intrinsic circadian rhythm, because the sleep-related secretion of growth hormone can be reversed acutely by sleep-wake reversal.[353] The sleep-related growth hormone release may be associated with slow-wave sleep (stages 3 and 4) defined polygraphically, but the mechanisms for this association have not been clearly defined. Growth hormone secretion during sleep can occur in the absence of slow-wave sleep, and slow-wave sleep can occur without sleep-related growth hormone release.

A number of attempts have been made to study the mechanism(s) of sleep-related growth hormone secretion. Neither noradrenergic[354] nor dopaminergic blockers[350] inhibits growth hormone release during sleep, and the role of serotonin (5-HT) is controversial because three different antiserotoninergic agents are reported to increase,[355] decrease,[356] or have no effect[357] on the sleep-related growth hormone release. A number of factors inhibit sleep-related growth hormone secretion, including imipramine, clomiphene, medroxyprogesterone, somatostatin, obesity, fatty acids, and chronic alcoholism. An anticholinergic agent, methscopolamine, may block the growth hormone surge during sleep without any effect on plasma prolactin or slow-wave sleep.[358] Neurotransmitters and metabolic factors thus appear to be involved in sleep-related growth hormone secretion.

Acute physical stress or exercise stimulate growth hormone release in many species, including man.[359,360] Physical trauma, electroshock therapy, and surgical operations result in a rise of growth hormone in humans, and growth hormone release is also stimulated by arterial puncture and pyrogen administration. The growth hormone response to insulin hypoglycemia may be due to stress, because growth hormone release is associated to some degree with the severity of side effects to insulin, such as sweating, palpitation, and generalized weakness. α-adrenergic blockers inhibit growth hormone release induced by stress. Growth hormone secretion in nonhuman primates is also stress responsive. A marked elevation of growth hormone is caused by stresses such as pain, loud noise, capture, ether inhalation, hemorrhage, or aversive conditioning.[143] Unlike release in primates, the amplitude of episodic growth hormone release in rats and mice is inhibited by stress, and increased somatostatin secretion appears to contribute to the stress-related inhibition of growth hormone release in rodents.[144,277]

SUMMARY

The large volume of data published thus far on the biological actions of growth hormone suggest a critical role not only in body growth but in maintenance of cellular function in a number of tissues of adult animals. Recent studies demonstrating the effects of growth hormone on cells of the immune system, cardiovascular system, bone, kidney, and more recently brain suggest that this hormone has an important role in maintaining cellular function within systems and coordinating the maintenance of cellular function between systems. Despite progress in identifying the biological actions of growth hormone, mechanisms responsible for the regulation of episodic growth hormone release have proceeded at a slower rate. Although it is clear that somatostatin and GHRH are necessary for episodic release, the diversity of hypothalamic peptides and the complex regulation of these peptides by neurotransmitters has complicated investigations. Nevertheless, the general consensus is that trough levels of growth hormone result from somatostatin secretion whereas peak levels are regulated by GHRH. The dynamic interaction between these peptides contributes to growth hormone secretory dynamics. Both neurotransmitter and neuropeptide levels regulate growth hormone through either inhibition or facilitation of somatostatin and GHRH secretion. Although much has been learned concerning the complex interrelationships between neurotransmitters, neuropeptides, and the secretion of somatostatin and GHRH, the specific mechanisms that interact to regulate these compounds remain unknown.

ACKNOWLEDGMENTS

This work was supported, in part, by the NIH grants AG07752 and AA08536.

REFERENCES

1. **Li, C. H., Evans, H. M., and Simpson, M. E.,** Isolation and properties of the anterior hypophysial growth hormone, *J. Biol. Chem.*, 159, 353, 1945.
2. **Utiger, R. D., Parker, M. L., and Daughaday, W.,** Studies on human growth hormone. I. A radioimmunoassay for human growth hormone, *J. Clin. Invest.*, 41, 254, 1962.
3. **Li, C. H., Dixon, J. S., and Liu, W. K.,** Human pituitary growth hormone. XIX. The primary structure of the hormone, *Arch. Biochem. Biophys.*, 133, 70, 1969.
4. **Niall, H. D.,** A revised primary structure for human growth hormone, *Nature*, 230, 90, 1971.
5. **Finkelstein, J., Roffwarg, H., Boyar, R., Kream, J., and Hellman, L.,** Age-related changes in the twenty-four hour spontaneous secretion of growth hormone, *J. Clin. Endocrinol. Metab.*, 35, 665, 1972.
6. **Martial, J. A., Baxter, J. D., and Goodman, H. M.,** Human growth hormone: complementary DNA cloning and expression in bacteria, *Science*, 205, 602, 1979.
7. **Li, C. H., Chung, D., Lahm, H. W., and Stein, S.,** The primary structure of monkey pituitary growth hormone, *Arch. Biochem. Biophys.*, 245, 287, 1986.
8. **Seeburg, P. H., Shine J., Martial J. A., Baxter, J. D., and Goodman, H. M.,** Nucleotide sequence and amplification in bacteria of structural gene for rat growth hormone, *Nature*, 270, 486, 1977.
9. **Linzer, D. I. H. and Talamantes F.,** Nucleotide sequence of mouse prolactin and growth hormone mRNAs and expression of these mRNAs during pregnancy, *J. Biol. Chem.*, 260, 9574, 1985.
10. **Frieden, E.,** Hormones of the anterior pituitary, in *Clinical Endocrinology*, Academic Press, New York, 1976, 111.
11. **Andrews, P.,** Molecular weight of prolactin and pituitary growth hormones estimated by gel filtration, *Nature*, 209, 155, 1966.
12. **Chen, W. Y., White, D. C., Wagner, T. E., and Kopchick, J. J.,** Expression of a mutated bovine growth hormone gene suppresses growth in transgenic mice, *Proc. Natl. Acad. Sci. U.S.A.*, 87, 5061, 1990.
13. **Chen, W. Y., White, D. C., Wagner, T. E., and Kopchick, J. J.,** Functional antagonism between endogenous mouse growth hormone (GH) and a GH analog results in dwarf transgenic mice, *Endocrinology*, 129, 1402, 1991.
14. **Lewis, U. J., Dunn, J. T., Bonewald L. F., Seavey, B. K., and van der Laan, W. P.,** A naturally occurring structural variant of human growth hormone, *J. Biol. Chem.*, 253, 2679, 1978.
15. **Lewis U. J., Bonewald, L. F., and Lewis, L. J.,** The 20,000-dalton variant of human growth hormone: location of the amino acid deletions, *Biochem. Biophys. Res. Commun.*, 92, 511, 1980.
16. **Estes, P. A., Cooke, N. E., and Liebhaber, S. A.,** A native RNA secondary structure controls alternative splice-site selection and generates two human growth hormone isoforms, *J. Biol. Chem.*, 267, 14903, 1992.
17. **Baumann, G.,** Growth hormone heterogeneity: genes, isoforms and binding variants, *Endocr. Rev.*, 12, 424, 1991.
18. **Sinha, Y. N. and Lewis, U. J.,** A lectin binding immunoassay indicates a possible glycosylated growth hormone in the human pituitary gland, *Biochem. Biophys. Res. Commun.*, 140, 491, 1986.
19. **Bollenger, F., Velkeniers, B., Hooghe-Peters, E., Mahler, A., and Vanhaelst, L.,** Multiple forms of rat prolactin and growth hormone in pituitary cell populations separated using Percoll gradient system: disulphide bridge dimers and glycosylated variants, *J. Endocrinol.*, 120, 201, 1989.
20. **Aramburo, C., Montiel, J. L., Proudman, J. A., Berghman, L. R., and Scanes C. R.,** Phosphorylation of prolactin and growth hormone, *J. Mol. Endocrinol.*, 8, 183, 1992.
21. **Liberti, J. P. and Joshi, G. S.,** Synthesis and secretion of phosphorylated growth hormone by rat pituitary glands *in vitro*, *Biochem. Biophys. Res. Commun.*, 137, 806, 1986.
22. **Tannenbaum, G. S. and Martin, J. B.,** Evidence for an ultradian rhythm governing growth hormone secretion in the male rat, *Endocrinology*, 98, 562, 1976.

23. **Hartman, M. L., Faria, A. C. S., Vance, M. L., Johnson, M. L., Thorner, M. O., and Veldhuis, J. D.,** Temporal structure of *in vivo* growth hormone secretory events in humans, *Am. J. Physiol.*, 260, E101, 1991.

24. **Eden, S.,** The secretory patterns of growth hormone, *Acta. Physiol. Scand.*, 104, 1, 1978.

25. **Tannenbaum, G. S.,** Somatostatin as a physiological regulator of pulsatile growth hormone secretion, *Horm. Res.*, 29, 70, 1988.

26. **Veldhuis, J. D., Lizarralde, G., and Iranmanesh, A.,** Divergent effects of short term glucocorticoid excess on the gonadotropic and somatotropic axes in normal men, *J. Clin. Endocrinol. Metab.*, 74, 96, 1992.

27. **Faria, A. C. S., Bekenstein, L. W., Booth, R. A., Vaccaro, V. A., Asplin, C. M., Veldhuis, J. D., Thorner, M. O., and Evans, W. S.,** Pulsatile growth hormone release in normal women during the menstrual cycle, *Clin. Endocrinol.*, 36, 591, 1992.

28. **Veldhuis, J. D., Blizzard, R. M., Rogol, A. D., Martha, P. M., Kirkland, J. L., and Sherman, B. M.,** Properties of spontaneous growth hormone secretory bursts and half-life of endogenous growth hormone in boys with idiopathic short stature, *J. Clin. Endocrinol. Metab.*, 74, 766, 1992.

29. **Martha, P. M., Goorman, K. M., Blizzard, R. M., Rogal, A. D., and Veldhuis, J. D.,** Endogenous growth hormone secretion and clearance rate in normal boys as determined by deconvolution analysis: relationship to age, pubertal status, and body mass, *J. Clin. Endocrinol. Metab.*, 74, 335, 1992.

30. **Carlsson, L. M. S., Rosberg, S., Vitangcol, R. V., Wong, W. L. T., and Albertsson-Kirkland, K.,** Analysis of 24-hour plasma profiles of growth hormone(GH)-binding protein, GH/GH binding protein complex, and GH in healthy children, *J. Clin. Endocrinol. Metab.*, 77, 356, 1993.

31. **Carlson, H. E., Gillin, J. C., Gorden, P., and Snyder, F.,** Absence of sleep related growth hormone peaks in aged normal subjects and in acromegaly, *J. Clin. Endocrinol. Metab.*, 34, 1102, 1972.

32. **Rudman, D., Vintner, M. H., Rogers, C. M., Lubin, M. F., Flemming, G. A., and Bain, R. P.,** Impaired growth hormone secretion in the adult population, *J. Clin. Invest.*, 67, 1361, 1981.

33. **Sonntag, W. E., Steger, R. W., Forman, L. J., and Meites, J.,** Decreased pulsatile release of growth hormone in old male rats, *Endocrinology*, 107, 1875, 1980.

34. **Steiner, R. A., Stewart, J. K., Barber, J., Koerker, D., Goodner, J. C., Brown, A., Illner, P., and Gale, C. C.,** Somatostatin: a physiologic role in the regulation of growth hormone secretion in the adolescent male baboon, *Endocrinology*, 102, 1587, 1978.

35. **Kaler, L. W., Gliessman, P., Craven, J., Hill, J., and Critchlow, V.,** Loss of enhanced nocturnal growth hormone secretion in aging rhesus males, *Endocrinology*, 119, 1281, 1986.

36. **Martin, J. B.,** Brain mechanisms for integration of growth hormone secretion, *Physiologist,* 22, 23, 1979.

37. **DeVos, A., Ultsch, M., and Kossiakoff, A. A.,** Human growth hormone and extracellular domain of its receptor: crystal structure of the complex, *Science*, 255, 306, 1992.

38. **Fuh, G., Cunningham, B. C., Fukunaga, R., Nagata, S., Goeddel, D. V., and Wells, J. A.,** Rationale design of potent antagonists to the human growth hormone receptor, *Science*, 256, 1677, 1992.

39. **Argetsinger, L. S., Campbell, G. S., Yang, X. J., Witthuhn, B. A., Silvennoline, O., Ihle, J. N., and Carter-Su, C.,** Identification of JAK2 as a growth hormone receptor- associated tyrosine kinase, *Cell*, 74, 237, 1993.

40. **Sotiropoulos, A., Perrot-Applanat, M., Dinerstein, H., Pallier, A., Postel-Vinay, M. C., Finidori, J., and Kelly, P.,** Distinct cytoplasmic regions of the growth hormone receptor are required for activation of JAK2, mitogen-activated protein kinase and transcription, *Endocrinology*, 135, 1292, 1994.

41. **Campbell, G. S., Pang, L., Miyasaka, T., Saltiel, A. R., and Carter-Su, C.,** Stimulation by growth hormone of MAP kinase activity in 3T3-F442A fibroblasts, *J. Biol. Chem.* 267, 6074, 1992.

42. **Moller, C., Hansson, A., Enberg, B., Lobie, P. E., and Norstedt, G.,** Growth hormone induction of tyrosine phosphorylation and activation of mitogen-activated kinases in cells transfected with rat GH receptor cDNA, *J. Biol. Chem.*, 267, 23403, 1992.

43. **Anderson, N. G.,** Growth hormone activates mitogen-activated protein kinase and S6 kinase and promotes intracellular tyrosine phosphorylation in 3T3-F442A preadipocytes, *Biochem. J.*, 284, 649, 1992.

44. **Weil, R.,** Pituitary growth hormone and intermediary metabolism. 1. The hormonal effect on the metabolism of fat and carbohydrate, *Acta Endocrinol. Suppl.*, 98, 1, 1965.

45. **Rabinowitz, D., Merimee, T. J., Maffezzolo, R., and Burgess, J. A.,** Patterns of hormonal release after glucose, protein and glucose plus protein, *Lancet,* 2, 434, 1966.

46. **Rabinowitz, D., Merimee, T. J., Nelson, J. K., Schultz, R. B., and Burgess, J. A.,** The influence of proteins and amino acids on growth hormone release in man, in *Growth Hormone,* Pecile, A. and Muller, E. E., Eds., Excerpta Medica, New York, 1968, 105.

47. **Schnure, J. J. and Lipman, R.,** Physiological studies of growth hormone secretion during sleep: nonsuppressibility by hyperglycemia and impairment in glucose tolerance, *Proc. 52nd Meet. Endocr. Soc.,* No. 214, 1970 (Abstract).

48. **Takano, K., Hizuka, N., Shikume, K., Asakawa, K., and Kogawa, M.,** Short-term study of biosynthesized hGH in man, *Endocrinol. Jpn.*, 30, 79, 1983.

49. **Bassett, J. M. and Wallace, A. L. C.,** Short-term effects of ovine growth hormone in plasma glucose, free fatty acids and ketones in sheep, *Metabolism*, 15, 933, 1966.

50. **Rudman, D., Feller, A. G., Nagraj, H. S., Gergans, G. A., Lalitha, P. Y., Goldberg, A. F., Schlenker, R. A., Conn, L., Rudman, I. W., and Mattson, D. E.,** Effects of growth hormone in men over 60 years old, *N. Engl. J. Med.*, 323, 1, 1990.

51. **Bodet, P. T., Rubenstein, D., McGarry, E. E., and Beck, J. C.,** Utilization of free fatty acids by diaphragm *in vitro*, *Am. J. Physiol.*, 203, 311, 1962.

52. **Goodman, H. M.,** Effects of chronic growth hormone treatment on lipogenesis by rat adipose tissue, *Endocrinology*, 72, 95, 1963.

53. **Knobil, E. and Hotchkiss, J.,** Growth hormone, *Annu. Rev. Physiol.*, 26, 47, 1964.

54. **Knobil, E.,** Direct evidence for fatty acid mobilization in response to growth hormone administration in rat, *Proc. Soc. Exp. Biol. Med.*, 101, 288, 1959.

55. **Raben, M. S. and Hollenberg, C. H.,** Growth hormone and the mobilization of fatty acids, *Ciba Found. Colloq. Endocrinol.*, 13, 89, 1959.

56. **Root, A. W.,** Chemical and biological properties of growth hormone, in *Human Pituitary Growth Hormone,* Charles C Thomas, Springfield, IL, 1972, 3.

57. **Franklin, M. J. and Knobil, E.,** The influence of hypophysectomy and of growth hormone administration on oxidation of palmitate-^{14}C by the unanesthetized rat, *Endocrinology*, 68, 867, 1961.

58. **Winkler, B., Steele, R., Altszuler, N., Dunn, A., and deBodo, R. C.,** Effects of growth hormone on free fatty acid metabolism, *Fed. Proc.*, 21, 198, 1962.

59. **Kinsell, L. W., Visintine, R. E., Michaels, G. D., and Walker, G.,** Effects of human growth hormone on lipid metabolism in diabetic subjects, *Metabolism*, 11, 136, 1962.

60. **Allen, A., Medes, G., and Weinhouse, S.,** A study of the effects of growth hormone on fatty acid metabolism *in vitro*, *J. Biol. Chem.*, 221, 333, 1956.

61. **Bauman, J. W., Hill, R., Nejad, N. S., and Chaikoff, L.,** Effect of bovine pituitary growth hormone on hepatic cholesterogenesis of hypophysectomized rats, *Endocrinology*, 65, 73, 1959.

62. **Greenbaum, A. L. and Glascock, R. F.,** The synthesis of lipids in the livers of rats treated with pituitary growth hormone, *Biochem. J.*, 67, 360, 1957.

63. **Noall, M. W., Riggs, T. R., Walker, L. M., and Christensen, H. N.,** Endocrine control of amino acid transfer. Distribution of an unmetabolizable amino acid, *Science*, 126, 1002, 1957.

64. **Riggs, T. R. and Walker, L. M.,** Growth hormone stimulation of amino acid transport into rat tissues *in vivo*, *J. Biol. Chem.*, 235, 3603, 1960.

65. **Kostyo, J. L., Hotchkiss, J., and Knobil, E.,** Stimulation of amino acid transport in isolated diaphragm by growth hormone added *in vitro*, *Science*, 130, 1653, 1959.

66. **Kipnis, D. M. and Reiss, E.,** The effect of cell structure and growth hormone on protein synthesis in striated muscle, *J. Clin. Invest.*, 39, 1002, 1960.

67. **Staehelin, M.,** Protein metabolism: influence of growth hormone, in *Anabolic Steroids and Nutrition in Health and Disease*, Querido, A., Ed., Springer-Verlag, Basel, 1962, 521.

68. **Kostyo, J. L.,** Rapid effects of growth hormone on amino acid transport and protein synthesis, *Ann. N.Y. Acad. Sci.*, 148, 389, 1968.

69. **Nutting, D. F.,** Ontogeny of sensitivity to growth hormone in rat diaphragm muscle, *Endocrinology*, 98, 1273, 1976.

70. **Nutting, D. F. and Coats, L. J.,** Hormonal alterations in the sensitivity of amino acid transport to growth hormone in muscle of young rats, *Proc. Soc. Exp. Biol. Med.*, 156, 446, 1977.

71. **Martinez, J. A., DelBarrio, A. S., and Larralde, J.,** Evidence of a short term effect of growth hormone on *in vivo* bone protein synthesis in normal rats, *Biochem. Biophys. Acta*, 1093, 111, 1991.

72. **Jorgensen, P. H., Andreassen, T. T., and Jorgensen, K. D.,** Growth hormone influences collagen deposition and mechanical strength of intact rat skin, *Acta Endocrinol.*, 120, 767, 1989.

73. **Barbul, A., Rettura, G., Levenson, S. M., and Seifter, F.,** Wound healing and thymotropic effects of arginine: a pituitary mechanism of action, *Am. J. Clin. Nutr.*, 37, 786, 1983.

74. **Jorgenson, P. H. and Andreassen, T. T.,** A dose response study of the effect of biosynthetic human growth hormone on formation and strength of granulation tissue, *Endocrinology*, 121, 1637, 1987.

75. **Strenfos, H. H., and Jansson, J. O.,** Growth hormone stimulates granulation tissue formation and insulin-like growth factor-1 gene expression of the the rat, *J. Endocrinol.*, 132, 293, 1992.

76. **Salmon, W. D., and Daughaday, W. H.,** A hormonally controlled serum factor which stimulates sulfate incorporation by cartilage *in vitro*, *J. Lab. Clin. Med.*, 49, 825, 1957.

77. **Van Wyk, J. J., Underwood, L. E., Hintz, R. L., Clemmons, D. R., Voina, S. J., and Weaver, R. P.,** The somatomedins: a family of insulin-like hormones under growth hormone control, *Recent Prog. Horm. Res.*, 22, 259, 1974.

78. **Shermer, J., Raizada, M. K., Masters, B. A., Ota, A., and LeRoith, D.,** Insulin-like growth factor-1 receptors in neural and glial cells. Characterization and biological effects in primary culture, *J. Biol. Chem.*, 262, 7693, 1987.

79. **Rinderknecht, E. and Humbel R. E.,** The amino acid sequence of insulin-like growth factor-1 and its structural homology with proinsulin, *J. Biol. Chem.*, 253, 2769, 1978.

80. **Rechler, M. M. And Nissley, P. S.,** The nature and regulation of the receptors for insulin-like growth factors, *Annu. Rev. Physiol.*, 47, 425, 1985.

81. **Daughaday, W. H. and Rotwein, P.,** Insulin-like growth factors I and II. Peptide, messenger ribonucleic acid and gene structures, serum and tissue concentrations, *Endocr. Rev.*, 10, 68, 1989.

82. **Binoux, M., Hossenloop, L., Hardouin, S., Seurin, D., Lassarre, C., and Gourmelen, M.,** Somatomedin (insulin-like growth factors)-binding proteins: molecular forms and regulation, *Horm. Res.*, 24, 141, 1986.

83. **Beach, R. K. and Kostyo, J. L.,** Effect of growth hormone on DNA content of muscles of young hypophysectomized rats, *Endocrinology*, 82, 882, 1968.

84. **Goldspink, D. F., and Goldberg, A. L.,** Influence of pituitary growth hormone on DNA synthesis in rat tissues, *Am. J. Physiol.*, 228, 302, 1975.

85. **Greenspan, F. S., Li, C. H., Simpson, M. E., and Evans, H. M.,** Bioassay of hypophyseal growth hormone: the tibia test, *Endocrinology*, 45, 455, 1949.

86. **Wilhelmi, A. E.,** Growth hormone measurement-bioassay, in *Methods in Investigative and Diagnostic Endocrinology*, Berson, S. A. and Yalow, R. S., Eds., North-Holland, Amsterdam, 1973, 296.

87. **Bates, P. C. and Pell, J. M.,** Action and interaction of growth hormone and the β-agonist, clenbuterol, on growth, body composition and protein turnover in dwarf mice, *Br. J. Nutr.*, 65, 115, 1991.

88. **Smeets, T. and van Buul-Offers, S.,** The influence of growth hormone, somatomedins, prolactin and thyroxine on the morphology of the proximal tibial epiphysis and growth plate of Snell dwarf mice, *Growth*, 47, 160, 1983.

89. **Gause, I., Eden, S., Jansson, J. O., and Isaksson, O.,** Effects of *in vivo* administration of antiserum to rat growth hormone on body growth and insulin-responsiveness in adipose tissue, *Endocrinology*, 112, 1559, 1983.

90. **Flint, D. J. and Gardner, M. J.,** Inhibition of neonatal rat growth and circulating concentrations of insulin-like growth factor-1 using an antiserum to rat growth hormone, *J. Endocrinol.*, 122, 79, 1989.

91. **Gardner, M. J. and Flint, D. J.,** Long-term reductions in GH, insulin-like growth factor-1 and body weight gain in rats neonatally treated with antibodies to rat growth hormone, *J. Endocrinol.*, 124, 381, 1990.

92. **Palmiter, R. D., Brinster, R. L., Hammer, R. E., Trumbauer, M. E., Rosenfeld, M. G., Birnberg, N. C., and Evans, R. M.,** Dramatic growth of mice that develop from eggs microinjected with metallothionein-growth hormone fusion genes, *Nature*, 300, 611, 1982.

93. **Palmiter, R. D., Norstedt, F. M., Gelinas, R. E., Hammer, R. E., and Brinster, R. L.,** Metallothionein-human GH fusion genes stimulate growth of mice, *Science*, 222, 809, 1983.

94. **Bengtsson, B. A., Eden S., Lonn, L., Kvist, H., Stokland, A., Lindstedt, G., Bosaens, I., Tolli, J., Sjostrom, L., and Isaksson, O. G. P.,** Treatment of adults with growth hormone (GH) deficiency with recombinant human GH, *J. Clin. Endocrinol. Metab.*, 76, 309, 1993.

95. **Binnerts, A., Swart, G. R., Wilson, J. H. P., Hoogerbrugge, N., Pols, H. A. P., Birkenhager, J. C., and Lamberts, S. W. J.,** The effect of growth hormone administration in growth hormone deficient adults on bone, protein, carbohydrate, and lipid homeostasis, as well as body composition, *Clin. Endocrinol.*, 37, 79, 1992.

96. **Antoniazzi, F., Radetti, G., Zamboni, G., Gambaro, G., Adami, S., and Tato, L.,** Effects of 1,25 dihydroxyvitamin D$_3$ and growth hormone therapy on serum osteocalcin levels in children with growth hormone deficiency, *Bone Miner.*, 21, 151, 1993.

97. **Marcus, R. G., Butterfield, L., Holloway, L., Gilliland, L., Baylink, D. J., Hintz, R. L., Sherman, B. M.,** Effects of short term administration of recombinant human growth hormone to elderly people, *J. Clin. Endocrinol. Metab.*, 70, 519, 1990.

98. **Burstein, S., Chen, I. W., and Tsang, R. C.,** Effects of growth hormone replacement therapy on 1,25 dihydroxyvitamin D and calcium metabolism, *J. Clin. Endocrinol. Metab.*, 56, 1246, 1983.

99. **Gertner, J. M., Tamborlane, W. V., Hintz, R. L., Horst, R. L., and Genel, M.,** The effects on mineral metabolism of overnight growth hormone infusion in growth hormone deficiency, *J. Clin. Endocrinol. Metab.*, 53, 818, 1981.

100. **Hirschberg, R. and Kopple, J.,** Increase in renal plasma flow and glomerular filtration rate during growth hormone treatment may be mediated by insulin-like growth factor-1, *Am. J. Nephrol.*, 8, 249, 1988.

101. **Christiansen, J. S., Gammelgaard, J., Orskov, H., Andersen, A. R., Telmer, S., and Parving, H. H.,** Kidney function and size in normal subjects before and during growth hormone administration for one week, *Eur. J. Clin. Invest.*, 11, 487, 1981.

102. **Malaisse, W. J., Malaisse-Lagae, F., King, S., and Wright, P. H.,** Effect of growth hormone on insulin secretion, *Am. J. Physiol.*, 215, 423, 1968.

103. **Sirek, A., Vranic, M., Sirek, O. V., Vigas, M., and Policova, Z.,** Effect of growth hormone on acute glucagon and insulin release, *Am. J. Physiol.*, 237, E107, 1979.

104. **Tai, T. Y. and Pek, S.,** Direct stimulation by growth hormone of glucagon and insulin release from isolated rat pancreas, *Endocrinology*, 99, 669, 1976.

105. **Colby, H. D., Caffrey, J. L., and Kitay, J. I.,** Interaction of growth hormone and ACTH in the regulation of adrenocortical secretion in rats, *Endocrinology*, 93, 188, 1973.

106. **Kramer, R. E., Greiner, J. W., and Colby, H. D.,** Sites of action of growth hormone on adrenocortical steroidogenesis in rats, *Endocrinology,* 101, 297, 1977.

107. **Sato, T., Suzuki, Y., Taketani, T., Ishiguro, K., Masuyama, T., Sano, M., Kawashima, H., Koizuma, S., and Nakajima, H.,** Enhanced peripheral conversion of thyroxine to triiodothyronine during hGH therapy in GH deficient children, *J. Clin. Endocrinol. Metab.,* 45, 324, 1977.

108. **Gelhoed-Durjvestyn, P. H. L. M., Roelfsema, F., Schroder-van der Elst, J., van Doorn, J., and van der Heide, D.,** Effect of administration of growth hormone on plasma and intracellular levels of thyroxine and triiodothyronine in thyroidectomized thyronine treated rats, *J. Endocrinol.,* 133, 45, 1992.

109. **Zipf, W. B., Payne, A. H., and Ketch, R. P.,** Prolactin, growth hormone, and luteinizing hormone in the maintenance of luteinizing hormone receptors, *Endocrinology,* 103, 595, 1978.

110. **Jia, X. C., Kalmijn, J., and Hseuh, A. J. W.,** Growth hormone enhances follicle stimulating hormone induced differentiation of cultured rat granulosa cells, *Endocrinology,* 118, 1401, 1986.

111. **Arsenijevic, Y., Wehrenberg, W. B., Conz, A., Eshkol, A., Sizonenko, P. C., and Aubert, M. L.,** Growth hormone deprivation induced by passive immunization against rat GH-releasing factor delays sexual maturation in the male rat, *Endocrinology,* 124, 3050, 1989.

112. **Norstedt, G., Wrange, O., and Gustafsson, J. A.,** Multihormonal regulation of the estrogen receptor in rat liver, *Endocrinology,* 108, 1190, 1981.

113. **Lax, E. R., Rumstadt, F., Plasczyk, H., Peetz, A., and Schriefers, H.,** Antagonistic action of estrogens, flutamide, and human growth hormone on androgen induced changes in the activities of some enzymes in hepatic steroid metabolism in the rat, *Endocrinology,* 113, 1043, 1983.

114. **Leakey, J. E. A., Bazare, J. J., Harmon, J. R., Feuers, R. J., Duffy, P. H., and Hart, R. W.,** Effects of long-term caloric restriction on hepatic drug-metabolizing enzyme activities in the Fischer 344 rat, in *Biological Effects of Dietary Restriction,* Fishbein, L., Ed., ISLI Monographs, Springer-Verlag, New York, 1991, 207.

115. **Rivier, J., Spies, J., Thorner, M., and Vale, W.,** Characterization of a growth hormone-releasing factor from a human pancreatic islet tumor, *Nature,* 300, 276, 1982.

116. **Ling, N., Esch, F., Bohlen, P., Brazeau, P., Wehrenberg, W. B., and Guillemin, R.,** Isolation, primary structure, and synthesis of human hypothalamic somatocrinin: growth hormone releasing factor, *Proc. Natl. Acad. Sci. U.S.A.,* 81, 4302, 1984.

117. **Brazeau, P., Vale, W., Burgus, R., Ling, N., Butcher, M., Rivier, J., and Guillemin, R.,** Hypothalamic polypeptide that inhibits the secretion of immunoreactive pituitary growth hormone, *Science,* 179, 77, 1973.

118. **Tannenbaum, G. S. and Ling, N.,** The interrelationships of growth hormone releasing factor and somatostatin in generation of the ultradian rhythm of growth hormone secretion, *Endocrinology,* 115, 1952, 1984.

119. **Krulich, L., Dhariwal, A. P. S., and McCann, S. M.,** Stimulatory and inhibitory effects of purified hypothalamic extract on growth hormone release from rat pituitary *in vitro, Endocrinology,* 83, 783, 1968.

120. **Vale, W., Brazeau, P., Grant, G., Nussey, A., Burgus, R., Rivier, J., Ling, N., and Guillemin, R.,** Premiers observations sur le mode d'action de la somatostatine un facteur hypothalamique, qui inhibe la secretion de l'hormone de croissance, *Comples Retidus Acad. Sci.,* 275, 2913, 1972.

121. **Guillemin, R.,** Hypothalamic hormones: releasing and inhibiting factors, in *Neuroendocrinology,* Krieger, D. T. and Hughes, J. C, Eds., Sinauer, Sunderland, MA, 1980, 23.

122. **Martin, J.,** Brain regulation of growth hormone secretion, in *Frontiers of Neuroendocrinology,* Martini, L. and Ganong, W., Eds., Raven Press, New York, 1976, 12.

123. **Vale, W., Rivier, C., and Brown, M.,** Regulatory peptides of the hypothalamus, *Annu. Rev. Physiol.,* 39, 473, 1977.

124. **Arimura, A., Smith, W. D., and Schally, A. V.,** Blockade of the stress-induced decrease in blood GH by antisomatostatin serum in rats, *Endocrinology,* 98, 540, 1976.

125. **Ferland, L., Labrie, F., Jobin, M., Arimura, A., and Schally, A. V.,** Physiological role of somatostatin in the control of growth hormone and thyrotropin secretion, *Biochem. Biophys. Res. Commun.,* 68,149,1976.

126. **Terry, L., Willoughby, J., Brazeau, P., Martin, J., and Patel, Y.,** Antiserum to somatostatin prevents stress-induced inhibition of growth hormone secretion in the rat, *Science,* 192, 565, 1976.

127. **Tannenbaum, G. S., Epelbaum, J., Colle, E., Brazeau, P., and Martin, J. B.,** Antiserum to somatostatin reverses starvation induced inhibition of growth hormone but not insulin secretion, *Endocrinology,* 102, 1909, 1978.

128. **Hall, R., Besser, G., Schally, A., Coy, D., Evered, D., Goldie, D., Kastin, A., McNeilly, A., Mortimer, C., Phenekas, C., Tunbridge, W., and Weightman, D.,** Action of growth hormone release inhibitory hormone in healthy men and in acromegaly, *Lancet,* 2, 581, 1973.

129. **Vale, W., Rivier, C., and Guillemin, R.,** Effects of somatostatin on the secretion of thyrotropin and prolactin, *Endocrinology,* 95, 968, 1974.

130. **Krulich, L., Illner, P., Fawcett, C., Quijada, M., and McCann, S. M.,** Dual hypothalamic regulation of growth hormone secretion, in *Growth and Growth Hormone,* Pecile, A. and Mueller, E., Eds., Excerpta Medica, Amsterdam, 1972, 112.

131. **Brownstein, M., Arimura, A., Sato, H., Schally, A. V., and Kizer, J.,** The regional distribution of somatostatin in the rat brain, *Endocrinology,* 96, 1456, 1975.

132. **Kizer, J., Palkovits, M., and Brownstein, M.,** Releasing factors of the circumventricular organs of the rat brain, *Endocrinology,* 98, 311, 1976.

133. **Palkovits, M., Brownstein, M., Arimura, A., Sato, H., Schally, A. V., and Kizer, J.,** Somatostatin content of the hypothalamic ventromedial and arcuate nuclei and the circumventricular organs in the brain, *Brain Res.,* 1091, 4301, 1976.

134. **Patel, Y., Weir, G., and Reichlin, S.,** Anatomic distribution of somatostatin in brain and pancreas islets by radioimmunoassay, Proc. 57th Annu Meet. Endocr. Soc., No. 127, 1975 (abstract).

135. **Hokfelt, T., Efendic, S., Johansson, O., Luft, R., and Arimura, A.,** Immunohistochemical localization of somatostatin (growth hormone release-inhibiting factor) in the guinea pig brain, *Brain Res.,* 80, 165, 1974.

136. **King, J. C., Gerall, A. A., Fishback, J., Elkind, K., and Arimura, A.,** Growth hormone-release inhibiting hormone (GHRIH) pathway of the rat hypothalamus revealed by the unlabeled antibody peroxidase-anti peroxidase method, *Cell Tissue Res.,* 160, 423, 1975.

137. **Stal, G., Vigh, S., Schally, A. V., Arimura, A., and Flerko, B.,** GH-RIH containing neural elements in the rat hypothalamus, *Brain Res.,* 90, 352, 1975.

138. **Pelletier, G., LeClerc, R., Dube, D., Arimura, A., and Schally, A. V.,** Immunohistochemical localization of luteinizing hormone-releasing hormone (LH-RH) and somatostatin in the organum vasculosum of the laminae terminalis of the rat, *Neuroscience,* 4, 27, 1977.

139. **Alpert, L., Brawer, J., Patel, Y., and Reichlin, S.,** Somatostatin neurons in anterior hypothalamus: immunocytochemical localization, *Endocrinology,* 98, 255, 1976.

140. **Elde, R. and Parsons, J.,** Immunocytochemical localization of somatostatin in cell bodies of the rat hypothalamus, *Am. J. Anat.,* 144, 541, 1975.

141. **Hokfelt, T., Efendic, E., Helimstrom, C., Johansson, O., Luft, R., and Arimura, A.,** Cellular localization of somatostatin in endocrine-like cells and neurons of the rat with special reference to the A cells of the pancreatic islets and to the hypothalamus, *Acta Endocrinol.,* 80, 1, 1975.

142. **Chihara, K., Arimura, A., Kubli-Garfias, C., and Schally, A. V.,** Enhancement of immunoreactive somatostatin release into hypophysial portal blood by electrical stimulation of the preoptic area in the rat, *Endocrinology,* 105, 1416, 1979.

143. **Martin, J. B.,** The role of hypothalamic and extrahypothalamic structures in the control of growth hormone secretion, in *Advances in Human Growth Hormone Research,* Raiti, S., Ed., National Institutes of Health, Washington, D.C., 1974, 223.

144. **Rice, R. W. and Critchlow, V.,** Extrahypothalamic control of stress induced inhibition of growth hormone secretion in the rat, *Endocrinology,* 99, 970, 1976.

145. **Millar, R. P., Dennis, P., Tobler, C., King, J. C., Schally, A. V., and Arimura, A.,** Presumptive prohormonal forms of hypothalamic peptide hormones, in *The Biology of Hypothalamic Neurosecretion,* Vincent, J. and Kordon, C., Eds., Centre National de la Recherche Scientifique, Bordeaux, France, 1977, 488.

146. **Sonntag, W. E., Gottschall, P. E., and Meites, J.,** Increased secretion of somatostatin-28 from hypothalamic neurons of aged animals, *Brain Res.,* 380, 229, 1986.

147. **Deuben, R. R. and Meites, J.,** Stimulation of pituitary growth hormone release by a hypothalamic extract *in vitro, Endocrinology,* 74, 408, 1964.

148. **Frohman, L. A. and Bernardis, L. L.,** Growth hormone and insulin levels in weanlings, *Endocrinology,* 82, 1125, 1968.

149. **Frohman, L., Bernardis, L., and Kant, K.,** Hypothalamic stimulation of growth hormone secretion, *Science,* 162, 580, 1968.

150. **Lin, D. H., Bollinger, J., Ling, N., and Reichlin, S.,** Immunoreactive growth hormone releasing factor in human stalk median eminence, *J. Clin. Endocrinol. Metab.,* 58, 1197, 1984.

151. **Bloch, B., Brazeau, P., Ling, N., Bohlen, P., Esch, F., Wehrenberg, W. B., Benoit, R., Bloom, F., and Guillemin, R.,** Immunohistochemical detection of growth hormone releasing factor in brain, *Nature,* 301, 607, 1983.

152. **Werner, H., Okon, E., Fridkin, M., and Koch, Y.,** Localization of growth hormone releasing hormone in the human hypothalamus and pituitary stalk, *J. Clin. Endocrinol. Metab.,* 63, 47, 1986.

153. **Ibata, Y., Okamura, H., Makino, S., Kawakami, F., Morimoto, N., and Chihara, K.,** Light and electron microscopic immunocytochemistry of GRF-like immunoreactive neurons and terminals in the rat hypothalamic arcuate nucleus and median eminence, *Brain Res.,* 370, 136, 1986.

154. **Frohman, L. A., Downs, T. R., Chomczynski, P., and Frohman, M. A.,** Growth hormone releasing hormone: structure, gene expression, and molecular heterogeneity, *Acta Pediatr. Scand.,* 367, 81, 1990.

155. **Chomczynski, P., Downs, T. R., and Frohman, L. A.,** Feedback regulation of growth hormone (GH) releasing hormone gene expression by GH in rat hypothalamus, *Mol. Endocrinol.,* 2, 236, 1988.

156. **Wehrenberg, W. B., Bloch, B., and Ling, N.,** Pituitary secretion of growth hormone in response to opioid peptides and opiates is mediated through growth hormone releasing factor, *Neuroendocrinology,* 41, 13, 1985.

157. **Gil-Ad, I., Laron, Z., and Koch, Y.,** Effect of acute and chronic administration of clonidine on hypothalamic content of growth hormone releasing hormone and somatostatin in the rat, *J. Endocrinol.*, 131, 381, 1991.

158. **Murakami, Y., Kato, Y., Koshiyama, H., Okimura, Y., Fujii, Y., Sato, M., Shakutsui, S., Watanabe, M., and Fujita, T.,** Effect of dopamine on immunoreactive growth hormone releasing factor and somatostatin secretion from rat hypothalamic slices perifused *in vitro, Brain Res.*, 407, 405, 1987.

159. **Kitajima, N., Chihara, K., Abe, H., Okimura, Y., Kajii, Y., Sato, M., Shakutsui, S., Watanabe, M., and Fujita, T.,** Effects of dopamine on immunoreactive growth hormone releasing factor and somatostatin secretion from rat hypothalamic slices perifused *in vitro, Endocrinology*, 124, 69, 1989.

160. **Aulakh, C. S., Hill, J. L., and Murphy, D. L.,** Attenuation of clonidine-induced growth hormone release following chronic glucocorticoid and 5-hydroxytryptamine uptake inhibiting antidepressant treatments, *Neuroendocrinology*, 59, 35, 1994.

161. **Shibasaki, T., Yamauchi, N., Hotta, M., Masuda, A., Imaki, T., Demura, H., Ling, N., and Shizume, K.,** *In vitro* release of growth hormone releasing factor from rat hypothalamus: effect of insulin-like growth factor-1, *Regulatory Peptides*, 15, 47, 1986.

162. **Yamaguchi, N., Shibasaki, T., Ling, N., and Demura, H.,** *In vitro* release of growth hormone releasing factor (GRF) from hypothalamus: somatostatin inhibits GRF release, *Regulatory Peptides*, 33, 71, 1991.

163. **Sugihara, H., Minami, S., and Wakabayashi, I.,** Post-somatostatin rebound secretion of growth hormone is dependent on growth hormone releasing factor in unrestrained female rats, *J. Endocrinol.*, 122, 583, 1989.

164. **Murakami, Y., Kato, Y., Kabayama, Y., Inoue, T., Koshiyama, H., and Imura, H.,** Involvement of hypothalamic growth hormone (GH) releasing factor in GH secretion induced by intracerebroventricular injection of somatostatin in rats, *Endocrinology*, 120, 311, 1987.

165. **Wehrenberg, W. B., Brazeau, P., Luben, R., Bohlen, P., and Guillemin, R.,** Inhibition of pulsatile secretion of growth hormone by monoclonal antibodies to the hypothalamic growth hormone releasing factor, *Endocrinology*, 111, 2147, 1982.

166. **Sato, M., Chihara, K., Kita, T., Kashio, Y., Okimura, Y., Kitajima, N., and Fujita, T.,** Physiologic role of somatostatin-mediated autofeedback regulation for growth hormone: importance of growth hormone in triggering somatostatin release during a trough period of pulsatile growth hormone release in conscious male rats, *Neuroendocrinology*, 50, 139, 1989.

167. **Magnan, E., Cataldi, M., Guillaume, V., Mazzocchi, L., Dutour, A., Razafindraibe, H., Sauze, N., Renard, M., and Oliver, C.,** Role of growth hormone (GH) releasing hormone and somatostatin in the mediation of clonidine induced GH release in the rat, *Endocrinology*, 134, 562, 1994.

168. **Zeitler, P., Tannenbaum, G. S., Clifton, D. K., and Steiner, R. A.,** Ultradian oscillations in somatostatin and growth hormone releasing hormone mRNAs in the brains of adult male rats, *Proc. Natl. Acad. Sci. U.S.A.*, 88, 8920, 1991.

169. **Casanueva, F. F., Popovic, V., and Leal-Cerro, A.,** The physiology of growth hormone secretion, in *Molecular and Clinical Advances in Pituitary Disorders,* Melmed, S., Ed., Endocrine Research and Education, Los Angeles, 1993, 145.

170. **Gaulden, E. C., Littlefield, D. C., Sutoff, O. E., and Seivert, A. L.,** Menstrual abnormalities associated with heroin addiction, *Am. J. Obstet. Gynecol.*, 90, 155, 1964.

171. **Hollister, L. E.,** Human pharmacology of drugs of abuse with emphasis on neuroendocrine effects, *Prog. Brain Res.*, 39, 373, 1973.

172. **Mendelson, J. H., Meyer, R. E., Ellingloe, J., Gurin, S. M., and McDougle, M.,** Effects of heroin and methadone on plasma cortisol and testosterone, *J. Pharmacol. Exp. Ther.*, 195, 296, 1975.

173. **Meites, J., Nicoll, S., Talwalker, P. K., and Hopkins, T. F.,** Induction and maintenance of mammary growth and lactation by neurohormones, drugs, nonspecific stresses, and hypothalamic tissue, in *Proc. 1st Int. Congr. Endocrinol.,* Excerpta Medica, Copenhagen, 1960, 280.

174. **Kokka, N., Garcia, J. F., George, R., and Elliott, H. H. W.,** Growth hormone and ACTH secretion: evidence for an inverse relationship in rats, *Endocrinology*, 90, 735, 1972.

175. **Dupont, A., Cusan, L., Garon, M., Labrie, F., and Li, C. H.,** β-endorphin: stimulation of growth hormone release *in vivo, Proc. Natl. Acad. Sci. U.S.A.*, 74, 358, 1977.

176. **Rivier, C., Vale, W., Ling, N., Brown, M., and Guillemin, R.,** Stimulation *in vivo* of the secretion of prolactin and growth hormone by β-endorphin, *Endocrinology,* 100, 238, 1977.

177. **Bruni, J. F., Van Vugt, D. A., Marshall, S., and Meites, J.,** Effects of naloxone, morphine and methionine enkephalin on serum prolactin, luteinizing hormone, follicle stimulating hormone, thyroid stimulating hormone and growth hormone, *Life Sci.,* 21, 461, 1977.

178. **Cusan, L., Dupont, A., Kiedzik, G. S., Labrie, F., Coy, D. H., and Schally, A. V.,** Potent prolactin and growth hormone releasing activity of more analogues of met-enkephalin, *Nature*, 268, 544, 1977.

179. **Shaar, C. J., Frederickson, R. C. A., Dininger, N. B., and Jackson, L.,** Enkephalin analogues and naloxone modulate the release of growth hormone and prolactin-evidence for regulation by an endogenous opioid peptide in brain, *Life Sci.,* 2, 853, 1977.

180. **Shaar, C. J. and Clemens, J. A.,** The effects of opiate agonists on growth hormone and prolactin release in rats, *Fed. Proc.*, 39, 2539, 1980.

181. **Martin, J. B., Tolis, G., Woods, I., and Guyda, H.,** Failure of naloxone to influence physiological growth hormone and prolactin secretion, *Brain Res.,* 168, 210, 1979.

182. **Tannenbaum, G. S., Panerai, A. E., and Friesen, H. G.,** Failure of β-endorphin antiserum, naloxone, and naltrexone to alter physiologic growth hormone and insulin secretion, *Life Sci.,* 25, 1983, 1979.

183. **Hulting, A. L., Meister, B., Carlsson, L., Hilding, A., and Isaksson, O.,** On the role of the peptide galanin in regulation of growth hormone secretion, *Acta Endocrinol.,* 125, 518, 1991.

184. **Simpkins, J. W., Millard, W. J., and Berglund, L. A.,** Effect of chronic stimulation or antagonism of opiate receptors on growth hormone secretion in male and female rats, *Life Sci.,* 52, 1443, 1993.

185. **Stubbs, W. A., Jones, A., Edwards, C. R. W., Delitalia, G., Jeffcoat, W. J., Rattner, S. J., and Bessner, G. M.,** Hormonal and metabolic responses to an enkephalin analogue in normal man, *Lancet,* 1, 1225, 1978.

186. **Lal, S., Nair, N. P. V., Cervantes, P., Pulman, J., and Guyda, H.,** Effects of naloxone and levallorphan on serum prolactin concentrations and apomorphine-induced growth hormone secretion, *Acta Psychiatr. Scand.,* 59, 173, 1979.

187. **Morley, J. E., Baranetsky, N. G., Wingert, T. O., Carlson, H. E., Hershmman, J. M., Melmed, S., Levin, S. R., Jamison, K. R., Weitzman, R., Chang, R. J., and Varrner, A. A.,** Endocrine effects of naloxone-induced opiate receptor blockade, *J. Clin. Endocrinol. Metab.,* 50, 251, 1980.

188. **Spiler, L. J. and Molitch, M. E.,** Lack of modulation of pituitary hormone stress response by neural pathways involving opiate receptors, *J. Clin. Endocrinol. Metab.,* 50, 516, 1980.

189. **Wakabayashi, I., Demura, R., Miki, N., Ohmura, E., Miypshi, H., and Shizume, K.,** Failure of naloxone to influence plasma growth hormone, prolactin, and cortisol secretions induced by insulin hypoglycemia, *J. Clin. Endocrinol. Metab.,* 50, 597, 1980.

190. **Chihara, K., Arimura, A., Coy, D. H., and Schally, A. V.,** Studies on the interactions of endorphins, substance P, and endogenous somatostatin in growth hormone and prolactin release in rats, *Endocrinology,* 102, 281, 1978.

191. **Ferland, L., Fuxe, K., Eneroth, P., Gustafsson, J. A., and Skett, P.,** Effects of methionine-enkephalin on prolactin release and catecholamine levels and turnover in the median eminence, *Eur. J. Pharmacol.,* 43, 89, 1977.

192. **Van Vugt, D. A., Bruni, J. F., Sylvester, P. W., Chen, H. T., Leiri, T., and Meites, J.,** Interaction between opiates and hypothalamic dopamine on prolactin release, *Life Sci.,* 24, 2361, 1979.

193. **Van Ree, J. M., Versteeg, D. H. G., Shaapen-Kok, W. B., and DeWied, D.,** Effects of morphine on hypothalamic noradrenalin and on pituitary-adrenal activity in rats, *Neuroendocrinology,* 22, 305, 1976.

194. **Haubrich, D. R. and Blake, D. E.,** Modification of serotonin metabolism in rat brain after acute or chronic administration of morphine, *Biochem. Pharmacol.,* 22, 2753, 1973.

195. **Yarbrough, G. G., Buxbaum, D. M., and Sanders-Bush, E.,** Increased serotonin turnover in the acutely morphine treated rat, *Life Sci.,* 10, 977, 1971.

196. **Van Loon, G. R. and DeSouza, E. B.,** Effects of β-endorphin on brain serotonin metabolism, *Life Sci.,* 23, 971, 1978.

197. **Martin, J. B., Audet, J., and Saunders, A.,** Effects of somatostatin and hypothalamic ventromedial lesions on GH release induced by morphine, *Endocrinology,* 96, 839, 1975.

198. **Casanueva, F., Betti, R., Frigerio, C., Cocchi, D., Mantegassa, P., and Mueller, E. E.,** Growth hormone-releasing effect of an enkephalin analogue in the dog: evidence for cholinergic mediation, *Endocrinology,* 106, 1239, 1980.

199. **Kato, Y., Katakami, H., Matsushita, N., Hiroto, S., Shimatsu, A., Waseda, N., and Imura, H.,** Monoaminergic involvement in growth hormone release induced by a synthetic enkephalin analogue in the rat, 62nd Annu Meet. Endocr. Soc., Abstr. 476, 1980.

200. **Meister, B., Scanlon, M. F., and Hokfelt, T.,** Occurrence of galanin-like immunoreactivity on growth hormone-releasing factor (GRF) containing neurons of the monkey (*Macaca fascicularis*) infundibular nucleus and median eminence, *Neurosci, Lett.,* 119, 136, 1990.

201. **Hyde, J. F., Engle, M. G., and Maley, B. E.,** Colocalization of galanin and prolactin within secretory granules of anterior pituitary cells in estrogen treated Fischer 344 rats, *Endocrinology,* 129, 270, 1991.

202. **Loche, S., Vista, N., Ghigo, E., Vanelli, S., Arvat, E., Benso, L., Corda, R., Cella, S. G., Muller, E. E., and Pintor, C.,** Evidence for involvement of endogenous somatostatin in the galanin-induced growth hormone secretion in children, *Pediatr. Res.,* 27, 405, 1990.

203. **Murakami, Y., Ohshima, K., Mochizuki, T., and Yanaihara, N.,** Effect of human galanin on growth hormone, prolactin and antidiuretic hormone secretion in normal men, *J. Clin. Endocrinol. Metab.,* 77, 1436, 1993.

204. **Arvat, E., Ghigo, E., Nicolosi, M., Boffano, G. M., Bellone, J., Yin-Zhang, W., Mazza, E., and Camanni, F.,** Galanin reinstates the growth hormone response to repeated growth hormone releasing hormone administration in man, *Clin. Endocrinol.,* 36, 347, 1992.

205. **Bauer, F. E., Venetikou, M., Burrin, J. M., Ginsberg, L., MacKay, D. J., and Bloom, S. R.,** Growth hormone release in man induced by galanin, a new hypothalamic peptide, *Lancet,* 2, 192, 1986.

206. **Cella, S. G., Locatelli, V., De Gennarro, V., Bondiolotti, G. P., Pintor, C., Loche, S., Provessa, M., and Mueller, E. E.,** Epinephrine mediates the growth hormone releasing effect of galanin in intact rats, *Endocrinology*, 122, 855, 1988.

207. **Maiter, D. M., Hooi, S. C., Koenig, J. L., and Martin, J. B.,** Galanin is a physiological regulator of spontaneous pulsatile secretion of growth hormone in the male rat, *Endocrinology*, 126, 1216, 1990.

208. **Murakami, Y., Kato, Y., Shimatsu, A., Koshiyama, H., Hattori, N., Yanaihara, N., and Imura, H.,** Possible mechanisms involved in growth hormone secretion induced by galanin in the rat, *Endocrinology*, 124, 1224, 1989.

209. **Negro-Vilar, A., Lopez, F., Merchenthaler, I., Liposits, Z., and Guistina, A.,** Neuropeptide regulation of growth hormone secretion, in *Molecular and Cellular Advances in Pituitary Tumors*, Melmed, S., Ed., Endocrine Research and Education, Los Angeles, CA, 1993, 62.

210. **Snyder, S. H.,** Brain peptides as neurotransmitters, *Science,* 209, 976, 1980.

211. **Rivier, C., Brown, M., and Vale, W.,** Effects of neurotensin, substance P and morphine sulfate on the secretion of prolactin and growth hormone in the rat, *Endocrinology*, 100, 751, 1977.

212. **Kato, Y., Chihara, K., Ohgo, S., Iwasaki, Y., Abe, H., and Imura, H.,** Growth hormone and prolactin release by substance P in rats, *Life Sci.*, 19, 441, 1976.

213. **Takahara, J. A., Arimura, A., and Schally, A. V.,** Effect of catecholamines on the TRH-stimulated release of prolactin and growth hormone from sheep pituitaries *in vitro*, *Endocrinology*, 95, 1490, 1974.

214. **Convey, E. M., Tucker, H. A., Smith, V. G., and Zolman, J.,** Bovine prolactin, growth hormone, thyroxine, and corticoid response to thyrotropin-releasing hormone, *Endocrinology*, 92, 471, 1973.

215. **Giannattasio, G., Zanini, A., Panerai, A. E., Meldolesi, J., and Mueller, E. E.,** Studies on rat pituitary homographs. Effects of thyrotropin-releasing hormone on *in vitro* biosynthesis and release of growth hormone and prolactin, *Endocrinology*, 104, 237, 1979.

216. **Strbak, V., Angyal, R., Jurcovicova, J., and Randoskova, A.,** Role of thyrotropin releasing hormone in thyroid stimulating hormone and growth hormone regulation during post-natal maturation in female wistar rats, *Biol. Neonate*, 50, 91, 1986.

217. **Mueller, E. E.,** Neural control of somatotropic function, *Physiol. Rev.*, 67, 962, 1987.

218. **McDonald, J. K., Koenig, J. E., Gibbs, D. M., Collins, P., and Noe, B. P.,** High concentrations of neuropeptide Y in pituitary portal blood of rats, *Neuroendocrinology*, 46, 538, 1987.

219. **McDonald, J. K., Lumpkin, M. D., Samson, W. K., and McCann, S. M.,** Neuropeptide Y affects secretion of luteinizing hormone and growth hormone in ovariectomized rats, *Proc. Natl. Acad. Sci. U.S.A.*, 82, 561, 1985.

220. **Catzeflis, C., Pierroz, D., Rohner-Jeanrenaud, F., Rivier, J. E., Sizonenko, P. C., and Aubert, M. L.,** Neuropeptide Y administered chronically into the lateral ventricle profoundly inhibits both the gonadotropic and somatotropic axes in the intact adult female rats, *Endocrinology,* 132, 224, 1993.

221. **Rettori, V., Milenkovic, L., Aguila, M. C., and McCann, S. M.,** Physiologically significant effect of neuropeptide Y to suppress growth hormone release by stimulating somatostatin discharge, *Endocrinology*, 126, 2296, 1990.

222. **Anastasia, A., Erspamer, V., and Bucci, H.,** Isolation and structure of bombesin and alytesin, analogous active peptides from the skin of the European amphibians, Bombena and Avtes, *Experientia*, 27, 166, 1971.

223. **Rivier, C., Rivier, J., and Vale, W.,** The effect of bombesin and related peptides on prolactin and growth hormone secretion in the rat, *Endocrinology*, 102, 519, 1978.

224. **Karashima, T., Okajima, T., Kato, K., and Ibayashi, H.,** Suppressive effects of cholecystokinin and bombesin on growth hormone and prolactin secretion in urethane anesthetized rats, *Endocrinol. Jpn.*, 31, 539, 1984.

225. **Houben, H. and Denef, C.,** Stimulation of growth hormone and prolactin release from rat pituitary cell aggregates by bombesin and ranatensin like peptides is potentiated by estradiol, 5α-dihydrotestosterone and dexamethazone, *Endocrinology*, 126, 2257, 1990.

226. **Westendorf, J. M. and Schonbrunn, A.,** Bombesin stimulates prolactin and growth hormone release by pituitary cells in culture, *Endocrinology*, 110, 352, 1982.

227. **Carraway, R. and Leeman, S. E.,** The isolation of a new hypotensive peptide, neurotensin, from bovine hypothalami, *J. Biol. Chem.*, 248, 6854, 1973.

228. **Rivier, C., Brown, M. and Vale, W.,** Effects of neurotensin, substance P and morphine sulfate on the secretion of prolactin and growth hormone in the rat, *Endocrinology*, 100, 751, 1977.

229. **Vijayan, E. and McCann, S. M.,** Effect of intraventricular injection of γ-aminobutyric acid (GABA) on plasma growth hormone and thyrotropin in conscious ovariectomized rats, *Endocrinology*, 103, 1888, 1978.

230. **Kato, Y., Dupre, J., and Beck, J. C.,** Plasma growth hormone in the anesthetized rat: effects of dibutyryl cyclic AMP, prostaglandin E, adrenergic agents, vasopressin, chlorpromazine, amphetamine, and L-DOPA, *Endocrinology*, 93, 135, 1973.

231. **Heidingsfelder, S. A. and Blackard, W. G.,** Adrenergic control mechanism for vasopressin-induced plasma growth hormone response, *Metabolism,* 17, 1019, 1968.

232. **Wilber, J. F., Nagel, T., and White, W. F.,** Hypothalamic growth hormone-releasing activity (GRA): characterization by the *in vitro* rat pituitary and radioimmunoassay, *Endocrinology*, 89, 1419, 1971.

233. **Franci, C. R., Anselmo-Franci, J. A., Kozlowski, G. P., and McCann, S. M.,** Actions of endogenous vasopressin and oxytocin on anterior pituitary hormone secretion, *Neuroendocrinology*, 57, 693, 1993.

234. **Emson, P. C., Fahrenkrug, J., DeMuckadell, O. B. S., Jessel, T. M., and Iverson, L. L.,** Vasoactive intestinal polypeptide (VIP): vesicular localization and potassium evoked release from rat hypothalamus, *Brain Res.,* 143, 174, 1978.

235. **Said, S. L. and Porter, J. C.,** Vasoactive intestinal polypeptide (VIP): evidence for secretion in hypophyseal portal blood, *Fed. Proc.*, 37, 482, 1978.

236. **Bluet-Pajot, M., Mounier, F., Leonard, J., Kordon, C., and Durand, D.,** Vasoactive intestinal peptide induces a transient release of growth hormone in the rat, *Peptides*, 8, 35, 1987.

237. **Kashio, Y., Chomczynski, P., Downs, T. R., and Frohman, L. A.,** Growth hormone and prolactin secretion in cultured somatomammotroph cells, *Endocrinology*, 127, 1129, 1990.

238. **Matsushita, N., Kato, Y., Katakami, H., Shimatsu, A., Yanaihara, N., and Imura, H.,** Stimulation of growth hormone release by vasoactive intestinal polypeptide from human pituiatry adenomas *in vitro, J. Clin. Endocrinol. Metab.*, 53, 1297, 1981.

239. **Chihara, K., Kaji, H., Minamitani, N., Kodama, H., Kita, T., Goto, B., Chiba, T., Coy, D., and Fujita, T.,** Stimulation of growth hormone by vasoactive interstinal polypeptide in acromegaly, *J. Clin. Endocrinol. Metab.*, 58, 81, 1984.

240. **Fischer, J. A., Tobler, P. H., Kaufman, M., Born, W., Henke, H., Cooper, P. E., Sagar, S. M., and Martin, J. B.,** Calcitonin: regional distribution of the hormone and its binding sites in the human brain and pituitary, *Proc. Natl. Acad. Sci. U.S.A.,* 78, 7801, 1981.

241. **Cantalamessa, L., Catania, A., Reschini, E., and Peracchi, M.,** Inhibitory effect of calcitonin on growth hormone and insulin secretion in man, *Metabolism*, 27, 987, 1978.

242. **Looij, B. J., Roelfsema, F., van der Heide, D., Frolich, M., Souverijn, M., and Nieuwenhuijen-Kruseman, A. C.,** The effect of calcitonin on growth hormone secretion in man, *Clin. Endocrinol.*, 29, 517, 1988.

243. **Ceda, G. P., Denti, L., Ceresini, G., Rastelli, G., Dotti, C., Cavatieri, S., Valenti, G., and Hoffman, A. R.,** Calcitonin inhibition of growth hormone releasing hormone induced growth hormone secretion in normal men, *Acta Endocrinol.*, 120, 416, 1989.

244. **Lengyel, A. M. J. and Tannenbaum, G. S.,** Mechanisms of calcitonin-induced growth hormone (GH) suppression: roles of somatostatin and GH releasing factor, *Endocrinology*, 120, 1377, 1987.

245. **Miyata, A., Arimura, A., Dahl, R. D., Minamino, N., Uehara, A., Jiang, L., Culler, M. D., and Coy, D. H.,** Isolation of a novel 38 residue hypothalamic polypeptide which stimulates adenylate cyclase in pituitary cells, *Biochem. Biophys. Res. Commun.*, 164, 567, 1989.

246. **Abe, H., Kato, Y., Iwasaki, Y., Chihara, K., and Imura, H.,** Central effects of somatostatin on the secretion of growth hormone in the anesthetized rat, *Proc. Soc. Exp. Biol. Med.*, 159, 346, 1978.

247. **Mueller, E. E., Pra, P. D., and Pecile, A.,** Influence of brain neurohumors injected into the lateral ventricle of the rat on growth hormone release, *Endocrinology*, 83, 893, 1968.

248. **Smythe, G. A., Brandstater, J. F., and Lazarus, L.,** Serotonergic control of rat growth hormone secretion, *Neuroendocrinology,* 17, 245, 1975.

249. **Chen, H. T., Mueller, G. P., and Meites, J.,** Effects of L-DOPA and somatostatin on suckling induced release of prolactin and GH, *Endocr. Res.*, 1, 283, 1974.

250. **Muller, E. E., Cocchi, D., Jalando, H., and Udeshini, G.,** Antagonistic role for norepinephrine and dopamine in the control of growth hormone secretion in the rat, *Endocrinology*, 92, A248, 1973.

251. **Mueller, G. P., Simpkins, J., Meites, J., and Moore, K. E.,** Differential effects of dopamine agonists and haloperidol on release of prolactin, thyroid stimulating hormone, growth hormone and luteinizing hormone in rats, *Neuroendocrinology*, 20, 121, 1976.

252. **Vijayan, E., Krulich, L., and McCann, S. M.,** Catecholaminergic regulation of TSH and growth hormone release in ovariectomized and ovariectomized, steroid-primed rats, *Neuroendocrinology*, 26, 174, 1978.

253. **Ruch, W., Jaton, A. L., Bucher, B., Marbach, P., and Doepfner, W.,** Alpha adrenergic control of growth hormone in adult male rat, *Experientia*, 32, 529, 1976.

254. **Tannenbaum, G. S. and Martin, J. B.,** Evidence for an endogenous ultradian rhythm governing growth hormone secretion in the rat, *Endocrinology*, 98, 540, 1976.

255. **Martin, J. B., Brazeau, P., Tannenbaum, G. S., Willoughby, J. O., Epelbaum, J., Terry, L. C., and Durand, D.,** Neuroendocrine organization of growth hormone regulation, in *The Hypothalamus*, Reichlin, S., Dessarin, R. I., and Martini, B., Eds., Raven Press, New York, 1978, 329.

256. **Willoughby, J. O., Terry, L. C., Brazeau, P., and Martin, J. B.,** Pulsatile growth hormone, prolactin, and thyrotropin secretion in rats with hypothalamic deafferentation, *Brain Res.*, 127, 137, 1977.

257. **Weiner, R. I., Shryne, J. E., Gorski, R. A., and Sawyer, C. H.,** Changes in the catecholaminergic content of the rat hypothalamus following deafferentation, *Endocrinology*, 90, 867, 1972.

258. **Nemeroff, C. B., Konkol, R. J., Bissette, G., Youngblood, W., Martin, J. B., Brazeau, P., Rone, M. S., Prange, A. J., Jr., Breese, G. R., and Kizer, J. S.,** Analysis of the disruption in hypothalamic pituitary regulation in rats treated neonatally with monosodium L-glutamate (MSG): evidence for the involvement of tubero infundibular cholinergic and dopaminergic systems in neuroendocrine regulation, *Endocrinology*, 101, 613, 1977.

259. **Wakabayashi, I., Miyazawa, H., Kanda, M., Miki, N., Demura, R., Demura, H., and Shizume, K.,** Stimulation of immunoreactive somatostatin release from hypothalamic synaptosomes by high (K+) and dopamine, *Endocrinol. Jpn.,* 24, 601, 1977.

260. **Negro-Vilar, A., Ojeda, S. R., Arimura, A., and McCann, S. M.,** Dopamine and norepinephrine stimulate somatostatin release by median eminence fragments *in vitro, Life Sci.,* 23, 1493, 1978.

261. **Martin, J. B., Durand, D., Gurd, W., Faille, G., Audet, J., and Brazeau, P.,** Neuropharmacological regulation of episodic growth hormone and prolactin secretion in the rat, *Endocrinology,* 102, 106, 1978.

262. **Schaub, C., Bluet-Pajot, M. T., Mouonier, F., Segalen, A., and Duhault, J.,** Effects of noradrenergic agonists and antagonists on growth hormone secretion under gamma-hydroxybutyrate narcoanalgesia in the rat, *Psychoneuroendocrinology,* 5, 139, 1980.

263. **Kato, Y., Dupre, J., and Beck, J. C.,** Plasma growth hormone in the anesthetized rat: effects of dibutyryl cyclic AMP, prostaglandin E, adrenergic agents, vasopressin, chlorpromazine, amphetamine and L-DOPA, *Endocrinology,* 93, 135, 1973.

264. **Takahashi, K., Tsushima, T., and Irie, M.,** Effect of catecholamines on plasma growth hormone in dogs, *Endocrinology,* 20, 323, 1973.

265. **Holland, F. J., Richards, G. E., Kaplan, S. L., Ganong, W. F., and Grumbach, M. M.,** The role of biogenic amines in the regulation of growth hormone and corticotropin secretion in the trained conscious dog, *Endocrinology,* 102, 1452, 1978.

266. **Steiner, R. A., Illner, P., Rolfs, A. D., Toivola, P. T. K., and Gale, C. C.,** Noradrenergic and dopaminergic regulation of GH and prolactin in baboons, *Neuroendocrinology,* 26, 15, 1978.

267. **Toivola, P. T. K. and Gate, C. C.,** Effect of temperature on biogenic amine infusion into hypothalamus of baboon, *Neuroendocrinology,* 6, 210, 1970.

268. **Toivola, P. T. K. and Gale, C. C.,** Stimulation of growth hormone release by microinjection of norepinephrine into hypothalamus of baboon, *Endocrinology,* 90, 895, 1974.

269. **Chambers, J. W. and Brown, G. M.,** Neurotransmitter regulation of growth hormone and ACTH in the rhesus monkey: effects of biogenic amines, *Endocrinology,* 98, 420, 1976.

270. **Marantz, R., Sachar, E. J., Weitzman, E., and Sassin, J.,** Cortisol and GH responses to D- and L-amphetamine in monkeys, *Endocrinology,* 99, 459, 1976.

271. **Boyd, A. E., Lebovitz, H. E., and Preiffer, J. B.,** Stimulation of human- growth-hormone secretion by L-DOPA, *N. Engl. J. Med.,* 283, 1425, 1970.

272. **Burrow, G. N., May, P. B., Spaulding, S. W., and Donabedian, R. K.,** TRH and dopamine interactions affecting pituitary hormone secretion, *J. Clin. Endocrinol. Metab.,* 45, 65, 1977.

273. **Leebau, W. F., Lee, L. A., and Woolf, P. D.,** Dopamine affects basal and augmented pituitary hormone secretion, *J. Endocrinol. Metab,* 47, 480, 1978.

274. **Collu, R., Fraschini, F., Visconti, P., and Martini, L.,** Adrenergic and serotonergic control of growth hormone secretion in adult male rats, *Endocrinology,* 90, 1231, 1972.

275. **Smythe, G. A. and Lazarus, L.,** Suppression of human growth hormone secretion by melatonin and cyproheptadine, *J. Clin. Invest.,* 54, 116, 1974.

276. **Smythe, G. A., Brandstater, J. F., and Lazarus, L.,** Serotonergic control of rat growth hormone secretion, *Neuroendocrinology,* 17, 245, 1975.

277. **Collu, R., Du Ruisseau, P., and Tache, Y.,** Role of putative neurotransmitters in prolactin, GH and LH response to acute immobilization stress in male rats, *Neuroendocrinology,* 28, 178, 1979.

278. **Arnold, M. A. and Fernstrom, J. D.,** Serotonin receptor antagonists block a natural, short-term surge in serum growth hormone levels, *Endocrinology,* 103, 1159, 1978.

279. **Eden, S., Bolle, P., and Modegh, K.,** Monoaminergic control of episodic growth hormone secretion in the rat: effects of reserpine, alpha-methyl-p-tyrosine, p-chlorophenylalanine, and haloperidol, *Endocrinology,* 105, 523, 1979.

280. **Mueller, E. E., Udeschini, G., Secchi, C., Zambotti, F., Panerai, A. E., Vicentini, L., Cocola, F., and Mantegazza, P.,** Inhibitory role of the serotonergic system in hypoglycemia-induced growth hormone release in the dog, *Acta Endocrinol,* 82, 71, 1976.

281. **Bivens, C. H., Lebovitz, H. E., and Feldman, J. M.,** Inhibition of hypoglycemia induced growth hormone secretion by the serotonin antagonists cyproheptadine and methysergide, *N. Engl. J. Med.,* 289, 236, 1973.

282. **Imura, H., Nakai, Y., and Yoshimi, T.,** Effect of 5-hydroxytryptophan (5-HTP) on growth hormone and ACTH release in man, *J. Clin. Endocrinol. Med.,* 36, 204, 1973.

283. **Nakai, Y., Imura, H., Sakurai, H., Kurahachi, H., and Yoshimi, T.,** Effect of cyproheptadine on human growth hormone secretion, *J. Clin. Endocrinol. Metab.,* 38, 446, 1974.

284. **Benkert, O., Laakman, G., Souvatzoglou, A., and Von Werder, K.,** Missing indicator function of growth hormone and luteinizing hormone blood levels for dopamine and serotonin concentration in the human brain, *J. Neural. Transm.,* 34, 291, 1973.

285. **Mueller, E. E., Brambilla, F., Cavagnini, F., Peracchi, M., and Panerai, A.,** Slight effect of L-tryptophan on growth hormone release in normal human subjects, *J. Clin. Endocrinol. Metab.,* 39, 1, 1974.

286. **Chihara, K., Kato, Y., Maeda, K., Matsukura, S., and Imura, H.,** Suppression by cyproheptidine of human growth hormone and cortisol secretion during sleep, *J. Clin. Invest.*, 57, 1392, 1976.

287. **Liuzzi, A., Panerai, A. E., Chiodini, P. G., Secchi, C., Cocchi, D., Botalla, L., Silvestrini, F., and Mueller, E. E.,** Neuroendocrine control of growth hormone secretion: experimental and clinical studies, in *Growth Hormone and Related Peptide*, Pecile, A. and Muller, E. E., Eds., Excerpta Medica, Amsterdam, 1976, 236.

288. **Sorrentino, S., Schatch, D. S., and Reiter, R. J.,** Environmental control of growth and growth hormone, in *Growth and Growth Hormone*, Pecile, A. and Muller, E. E., Eds., Excerpta Medica, Princeton, NJ, 1972, 330.

289. **Smythe, G. A. and Lazarus, L.,** Growth hormone regulation by melatonin and serotonin, *Nature*, 244, 230, 1973.

290. **Anton-Tay, F., Chow, C., Anton, S., and Wurtman, R. J.,** Brain serotonin concentration: elevation following intraperitoneal administration of melatonin, *Science*, 162, 277, 1968.

291. **Ronnelkeiv, O. K. and McCann, S. M.,** Growth hormone release in conscious pinealectomized and sham-operated male rats, *Endocrinology*, 102, 1694, 1978.

292. **Willoughby, J. O.,** Pinealectomy mildly disturbs the secretory patterns of prolactin and growth hormone in the unstressed rat, *J. Endocrinol.*, 86, 101, 1980.

293. **Smythe, G. A. and Lazarus, L.,** Growth hormone response to melatonin in man, *Science*, 184, 1373, 1974.

294. **Baldessarrini, R. J. and Karobath, M.,** Biochemical physiology of central synapses, *Annu. Rev. Physiol.*, 35, 273, 1973.

295. **Fioretti, P., Melis, G. B., Paoletti, M., Parodo, G., Caminiti, F., Corsini, G. U., and Martini, L.,** Gamma-amino-β-hydroxybutyric acid stimulates prolactin and growth hormone release in normal women, *J. Clin. Endocrinol. Metab.*, 47, 1336, 1978.

296. **Takahara, J., Yunoki, S., Yakushiji, W., Yamauchi, J., Yamane, Y., and Ofuji, T.,** Stimulatory effects of gamma-hydroxybutyric acid on growth hormone and prolactin release in humans, *J. Clin. Endocrinol. Metab.*, 44, 1014, 1977.

297. **Cavagnini, F., Invitti, C., Pinto, M., Maraschini, C., Di Landro, A., Dubini, A., and Marelli, A.,** Effect of acute and repeated administration of gamma aminobutyric acid (GABA) on growth hormone and prolactin secretion in man, *Acta Endocrinol.*, 93, 149, 1980.

298. **Abe, H., Kato, Y., Chihara, K., Ohgo, S., Iwasaki, Y., and Imura, H.,** Growth hormone release by gamma-aminobutyric acid (GABA) and gamma- amino-β-hydroxybutyric acid (GABOB) in the rat, *Endocrinol. Jpn.*, 24, 229, 1977.

299. **Takahara, J., Yunoki, S., Hosogi, H., Yakushiji, W., Kageyama, J., and Ofuji, T.,** Concomitant increases in serum growth hormone and hypothalamic somatostatin in rats after injection of gammaaminobutyric acid, aminooxyacetic acid, or gamma-hydroxybutyric acid, *Endocrinology*, 106, 343, 1980.

300. **Vijayan, E. and McCann, S. M.,** Effects of intraventricular injection of gamma-aminobutyric acid on plasma growth hormone and thyrotropin in conscious ovariectomized rats, *Endocrinology*, 103, 1888, 1978.

301. **Casanueva, F., Betti, R., Frigerio, C., Cocchi, D., Mantegazza, P., and Mueller, E. E.,** Growth hormone-releasing effect of an enkephalin analog in the dog: evidence for cholinergic mediation, *Endocrinology*, 106, 1239, 1980.

302. **Bruni, J. F. and Meites, J.,** Effects of cholinergic drugs on growth hormone release, *Life Sci.*, 23, 1351, 1978.

303. **Locatelli, V., Tosello, A., Redaelli, M., Ghigo, E., Massara, F., and Mueller, E. E.,** Cholinergic agonist and antagonist drugs modulate the growth hormone response to growth hormone releasing hormone in the rat: evidence for mediation by somatostatin, *J. Endocrinol.*, 111, 271, 1986.

304. **Bruni, J. F. and Meites, J.,** Effects of cholinergic drugs on growth hormone release, *Life Sci.*, 23, 1351, 1978.

305. **Mukherjee, A., Snyder, A. G., and McCann, S. M.,** Characterization of muscarinic cholinergic receptors on intact rat anterior pituitary cells, *Life Sci.*, 27, 475, 1980.

306. **Ross, R. J., Ttsagarakis, S., Grossman, A., Nhagafoong, L., Touzel, R. J., Rees, L. H., and Besser, G. M.,** GH feedback occurs through modulation of hypothalamic somatostatin under cholinergic control: studies with pyridostigmine and GHRH, *Clin. Endocrinol.*, 27, 727, 1988.

307. **Massara, F., Ghigo, E., Goffi, S., Molinatti, G. M., Mueller, E. E., and Camanni, F.,** Blockade of hp-GRF-40 induced GH release in normal men by a cholinergic muscarinic antagonist, *J. Clin. Endocrinol. Metab.*, 59, 1025, 1984.

308. **Jordon, V., Dieguez, C., Lafaffian, I., Rodriguez-Arano, M. D., Gomez-Pan, A., Hall, R., and Scanlon, M. F.,** Influence of dopaminergic, adrenergic, and cholinergic blockade and TRH administration on GH responses to GRF 1-29, *Clin. Endocrinol*, 24, 291, 1986.

309. **Taylor, B. J., Smith, P. J., and Brook, C. G. D.,** Inhibition of physiologic growth hormone secretion by atropine, *Clin. Endocrinol.*, 22, 497, 1985.

310. **Casanueva, F. F., Villanueva, L., Dieguez, C., Cabranes, J. A., Diaz, Y., Szoke, B., Scanlon, M. F., Schally, A. V., and Fernandez-Cruz, A.,** Atropine blockade of growth hormone (GH)-releasing hormone induced GH secretion in man is not exerted at pituitary level, *J. Clin. Endocrinol. Metab.*, 62, 186, 1986.

311. **Delitala, G., Grossman, A., and Besser, G. M.,** Opiate peptides control growth hormone secretion through a cholinergic mechanism in man, *Clin. Endocrinol.*, 18, 401, 1983.

312. **Peters, J. R., Evans, P. J., Page M. D., Hall, R., Gibbs, J. T., Dieguez, C., and Scanlon, M. F.,** Cholinergic muscarinic receptor blockade with pirenzepine abolishes slow-wave sleep related growth hormone release in normal adult males, *Clin. Endocrinol.*, 25, 213, 1986.

313. **Arvat, E., Cappa, M., Casanueva, F. F., Diegues, C., Ghigo, E., Nicolosi, M., Valcavi, R., and Zini, M.,** Pyridostigmine potentiates growth hormone (GH) releasing hormone induced GH release in both men and women, *J. Clin. Endocrinol. Metab.*, 76, 374, 1993.

314. **Penalva, A., Carballo, A., Pombo, M., Casanueva, F. F., and Dieguez, C.,** Effect of growth hormone (GH) releasing hormone (GHRH), atropine, pyridostigmine or hypoglycemia on GHRP-6 induced GH secretion in man, *J. Clin. Endocrinol. Metab.*, 76, 168, 1993.

315. **Delitala, G., Frulio, T., Pacifico, A., and Maioli, M.,** Participation of cholinergic muscarinic receptors in glucagon and arginine mediated growth hormone secretion in man, *J. Clin. Endocrinol. Metab.*, 55, 1231, 1982.

316. **Delitala, G., Maioli, M., Pacifico, A., Brianda, S., Palermo, M., and Mannelli, M.,** Cholinergic receptor control mechanisms for Ldopa, apomorphine, and clonidine induced growth hormone secretion in man, *J. Clin. Endocrinol. Metab.*, 57, 1145, 1983.

317. **Rudolph, C., Richards, G. E., Kaplan, S., and Ganong, W. F.,** Effect of intraventricular histamine on growth hormone secretion in dogs, *Neuroendocrinology*, 29, 169, 1979.

318. **Watkins, J. C. and Evans, R. H.,** Excitatory amino acid transmitters, *Annu. Rev. Pharmacol. Toxicol.*, 21, 165, 1981.

319. **Meeker, R. B., Swanson, D. J., and Hayward, J. N.,** Ultrastructural distribution of glutamate immunoreactivity within neurosecretory endings and pituicytes of the rat neurohypophysis, *Brain Res.*, 564, 181, 1991.

320. **Mason, G. A., Bissette, G., and Nemeroff, C. B.,** Effects of excitotoxic amino acids on pituitary hormone secretion in the rat, *Brain Res.*, 289, 366, 1983.

321. **Gay, V. L. and Plant, T. M.,** N-Methyl-D,L-aspartate elicits hypothalamic gonadotropin releasing hormone release in prepubertal male rhesus monkeys (*Macaca mulatta*), *Endocrinology*, 120, 2289, 1987.

322. **Estienne, M. J., Schillo, K. K., Green, M. A., Hileman, S. M., and Boling, J. A.,** N-Methyl-D,L-aspartate stimulates growth hormone but not luteinizing hormone secretion in the sheep, *Life Sci.*, 44, 1527, 1989.

323. **Acs, Z., Lonart, G., and Makara, G. B.,** Direct effects of excitatory amino acids on pituitary growth hormone release, *Neuroendocrinology*, 52, 156, 1990.

324. **Niimi, M., Sato, M., Murao, K., Takahara, J., and Kawanishi, K.,** Effect of excitatory amino acid receptor agonists on secretion of growth hormone as assessed by the reverse hemolytic plaque assay, *Neuroendocrinology*, 60, 173, 1994.

325. **Root, R. W.,** Amino acids increase growth hormone secretion in man, *J. Endocrinol. Invest.*, 12, 3, 1989.

326. **Alba-Roth, J., Muller, O. A., and Schopohl, J.,** Excitatory amino acids increase growth hormone secretion by inhibiting somatostatin, *J. Clin. Endocrinol. Meta.*, 67, 1186, 1988.

327. **Reichlin, S.,** Regulation of somatotrophic hormone secretion, in *The Pituitary Gland,* Harris, G. W. and Donovan, T., Eds., Butterworths, London, 1966, 270.

328. **Peake, G. T., Birge, C. A., and Daughaday, W. H.,** Alterations of radioimmuno-assayable growth hormone and prolactin during hypothyroidism, *Endocrinology*, 92, 487, 1973.

329. **Hervas, F., Morreale de Escobar, G., and Escobar del Rey, F.,** Rapid effects of single small doses of thyroxine and triiodo-L-thyronine on growth hormone, as studied in the rat by radioimmunoassay, *Endocrinology*, 97, 91, 1975.

330. **Takuchi, A., Suzuki, M., and Tsuchiya, S.,** Effects of thyroidectomy on the secretory profiles of growth hormone, thyrotropin and corticosterone in the rat, *Endocrinol. Jpn.*, 25, 381, 1978.

331. **Coiro, V., Braverman, L. E., Christianson, D., Fang, S., and Goodman, H. M.,** Effect of hypothyroidism and thyroxine replacement on growth hormone in the rat, *Endocrinology*, 105, 641, 1979.

332. **Samuels, H. H., Tsai, J. S., and Clinton, R.,** Thyroid hormone action: a cell-culture system responsive to physiological concentrations of thyroid hormones, *Science*, 181, 1253, 1973.

333. **Tsai, J. S. and Samuels, H. H.,** Thyroid hormone action: stimulation of growth hormone and inhibition on prolactin secretion in cultured pituitary cells, *Biochem. Biophys. Res. Commun.*, 59, 420, 1974.

334. **Iwatsubo, H., Omori, K., Okada, Y., Fukuchi, M., Miyai, K., Abe, H., and Kumahara, Y.,** Human growth hormone secretion in primary hypothyroidism before and after treatment, *J. Clin. Endocrinol. Metab.*, 27, 1751, 1967.

335. **Kato, H. P., Youlton, R., Kaplan, S. L., and Grumbach, M. M.,** Growth and growth hormone: growth hormone release in children with primary hypothyroidism and thyrotoxicosis, *J. Clin. Endocrinol. Metab.*, 29, 346, 1969.

336. **MacGillivray, M. H., Aceto, T., Jr., and Frohman, L. A.,** Plasma growth hormone responses and growth retardation in hypothyroidism, *Am. J. Dis. Child.*, 115, 273, 1968.

337. **Dupont, A., Merand, Y., and Barden, N.,** Effect of propylthiouracil and thyroxine on the inactivation of somatostatin by rat hypothalamus, *Life Sci.*, 23, 2007, 1978.

338. **Dickerman, E., Dickerman, S., and Meites, J.,** Influence of age, sex, and estrous cycle on pituitary and plasma GH levels in rats, in *Growth and Growth Hormone*, Meites, J., Ed., Excerpta Medica, Milan, 1971, 252.

339. **Malacara, J. M., Valverde, R., and Reichlin, S.,** Elevation of plasma radioimmunoassayable growth hormone in the rat induced by porcine hypothalamic extract, *Endocrinology*, 91, 1189, 1972.
340. **Frantz, A. G. and Rabkin, M. T.,** Effects of estrogen and sex difference on secretion of human growth hormone, *Endocrinol. Metab.*, 25, 1470, 1965.
341. **Merimee, T. J., Fineberg, S. E., and Tyson, J. E.,** Fluctuation of human growth hormone secretion during menstrual cycle: response to arginine, *Metabolism*, 18, 606, 1969.
342. **Illig, R. and Prader, A.,** Effect of testosterone on growth hormone secretion in patients with anorexia and delayed puberty, *Clin. Endocrinol. Metab*, 30, 615, 1970.
343. **Finkelstein, J. W., Roffwarg, H. P., Boyar, R. M., Kream, J., and Hellman, L.,** Age-related changes in the twenty four hour spontaneous secretion of growth hormone, *J. Clin. Endocrinol. Metab.*, 35, 655, 1972.
344. **Simon, S. M., Schiffer, M., Glick, S. M., and Schwartz, E.,** Effect of medroxy-progesterone acetate upon stimulated release of growth hormone in men, *J. Clin. Endocrinol. Metab.*, 27, 1633, 1967.
345. **Lucke, C. and Glick, S. M.,** Effect of medroxyprogesterone acetate on the sleep-induced peak of growth hormone secretion, *J. Clin. Endocrinol. Metab.*, 33, 851, 1971.
346. **Lawrence, A. M. and Kirsteins, L.,** Progestins in the medical management of active acromegaly, *J. Clin. Endocrinol. Metab.*, 30, 646, 1970.
347. **Frantz, A. G. and Rabkin, M. T.,** Human growth hormone: clinical measurement response to hypoglycemia and suppression by corticosteroids, *N. Engl. J. Med.*, 271, 1375, 1964.
348. **Hartog, M., Graafar, M. A., and Fraser, R.,** Effect of corticosteroids on serum growth hormone, *Lancet*, 2, 376, 1964.
349. **Krieger, D. T. and Glick, S. M.,** Growth hormone and cortisone responsiveness in Cushing's syndrome: relation to a possible central nervous system etiology, *Am. J. Med.*, 52, 25, 1972.
350. **Takahashi, K., Kipnis, D. M., and Daughaday, W. H.,** Growth hormone secretion during sleep, *J. Clin. Invest.*, 47, 2079, 1968.
351. **Honday, Y., Takahashi, K., Takahashi, S., Azimi, K., Irie, M., Sakuma, M., Tsushima, T., and Shizume, K.,** Growth hormone secretion during nocturnal sleep in normal subjects, *J. Clin. Endocrinol. Metab.*, 29, 20, 1969.
352. **Parker, D. C., Sassin, J. F., Mace, J. W., Gotlin, R. W., and Rossman, L. G.,** Human growth hormone release during sleep: electroencephalographic correlation, *J. Clin. Endocrinol. Metab.*, 29, 871, 1969.
353. **Sassin, J. F., Parker, D. C., Mace, J. W., Gotlin, R. W., Johnson, L. C., and Rossman, L. G.,** Human growth hormone release: relation to slow-wave sleep and sleep-waking cycles, *Science*, 165, 513, 1969.
354. **Lucke, C. and Glick, S. M.,** Experimental modification of the sleep-induced peak of growth hormone secretion, *J. Clin. Endocrinol. Metab.*, 32, 729, 1971.
355. **Mendelson, W. B., Jacobs, L. S., Reichman, J. D., Othmer, E., Cryer, P. E., Trivedi, B., and Daughaday, W. H.,** Methysergide: suppression of sleep-related prolactin secretion and enhancement of sleep-related growth hormone secretion, *J. Clin. Invest.*, 56, 690, 1975.
356. **Chihara, K., Kato, Y., Maeda, K., Matsukura, S., and Imura, H.,** Suppression by cyproheptadine of pulsatile growth hormone and cortisol secretion during sleep, *J. Clin. Invest.*, 57, 1393, 1976.
357. **Malarkey, W. B. and Mendell, J. R.,** Failure of a serotonin inhibitor to affect nocturnal GH and prolactin secretion in patients with Duchenne muscular dystrophy, *J. Clin. Endocrinol. Metab.*, 43, 889, 1976.
358. **Mendelson, W. B., Sitaram, N., Wyatt, R. J., Gillin, J. C., and Jacobs, L. S.,** Methscopolamine inhibition of sleep related growth hormone secretion, *J. Clin. Invest.*, 61, 1683, 1978.
359. **Reichlin, S.,** Regulation of somatotropic hormone secretion, in *Handbook of Physiology,* Section 7, Endocrinology, VoI. 4, Part 2, Greep, P. and Astwood, E. B., Eds., American Physiological Society, Williams & Wilkins, Baltimore, 1975, 405.
360. **Martin, J. B., Reichlin, S., and Brown, G. M.,** Eds., Regulation of growth hormone secretion and its disorders, in *Clin. Neuroendocrinol.,* F. A. Davis, Philadelphia, 1977, 147.

Chapter 7

PROLACTIN

Charles A. Hodson

CONTENTS

This review is a general survey of the chemistry and physiological regulation of prolactin in man and experimental animals. In animals the review focuses on the rat. In some cases review articles are cited. For more comprehensive reviews the reader is referred to the recent discussions by Cooke,[1] Neill and Nagy,[2] and Yen.[3]

HISTORY

In 1928, Stricker and Grueter[4] isolated a lactogenic substance from the pituitary gland that stimulated milk secretion when it was given to pseudopregnant rabbits. This substance was named prolactin by Riddle et al.,[5] who had further purified the hormone and developed the pigeon crop-sac method of bioassay. In 1954, Everett[6] established that prolactin secretion was under inhibitory control by the hypothalamus. Everett showed that transplanted pituitary gland tissue could maintain corpus luteum function in a hypophysectomized rat. In 1970, Li et al.[7] reported the primary structure of ovine prolactin, and in 1972, Hwang et al.[8] isolated human prolactin. The discovery of prolactin in the human was delayed for many years because of difficulty in developing bioassays, the close similarity between growth hormone and prolactin, and the low concentrations of prolactin in the pituitary gland.[9]

After radioimmunoassays for prolactin were developed, considerable progress was made in determining the neural, pharmacological, and physiological regulation of prolactin secretion during the 70s and 80s.[10-12] The subsequent development of molecular biology techniques allowed rapid advances in our knowledge of the prolactin gene. The structure of the prolactin gene was reported in 1980.[13,14] The techniques of molecular biology have also been useful for determining the structure of the prolactin receptor.[15-18] The gene for the prolactin receptor was cloned in 1988.[19]

Early studies on the function of prolactin were directed toward its lactogenic[20] and gonadotropic properties.[6] Prolactin, however, has a wide variety of functions in mammals and non-mammalian vertebrates.[21] Riddle[22] suggested that prolactin is a general metabolic hormone. With the development of the prolactin radioreceptor assay (RRA), receptors for prolactin were found in a variety of nonreproductive tissues.[17,18] We are now beginning to understand how prolactin acts in these organs.[18]

Recently a system of neurons that are immunoreactive has been traced in the central nervous system.[23] These fibers originate in the lateral hypothalamus and terminate in several brain reigons, including hypothalamus, midline thalamus, stria terminalis, raphe dorsalis, and locus coeerulus. Hypophysectomy does not affect these neurons and their function is not known.

ASSAYS

The pigeon crop-sac test is the oldest bioassay for prolactin.[5] Prolactin stimulates the crop of pigeons and doves. Prolactin causes the crop-sac wall to thicken and the apical cells to desquamate. The thick, milky secretion of desquamated cells is called crop milk. In the original crop-sac assay, prolactin was given by systemic injection and the increase in crop-sac weight was measured. More sensitive variations of this test have employed visual determination of the minimal amount of prolactin capable of stimulating the crop.[24] In the "local crop-sac" methods, prolactin is given by intradermal injection directly over the crop-sac and the area of crop-sac stimulated to secrete is measured.

Newer bioassays for prolactin include the *in vitro* mouse mammary gland assays.[25,26] In these tests, mammary tissue from mice in mid-pregnancy is incubated in insulin-rich culture media. The cultures are then exposed to test agents or prolactin and an aspect of milk synthesis, such as the formation of casein or lactose or histologic changes, in the cultured cells is examined. *In vivo* bioassays for prolactin include litter weight gains during the course of lactation or weight gains by litters during nursing trials.[27] These assays are not very sensitive or specific. *In vivo* methods for prolaction bioassay also include studying the response of the mammary gland to intraductal injections of prolactin,[28] or induction of lactation in estrogen-primed rat ovariectomized rats.[29] Because of the diverse actions of prolactin, new *in vitro* bioassays utilizing other types of tissue have been developed such as the mouse lymphoma cell cultures.[30]

Prolactin is commonly measured by radioimmunoassay (RIA) or by RRA and numerous methods and antibodies for various species are available. Discrepancy between RIA and bioassay measurements of prolactin was first extensively discussed by Nicoll.[31] Nicoll suggested that structural differences in the prolactin molecule caused the differences in assay results. Recent studies indicate that there is considerable variation in the structure of the prolactin molecule[32] (see Table 1). Because many forms of prolactin are biologically inactive or have reduced biological activity, a bioassay or RRA gives a better measurement of the amount of biologically active prolactin in a sample than a RIA measurement. Conversely, there are forms of prolactin with reduced immunoactivity that are missed by RIA. Because multiple forms of prolactin originate from posttranslational processing and cleavage in target tissues there is no "best assay" for all forms of the prolactin molecule. The sensitivity of RIAs and the speed at which these tests can be done make them ideal for routine serum prolactin assays and for studies on the physiological regulation of prolactin. Immunoassay machines that employ fluorescent or photometric detection now allow automated measurement of prolactin for clinical purposes.

TABLE 1
Relative Proportion of Some of The Variants of Prolactin
in the Pituitary Gland and Plasma

Prolactin Variants	Pituitary (% of total)	Plasma (% of total)
23 K	40–80	Detected in plasma
21 K	20–40	—
25 K	3–15	Detected in plasma
Cleaved	<1	—
Deamidated	5	—
Phosphorylated	—	40–75
Glycosylated	5–40	—
Sulgated	—	—
Dimers, noncovalent	5	—
Dimers, disulfide	5	—
Oligomers	?	10–20
Binding protein bound	—	30–40

Note: In humans, existence of only the 23-K, glycosylated, and oligomeric forms is convincingly established; evidence for the occurrence of the cleaved, deamidated, and 21-K variants is suggestive in nature, and the other forms have not yet been reported. *(From Sinha, Y. N., Trends Endocrinol. Metab., 3(3), 101, 1992. With permission.)*

Hemolytic plaque assay can be used to measure prolactin production by single cells *in vitro*. This method has been very useful for the study of prolactin production. Problems such as identifying peptides or hormones that are co-secreted with prolactin have been studied.[33,34] In addition, the technique has been used to study recruitment of cells within the pituitary gland during pregnancy and lactation.[35-37] With new imaging methods, such as confocal laser microscopy and atomic force microscopy, the examination of cells identified by the hemolytic plaque assay should be even more productive. In a hemolytic plaque assay prolactin antiserum compliment and red cells are added to cultured cells on petri plates. The lysis of the red cells around the cells producing prolactin identifies them. The size of the hemolysis zone or plaque can be measured to indicate the amount of prolactin produced.

CHEMISTRY OF PROLACTIN

The primary structure of the ovine prolactin molecule was determined in 1970. It has a molecular weight of about 23-kDa and consists of 199 amino acids in a single chain.[38,39] There are three disulfide bridges in the prolactin molecule, forming two small loops and one large loop in the molecule (see Figure 1).[32] The primary structures of prolactin from many species have been determined and all are similar to ovine prolactin. In mice and rats the prolactin molecule contains 197 amino acids, and in other species 199 amino acids. Prolactin, placental lactogens, and growth hormone all have the same basic structure. These hormones were derived from a common ancestral gene through gene duplication before bony fish evolved.[40,41]

The structure of the human prolactin gene was determined in 1981.[13,14] This gene is located on chromosome 6. It consists of 5 exons and 4 introns. There is only one form of the prolactin gene in the pituitary gland, and all variations in the prolactin molecule originate by posttranslational processing.[32] In contrast, there are several genes for placental lactogen, and different forms of placental lactogen appear at different times during pregnancy.[42]

Human prolactin and the prolactins in other species have been found in the circulation in three forms with different molecular sizes. These forms of prolactin were originally determined by elution from Sephadex columns.[43] "Small" prolactin has a molecular weight

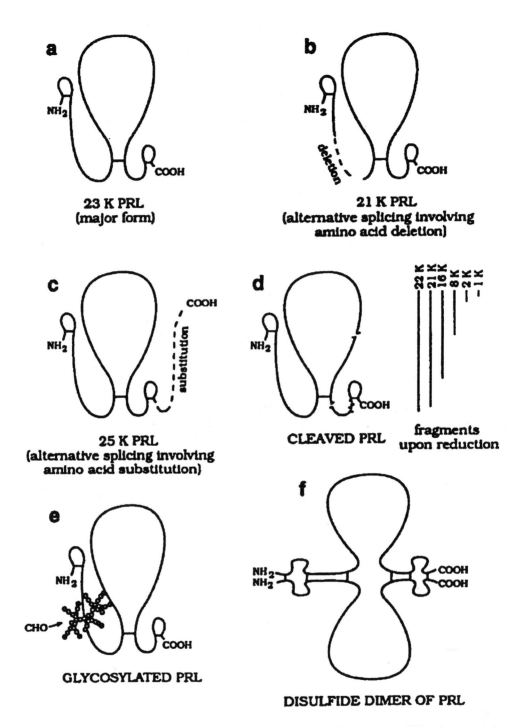

FIGURE 1. Schematic showing the structural variation in the prolactin (PRL) molecule. CHO refers to carbohydrate moiety attachment at amino acid position 31 (e). Broken lines indicate deletions or substitutions (b, c). Nicks indicate cleavage points producing the prolactin fragments (d). (f) The disulfide dimer of prolactin. *(From Sinha, Y. N.,* Trends Endocrinol. Metab., *3(3), 101, 1992. With permission.)*

of 23 kDa and is the monomeric form of the molecule. "Big" prolactin has a molecular weight of 56 kDa and is a disulfide-linked dimer of prolactin. There is a third, even larger molecule, "big-big" prolactin, which is a prolactin antibody complex of at least 100 kDa.

Prolactins of different size and structures have also been characterized on the basis of their electrophoretic mobility. These modified "prolactins" result from posttranslational processing of the prolactin molecule. Table 1 lists the isoforms of prolactin by weight, and their abundance, as determined in electrophoretic mobility studies.[32] The predominant form of prolactin found in the pituitary gland and in the circulation is the 23-kDa monomeric form.

Monomeric prolactin can have chemical substitutions (see Figure 1 and Table 1).[32] Prolactin can be glycosylated at its serine and threonine residues. The relative abundance of glycosylated and nonglycosylated prolactin varies between species. Glycosylated prolactin has increased activity in the crop-sac assay and subnormal activity in other assays. The immunoreactivity of glycosylated prolactin is also reduced. The threonine and/or serine residues of prolactin can be phosphorylated. Phosphorylation reduces the biological activity of the prolactin molecule. Prolactin can be sulfated. Sulfur is incorporated on tyrosine or the carbohydrate moieties of glycosylated prolactin.

Prolactin is cleaved into smaller molecules in target tissues and these fragments may have biological activity. The 16-kDa fragment of prolactin produces a weak stimulation of NB2 lymphoma cell proliferation[44] and casein synthesis in mammary gland explants. The 16-kDa fragment decreases angiogenesis *in vitro*.[45] The 8-kDa fragment can stimulate endothelial cell proliferation. These observations suggest reduced activity when prolactin is cleaved[46] and contrast with growth hormone where cleavage can increase biological activity. Prolactin can be deamidated. In this process, ammonia is removed from the asparginine and glutamine residues of prolactin. Deamidation reduces the biological and immunological activities of prolactin.

THE LACTOTROPH

Prolactin is secreted by acidophilic cells called lactotrophs or mammotrophs in the anterior pituitary gland.[47,48] In the rat these cells are polygonal in shape and are uniformly distributed throughout the pituitary gland. In humans these cells account for 10 to 30% of the secretory cells in the anterior pituitary gland. They are concentrated in the posterior-lateral margin of the gland in humans. There are relatively few lactotrophs in human males. There are more lactotrophs in human females and the number of cells in females increases during pregnancy and lactation. Estrogen treatment can increase the number of lactotrophs in the pituitary gland. Increased estrogen secretion during pregnancy can cause "recruitment" or increase the number of cells secreting prolactin. Porter et al. have shown that growth hormone-producing cells can be transformed to produce prolactin during lactation and that these cells revert to growth hormone-secreting cells after weaning.[37]

Prolactin is synthesized in the endoplasmic reticulum as a prehormone.[1] A 30-amino acid leader peptide sequence is cleaved from the prolactin prehormone when the molecule enters the lumen of the endoplasmic reticulum. Prolactin is then transported to the golgi where it is packaged in secretory vesicles or granules. Within the prolactin granules there is further concentration of the hormone. Chemical bonding between the prolactin molecules within a granule, perhaps by sulfation, facilitates the concentration of prolactin. "Older" prolactin granules can coalesce into larger granules.[48] It is thought that these large granules are destined for degradation by lysosomal activity in a process called crinophagy.

Lactotrophs have receptors for numerous substances including estrogens, dopamine, thyrotropin-releasing hormone (TRH), vasoactive intestinal polypeptide (VIP), and progesterone.[49] Estrogens act on the mammotrophs to promote prolactin synthesis and they increase the formation of prolactin messenger RNA.[50] Under estrogenic stimulation, there is also proliferation of the endoplasmic reticulum and an initial increase followed by a decrease in the number of secretory granules in the lactotrophs. Progesterone in part counteracts the stimulatory effects of estrogens on prolactin synthesis and secretion,[50] but during pregnancy there is considerable growth of the pituitary gland.

Estrogens have mitogenic effects on the mammotrophs. During prolonged estrogenic stimulation, the number of mammotrophs is increased. In rodents, prolonged estrogen treatment induces the formation of pituitary adenomas.[51] These tumors result in part from disruption of the vascular supply to the pituitary gland, which produces islands of tissue that do not receive inhibitory input from the hypothalamus.[52] In rats there is a strain difference in this susceptiblilty to the effect of estrogen. Prolactin-secreting adenomas are the most common type of pituitary tumor in humans and are a major cause of infertility.[53] In many cases these tumors are microadenomas. The cause of the high incidence of prolactin-secreting tumors in humans is not apparent.

Integrity of mammotrophs is dependent on thyroid hormones. The decrease in thyroid hormones resulting from thyroidectomy causes atrophy of prolactin cells and their organelles. Thyroid hormone replacement can restore the mammotroph to normal in a thyroidectomized animal.[54] Thyroidectomy can block also stress-induced prolaction secretion.[55]

PROLACTIN SECRETION IN MAMMALS

Prolactin is secreted from the pituitary gland in response to nursing, stress, mating, ovulation, estrogen treatment, and eating. Between these events, prolactin is secreted in a pulsatile manner.[56,57] The anterior pituitary cells have an intrinsic pulsatile pattern of prolactin release as well.[58]

In humans serum prolactin levels increase gradually during pregnancy.[59] In rats and most other species serum prolactin concentrations in the circulation are low until the time of parturition.[60-62] Pituitary gland prolactin stores are increased during pregnancy.[59] This increase in prolactin results from increased estrogens produced by the corpus luteum or in the placenta.[63] In some species placental lactogens exert a feedback on the hypothalamus to increase dopamine turnover and which prevents an increase in serum prolactin.[64]

Prolactin is released in response to the suckling stimulus during lactation.[65] This response becomes conditioned in rodents. After a dam has experienced lactation, exposure to nursing rat pups or the sounds of suckling can induce prolactin secretion.[66]

The release of prolactin in response to nursing is greatest early in lactation. The amount of prolactin produced in response to suckling and prolactin levels in the circulation decrease as lactation progresses in the human.[3,67] These decreases are correlated with reduced nursing frequency as lactation progresses. The decline in circulating prolactin is apparently offset by changes in the receptor fields in the mammary gland because milk production increases in the latter stages of lactation. Prolactin produced during lactation also decreases fertility and plays a role in the genesis of lactational anestrus[68] or lactational amenorrhea in humans.[53,69] In the rat suckling can cause an apparent depletion of pituitary gland prolactin content within 1–2 min.[70] The appearance of prolactin in the serum following suckling is delayed and requires 10–20 min to reach maximal concentration.[71] The transformed production is apparently aggregated in pituitary cells and is not detectable by RIA. The prolactin is eventually converted to its original form.

Prolactin is secreted in response to all stressful stimuli including heat, physical restraint, noise, hypoglycemia, inflammation, and pain. In man, physical and psychogenic stresses also induce release of prolactin. The function of stress-induced prolactin secretion is unclear at present.[72-75] Prolactin does have a role in mediating the immune response and stress-induced prolactin may regulate this system.

Prolactin is secreted in response to the stimulus of mating.[76] In rodents mating-induced release of prolactin maintains the corpus luteum. In pregnant or pseudopregnant rats, prolactin is secreted in episodic diurnal and nocturnal surges.[77-79] They are triggered by mating and once initiated they continue until placental lactogen is produced[64] or there is involution of the corpus luteum.[76] In human females, but not in males, prolactin is secreted in response to orgasm. The function of the prolactin secreted at orgasm is unknown.[80]

Prolactin is also secreted at ovulation, concurrently with the luteinizing hormone (LH) and follicle-stimulating hormone (FSH) surges in all mammalian species.[12,53,60,81,82] The prolactin surge at ovulation is facilitated by the increased preovulatory estrogen secretion that occurs as the dominant ovarian follicle develops. The increase in estrogen increases prolactin levels in the pituitary gland and sensitizes the lactotrophs to many substances that can stimulate prolactin.[83,84] Paracrine interactions between the gonadotrophs and the lactotrophs may facilitate this release of prolactin during the LH surge.[85,86] The function of the increase in prolactin secretion at the time of ovulation is not known for most species. In rats the ovulatory surge of prolactin may serve as a luteolytic signal.[87]

Prolactin secretion is induced by eating, and prolactin levels are increased following meals by humans and experimental animals. Feeding-induced prolactin release is mediated by cholecystokinin, which is released from the gut following a meal.[88-91] The vagus nerve may also play a role in mediating prolactin release in response to food ingestion but its role is not clear at present.

During the menstrual cycle and estrous cycles of primates prolactin is secreted in a pulsatile manner. Many prolactin pulses are coincident with LH pulses.[57,92,93] The prolactin pulses are thought to originate from LH-releasing hormone (LHRH) action in the pituitary gland and they are blocked by LHRH antagonists. In the pituitary gland LHRH may act through gonadotrophs to promote prolactin secretion.[85,94-97] The gonadotrophs may release a substance(s) in addition to LH that stimulates the lactotrophs in a paracrine manner to promote prolactin secretion. Several substances may serve as paracrine mediators of prolactin secretion. The substances include VIP, angiotensin-II[97,98] from gonadotrophs, and perhaps acetylcholine and αMSH. Further research will clarify the roles of these agents as paracrine regulators of the lactotrophs (see Table 2).

ACTIONS OF PROLACTIN

The effects of prolactin in mammals are exerted primarily on the organs of reproduction. Prolactin is also an important factor in the regulation of the immune system,[99] pancreatic development,[100] and metabolism.

With regard to reproduction prolactin stimulates the secretion of milk during lactation and promotes the growth of the mammary glands during pregnancy.[101-103] Prolactin can induce lactogenesis in ovariectomized, adrenalectomized, and hypophysectomized rats and mice when it is given in combination with an adrenal corticosteriod.[104,105]

Prolactin induces polarity in mammary gland cells[106] and the appearance of golgi vesicles which contain casein. In vitro prolactin can induce casein synthesis,[107-109] α-lactalbumin,[110,111] lactose, and milk fat synthesis.[112,113]

In rodents, prolactin activates the corpus luteum and acts as part of a luteotropic complex with LH to maintain corpus luteum function.[114] In other species prolactin is not a factor in the regulation of the corpus luteum, but prolactin may be trophic to the regulation of granulosa cell function in the human ovary.[115,116] Prolactin also acts on the testes, stimulating gonadotropin binding and increasing testosterone production.[117,118] Prolactin acts on the prostate gland and increases prostatic secretions. Prolactin receptors have been demonstrated in the prostate gland.[119] Prolactin can stimulate growth and differentiation of prostate cells *in vitro*.[120]

At high concentrations, prolactin is antigonadotropic. Prolactin has a direct inhibitory effect on the hypothalamus and prevents gonadotropin secretion.[117,121] Studies in rodents show that prolactin can prevent the release of gonadotropins in response to gonadectomy.[122,123] More recently, it has been shown that prolactin can reduce LHRH secretion from cultured LHRH cells *in vitro*.[44] These results suggest that hyperprolactinemia can prevent hypothalamic LHRH release. Prolactin also has direct antigonadal effects. It can be luteolytic in the rat. At high levels, prolactin reduces 20α-hydroxysteroid dehydrogenase activity in the ovary.[124,125]

TABLE 2
Agents Affecting Prolactin Secretion

Agent	Systemic/CNS Action[a]	Pituitary Action[a]	Comments[b]
Melanocyte-stimulating hormone (α-MSH)		+[256]	E2 induced increases in the number of PRL cells were blocked by αMSH antiserum.
	-[255]		Reduces suckling-induced PRL release in rats.
Acetylcholine		-[258]	
		-[259]	May be a paracrine PRL inhibitor.
	-[201]		Atropine given ICV increases PRL.
	-[202]		
	-[257]		
	-[175]		Nicotine given ICV increases PRL.
Angiotensin-II		+[95]	
		+[98]	Paracrine role mediating LHRH-induced PRL release.
		+[189]	
		+[190]	
	+[260]		
Ascorbate		-[261]	May act in a paracrine manner to augment DA. Ascorbate-deficient rats are more responsive to stress.
Atrial natriuretic hormone (ANH)	-[262]	NE[262]	Inhibits PRL when given ICV.
	-[263]		ANH affects prolactin via DA receptors.
Bombesin	+[232]		
		+[265]	Bombesin stimulates PRL secretion *in vitro.*
	-[264]		Bombesin blocks E2-induced PRL surges.
Bradykinin	-[266]	NE[266]	
Calcitonin		-[267]	Antisera to calcitonin increases PRL production *in vitro* and calcitonin decreases PRL.
Calcitonin gene-related peptide (CGRP)		-[268]	Decreases TRH induced PRL secretion.
Catecholamines			
Epinephrine		-[164]	Weak inhibition of PRL *in vitro.*
		-[174]	
Dopamine		-[174]	
		-[269]	
		+[270]	Cytosolic calcium and PRL are increased.
	±[152]		Low doses of DA increase PRL in α-methyltyrosine-treated rats; high doses decreased PRL.
		±[271]	High doses reduce PRL and low doses increase PRL.
		+[272]	Low doses of D_2 agonists stimulate PRL secretion *in vitro.*
Norepinephrine	+[62]		
	+[224]		
	-[174]		Reduces suckling induced PRL secretion.
		-[164]	Weak inhibitor of PRL secretion *in vitro.*
Cholecystokinin	+[273]		Progumide increases PRL.
	+[274]	+[274]	
		+[275]	
Endothelins		-[166]	Inhibits PRL in serum-free media.
		+[166]	Stimulates PRL in serum-enriched media.
		-[167]	
Estrogen	+[276]		Estradiol treatment induces daily PRL surges.
	+[277]		
		+[278]	
		+[83]	

TABLE 2 (continued)
Agents Affecting Prolactin Secretion

Agent	Systemic/CNS Action[a]	Pituitary Action[a]	Comments[b]
γ-Aminobutyric acid (GABA)	−[207]		
	+[227]		
	+[279]		Baclofen given by iv injection increases PRL.
		−[228]	Baclofen decreases PRL *in vitro* and a GABA antagonist reverses the effect of baclofen.
		−[229]	
		−[230]	
		−[280]	
Galanin		+[281]	Galanin antiserum reduces the latter half of the preovulatory PRL surge.
Gastrin	−[282]		
Histamine	+[206]		
Histidyl-proline-diketopiperazine		−[283]	
		−[284]	
		−[285]	
		−[286]	
LHRH		+[287]	Paracrine action evoking PRL release.
		+[98]	Angiotensin-II mediates paracrine effect.
		+[85]	Stimulation of PRL in *in vitro* coculture of lactotrophs and gonadotrophs.
Neurohypophyseal peptides			
Arginine vasopressin	+[232]		
Oxytocin	+[288]		Reduces stress-induced PRL.
	+[289]		
Vasotocin	+[290]		
Vasopressin	+[291]		Antiserum reduces suckling-induced PRL.
	−[288]		
	+[292]		
Neurotensin	−[234]		Neurotensin reduces PRL when given ICV.
	+[192]		
Opioid peptides	+[293]		Increases PRL in pseudopregnant rats.
	+[294]		
	+[205]		
	+[218]		
Pituitary adenylate cyclase activating polypeptide (PACAP)		+[295]	Stimulates PRL gene transcription in GH$_3$ cells.
Peptide histidine-isoleucine (PHI)	+[296]	+[296]	
Amines			
Octopamine	−[297]	−[297]	The amines act by DA receptors to reduce PRL.
Phenyl ethylamine	−[297]	NE[297]	
Tyramine		−[297]	
Serotonin	+[203]		5-HT stimulates PRL surges at proestrus.
	+[214]		5-HT neurons mediate stresses-induced PRL release.
	+[298]		
		+[215]	
Substance P	+[192]		
	+[299]		
	+[300]	+[300]	

TABLE 2 (continued)
Agents Affecting Prolactin Secretion

Agent	Systemic/CNS Action[a]	Pituitary Action[a]	Comments[b]
Thyroid hormone		+[54]	Thyroidectomy causes atrophy of PRL cells.
		+[55]	Thyroidectomy blocks stress-induced PRL increase.
Tumor necrosis factor		+[301]	Stimulates PRL *in vitro*.
α (TNF α)		+[302]	Effect is Ca[++] mediated.
Transforming growth factor β (TGF β)		−[303]	
Thyrotropin-releasing hormone (TRH)		+[191]	
		+[192]	
		+[64]	
		+[172]	
		NE+[193]	TRH did not stimulate basal or peak PRL in pseudopregnant rats. Blockade of DA receptors allowed TRH stimulation.
Vasoactive intestinal polypeptide (VIP)	+[304]	+[304]	E2 is needed for VIP stimulation of PRL.
		+[310]	Autocrine stimulation.
	+[305]		
	+[306]		
	+[307]		Hypothalamic VIP changes during suckling.
	+[308]		
	+[309]		
		+[229]	
Amino acids			
Tyrosine	+[88]		Acts by increasing catecholamines.
	+[311]		
Tryptophan	+[312]		Acts by increasing serotonin.
	+[212]		
Taurine	+[313]		Increases PRL when given by ICV injection. May be mediated by opioids.
N-Methyl-D-aspartic acid (NMA)		+[314]	

[a] +, stimulation; −, inhibition; NE, no effect; ±, increase and decrease.
[b] E2, estradiol; PRL, prolatin; ICV, intracerebroventricular injection; LHRH, luteinizing hormone-releasing hormone; DA, dopamine; ANH, atrial natriuretic hormone; 5-HT, 5-hydroxytryptamine.

These antigonadotropic effects of prolactin occur both during lactation and in disorders of prolactin secretion.[53]

Prolactin has a major role in regulating the immune system. Hypophysectomy decreases immunocompetence, and prolactin treatment reverses this effect.[126,127] When hypophysectomized rats are treated with prolactin antiserum they die of anemia.[128] Apparently, residual prolactin or a prolactin-like peptide is stimulatory to hematopoiesis. Prolactin is produced by some lymphocytes and other cells in the immune sysytem.[44,129] Lymphocytes contain prolactin receptors[130] and prolactin stimulates lymphocyte activity and also acts as a mitogen.[131,132] Prolactin treatment increases inflammatory responses to irritants.[133]

Prolactin stimulates the pancreas, causing development of pancreatic islet tissue.[100,134] Placental lactogen can also stimulate the growth of pancreatic islets.[100,135]

Prolactin has general metabolic effects in mammals which are superficially similar to those of the growth hormone. Prolactin can stimulate weight gain in female rats. Prolactin treatment increases body fat whereas growth hormone decreases fat.[136,137] Both hormones promote nitrogen retention, but growth hormone is specific in this regard. Prolactin does not have a specific effect on visceral growth as was suggested by Riddle.[22] Prolactin does stimulate food intake acting on CNS neurons.[136]

Receptors for prolactin have been found in mammalian kidneys and there are reports indicating that prolactin participates in salt regulation.[138,139] In other vertebrate classes, the actions of prolactin are very diverse and have been discussed in prior reviews.[21]

HYPOTHALAMIC CONTROL OF PROLACTIN SECRETION

In mammals, prolactin secretion is tonically inhibited.[140] Prolactin secretion is increased when the pituitary is transplanted or when the median eminence of the hypothalamus is destroyed.[141-143] Removal of the posterior lobe of the pituitary gland also results in an increase in basal prolactin secretion, indicating that it is also a source of dopamine.[144,145]

Prolactin secretion is inhibited by dopamine or by an unidentified prolactin-inhibiting factor (PIF).[97,146,147] Dopamine is carried from the median eminence to the mammotrophs in the long hypophyseal portal vessels and from the posterior lobe of the pituitary gland in the short portal vessel.[148,149] In the pituitary gland dopamine acts on the mammotrophs to inhibit secretion of prolactin. Dopamine acts on D_2 dopamine receptors causing inhibition of adenyl cyclase activity.[150] Dopamine inhibits prolactin at concentrations between 10^{-7} and $10^{-9} M$. At lower concentrations ($10^{-10} M$ or less) dopamine stimulates prolactin secretion *in vitro*.[151,152] The action of dopamine is antagonized in part by estrogen, which stimulates the secretion of prolactin by the mammaotrophs.[101,153-155] Dopamine has been detected and its concentration has been measured in hypophyseal portal blood.[156-158] When dopamine is infused at these concentrations prolactin secretion is inhibited. The dopamine in the long hypophysial portal vessels is released from the tuberoinfundibular system of the hypothalamus. The dopamine in the short portal vessels is released from the tuberohypophyseal system. The two dopamine systems are independently regulated, and Moore and Demarest[159] have indicated that the tuberohypophyseal system is not a site for short loop feedback regulation of prolactin secretion. When catecholamine synthesis is blocked by α-methyl-apra-tyrosine, a prompt increase in prolactin secretion takes place.[160] In addition, administration of dopamine antagonists increases prolactin secretion.[161] When dopamine agonists like the ergots are administered, prolactin secretion is decreased.[143,162] Dopamine agonists can inhibit secretion of prolactin in response to suckling, during pseudopregnancy, and during the afternoon of proestrus in the rat.[153,163] Collectively, these observations suggest that prolactin secretion is physiologically inhibited by dopamine.

As yet there is no sound physiological evidence for a PIF distinct from dopamine but the list of potential candidates is growing (see Table 2). Some of these substances may act to augment the effect of dopamine in inhibiting prolactin secretion. γ-Aminobutyric acid (GABA), epinephrine, and norepinephrine can inhibit prolactin secretion by the mammotrophs. The role of epinephrine and norepinephrine as physiological inhibitors of prolactin secretion is doubtful because they are much less potent than dopamine in inhibiting prolactin secretion and they are not present in portal blood in concentrations sufficient to inhibit prolactin.[164,165] GABA is secreted into portal blood but it is less potent than dopamine and it is not likely to be a PIF.[2] Endothelins also inhibit prolactin secretion from the pituitary gland directly and they are found in the short portal vessels. The endothelins may have a paracrine or autocrine role in inhibiting prolactin secretion in the lactating animal but further work is needed to clarify their role.[166,167]

Prolactin acts on the hypothalamus to inhibit its own secretion.[168-171] Prolonged hyperprolactinemia resulting from transplantable prolactin-secreting tumors results in reduced *in situ* pituitary prolactin content. The reduction can be reversed by the blockade of hypothalamic catecholamine synthesis.[123,172-174]

Prolactin can increase dopamine turnover in the tuberoinfundibular system, and dopamine concentrations in hypophyseal portal blood are increased when the tuberoinfundibular system is active.[159,175-178] Injections of ovine prolactin can prevent stress-induced prolactin release in rats.[179] Implants of prolactin in the median eminence in rats can interrupt pseudopregnancy.[147]

During conditions of stress, suckling during lactation, or pseudopregnancy, prolactin is rapidly secreted and surges in serum concentrations take place.[2] It is not known whether inhibition of the tuberoinfundibular dopamine system or the release of a prolactin-releasing factor (PRF) evokes these surges in prolactin secretion.[163,166,180-184] As previously mentioned, dopamine has a dual action on prolactin secretion. At high concentrations dopamine is inhibitory and at low concentrations it stimulates prolactin secretion. Therefore decreased dopamine tone should stimulate prolactin surges. The administration of dopamine agonists, however, can prevent prolactin release during these events, perhaps masking a stimulatory effect of dopamine or overriding the action of a PRF.[185]

There are numerous candidates for a PRF; VIP, TRH, oxytocin, and angiotensin-II are possible candidates (see Table 2). The posterior lobe may be the source of the PRF because its removal disrupts suckling-induced prolactin release.[186,187] A PRF is believed to stimulate prolactin release during suckling, stress,[180] and the proestrous LH surge.[186] Antisera to VIP and oxytocin attenuate suckling-induced prolactin release in rats. Oxytocin antagonists can also attenuate suckling-induced prolactin release.[71,188] Collectively, these observations suggest that a neuropeptide serves as a PRF.

There is sound evidence that angiotensin-II serves as a paracrine PRF stimulating pulsatile prolactin secretion. Angiotensin-II is produced in gonadotrophs and is secreted by the gonadotrophs in response to LHRH stimulation.[95,98,189,190]

TRH produces prolactin release from *in vitro* cultures of pituitary tissue and when given systemically.[191-196] Because prolactin and thyroid-stimulating hormone (TSH) are not necessarily released concurrently (i.e., during conditions of heat and cold stress), it is not likely that TRH is the PRF.[197,198] The action of TRH on the mammotrophs is altered by estrogen and dopamine. TRH action is facilitated by estrogen and inhibited by dopamine and its agonists.[16,193,199,200]

Other hypothalamic neurotransmitters or putative neurotransmitters that influence prolactin secretion include acetylcholine, which probably inhibits prolactin secretion via the tuberoinfundibular dopamine system,[201,202] and serotonin,[203] melatonin,[204] endorphins, enkephalins,[205] histamine,[206] norepinephrine,[62] and GABA.[207,208] These substances influence prolactin secretion by acting in the hypothalamus through a PRF or by decreasing dopamine. The effect of these agents and references are cited in Table 2.

Acetylcholine injection into the ventricles of the brain or systemic injection of acetylcholine agonists reduces prolactin secretion.[201,209] The inhibitory effects of acetylcholine on prolactin secretion are apparently mediated by catecholamines, because acetylcholine cannot prevent prolactin release when hypothalamic catecholamine activity is inhibited.[202,210] A role of acetylcholine in the control of prolactin secretion is suggested because the acetylcholine agonist pilocarpine prevents stress and suckling-induced prolactin release.[209]

Serotonin, its precursors 5-hydroxytryptophan and tryptophan, or its metabolite melatonin stimulates prolactin release.[204,211,212] Blockade of serotonin receptors or its synthesis prevents the release of prolactin in response to the stimuli of suckling or estrogen injection.[213,214] Serotonin has no direct stimulatory effect on pituitary prolactin release *in vitro*, but it can increase prolactin secretion in rats bearing ectopic pituitary gland tissue.[215] Serotoninergic neurons may increase release of a PRF, because serotonin agonists induce prolactin release more rapidly than blockade of the brain catecholaminergic systems.[216]

The endogenous opiates (enkephalins and endorphins) and morphine also cause a rapid increase in prolactin secretion when they are given by systemic or intraventricular injection. Administration of opiate antagonists, such as naloxone or naltrexone, prevent prolactin release in response to stress or suckling and reduce basal prolactin secretion.[205,217,218] The endogenous opiates do not act directly on the pituitary gland. They may inhibit the activity of the tuberoinfundibular dopamine system or act through a PRF.[219] Recent data suggest that endorphins are colocalized in the neurons of the tuberoinfundibular dopamine system.

Norepinephrine can stimulate prolactin release by a hypothalamic action, distinct from its inhibitory effect in the pituitary gland.[160] In the pituitary, norepinephrine binds to dopamine receptors on the mammotrophs and blocks prolactin release. *In vivo* administration of L-DOPA, which increases brain norepinephrine content, results in increased prolactin secretion.[220] Administration of clonidine, an α_2-adrenergic agonist, at high doses results in an increased prolactin secretion, as do intraventricular injections of norepinephrine.[221] Administration of disulfiram, an inhibitor of norepinephrine synthesis, or 6-hydroxydopamine, which causes selective destruction of noradrenergic neurons, results in reduced prolactin secretion.[222,223] These results suggest that noradrenergic neurons stimulate prolactin release, although the role of these neurons is not resolved.[224]

Histamine given by intraventricular injection causes increased prolactin secretion whereas blockade of histamine receptors inhibits release of prolactin in response to stress or suckling.[225,226] These effects suggest a stimulatory role of histamine-containing neurons in the regulation of prolactin secretion that does not involve the tuberoinfundibular system.[206]

GABA has been reported both to stimulate and to inhibit prolactin secretion in the rat. Administration of GABA into the ventricular system of the rat brain stimulates prolactin secretion.[227] At high concentrations, GABA can prevent prolactin release from pituitary glands *in vitro*.[228-230] GABA is probably not a physiologic PIF because the concentrations of GABA required to inhibit prolactin release *in vitro* are higher than the concentrations found in portal blood.[231] A physiological role for GABA in the regulation of prolactin has not been demonstrated.

Many peptides and alter the secretion of prolactin acting in the hypothalamus (see Table 2). including substance P,[192] bombesin,[232,233] neurotensin,[192,234] and VIP.[235-237] The role of these peptides in the regulation of prolactin secretion is not clear.

MECHANISM OF PROLACTIN ACTION

Membrane-bound receptor molecules for prolactin have been demonstrated in mammals in a variety of tissues, including liver, kidney, adrenal, ovary, testes, uterus, prostate, seminal vesicle, mammary gland, and tumors.[238-240] The number of receptors in these tissues varies in different mammalian species. The prolactin receptor gene has been isolated and cloned and the structure of the prolactin receptor has been determined. There are apparently two forms of the prolactin receptor: a short form, which consists of about 300 amino acids, and a long form, which contains about 600 amino acids. Both of these molecules are single-chain proteins with one transmembrane spanning domain. Analysis of their amino acid sequences indicates that there is no recognizable sequence in either molecule that is known to mediate intracellular signaling.[19,241,242] It has also been proposed that the prolactin receptors in different tissues are distinct.[17]

The binding of prolactin to its receptors is modulated by hormones. For example, in the rat liver, estrogens stimulate prolactin binding whereas ovariectomy results in decreased prolactin binding. Hypophysectomy reduces prolactin binding in the liver, an effect that can be reversed by prolactin injection. Prolactin receptors in liver and mammary glands are both up- and down-regulated by prolactin. When prolactin is first dissociated from its receptors with $MgCL_2$, or if prolactin secretion is blocked by ergot treatment, receptor fields in the mammary gland and liver are opened. When prolactin is administered, down-regulation of the receptor field (i.e., reduction in prolactin receptors) takes place within 15 min. After this rapid down-regulation, gradual up-regulation (increased numbers of available prolactin receptors) takes place and within 24 h the number of available prolactin receptors is restored.[18,239]

After the initial binding of prolactin to its receptor, prolactin is internalized in the target cells. Prolactin is found in the Golgi apparatus of rat livers,[243] in mammary gland tissue, and in milk.[244] Whether internalization of prolactin represents a degradation of the hormone receptor complex inside the cell or a control signal is unknown. The prolactin molecule is cleaved in target tissues, and this may facilitate its action.[245]

Studies conducted primarily by Rillema and colleagues[109,246] on mouse mammary gland explants suggest that the intracellular effects of prolactin after its initial binding to membrane receptors could be mediated by a variety of messengers, including cyclic nucleotides, prostaglandins, and polyamines. This inference is based on the stimulation of these mediators by prolactin in *in vitro* cultures. Some of these mediators can stimulate various aspects of milk formation. The effect of prolactin on milk synthesis is partially mediated by cyclic GMP (cGMP). Levels of cGMP rise and cyclic AMP levels decrease in the mammary gland when lactation is initiated.[247,248] Moreover, cGMP will mimic the effect of prolactin on mammary gland RNA synthesis.[249] In contrast, dibutyl cAMP or theophylline treatment reduces DNA, RNA, and fat synthesis in mammary gland tissue.[250] Prostaglandin $F_2\alpha$ stimulates the induction of lactation in the rat. In tissue cultures, arachidonic acid and prostaglandins increase RNA synthesis, but do not increase casein synthesis. Indomethacin, which blocks prostaglandin synthesis, reduces the stimulating effect of prolactin on both casein and RNA synthesis in mouse mammary gland explants.[251,252]

Polyamine levels are elevated in the lactating mammary gland. Prolactin treatment promptly elevates ornithine decarboxylase activity in cultured mammary glands. Blockage of polyamine synthesis inhibits prolactin-stimulated milk protein synthesis *in vitro*.[253,254]

SUMMARY

Prolactin has more diverse actions than any other pituitary hormone. Some progress has been made in understanding the mechanism of its action at the intracellular level. The second messenger for prolactin has not been determined. We still do not know if a unified mechanism governs the effects of prolactin in its diverse actions.

Much progress has been made in understanding the physiology of prolactin receptors and their regulation, which is dependent on both the concentration of hormone in the circulation and the available receptor field.

A great deal of progress has been made regarding the regulation of prolactin secretion by the hypothalamus. The identity of the prolactin-releasing hormone, if one exists, and a complete uderstanding of paracrine and autocrine regulation of prolactin secretion within the pituitary gland need to be established.

REFERENCES

1. **Cooke, N. E.,** Prolactin: normal synthesis, regulation, and actions, in *Endocrinology*, Vol. 1, 2nd ed., DeGroot, L. J., Besser, G. M., Cahill, G. F., Marshall, J. C., Nelson, D. H., Odell, W. D., Potts, J. T., Rubenstein, A. H., Steinberger, E., and Martini, L., Eds., W. B. Saunders, Philadelphia, 1989, 384.
2. **Neill, J. D. and Nagy, G. M.,** Prolactin secretion and its control, in *The Physiology of Reproduction*, Vol. 2, 2nd ed, Knobil, E. and Neill, J. D., Eds., Raven Press, New York, 1994, 1833.
3. **Yen, S. S. C.,** Prolactin in human reproduction, in *Reproductive Endocrinology*, 3rd ed., Yen, S. S. C. and Jaffe, R. B., Eds., W. B. Saunders, Philadelphia, 1991, 357.
4. **Stricker, S. and Grueter, F.,** Action du lobe anterieur de l'hypophyse sur la montee laiteuse, *C. R. Soc. Biol.*, 99, 1978, 1928.
5. **Riddle, O., Bates, R. W., and Dykshorn, S.,** The preparation, identification, and assay of prolactin—a hormone of the anterior pituitary, *Am. J. Physiol.*, 105, 191, 1933.
6. **Everett, J. W.,** Luteotropic function of autografts of the rat hypophysis, *Endocrinology*, 54, 685, 1954.
7. **Li, C. H., Dixon, J. S., Lo, T. B., Schmidt, K. D., and Pankov, Y. A.,** Studies on pituitary lactogenic hormone, 30. The primary structure of the sheep hormone, *Arch. Biochem. Biophy.*, 141, 705, 1970.
8. **Hwang, P., Guyda, H., and Friesen, H. G.,** Purification of human prolactin, *J. Biol. Chem.*, 247, 1955, 1972.

9. **Kleinberg, D. L. and Frantz, A. G.,** Human prolactin, measurment by in vitro bioassay, *J. Clin. Invest.,* 50, 1557, 1971.

10. **Meites, J., Simpkins, J., Bruni, J., and Advis, J.,** Role of biogenic amines in control of anterior pituitary hormones, *IRCS J. Med. Sci.,* 5, 1, 1977.

11. **McCann, S. M., Kalra, P. S., Kalra, S. P., Donoso, A. O., Bishop, W., Schneider, H. P. G., Fawcett, C. P., and Krulich, L.,** The role of monoamines in the control of gonadotropin and prolactin secretion, in *Gonadotropins,* Soxana, B. B., Geling, C. G., and Gandy, H. M., Eds., Wiley, New York, 1972, 49.

12. **Neill, J. D.,** Neuroendocrine regulation of prolactin secretion, *Frontiers in Neuroendocrinology,* Vol. 6, Ganong, W. F. and Martini, L., Eds., Raven Press, New York, 1980, 129.

13. **Chien, Y. H. and Thompson, B. E.,** Genomic organization of rat prolactin and growth hormone genes, *Proc. Natl. Acad. Sci. U.S.A.,* 77, 4583, 1980.

14. **Truong, A. T., Duez, C., Belayew, A., Renard, A., Pictet, R., Bell, G. I., and Martial, J. A.,** Isolation and characterization of the human prolactin gene, *EMBO J.,* 3, 429, 1984.

15. **Leong, D. A., Frawley, S. L., and Neill, J. D.,** Neuroendocrine control of prolactin secretion, *Annu. Rev. Physiol.,* 45, 109, 1983.

16. **Plotsky, P. M. and Neill, J. D.,** Interactions of dopamine and thyrotropin releasing hormone (TRH) in the regulation of prolactin release in lactating rats, *Endocrinology,* 111, 168, 1982.

17. **Kelly, P. A., Djiane, J., and Edery, N.,** Different forms of the prolactin receptor: insights into mechanisms of prolactin action, *Trends Endocrinol. Metab.,* 3, 54, 1992.

18. **Kelly, P. A., Djiane, J., Postel-Vinay, M. C., and Edery, M.,** The prolactin/growth hormone receptor family, *Endocr. Rev.,* 12, 235, 1991.

19. **Boutin, J. M., Jolicoeur, C., Okamura, H., Gagnon, J., Edery, M., Shirota, M., Banville, D., Dusanter-Fourt, I., Djiane, J., and Kelly, P. A.,** Cloning and expression of the rat prolactin receptor, a member of the growth hormone/prolactin receptor gene family, *Cell,* 53, 69, 1988.

20. **Meites, J. and Turner, C. W.,** Studies concerning the induction and maintenance of lactation. I. The mechanism controlling the initiation of lactation at parturition, *Mo. Agric. Exp. Stn. Res. Bull.,* 415, 1, 1948.

21. **Nicoll, C. S.,** Physiological actions of prolactin, in *Handbook of Physiology. Section 7: Endocrinology,* Vol. 4, Part 2, Greep, R. O., Astwood, E. B., Knobil, E., Sawyer, W. H., and Geiger, S. R., Eds., American Physiological Society, Washington, D. C., 1974, 253.

22. **Riddle, O.,** Prolactin in vertebrate function and organization, *J. Nat. Cancer Inst.,* 31, 1039, 1963.

23. **Paut-Pagano, L., Roky, R., Valatx, J. L., Kitahama, K., and Jouvet, M.,** Anatomical distribution of prolactin-like immunoreactivity in the rat brain, *Neuroendocrinology,* 58, 682, 1993.

24. **Reece, R. P. and Turner, C. W.,** The lactogenic and thyrotropic hormone content of the anterior lobe of the pituitary, *Mo. Agric. Exp. Stn. Res. Bull.,* 266, 1937.

25. **Elias, T.,** Cultivation of adult mouse mammary gland in hormone-enriched synthetic medium, *Science,* 126, 842, 1957.

26. **Turkington, R. W.,** Molecular biological aspects of prolactin, in *Lactogenic Hormones,* Wolstenholme, G. E. W. and Knight, J., Eds., Churchill Livingston, Edinburgh, 1972, 111.

27. **Turner, C. W.,** Hormones influencing intensity of milk secretion in the rat, *Mo. Agric. Exp. Stn. Res. Bull.,* 982, 1971.

28. **Lyons, W. R.,** The direct mammotrophic action of lactogenic hormone, *Proc. Soc. Exp. Biol. Med.,* 58, 308, 1942.

29. **Meites, J. and Turner, C. W.,** Studies concerning the induction and maintenance of lactation. II. The normal maintenance and experimental inhibition and augmentation of lactation, *Mo. Agric. Exp. Stn. Res. Bull.,* 416, 1, 1948.

30. **Rao, Y. P., Olson, M. D., Buckley, D. J., and Buckley, A. R.,** Nuclear colocalization of prolactin and the prolactin receptor in rat Nb2 node lymphoma cells, *Endocrinology,* 133, 3062, 1993.

31. **Nicoll, C. S.,** Radioimmunoassay and radioreceptor assays for prolactin and growth hormone: a critical appraisal, *Am. Zool.,* 15, 881, 1975.

32. **Sinha, Y. N.,** Prolactin variants, *Trends Endocrinol. Metab.,* 3, 100, 1992.

33. **Frawley, L. S. and Boockfor, F. R.,** Mammosomatotropes: presence and functions in normal and neoplastic pituitary tissue, *Endocr. Rev.,* 12, 337, 1991.

34. **Porter, T. E., Wiles, C. D., and Frawley, L. S.,** Lactotrope differentiation in rats is modulated by a milk-borne signal transferred to the neonatal circulation, *Endocrinology,* 133, 1284, 1993.

35. **Boockfor, F. R., Hoeffler, J. P., and Frawley, L. C.,** Cultures of GH3 cells are functionally heterogeneous: thyrotropin releasing hormone, estradiol, and cortisol cause reciprocal shifts in the proportions of growth hormone and prolactin secretors, *Endocrinology,* 117, 418, 1985.

36. **Boockfor, F. R. and Frawley, L. S.,** Functional variations among prolactin cells from different pituitary regions, *Endocrinology,* 120, 874, 1987.

37. **Porter, T. E., Wiles, C. D., and Frawley, L. S.,** Evidence for bidirectional interconversion of mammotropes and somatotropes: rapid reversion of acidophilic cell types to pregestational proportions after weaning, *Endocrinology,* 129, 1215, 1991.

38. **Li, C. H.,** Chemistry of ovine prolactin, in *Handbook of Physiology. Section 7: Endocrinology*, Vol. 4, Knobil, E. and Sawyer, W. H., Eds., American Physiological Society, Washington, D. C., 1974, 103.

39. **Li, C. H.,** Studies on pituitary lactogenic hormone: the primary structure of the porcine hormone, *Int. J. Pep. Protein Res.*, 8, 205, 1976.

40. **Cooke, N. E., Coit, D., Shine, J., Baxter, J. D., and Martial, J. A.,** Human prolactin cDNA structural analysis and evolutionary comparisons, *J. Biol. Chem.*, 256, 4007, 1981.

41. **Miller, W. and Eberhardt, N. L.,** Structure and evolution of the growth hormone gene family, *Endocr. Rev.*, 4, 97, 1983.

42. **Soares, M. J., Faria, T. N., Roby, K. F., and Deb, S.,** Pregnancy and the prolactin family of hormones: coordination of anterior pituitary, uterine, and placental expression, *Endocr. Rev.*, 12, 402, 1991.

43. **Suh, H. K. and Frantz, A. G.,** Size heterogeneity of human prolactin in plasma and pituitary extracts, *J. Clin. Endocrinol. Metab.*, 39, 928, 1974.

44. **Witorsch, R. J., Day, E. B., LaVoie, H. A., Hashemi, N., and Taylor, J. K.,** Comparison of glucocorticoid-induced effects in prolactin-dependent and autonomous rat Nb2 lymphoma cells, *Proc. Soc. Exp. Biol. Med.*, 203, 454, 1993.

45. **Ferrara, N., Clapp, C., and Weiner, R.,** The 16 K fragment of prolactin specifically inhibits basal or fibroblast growth factor stimulated growth of capillary endothelial cells, *Endocrinology*, 129, 896, 1991.

46. **Clapp, C., Martial, J. A., Guzman, R. C., Rentier-Delure, F., and Weiner, R. I.,** The 16 kilodalton N-terminal fragment of human prolactin is a potent inhibitor of angiogenesis, *Endocrinology*, 133, 1292, 1993.

47. **Costoff, A.,** *Ultrastructure of Rat Adenohypophysis: Correlation with Function*, Academic Press, New York, 1973.

48. **Tixier-Vidal, A. and Farquhar, M. G.,** *The Anterior Pituitary*, Academic Press, New York, 1975.

49. **Lamberts, S. W. J. and MacLeod, R. M.,** Regulation of prolactin secretion at the level of the lactotroph, *Physiol. Rev.*, 70, 279, 1990.

50. **Cho, B. N., Suh, Y. H., Yoon, Y. D., Lee, C. C., and Kim, K.,** Progesterone inhibits the estrogen-induced prolactin gene expression in the rat pituitary, *Mol. Cell. Endocrinol.*, 93, 47, 1993.

51. **Furth, J. and Clifton, K. H.,** Experimental pituitary tumors, *The Pituitary Gland*, Vol. 2, Harris, G. W. and Donovan, B. T., Butterworths, London, 1966, 460.

52. **Elias, K. A. and Weiner, R. I.,** Direct arterial vascularization of estrogen-induced prolactin-secreting pituitary tumors, *Proc. Nat. Acad. Sci. U.S.A.*, 81, 4549, 1984.

53. **Frantz, A. G.,** Prolactin, *Endocrinology*, Vol. 1, DeGroot, L. J., Cahill, G. F., Odell, W. D., Martini, L., Potts, J. T., Nelson, D. H., Steinberger, E., and Winegrad, A. I., Eds., Grune & Stratton, New York, 1979, 153.

54. **Ozawa, H. and Kurosumi, K.,** Morphofunctional study on prolactin-producing cells of the anterior pituitaries in adult male rats following thyroidectomy, thyroxine treatment and/or thyrotropin-releasing hormone treatment, *Cell Tissue Res.*, 272, 41, 1993.

55. **Ramalho, M. J., Reis, L. C., Antunes-Rodrigues, J., and De Castro e Silva, E.,** Throidectomy blocks stress-induced prolactin rise in rats: role of the central serotonergic system, *Horm. Metab. Res.*, 24, 462, 1992.

56. **Yen, S. S. C., Tsai, C. C., Naftolin, F., Vandenberg, G., and Ajabor, L.,** Pulsatile patterns of gonadotropin release in subjects with and without ovarian function, *J. Clin. Endocrinol. Metab.*, 34, 671, 1972.

57. **Cetel, N. S. and Yen, S. S. C.,** Concomitant pulsatile release of prolactin and luteinizing hormone in hypogonadal women, *J. Clin. Endocrinol. Metab.*, 56, 1313, 1985.

58. **Shin, S. H. and Reifel, C. W.,** Adenohypophysis has an inherent property for pulsatile prolactin secretion, *Neuroendocrinology*, 32, 139, 1981.

59. **Tyson, J. E., Hwang, P., Guyda, H., and Friensen, H. G.,** Studies of prolactin secretion in human pregnancy, *Am. J. Obstet. Gynecol.*, 113, 14, 1972.

60. **Linkie, D. M. and Niswender, G. D.,** Serum levels of prolactin, luteinizing hormone and follicle stimulationg hormone during pregnancy in the rat, *Endocrinology*, 90, 632, 1972.

61. **Amenomori, Y., Chen, C. L., and Meites, J.,** Serum prolactin levels in rats in different reproductive states, *Endocrinology*, 86, 506, 1970.

62. **Vines, D. T., Convey, E. M., and Tucker, H. A.,** Serum prolactin and growth hormone responses to thyrotropin releasing hormone in postpubertal cattle, *J. Dairy Sci.*, 60, 1949, 1977.

63. **Meites, J.,** Neuroendocrine control of prolactin in experimental animals, *Clin. Endocrinol. (Suppl.)*, 6, 95, 1977.

64. **Arbogast, L. A., Soares, M. J., Tomogane, H., and Voogt, J. L.,** A trophoblast-specific factor(s) suppresses circulating prolactin levels and increases tyrosine hydroxylase activity in tuberoinfundibular dopaminergic neurons, *Endocrinology*, 131, 105, 1992.

65. **Grosvenor, C. E. and Turner, C. W.,** Release and restoration of pituitary lactogen in response to nursing stimuli in lactating rats, *Proc. Soc. Exp. Biol. Med.*, 96, 723, 1957.

66. **Grosvenor, C. E., Maiweg, H., and Mena, F.,** Observations on the development and retention during lactation of the mechanism for prolactin release by exteroceptive stimulation in the rat, in *Lactogenesis: The Initiation of Milk Secretion at Parturition*, Reynolds, M., and Folley, S. J. J., Eds., University of Pennsylvania Press, Philadelphia, 1969, 181.

67. **Tucker, H. A.,** Lactation and its hormonal control, in *The Physiology of Reproduction*, Vol. 2, 2nd ed., Knobil, E. and Neill, J. D., Eds., Raven Press, New York, 1994, 1065.

68. **Smith, S.,** Role of prolactin in regulating gonadotropin secretion and gonad function in female rats, *Fed. Proc.*, 39, 2571, 1980.

69. **McNeilly, A. S.,** Suckling and the control of gonadotropin secretion, in *The Physiology of Reproduction*, Vol. 2, 2nd ed., Knobil, E. and Neill, J. D., Eds., Raven Press, New York, 1994, 1179.

70. **Mena, F., Martinez-Escalera, G., Clapp, C., Aguayo, D., Forray, C., and Grosvenor, C. E.,** A solubility shift occurs during depletion-transformation of prolactin within the lactating rat pituitary, *Endocrinology*, 111, 1086, 1982.

71. **Grosvenor, C. E. and Mena, F.,** Regulating mechanisms for oxytocin and prolactin secretion during lactation, in *Neuroendocrine Perspectives*, Muller, E. E. and MacLeod, R. M., Eds., Elsevier Biomedical Press, Amsterdam, 1982, 69.

72. **Gala, R. R.,** Minireview: the physiology and mechanisms of the stress-induced changes in prolactin secretion in the rat, *Life Sci.*, 46, 1407, 1990.

73. **Noel, G. L., Suh, H. K., Stone, J. G., and Frantz, A. G.,** Human prolactin release during surgery and other conditions of stress, *J. Clin. Endocrinol. Metab.*, 35, 840, 1972.

74. **Neill, J. D.,** Effect of stress on serum prolactin and luteinizing hormone levels during the estrous cycle of the rat, *Endocrinology*, 87, 1192, 1970.

75. **Nagy, I., Kurcz, M., Kiss, C. S., Baranyai, P., Mosonyi, L., and Halmy, L.,** The effect of suckling, stress and drugs on pituitary prolactin content in the rat, *Acta Physiol. Acad. Sci. Hung.*, 38, 371, 1970.

76. **Gunnet, J. W. and Freeman, M. E.,** The mating induced release of prolactin: a unique neuroendocrine response, *Endocr. Rev.*, 1, 44, 1983.

77. **Freeman, M. E. and Neill, J. D.,** The pattern of prolactin secretion during pseudopregnancy in the rat: a daily nocturnal surge, *Endocrinology*, 90, 1292, 1972.

78. **Freeman, M. E. and Banks, J. A.,** Hypothalamic sites which control the surges of prolactin secretion induced by cervical stimulation, *Endocrinology*, 160, 668, 1980.

79. **Freeman, M. E.,** The ovarian cycle of the rat, in *The Physiology of Reproduction*, Knobil, E. and Neill, J. D., Eds., Raven Press, New York, 1988, 1893.

80. **Stearns, E. L., Winter, J. S. D., and Faiman, C.,** Effects of coitus on gonadotropin, prolactin and sex steroid levels in man, *J. Clin. Endocrinol. Metab.*, 37, 687, 1973.

81. **Neill, J. D.,** Prolactin: its secretion and control, *Handbook of Physiology. Section 7: Endocrinology,* Vol. 4, Sawyer, W. H. and Geiger, S. R., Eds., American Physiological Society, Washington, D. C., 1974, 469.

82. **Wildt, L., Hausler, A., Marshall, G., and Knobil, E.,** GnRH has prolactin releasing activity, *Fed. Proc.*, 39, 372 (abstr.), 1980.

83. **Chen, C. L. and Meites, J.,** Effects of estrogen and progesterone on serum and pituitary prolactin levels in ovariectomized rats, *Endocrinology*, 86, 503, 1970.

84. **Nagasawa, H., Chen, C.-L., and Meites, J.,** Effects of estrogen implant in median eminence on serum and pituitary prolactin levels in the rat, *Proc. Soc. Exp. Biol. Med.*, 132, 859, 1969.

85. **Denef, C.,** LHRH stimulates prolactin release from rat pituitary lactotrophs co-cultured with a highly purified population of gonadotrophs, *Ann. Endocrinol. (Paris)*, 42, 65, 1981.

86. **Denef, C. and Andries, M.,** Evidence for paracrine interaction between gonadotrophs and lactotrophs in pituitary cell aggregates, *Endocrinology*, 112, 813, 1983.

87. **Malven, P. V.,** Luteotrophic and luteolytic responses to prolactin in hypophysectomized rats, *Endocrinology*, 84, 1224, 1969.

88. **Ishizuka, B., Quigley, M. E., and Yen, S. S. E.,** Pituitary hormone release in response to food ingestion: evidence for neuroendocrine signals from gut to brain, *J. Clin. Endocrinol. Metab.*, 57, 1111, 1983.

89. **Quigley, M. E., Ishizuka, B., Ropert, J. F., and Yen, S. S. C.,** The food-entrained prolactin and cortisol release in late pregnancy and prolactinoma patients, *J. Clin. Endocrinol. Metab.*, 54, 1109, 1982.

90. **Quigley, M. E., Ropert, J. F., and Yen, S. S. C.,** Acute prolactin release triggered by feeding, *J. Clin. Endocrinol. Metab.*, 52, 1043, 1981.

91. **Reid, R. L. and Yen, S. S. C.,** The effect of β-endorphin on arginine-induced growth hormone and prolactin release, *Life Sci.*, 29, 2641, 1981.

92. **Yen, S. S. C., Hoff, J. D., Lasley, B. L., Casper, R. F., and Sheehan, K.,** Induction of prolactin release by LRF and LRF-agonist, *Life Sci.*, 26, 1963, 1980.

93. **Casper, R. F. and Yen, S. C. C.,** Simultaneous pulsatile release by prolactin and luteinizing hormone induced by luteinizing hormone releasing factor agonist, *J. Clin. Endocrinol. Metab.*, 52, 943, 1981.

94. **Denef, C. and Andries, M.,** Evidence for paracrine interaction between gonadotrophs and lactotrophs in pituitary cell aggregates, *Endocrinology*, 112, 813, 1983.

95. **Schramme, C. and Denef, C.,** Stimulation of prolactin release by angiotensin II in superfused rat anterior pituitary aggregates, *Neuroendocrinology*, 36, 483, 1983.

96. **Robberecht, W., Andries, M., and Denef, C.,** Stimulation of prolactin secretion from rat pituitary by luteinizing hormone releasing hormone: evidence against mediation by angiotensin II acting through a (Sar1-Ala8)-angiotensin II-sensitive receptor, *Neuroendocrinology*, 56, 185, 1992.

97. **Denef, C., Baes, M., and Schramme, C.,** Paracrine actions in the anterior pituitary: role in the regulation of prolactin and growth hormone secretion, in *Frontiers in Neuroendocrinology*, Vol. 9, Ganong, W. F. and Martini, L., Eds., Raven Press, New York, 1986, 115.

98. **Becu-Villalobos, D., Lacau-Mengido, I. M., Thyssen, S. M., Diaz-Torga, G. S., and Libertun, C.,** Effects of LHRH and ANG II on prolactin stimulation are mediated by hypophysial AT1 receptor subtype, *Am. J. Physiol.*, 266, E274, 1994.

99. **Berczi, I. and Nagy, E.,** The effect of prolactin and growth hormone on hemolymphopoietic tissue and immune function, in *Hormones and Immunity*, Berczi, I. and Kovacs, K., Eds., MTP Press Ltd, Lancaster, England, 1987, 145.

100. **Brelje, T. C., Parsons, J. A., and Sorenson, R. L.,** Regulation of islet beta-cell proliferation by prolactin in rat islets, *Diabetes*, 43, 263, 1994.

101. **Meites, J.,** Relation of prolactin and estrogen to mammary tumorigenesis in the rat, *J. Nat. Cancer Inst.*, 48, 1217, 1972.

102. **Meites, J.,** Maintenance of the mammary lobulo-alveolar system in rats after adreno-orchidectomy by prolactin and growth hormone, *Endocrinology*, 76, 1220, 1965.

103. **Meites, J. and Hopkins, T. F.,** Induction of lactation and mammary growth by pituitary grafts in intact and hypophysectomized rats, *Proc. Soc. Exp. Biol. Med.*, 104, 263, 1960.

104. **Kaplan, N. M.,** Successful pregnancy following hypophysectomy during the 12th week of gestation, *J. Clin. Endocrinol. Metab.*, 21, 1139, 1961.

105. **Gomez, E. T. and Turner, C. W.,** The adrenotrophic principle of the pituitary in relation to lactation, *Proc. Soc. Exp. Biol. Med.*, 36, 78, 1937.

106. **Mills, E. S. and Topper, Y. J.,** Some ultrastructural effects of insulin, hydrocortisone and prolactin on mammary gland explants, *J. Biol. Chem.*, 44, 310, 1970.

107. **Rosen, J. M., Woo, S. L. C., and Comstock, J. P.,** Regulation of casein messenger RNA during the development of the rat mammary gland, *Biochemistry*, 14, 2895, 1975.

108. **Hallowes, R. C., Wang, D. Y., and Lewis, D. J.,** The lactogenic effects of prolactin and growth hormone on mammary gland explants from virgin and pregnant Sprague Dawley rats, *J. Endocrinol.*, 57, 253, 1973.

109. **Rillema, J. A., Wing, L. Y. C., and Cameron, C. M.,** Effect of various concentrations of prolactin and growth hormone on the magnitude and stimulation of RNA synthesis, casein synthesis, and ornithine decarboxylase activity in mouse mammary gland explants, *Horm. Res.*, 15, 133, 1981.

110. **Vonderhaar, B. K., Owens, I. S., and Topper, Y. J.,** An early effect of prolactin on the formation of alpha-lactalbumin by mouse mammary epithelial cells, *J. Biol. Chem.*, 248, 467, 1973.

111. **Sankaran, L. and Topper, Y. J.,** Prolactin-induced α-lactalbumin activity in mammary gland explants from pregnant rabbits, *Biochem. J.*, 217, 833, 1984.

112. **Forsyth, I. A., Strong, C. R., and Dils, R.,** Interactions of insulin, corticosterone and prolactin in promoting milk fat syntheisis by mammary gland explants from pregnant rabbits, *Biochem. J.*, 129, 929, 1972.

113. **Collier, R. J., Bauman, D. E., and Hays, R. L.,** Lactogenesis in explant cultures of mammary tissue from pregnant cows, *Endocrinology*, 100, 1192, 1977.

114. **Rothchild, I.,** Interrelations between progesterone and the ovary, pituitary, and central nervous system in the control of ovulation and the regulation of progesterone secretion, *Vitam. Horm.*, 23, 209, 1965.

115. **Clifton, D. K. and Sawyer, C. H.,** Positive and negative feedback effects of ovarian steroids on luteinizing hormone release in ovariectomized rats following chronic depletion of hypothalamic norepinephrine, *Endocrinology*, 106(4), 1099, 1980.

116. **Sawyer, C.,** Some recent developments in brain-pituitary-ovarian physiology, *Neuroendocrinology*, 17, 97, 1975.

117. **Bartke, A., Smith, M. S., Michael, S. D., Peron, F. G., and Dalterio, S.,** Effects of experimentally-induced chronic hyperprolactinemia on testosterone and gonadotropin levels in male rats and mice, *Endocrinology*, 100, 182, 1977.

118. **Bartke, A.,** The role of prolactin in reproduction in male mammals, *Fed. Proc.*, 39, 2577, 1980.

119. **Costello, L. C. and Franklin, R. B.,** Effect of prolactin on the prostate, *Prostate*, 24, 162, 1994.

120. **Romero, L., Munoz, C., Lopez, A., and Vilches, J.,** Effects of prolactin on explant cultures of rat ventral prostate: morphological and immunohistochemical study, *Prostate*, 22, 1, 1993.

121. **Futterweit, W. and Krieger, D. T.,** Pituitary tumors associated with hyperprolactinemia and polycystic ovarian disease, *Fertil. Steril.*, 31, 608, 1979.

122. **Grandison, L., Hodson, C. A., Chen, H. T., Advis, J., Simpkins, J., and Meites, J.,** Inhibition by prolactin of post-castration rise in LH, *Neuroendocrinology*, 23, 312, 1977.

123. **Hodson, C. A., Simpkins, J. W., Pass, K. A., Aylsworth, C. F., Steger, R. W., and Meiters, J.,** Effects of a prolactin-secreting pituitary tumor on hypothalamic, gonadotropic and testicular function in male rats, *Neuroendocrinology*, 30, 7, 1980.

124. **Torjesen, P. A., Dahlin, R., Haug, E and Aakvaag, A.,** Prolactin and the regulation of 20α-dihydroproges-terone secretion of the super-luteinized rat ovary during luteolysis induced by a prostaglandin $F_{2α}$ analogue, *Acta Endocrinol.*, 87, 625, 1978.

125. **Zimgrod, A., Lindner, H. R., and Lamprecht, S. A.,** Reductive pathways of progesterone metabolism in the rat ovary, *Acta Endocrinol.,* 69, 141, 1972.

126. **Nagy, E. and Berczi, I.,** Immunodeficiency in hypophysectomized rats, *Acta Endocrinol.,* 89, 530, 1978.

127. **Berczi, I. and Nagy, E.,** Effects of hypophysectomy on immune function, in *Psychoneuroimmunology II*, Ader, R., Felton, D. L., and Cohen, N., Eds., Academic Press, New York, 1991, 339.

128. **Nagy, E. and Berczi, I.,** Hypophysectomized rats depend on residual prolactin for survival, *Endocrinology,* 128, 2776, 1991.

129. **Gala, R. R. and Shevach, E. M.,** Evidence for the release of a prolactin-like substance by mouse lymphocytes and macrophages, *Proc. Soc. Exp. Biol. Med.,* 205, 12, 1994.

130. **Shin, R. P. C., Elsholtz, H. P., Tanake, T., Friesen, H. G., Gout, P. W., Geer, C. T., and Noble, R. L.,** Receptor mediated mitogenic action of prolactin in a rat lymphoma cell line, *Endocrinology,* 113, 159, 1983.

131. **Spangelo, B. L., Hall, N. R., Ross, R., and Goldstein, A. L.,** Stimulation of in vivo antibody production and concanavalin A-induced mouse spleen cell mitogenesis by prolactin, *Immunopharmacology,* 14, 11, 1987.

132. **Hiestand, P. C., Mekler, P., Nordmann, R., Greider, A., and Permmongkol, C.,** Prolactin as a modulator of lymphocyte responsivness provides a possible mechanism of action for cyclosporin, *Proc. Nat. Acad. Sci. U.S.A.,* 83, 2599, 1986.

133. **Di Carlo, R., Meli, R., and Muccioli, G.,** Effects of prolactin on rat paw oedema induced by different irritants, *Agents Actions*, 36, 87, 1992.

134. **Sinha, Y. N. and Sorenson, R. L.,** Differential effects of glycosylated and nonglycosylated prolactin on islet cell division and insulin secretion, *Proc. Soc. Exp. Biol. Med.,* 503, 123, 1993.

135. **Brelje, T. C., Scharp, D. W., Lacy, P. E., Ogren, L., Talamantes, F., Robertson, M., Friesen, H. G., and Sorenson, R. L.,** Effect of homologous placental lactogens, prolactins, and growth hormones on islet B-cell division and insulin secretion in the rat, mouse, and human islets: implication for placental lactogen regulation of islet function during pregnancy, *Endocrinology,* 132, 879, 1993.

136. **Noel, M. B. and Woodside, B.,** Effects of systemic and central prolactin injections on food intake, weight gain, and estrous cyclicity in female rats, *Physiol. Behav.*, 54, 151, 1993.

137. **Byatt, J. C., Staten, N. R., Salsgiver, W. J., Kostelc, J. G., and Collier, R. J.,** Stimulation of food intake and weight gain in mature female rats by bovine prolactin and bovine growth hormone, *Am. J. Physiol.,* 264, E986, 1993.

138. **Donatsch, P. and Richardson, B. P.,** Localization of prolactin in rat kidney tissue using a double antibody technique, *J. Endocrinol.,* 66, 101, 1975.

139. **Horrobin, D. F.,** Prolactin as a regulator of fluid and electrolyte metabolism in mammals, *Fed. Proc.,* 39, 2567, 1980.

140. **Everett, J. W.,** Luteotrophic function of autografts of the rat hypophysis, *Endocrinology,* 54, 685, 1954.

141. **McCann, S. M. and Friedman, H. M.,** The effect of hypothalamic lesions on the secretion of luteotrophin, *Endocrinology,* 67, 597, 1960.

142. **Welsch, C. W., Nagasawa, H., and Meites, J.,** Increased incidence of spontaneous mammary tumors in female rats with induced hypothalamic lesions, *Cancer Res.*, 30, 2310, 1970.

143. **Welsch, C. W., Squiers, M. D., Cassell, E., Chen, C. L., and Meites, J.,** Median eminence lesions and serum prolactin: influence of ovariectomy and ergocornine, *Am. J. Physiol.,* 221, 1714, 1971.

144. **Peters, L., Hoefer, M. T., and Ben-Jonathan, N.,** The posterior pituitary: regulation of anterior pituitary prolactin secretion, *Science*, 213, 659, 1981.

145. **Ben-Jonathan, N.,** Dopamine, a prolactin-inhibiting hormone, *Endocr. Rev.*, 6, 564, 1985.

146. **Pasteels, J. L.,** Secretion de prolactine par l'hypophyse en culture de tissus, *C. R. Soc. Biol.*, 253, 2140, 1961.

147. **Meites, J., Nicoll, C. S., and Talwalker, P. K.,** The central nervous system and the secretion and release of prolactin, in *Advances in Neuroendocrinology*, Nalbandov, A. V., Ed., University of Illinois Press, Urbana, 1963, 238.

148. **Harris, G. W.,** *Neural Control of the Pituitary Gland*, Edward Arnold, London, 1955, pp. 7, 8.

149. **Peters, L. A., Hoefer, M. T., and Ben-Jonathan, N.,** The posterior pituitary: regulation of anterior pituitary prolactin secretion, *Science*, 213, 659, 1981.

150. **Burris, T. P., Stringer, L. C., and Freeman, M. E.,** Pharmacologic evidence that a D_2 receptor subtype mediates dopaminergic stimulation of prolactin secretion from the anterior pituitary gland, *Neuroendocri-nology*, 54, 175, 1991.

151. **Burris, T. P., Nguyen, D. N., Smith, S. G., and Freeman, M. E.,** The stimulatory and inhibitory effects of dopamine on prolactin secretion involve different G-proteins, *Endocrinology*, 130, 926, 1992.

152. **Arey, B. J., Burris, T. P., Basco, P., and Freeman, M. E.,** Infusion of dopamine at low concentration increases release of prolactin from α-methyl-p-tyrosine-treated rats, *Proc. Soc. Exp. Biol. Med.,* 203, 60, 1993.

153. **Heiman, M. L. and Ben-Jonathan, N.,** Rat anterior pituitary dopaminergic receptors are regulated by estradiol and during lactation, *Endocrinology*, 111, 1057, 1982.

154. **Nicoll, C. S. and Meites, J.,** Estrogen stimulation of prolactin production by rat adenohypophysis in vitro, *Endocrinology,* 70, 272, 1962.

155. **Ratner, A., Talwalker, P. K., and Meites, J.,** Effect of estrogen administration in vivo on prolactin release by rat pituitary in vitro, *Proc. Soc. Exp. Biol. Med.,* 112, 12, 1963.

156. **Gibbs, D. M. and Neill, J. D.,** Dopamine levels in hypophysial stalk blood in the rat are sufficient to inhibit prolactin secretion in vivo, *Endocrinology,* 102, 1895, 1978.

157. **Ben-Jonathan, N., Oliver, C., Weiner, H. J., Mical, R. S., and Porter, J. C.,** Dopamine in hypophysial portal plasma of the rat during the estrous cycle and throughout pregnancy, *Endocrinology,* 100, 452, 1977.

158. **Ben-Jonathan, N., Oliver, C., Weiner, H. J., Mical, R. S., and Porter, J. C.,** Dopamine in hypophysial portal plasma of the rat during the estrous cycle and throughout pregnancy, *Endocrinology,* 100, 452, 1977.

159. **Moore, K. E. and Demarest, K. T.,** Tuberoinfundibular and tuberohypophyseal dopaminergic neurons, in *Frontiers in Neuroendocrinology,* Ganong, W. F. and Martini, L., Eds., Raven Press, New York, 1982, 161.

160. **MacLeod, R. M.,** Influence of norepinephrine and catecholamine depleting agents on the synthesis and release of prolactin and growth hormone, *Endocrinology,* 85, 916, 1969.

161. **Gudelsky, G. A. and Moore, K. E.,** A comparison of the effects of haloperidol on dopamine turnover in the striatum, olfactory tubercle and median eminence, *J. Pharmacol. Exp. Ther.,* 202, 149, 1977.

162. **Nagasawa, H. and Meites, J.,** Suppression by ergocornine and iproniazid of carcinogen-induced mammary tumors in rats; effects on serum and pituitary prolactin levels, *Proc. Soc. Exp. Biol. Med.,* 135, 469, 1970.

163. **Arbogast, L. A., Murai, I., and Ben-Jonathan, N.,** Differential alterations in dopamine turnover rates in the stalk-median eminence and posterior pituitary during the preovulatory prolactin surge, *Neuroendocrinology,* 49, 525, 1989.

164. **Shaar, C. J. and Clemens, J. A.,** The role of catecholamines in release of anterior pituitary prolactin in vitro, *Endocrinology,* 95, 1202, 1974.

165. **Clemens, J. A.,** *Neuropharmacological Aspects of the Neural Control of Prolactin Secretion,* Plenum Press, New York, 1976.

166. **Dymshitz, J., Laudon, M., and Ben-Jonathan, N.,** Endothelin-induced biphasic response of lactotrophs cultured under different conditions, *Neuroendocrinology,* 55, 724, 1992.

167. **Domae, M., Yamada, K., Hanabusa, Y., and Furukawa, T.,** Inhibitory effects of endothelin-1 and endothelin-3 on prolactin release: possible involvement of endogenous endothelin isopeptides in the rat anterior pituitary, *Life Sci.,* 50, 715, 1992.

168. **Milenkovic, L., Parlow, A. F., and McCann, S. M.,** Physiological significance of the negative short-loop feedback of prolactin, *Neuroendocrinology,* 52, 389, 1990.

169. **Perkins, N. A., Westfall, T. C., Paul, C. V., MacLeod, R., and Rogol, A. D.,** Effect of prolactin on dopamine synthesis in medial basal hypothalamus: evidence for a short loop feedback, *Brain Res.,* 160, 431, 1979.

170. **Seiden, G. and Brodish, A.,** Physiological evidence for 'short-loop' feedback effects of ACTH on hypothalamic CRF, *Neuroendocrinology,* 8, 154, 1971.

171. **Hodson, C. A.,** Evidence of prolactin short loop feedback in the postpartum lactating rat, *Proc. Soc. Exp. Biol. Med.,* 173, 441, 1983.

172. **Mezey, E. and Palkovits, M.,** Two-way transport in the hypothalamo-hypophyseal system, in *Frontiers in Neuroendocrinology,* Vol. 9, Ganong, W. F. and Martini, L., Eds., Raven Press, New York, 1982, 1.

173. **MacLeod, R. M., Fontham, E. H., and Lehmeyer, J. E.,** Prolactin and growth hormone production as influenced by catecholamines and agents that affect brain catecholamines, *Neuroendocrinology,* 6, 283, 1970.

174. **Macleod, R. M.,** Regulation of prolactin secretion, in *Frontiers in Neuroendocrinology,* Vol. 4, Martini, L. and Ganong, W. F., Eds., Raven Press, New York, 1976, 1969.

175. **Matta, S. G. and Sharp, B. M.,** The role of the fourth cerebroventricle in nicotine-stimulated prolactin release in the rat: involvement of catecholamines, *J. Pharmacol. Exp. Ther.,* 260, 1285, 1992.

176. **Gudelsky, G. A., Simpkins, J., Mueller, G. P., Meites, J., and Moore, K. E.,** Selective actions of prolactin on catecholamine turnover in the hypothalamus and on serum LH and FSH, *Neuroendocrinology,* 22, 206, 1976.

177. **Fuxe, K., Hökfelt, T., and Nilsson, O.,** Castration, sex hormones, and tuberoinfundibular dopamine neurons, *Neuroendocrinology,* 5, 107, 1969.

178. **Hokfelt, T. and Fuxe, K.,** Effects of prolactin and ergot alkaloids on the tuberoinfundibular dopamine (DA) neurons, *Neuroendocrinology,* 9, 100, 1971.

179. **Advis, J. P., Hall, T. R., Hodson, C. A., Mueller, G. P., and Meites, J.,** Temporal relationship and role of dopamine in "short-loop" feedback of prolactin, *Proc. Soc. Exp. Biol. Med.,* 155, 567, 1977.

180. **Shin, S. H.,** Prolactin secretion in acute stress is controlled by prolactin releasing factor, *Life Sci.,* 25, 1829, 1979.

181. **Kehoe, L., Janik, J., and Callahan, P.,** Effects of immobilization stress on tuberoinfundibular dopaminergic (TIDA) neuronal activity and prolactin levels in lactating and non-lactating female rats, *Life Sci.,* 50, 55, 1991.

182. **Gala, R. R. and Haisenleder, D. J.,** Restraint stress decreases afternoon plasma prolactin levels in female rats. Influence of neural antagonists and agonists on restraint-induced changes in plasma prolactin and corticosterone, *Neuroendocrinology,* 43, 115, 1986.

183. **Hyde, J. F. and Ben-Jonathan, N.,** Characterization of prolactin-releasing factor in the rat posterior pituitary, *Endocrinology*, 122, 2533, 1986.

184. **Hyde, J. F., Murai, I., and Ben-Jonathan, N.,** The rat posterior pituitary contains a potent prolactin-releasing factor: studies with perifused anterior pituitary cells, *Endocrinology*, 121, 1531, 1987.

185. **Voogt, J. L. and Carr, L. A.,** Potentiation of suckling-induced release of prolactin by inhibition of brain catecholamine synthesis, *Endocrinology*, 97, 891, 1975.

186. **Murai, I., Reichlin, S., and Ben-Jonathan, N.,** The peak phase of the proestrous prolactin surge is blocked by either posterior pituitary lobectomy or antisera to vasoactive intestinal peptide, *Endocrinology*, 124, 1050, 1989.

187. **Murai, I. and Ben-Jonathan, N.,** Posterior pituitary lobectomy abolishes the suckling-induced rise in prolactin (PRL): evidence for a PRL-releasing factor in the posterior pituitary, *Endocrinology*, 121, 205, 1987.

188. **Samson, W. K., McDonald, J. K., and Lumpkin, M. D.,** Naloxone-induced dissociation of oxytocin and prolactin releases, *Neuroendocrinology*, 40, 68, 1985.

189. **Kubota, T., Judd, A. M., and MacLeod, R. M.,** The paracrine role of angiotensin in gonadotrophin-releasing hormone-stimulated prolactin release in rats, *J. Endocrinol.*, 125, 225, 1990.

190. **Aguilera, G., Hyde, C. L., and Catt, K. J.,** Angiotensin II receptors and prolactin release in pituitary lactotrophs, *Endocrinology*, 111, 1045, 1982.

191. **Bowers, C. Y., Friesen, H. G., Hwang, P., Guyda, H. J., and Folkers, K.,** Prolactin and thyrotropin release in man by synthetic pyroglutamyl-histidyl-prolinamide, *Biochem. Biophys. Res. Commun.*, 45, 1033, 1971.

192. **Rivier, C., Brown, M., and Vale, W.,** Effect of neurotensin, substance P and morphine sulfate on secretion of prolactin and growth hormone in the rat, *Endocrinology*, 100, 751, 1977.

193. **Schuiling, G. A., Valkhof, N., Moes, H., and Koiter, T. R.,** Dopamine and TRH-induced prolactin secretion in pseudopregnant rats, *Life Sci.*, 53, 357, 1993.

194. **Tashjian, A. H. J., Barowsky, N. J., and Jensen, D. K.,** Thyrotropin releasing hormone: direct evidence for stimulation of prolactin production by pituitary cells in culture, *Biochem. Biophys. Res. Commun.*, 43, 516, 1971.

195. **Boyd, A. E. and Sanchez-Franco, F.,** Changes in the prolactin response to thyrotropin-releasing hormone (TRH) during the menstrual cycle of normal women, *J. Clin. Endocrinol. Metab.*, 44, 985, 1977.

196. **Shin, S. H.,** Thyrotropin-releasing hormone (TRH) is not the physiological prolactin-releasing factor (PRF) in the male rat, *Life Sci.*, 23, 1813, 1978.

197. **Deeter, W. T. and Mueller, G. P.,** Differential effects of warm- and cold-ambient temperature on blood levels of β-endorphin and prolactin in the rat, *Proc. Soc. Exp. Biol. Med.*, 168, 369, 1981.

198. **Mueller, G. P., Chen, H. T., Dibbet, J. A., Chen, H. J., and Meites, J.,** Effects of warm and cold temperatures on release of TSH, GH and prolactin in rats, *Proc. Soc. Exp. Biol. Med.*, 147, 698, 1974.

199. **Judd, S. J., Rigg, L. A., and Yen, S. S. C.,** The effects of ovariectomy and estrogen treatment on the dopamine inhibition of gonadotropin and prolactin release, *J. Clin. Endocrinol. Metab.*, 49, 182, 1979.

200. **Martinez de la Escalera, G., Guthrie, J., and Weiner, R. I.,** Transient removal of dopamine potentiates the stimulation of PRL release by TRH but not VIP: stimulation via Ca^{2+}/protein kinase C pathway, *Neuroendocrinology*, 47, 38, 1988.

201. **Libertun, C. and McCann, S. M.,** Blockade of the release of gonadotropins and prolactin by subcutaneous or intraveneous injection of atropine in male and female rats, *Endocrinology*, 92, 1714, 1973.

202. **Donoso, A. O. and Bacha, J. C.,** Acetylcholine induced responses of plasma LH and prolactin in normal and 6-hydroxydopamine-treated rats, *J. Neural Transm.*, 37, 193, 1975.

203. **Tanaka, E., Baba, N., Toshida, K., and Suzuki, K.,** Evidence for 5-HT2 receptor involvement in the stimulation of preovulatory LH and prolactin release and ovulation in normal cycling rats, *Life Sci.*, 52, 669, 1993.

204. **Kamberi, L. A., Mical, R. S., and Porter, J. C.,** Effects of melatonin and serotonin on the release of FSH and prolactin, *Endocrinology*, 88, 1288, 1971.

205. **Bruni, J. F., VanVugt, D. A., Marshall, S., and Meites, J.,** Effects of naloxone, morphine and methionine enkephalin on serum prolactin, luteinizing hormone, follicle stimulating hormone, thyroid stimulating hormone and growth hormone, *Life Sci.*, 21, 461, 1977.

206. **Fleckenstein, A. E., Lookingland, K. J., and Moore, K. E.,** Evidence that histamine-stimulated prolactin secretion is not mediated by an inhibition of tuberoinfundibular dopaminergic neurons, *Life Sci.*, 51, 741, 1992.

207. **Racagni, G., Apud, J. A., Locatelli, V., Cocchi, D., Nistico, G., di Giorgio, R. M., and Müller, E. E.,** GABA of CNS origin in the rat anterior pituitary inhibits prolactin secretion, *Nature*, 281, 575, 1979.

208. **Grandison, L. and Guidotti, A.,** γ-Aminobutyric acid receptor function in rat anterior pituitary: evidence for control of prolactin release, *Endocrinology*, 105, 754, 1979.

209. **Grandison, L., Gelato, M., and Meites, J.,** Inhibition of prolactin secretion by cholinergic drugs, *Proc. Soc. Exp. Biol. Med.*, 145, 1236, 1974.

210. **Grandison, L. and Meites, J.,** Evidence for adrenergic mediation of cholinergic inhibition of prolactin release, *Endocrinology*, 99, 775, 1976.

211. **Lu, K.-H. and Meites, J.,** Effects of serotonin precursors and melatonin on serum prolactin release in rats, *Endocrinology*, 93, 152, 1973.

212. **Mueller, G. P., Twohy, C. P., Chen, H. T., Advis, J. P., and Meites, J.,** Effects of L-tryptophan and restraint stress on hypothalamic and brain serotonin turnover, and pituitary TSH and prolactin release in rats, *Life Sci.*, 18, 715, 1976.

213. **Kordon, C., Blake, C. A., Terkel, J., and Sawyer, C. H.,** Participation of serotonin-containing neurons in the suckling-induced rise in plasma prolactin levels in lactating rats, *Neuroendocrinology*, 13, 213, 1974.

214. **Jorgensen, H., Knigge, U., and Warberg, J.,** Effect of serotonin 5-HT1, 5-HT2, and 5-HT3 receptor antagonists on the prolactin response to restrain and ether stress, *Neuroendocrinology*, 56, 371, 1992.

215. **Stobie, K. M. and Shin, S. H.,** Serotonin stimulates prolactin secretion in the hypophysectomized adeno-hypophyseal grafted rat, *Acta Endocrinol.*, 102, 511, 1983.

216. **Clemens, J. A., Sawyer, B. D., and Cerimele, B.,** Further evidence that serotonin is a neurotransmitter involved in the control of prolactin secretion, *Endocrinology*, 100, 692, 1977.

217. **Shaar, C. J., Frederickson, R. C. A., Dinger, N. B., and Jackson, L.,** Enkephalin analogues and naloxone modulate the release of growth hormone and prolactin—evidence for regulation by an endogenous opioid peptide in brain, *Life Sci.*, 21, 853, 1977.

218. **Van Vugt, D. A., Bruni, J. F., and Meites, J.,** Naloxone inhibition of stress-induced increase in prolactin secretion, *Life Sci.*, 22, 85, 1978.

219. **Van Vugt, D. A., Bruni, J. F., Sylvester, P. W., Chen, H. T., Ieiri, T., and Meites, J.,** Interaction between opiates and hypothalamic dopamine on prolactin release, *Life Sci.*, 24, 2361, 1979.

220. **Donoso, A. O., Bishop, W., Fawcett, C. P., Krulich, L., and McCann, S. M.,** Effects of drugs that modify monoamine concentrations on plasma gonadotropin and prolactin levels in the rat, *Endocrinology*, 89, 774, 1971.

221. **Lawson, D. M. and Gala, R. R.,** The influence of adrenergic, dopaminergic, cholinergic and serotonergic drugs on plasma gonadotropin and prolactin levels in ovariectomized, estrogen treated rats, *Endocrinology*, 96, 313, 1975.

222. **Donoso, A. O., Bishop, W., and McCann, S. M.,** The effect of drugs which modify catecholamine synthesis on serum prolactin in rats with median eminence lesions, *Proc. Soc. Exp. Biol. Med.*, 143, 360, 1973.

223. **Fenske, M. and Wuttke, W.,** Effects of intraventricular 6-hydroxydopamine injections on serum prolactin and gonadotropin release, *Brain Res.*, 104, 68, 1976.

224. **Carr, L. A., Conway, P. M., and Voogt, J. L.,** Role of norepinephrine in the release of prolactin induced by suckling and estrogen, *Brain Res.*, 133, 305, 1977.

225. **Libertun, C. and McCann, S. M.,** The possible role of histamine in the control of prolactin and gonadotropin release, *Neuroendocrinology*, 20, 110, 1976.

226. **Arakelian, M. C. and Libertun, C.,** H1 and H2 histamine receptor participation in the brain control of prolactin secretion in lactating rats, *Endocrinology*, 100, 890, 1972.

227. **Mioduszewski, R., Grandison, L., and Meites, J.,** Stimulation of prolactin release in rats by GABA, *Proc. Soc. Exp. Biol. Med.*, 151, 44, 1976.

228. **Lux-Lantos, V., Rey, E., and Libertun, C.,** Activation of GABA B receptors in the anterior pituitary inhibits prolactin and luteinizing hormone secretion, *Neuroendocrinology*, 56, 687, 1992.

229. **Matsushita, N., Kato, Y., Shimatsu, A., Katakami, H., Yanaihara, N., and Imura, H.,** Effects of VIP, TRH, GABA, and dopamine on prolactin release from superfused rat anterior pituitary cells, *Life Sci.*, 32, 1263, 1983.

230. **Grossman, A., Delitala, G., Yeo, T., and Besser, G. M.,** GABA and muscimol inhibit the release of prolactin from dispersed rat anterior pituitary cells, *Neuroendocrinology*, 32, 145, 1981.

231. **Mitchell, R., Grieve, G., Dow, R., and Fink, G.,** Endogenous GABA receptor ligand in hypophysial portal blood, *Neuroendocrinology*, 37, 169, 1983.

232. **Buydens, P., Govaerts, J., Velkeniers, B., Finne, E., and Vanhaelst, L.,** The effect of bombesin on basal, alpha-methyl-p-tyrosine, haloperidol, morphine, bremazocine and stress-induced prolactin secretion, *Life Sci.*, 43, 1755, 1988.

233. **Seyler, L. E. J. and Reichlin, S.,** Luteinizing hormone release in the rat induced by blood volume depletion, *Endocrinology*, 92, 295, 1973.

234. **Pan, J. T., Tian, Y., Lookingland, K. J., and Moore, K. E.,** Neurotensin-induced activation of hypothalamic dopaminergic neurons is accompanied by a decrease in pituitary secretion of prolactin and alpha-melanocyte-stimulating hormone, *Life Sci.*, 50, 2011, 1992.

235. **Ruberg, M., Rotsztejn, W. H., Arancibia, S., Besson, J., and Enjalbert, A.,** Stimulation of prolactin release by vasoactive intestinal peptide, *Eur. J. Pharmacol.*, 51, 319, 1978.

236. **Abe, H., Engler, D., Molitch, M. E., Bollinger-Gruber, J., and Reichlin, S.,** Vasoactive intestinal peptide is a physiological mediator of prolactin release in the rat, *Endocrinology*, 116, 1383, 1985.

237. **Frawley, L. S. and Neill, J. D.,** Stimulation of prolactin secretion in rhesus monkeys by vasoactive intestinal peptide, *Neuroendocrinology*, 33, 79, 1981.

238. **Shiu, R. P. C. and Freisen, H. G.,** Properties of prolactin receptor from the rabbit mammary gland, *Biochem. J.,* 140, 301, 1974.

239. **Kelly, P. A. and Labrie, F.,** Endocrine control of prolactin receptors, in *Progress in Prolactin Physiology and Pathology,* Robyn, C. and Harter, M., Eds., Elsevier, Amsterdam, 1978, 59.

240. **Posner, B. I., Kelly, P. A., and Friesen, H. G.,** Prolactin receptor in rat liver: possible induction by prolactin, *Science,* 188, 57, 1978.

241. **Boutin, J. M., Edery, M., Shirota, M., Jolicouer, C., Lesueur, L., Ali, S., Gould, D., Djiane, J., and Kelley, P. A.,** Identification of a cDNA encoding a long form of PRl receptor in human hepatome and breast cancer, *Mol. Endocrinol.,* 3, 1455, 1989.

242. **Shirota, M., Banville, D., Joieveur, C., Boutin, J. M., Edery, M., Djiane, J., and Kelly, P. A.,** Two forms of prolactin receptor are present in rat ovary and liver, *Mol. Endocrinol.,* 4, 1136, 1990.

243. **Josefsberg, Z., Posner, B. I., Patel, B., and Bergeron, J. M.,** The uptake of prolactin into female rat liver, *J. Biol. Chem.,* 140, 301, 1979.

244. **Nolin, J. M. and Witorsch, R. J.,** Detection of endogenous immunoreactive prolactin in rat mammary epithelial cells during lactation, *Endocrinology,* 99, 949, 1976.

245. **Witorsch, R. J. and Kitay, J. I.,** Pituitary hormones affecting adrenal 5α-reductase activity: ACTH, growth hormone and prolactin, *Endocrinology,* 91, 764, 1972.

246. **Rillema, J. A.,** Mechanism of prolactin action, *Fed. Proc.,* 39, 2593, 1980.

247. **Rilema, J. A.,** Cyclic AMP, adenylate cyclase and cyclic AMP phospohdiesterase in mammary glands from pregnant and lactating mice, *Proc. Soc. Exp. Biol. Med.,* 151, 748, 1976.

248. **Sapag-Hagar, M. and Greenbaum, A. L.,** Changes in the activity of adenylate cyclase and cAMP-phosphodiesterase and of the level of 3′,5′-cyclic adenosine monophosphate in rat mammary gland during pregnancy and lactation, *Biochem. Biophys. Res. Commun.,* 53, 982, 1973.

249. **Rillema, J. A.,** Evidence suggesting that the cyclic nucleotides may mediate metabolic effects of prolactin in mouse mammary gland, *Horm. Metab. Res.,* 7, 45, 1975.

250. **Sapag-Hagar, M., Greenbaum, A. C., Lewis, D. J., and Hallowes, R. C.,** The effects of di-butyrl cAMP on enzymatic and metabolic changes in explants of rat mammary tissue, *Biochem. Biophys. Res. Commun.,* 59, 261, 1974.

251. **Vermouth, N. T. and Deis, R. P.,** Inhibitory effect of progesterone on the lactogenic and abortive effect of prostaglandin F$_2\alpha$, *J. Endocrinol.,* 66, 21, 1975.

252. **Rillema, J. A.,** Effects of prostaglandins on RNA and casein synthesis in mammary gland explants of mice, *Endocrinology,* 99, 490, 1976.

253. **Oka, T., Perry, J. W., and Kano, K.,** Hormone regulation of spermine synthetase during the development of mouse mammary epithelium in vitro, *Biochem. Biophys. Res. Commun.,* 63, 292, 1977.

254. **Richards, J. F.,** Ornithine decarboxylase activity in tissues of prolactin treated rats, *Biochem. Biophys. Res. Commun.,* 63, 292, 1975.

255. **Hill, J. B., Lacy, E. R., Nagy, G. M., Gorcs, J. T., and Frawley, L. S.,** Does alpha-melanocyte-stimulating hormone from the pars intermedia regulate suckling-induced prolactin release? Supportive evidence from morphological and functional studies, *Endocrinology,* 133, 2991, 1993.

256. **Ellerkman, E., Nagy, G. M., and Frawley, L. S.,** Alpha-melanocyte-stimulating hormone is a mammotrophic factor released by neurointermediate lobe cells after estrogen treatment, *Endocrinology,* 130, 133, 1992.

257. **Vijayan, E. and McCann, S. M.,** Effect of blockade of dopaminergic receptors on acetylcholine (Ach)-induced alterations of plasma gonadotropin and prolactin (Prl) in conscious ovariectomized rats, *Brain Res. Bull.,* 5, 23, 1980.

258. **Rudnick, M. S. and Dannies, P. S.,** Muscarinic inhibition of prolactin production in cultures of rat pituitary cells, *Biochem. Biophys. Res. Commun.,* 101, 689, 1981.

259. **Schaeffer, J. M. and Hsueh, A. J. W.,** Acetylcholine receptors in the rat anterior pituitary gland, *Endocrinology,* 106, 1377, 1980.

260. **Steele, M. K., Negro-Vilar, A., and McCann, S. M.,** Effect of angiotensin II on in vivo and in vitro release of anterior pituitary hormones in the female rat, *Endocrinology,* 109, 893, 1981.

261. **Kawaguchi, M., Hayakawa, F., Kamiya, Y., Fujii, T., Ito, J., Sakuma, N., and Fujinami, T.,** Effect of ascorbic acid on pituitary prolactin secretion in the non-ascorbate synthesizing Osteogenic Disorder Shionogi (ODS) rat, *Life Sci.,* 52, 975, 1993.

262. **Franci, C. R., Anselmo-Franci, J. A., and McCann, S. M.,** The role of endogenous atrial natriuretic peptide in resting and stress-induced release of corticotropin, prolactin, growth hormone and thyroid-stimulating hormone, *Proc. Nat. Acad. Sci. U.S.A.,* 89, 11391, 1992.

263. **Samson, W. K., Bianchi, R., and Mogg, R.,** Evidence for a dopaminergic mechanism for the prolactin inhibitory effect of atrial natriuretic factor, *Neuroendocrinology,* 47, 268, 1988.

264. **Mai, L. M. and Pan, J. T.,** Central administration of bombesin blocks the estrogen-induced afternoon prolactin surge, *Neuroendocrinology,* 57, 40, 1993.

265. **Westendorf, J. M. and Schonbrunn, A.,** Bombesin stimulates prolactin and growth hormone release by pituitary cells in culture, *Endocrinology*, 110, 352, 1982.

266. **Steele, M. K., Negro-Villar, A., and McCann, S. M.,** Effect of central injection of bradykinin and bradykinin-potentiating factor upon release of anterior pituitary hormones in ovariectomized female rats, *Peptides*, 1, 201, 1980.

267. **Shah, G. V., Deftos, L. J., and Crowley, W. R.,** Synthesis and release of calcitonin-like immunoreactivity by anterior pituitary cells: evidence for a role in paracrine regulation of prolactin secretion, *Endocrinology*, 132, 1367, 1993.

268. **Martin, T. F. J.,** Calcitonin peptide inhibition of TRH-stimulated prolactin secretion: additional evidence for inhibitory regulation of phospholipase C, *Trends Endocrinol. Metab.*, 3, 82, 1992.

269. **Shimatsu, A., Kato, Y., Matsushita, N., Katakami, H., Yanaihara, N., and Imura, H.,** Immunoreactive vasoactive intestinal polypeptide in rat hypophysial portal blood, *Endocrinology*, 108, 395, 1981.

270. **Burris, T. P. and Freeman, M. E.,** Low concentrations of dopamine increase cytosolic calcium in lactotrophs, *Endocrinology*, 133, 63, 1993.

271. **Parker, P. and Lawson, D.,** Does dopamine inhibit or stimulate prolactin release in vitro? The effects of dopamine concentration and duration of in vivo estradiol treatment, *Proc. Nat. Acad. Sci. U.S.A.*, 202, 451, 1993.

272. **Niimi, M., Takahara, J., Sato, M., Murao, K., and Kawanishi, K.,** The stimulatory and inhibitory effects of quinpirole hydrochloride, D_2-dopamine receptor agonist, on secretion of prolactin as assessed by the reverse hemolytic plaque assay, *Life Sci.*, 53, 305, 1993.

273. **Vijayan, E. and McCann, S. M.,** The effects of the cholecystokinin antagonist, proglumide, on prolactin secretion in the rat, *Life Sci.*, 40, 629, 1987.

274. **Vijan, E., Samspn, W. K., Said, S. I., and McCann, S. M.,** In vivo and in vitro effects of cholecystokinin on gonadotropin, prolactin, growth hormone and thyrotropin release in the rat, *Brain Res.*, 172, 295, 1979.

275. **Malarkey, W. B., O'Donsio, T. M., Kennedy, M., and Cataland, S.,** The influence of vasoactive intestinal polypeptide and cholecystokinin on prolactin release in rat and human monolayer cultures, *Life Sci.*, 28, 2489, 1981.

276. **Lawson, D. M. and Gala, R. R.,** The influence of surgery, time of day, blood volume reduction and anaesthetics on plasma prolactin in ovariectomized rats, *J. Endocrinol.*, 62, 75, 1974.

277. **Caligaris, L., Astrada, J. J., and Taleisnik, S.,** Oestrogen and progesterone influence on the release of prolactin in ovariectomized rats, *J. Endocrinol.*, 60, 205, 1974.

278. **Meites, J.,** Relation of estrogen to prolactin secretion in animals and man, *Adv. Biosci.*, 15, 195, 1974.

279. **Kimura, F., Jinnai, K., and Funabashi, T.,** A GABA B-receptor mechanism is involved in the prolactin release in both male and female rats, *Neurosci. Lett.*, 155, 183, 1993.

280. **Libertun, C., Arakelian, M. C., Larrea, G. A., and Foglia, V. G.,** Inhibition of prolactin secretion by GABA in female and male rats, *Proc. Soc. Exp. Biol. Med.*, 161, 28, 1979.

281. **Lopez, F. J., Meade, E. H. J., and Negro-Vilar, A.,** Endogenous galanin modulates the gonadotropin and prolactin proestrous surges in the rat, *Endocrinology*, 132, 795, 1993.

282. **Vijayan, E., Samson, W. K., and McCann, S. M.,** Effects of intraventricular injection of gastrin on release of LH, prolactin, TSH and GH in conscious ovariectomized rats, *Life Sci.*, 23, 2225, 1978.

283. **Bauer, K., Graf, K. J., Faivre-Bauman, A., Beier, S., Tixier-Vidal, A., and Kleinauf, H.,** Inhibition of prolactin secretion by histidyl-proline-diketopiperazine, *Nature*, 274, 174, 1978.

284. **Enjalbert, A., Ruberg, M., Arancibia, S., Priam, M., Bauer, K., and Kordon, C.,** Inhibition of in vitro prolactin secretion by histidyl-proline-diketopiperazine, a degradation product of TRH, *Eur. J. Pharmacol.*, 58, 97, 1979.

285. **Lamberts, S. W. and Visser, T. J.,** The effect of histidyl-proline-diketopiperazine, a metabolite of TRH, on prolactin release by the rat pituitary gland in vitro, *Eur. J. Pharmacol.*, 71, 337, 1981.

286. **Melmed, S., Carlson, H. E., and Hershman, J. M.,** Histidyl-proline diketopiperazine suppresses prolactin secretion in human pituitary cell cultures, *Clin. Endocrinol.*, 16, 97, 1982.

287. **Rodriguez, T., Bordiu, E., Rubio, J. A., Duran, A., and Charro, A. L.,** Effect of pulse frequency and amplitude of D-Trp6-luteinizing hormone-releasing hormone on the pulsatile secretion of prolactin and LH, *J. Endocrinol. Invest.*, 16, 601, 1993.

288. **Mormede, P., Vincent, J. D., and Kerdelhue, B.,** Vasopressin and oxytocin reduce plasma prolactin levels of conscious rats in basal and stress conditions: study of the characteristics of the receptor involved, *Life Sci.*, 39, 1737, 1986.

289. **McCann, S. M., Mack, R., and Gale, C.,** The possible role of oxytocin in stimulating the release of prolactin, *Endocrinology*, 64, 870, 1959.

290. **Shin, S. H.,** Vasopressin has a direct effect on prolactin release in male rats, *Neuroendocrinology*, 34, 55, 1982.

291. **Nagy, G. M., Gorcs, T. J., and Halasz, B.,** Attenuation of the suckling-induced prolactin release and the high afternoon oscillations of plasma prolactin secretion of lactating rats by antiserum to vasopressin, *Neuroendocrinology*, 54, 566, 1991.

292. **Nagy, G. M., Mulchahey, J. J., Smyth, D. G., and Neill, J. D.,** The glycopeptide moiety of vasopressin-neurophysin precursor is neurohypophysial prolactin releasing factor, *Biochem. Biophys. Res. Commun.,* 151, 524, 1988.

293. **Sagrillo, C. A. and Voogt, J. L.,** Time-dependent changes in beta-endorphin stimulated prolactin release during pregnancy, *Neuroendocrinology,* 56, 246, 1992.

294. **Schwinn, G., von zur Muklen, A., and Warnecke, U.,** Effects of dexamethasone on thyrotrophin and prolactin plasma levels in rats, *Acta. Endocrinol. (Copenhagen),* 82, 486, 1976.

295. **Coleman, D. T. and Bancroft, C.,** Pituitary adenylate cyclase-activating polypeptide stimulates prolactin gene expression in a rat pituitary cell line, *Endocrinology,* 133, 2736, 1993.

296. **Werner, S., Hulting, A. L., Hokfelt, T., Eneroth, P., Tatemoto, K., Mutt, V., Maroder, L., and Wusch, E.,** Effect of peptide PHI-27 on prolactin release in vitro, *Neuroendocrinology,* 37, 467, 1983.

297. **Becu-Villalobos, D., Thyssen, S. M., Rey, E. B., Lux-Lantos, V., and Libertun, C.,** Octopamine and phenylethylamine inhibit prolactin secretion both in vivo and in vitro, *Proc. Soc. Exp. Biol. Med.,* 199, 230, 1992.

298. **Lamberts, S. W. J. and MacLeod, R. M.,** The interaction of sertonergic and dopaminergic neurons on prolactin secretion in the rat, *Endocrinology,* 78, 287, 1978.

299. **Kato, Y., Chihara, K., Ohgo, S., Iwasaki, Y., Abe, H., and Imur, H.,** Growth hormone and prolactin release by substance P in rats, *Life Sci.,* 19, 441, 1976.

300. **Vijayan, E. and McCann, S. M.,** In vivo and in vitro effects of substance P and neurotensin on gonadotropin and prolactin release, *Endocrinology,* 105, 64, 1979.

301. **Koike, K., Hirota, K., Ohmichi, M., Kadowaki, K., Ikegami, H., Yamaguchi, M., Miyake, A., and Tanizawa, O.,** Tumor necrosis factor alpha increases release of arachidonate and prolactin from rat anterior pituitary cells, *Endocrinology,* 128, 2791, 1991.

302. **Koike, K., Masumoto, N., Kasahara, K., Yamaguchi, M., Tasaka, K., Hirota, K., Miyake, A., and Tanizawa, O.,** Tumor necrosis factor alpha stimulates prolactin release from anterior pituitary cells: a possible involvement of intracellular calcium mobilization, *Endocrinology,* 128, 2785, 1991.

303. **Murata, T. and Ying, S. Y.,** Transforming growth factor β and activin inhibit basal secretion of prolactin in a pituitary monolayer culture system, *Proc. Soc. Exp. Biol. Med.,* 198, 599, 1991.

304. **Pizzi, M., Rubessa, S., Simonazzi, E., Zanagnolo, V., Falsetti, L., Memo, M., and Spano, P. F.,** Requirement of oestrogens for the sensitivity of prolactin cells to vasoactive intestinal peptide in rats and man, *J. Endocrinol.,* 132, 311, 1992.

305. **Said, S. I. and Porter, J. C.,** Vasoactive intestinal polypeptide; release into hypophysial portal blood, *Life Sci.,* 24, 227, 1979.

306. **Lam, K. S. L.,** Vasoactive intestinal peptide in the hypothalamus and pituitary, *Neuroendocrinology,* 53, 45, 1991.

307. **Chiocchio, S. R., Parisi, M. N., Vitale, M. L., and Tramezzani, J. H.,** Suckling-induced changes of vasoactive intestinal peptide concentrations in hypothalamic areas implicated in the control of prolactin release, *Neuroendocrinology,* 54, 77, 1991.

308. **Frawley, L. S. and Neill, J. D.,** Stimulation of prolactin secretion in rhesus monkeys by vasoactive intestinal polypeptide, *Neuroendocrinology,* 33, 79, 1981.

309. **Kato, Y., Iwasaki, Y., Iwasaki, J., Abe, H., Yanaihara, N., and Imura, H.,** Prolactin release by vasoactive intestinal polypeptide in rats, *Endocrinology,* 103, 554, 1978.

310. **Tatemoto, K. and Mutt, V.,** Isolation and characterization of intestinal peptide porcine PHI (PHI-27), a new member of glucagon-secretin family, *Proc. Natl. Acad. Sci. U.S.A.,* 78, 6603, 1981.

311. **Rasmussen, D. D., Ishizuka, B., Quigley, M. E., and Yen, S. S. C.,** Effects of tyrosine and tryptophan ingestion on plasma catecholamine and 3,4-dihydroxyphenylacetic acid concentrations, *J. Clin. Endocrinol. Metab.,* 57, 760, 1983.

312. **MacIndoe, J. H. and Turkington, R. W.,** Stimulation of human prolactin secretion by intravenous infusion of L-tryptophan, *J. Clin. Invest.,* 52, 1972, 1973.

313. **Ikuyama, S., Okajima, T., Kato, K.-I., and Ibayashi, H.,** Effect of taurine on growth hormone and prolactin secretion in rats: possible interaction with opioid peptidergic system, *Life Sci.,* 43, 807, 1988.

314. **Arslan, M., Pohl, C. R., Smith, M. S., and Plant, T. M.,** Studies of the role of the N-methyl-D-aspartate (NMDA) receptor in the hypothalamic control of prolactin secretion, *Life Sci.,* 50, 295, 1992.

Chapter 8

THYROID AND PARATHYROID IMAGING

Brahm Shapiro and Milton D. Gross

CONTENTS

0-8493-9429-5/96/$0.00+$.50

INTRODUCTION

At various times almost every medical imaging modality has been applied to the thyroid and parathyroid glands. Many of these studies are of historical interest only or are used occasionally under specific circumstances.[1] Thyroid scintigraphy and ultrasound remain the most important and frequently performed techniques and will be covered in greatest detail.[1,2] It is nevertheless essential to emphasize that the clinical examination, particularly careful palpation of the neck, remains a most important technique in studying the thyroid gland. The palpatory findings must always be correlated with the imaging results.[1-4]

The widespread availability of highly specific and sensitive tests of thyroid function (particularly the third-generation thyroid-stimulating hormone [TSH] assay and free thyroxine measurements) have essentially eliminated radiopharmaceutical studies for the diagnosis of hyper- and hypothyroidism, although these tests retain some importance in the categorization of the etiology of disordered thyroid function.[1-3] This is particularly important prior to the therapy of hyperthyroidism with radioiodine. The development of sensitive serum thyroglobulin assays has provided an additional means to study thyroid cancer patients that is complementary to whole-body I-131 scintigraphy and perhaps partly replaced it.[2,4-6]

The extensive use of fine-needle aspiration biopsy of thyroid nodules and the development of well-defined, strict, cytopathological criteria for the diagnosis of thyroid diseases, particularly thyroid cancer, has greatly reduced the referral of patients for thyroid imaging as a means to categorize the nature of thyroid nodules.[1,2,7-10]

The parathyroid glands are not accessible to clinical examination and many techniques have been used to locate the lesion(s) causing hyperparathyroidism, including ultrasound, subtraction scintigraphy, venography and venous sampling with parathyroid hormone assay, arteriography, computed tomography (CT) and magnetic resonance imaging (MRI).[2,11-17] Nevertheless, the key to successful clinical location and resection of the lesions causing hyperparathyroidism is surgical exploration by a highly experienced surgeon who pays special attention to the embryologically determined potential sites of gland location.[16-19] Preoperative location may have a role in speeding initial surgery but becomes particularly important in cases requiring reoperation for recurrent or persistent hyperparathyroidism.[2,11,18-20]

EMBRYOLOGY AND ANATOMY

A knowledge of the relevant embryological origins and development of the thyroid and parathyroid glands and the anatomical relationships, cross-sectional anatomy, and vascular anatomy is necessary for the correct interpretation of the medical imaging procedures utilized to depict these organs.[21]

THE THYROID GLAND

At four weeks of gestation the thyroid anlage arises from the midline endoderm of the tongue anlage and migrates caudally to lie in front of the trachea by the seventh week.[21] The thyroid anlage divides into two lobes joined by an isthmus, the extent of which can be highly variable. This process of migration can give rise to many anatomical variants.[21] The most common, being present in up to 50% of subjects, is a pyramidal lobe extending from the isthmus (most often the left side) superiorly along the route of migration.[21] Abnormal sites of thyroid migration include complete failure of descent leading to a lingual thyroid; partial failure of descent with the gland coming to lie above or below the hyoid bone; excessive descent giving rise to an intrathoracic thyroid, usually in the superior mediastinum but rarely as caudal as the aortic arch or even the heart.[21,22] Epithelium-lined cysts (thyroglossal duct cysts) may also occur at any point along the embryological route of thyroid migration and these may or may not contain functioning thyroid tissue.[21,22]

The thyroid gland lies within the pretracheal fascia, which is attached to the hyoid bone, and thus the gland moves up with swallowing.[21] The isthmus overlies the second and third tracheal rings and the lobes lie lateral to the trachea and the lower portion of the larynx and anteromedial to the common carotid arteries, internal jugular veins, vagus nerves, and cervical sympathetic chains.[21]

The thyroid gland is among the most vascular of tissues and is fed by the superior and inferior thyroid arteries.[21] The former arise from the common or external carotid arteries and lie in close relationship to the external branch of the superior laryngeal nerve. The inferior thyroid arteries may be quite variable but most often arise from the thyrocervical trunk and the vessels cross over the ascending branch of the recurrent laryngeal nerve. In up to 10% of persons a thyroid ima artery may run in the midline, having most often arisen on the right.[21]

The thyroid venous drainage is even more variable than the arteries. The superior and inferior thyroidal veins run with the arteries.[21] A middle thyroid vein may be present in more than 50% of persons.[21]

THE PARATHYROID GLANDS

The parathyroid glands originate from the third and fourth branchial pouches, the inferior glands from the third and the superior glands from the fourth.[2,17,21,23] There are normally four glands, but in 6% of persons one or more additional glands may be present. The caudal migration of the inferior glands occurs with the thymus and they may be found with or within this organ. Variant sites of parathyroid migration may occur anywhere between the base of the skull and the heart. These include the tracheoesophageal groove, superior and posterior mediastinum, within the substance of the thyroid, within the carotid sheath, behind the innominate vein, along the arch of the aorta, the ascending aorta, or within the pericardium.[2,17,21,23]

The normal parathyroid gland weighs between 20 and 40 mg and is seldom more than 6 mm in largest dimensions.[17,21] The vascular anatomy is highly variable and depends on the location of the gland. In general the blood supply is derived from the nearest adjacent thyroidal artery. Venous drainage is commonly via the inferior thyroidal veins, but in the case of ectopic glands or prior surgery it may be to the vertebral, innominate, thymic, azygous, hemiazygous, or lateral accessory veins or directly into the superior vena cava.[2,17,21,23]

MEDICAL IMAGING TECHNIQUES: BASIC PRINCIPLES

The basic underlying physical principles used in the various major medical imaging modalities—radiography, ultrasound, MRI, and nuclear medicine imaging—are compared in Table 1.

THYROID IMAGING AND UPTAKE MEASUREMENTS

Nuclear medicine techniques depend on the administration of a suitable radiopharmaceutical which traces an appropriate physiological or metabolic pathway. Such an agent should be labeled with a radionuclide that has a moderate half-life (hours to a few days) and moderate gamma ray energy (approximately 100–250 keV) with a high photon yield and few particulate emissions (e.g., beta particles and Auger electrons which cannot be imaged but contribute to the radiation dose).

TABLE 1
Principles Underlying Medical Imaging Procedures

Procedure	Physical Principles	Refinements
Radiography	Attenuation of x-ray beam passed through patient (dependent on mass and atomic number of matter in x-ray path)	1. Image on film—standard radiography. 2. X-ray source and film moved together—laminography, tomography to blur all but selected planes. 3. Digital detector array—digital radiography, digital angiography, etc. 4. Introduction of high atomic number contrast into various anatomical spaces—angiography, venography, barium swallow, etc. 5. Quantification of attenuation of x-ray beam passed through patient at multiple angles with image reconstruction by backprojection—CAT (computed axial tomography).
Ultrasonography	Absorption and reflection of ultrasound beam by tissue	1. Images are intrinsically tomographic. 2. Real-time imaging. 3. Echogenic contrast media (e.g., intravenous injections of microbubbles). 4. Application of Doppler principle (e.g., color Doppler depiction of blood flow).
Magnetic resonance imaging (MRI)	Emission of radiofrequency signal by paramagnetic nuclei (e.g., protons) when placed in magnetic field and interrogated by radiofrequency signal stimulus	1. Images are intrinsically tomographic in any chosen plane. 2. Partial tissue characterization possible by application of appropriate signal sequence—proton density, chemical shift, etc. 3. Flowing blood gives signal void. 4. Paramagnetic contrast agents may be introduced into various anatomical spaces—gadolinium-EDTA intravenously, iron solutions in the gut.
Nuclear medicine imaging	Metabolism or pathophysiology traced *in vivo* by administration of suitable radiopharmaceutical (possible without pharmacological effect)	1. Rapidly acquired digital frames can be shown in cine mode—nuclear angiography. 2. Multiple projections can be reconstructed as tomographic sections—emission computed axial tomography (ECAT), single-photon emission computed tomography (SPECT). 3. *In vivo* quantification of regions of interest—quantitation of uptake. 4. Serial *in vivo* quantification of activity—time-activity curves. 5. Simultaneous detection of annihilation photons emitted at 180° to each other—positron emission tomography (PET). 6. Studies performed in the face of pharmacological or other interventions—T_3 suppression test, perchlorate discharge.

The *in vivo* detection of the radiopharmaceutical may be by means of highly sensitive detectors which permit quantification but which cannot depict the spatial distribution of the tracer in the gland (e.g., thyroid uptake measurements). Alternatively, imaging devices such as scanners or cameras can be used to produce *in vivo* maps of radiopharmaceutical distribution. Although less sensitive than the nonimaging devices, quantification is nevertheless possible when the device is interfaced to suitable nuclear medicine computers.

RADIOPHARMACEUTICALS

Radioiodine studies of the thyroid go back to the very origin of nuclear medicine, and it is a tribute to the unique functional data which such studies provide that the radioiodine uptake is still an essential part of the nuclear endocrinology armamentarium more than 50 years after its inception.[24,25] A wide range of other radiopharmaceuticals has been introduced to permit the noninvasive *in vivo* study of a range of physiological functions (see Table 2).

TABLE 2a
Clinically Useful Radioisotopes and Radiopharmaceuticals for Thyroid Scintigraphy

Agent	Mechanism(s) of Uptake	Clinical Utility
Radioiodide		
I-131[a]	Trapped and organified by follicular	Imaging[a,b,c]
I-123[b]	cells for biosynthesis of tri- or	Functional assessment—24-h uptake[a,b]
I-124[c]	tetraiodothyronine	Therapy
Tc-99m-O_4	Trapped by follicular cells, not organified	Imaging
		Functional assessment—uptake
Thallium (Tl)-201 chloride	Uptake proportional to blood flow (Na-K pump)	Imaging (not much affected by TSH)
Tc-99m-sestamibi	Uptake proportional to blood flow	Imaging (not much affected by TSH)
Gallium-67 citrate	Transferin bound in circulation Ferritin bound in lesions	Imaging (identification of inflammation, infection, anaplastic tumors, lymphoma)
Indium-111 pentetreotide	Binds to somatostatin receptors	Imaging of medullary carcinoma of the thyroid (MCT)
I-131 or I-123 metaiodo-benzylguanidine (MIBG)	Active amine uptake I mechanism	Imaging of MCT
Tc-99m dimercaptosuccinic acid (DMSA-V)	Unknown	Imaging of MCT
Anti-carcinoembryonic antigen (CEA) monoclonal antibodies	Binding to cellular antigen	Imaging of MCT
Fluorine-18 fluorodeoxy-glucose (F-18-FDG)	Glucose uptake and phosphorylation; glycolysis increased in tumors	Positron emission tomography (PET) (benign vs. malignant masses)

[a]   Planar imaging and 24-h uptake therapy.
[b]   Planar imaging and SPECT imaging and 24-h uptake.
[c]   Positron emission tomographic (PET) imaging.

Radioactive Iodines

Iodide subserves a unique role in human trace element metabolism.[1] There is only one stable isotope of iodine (I-127) and multiple radioisotopes are available, several of which (I-123, I-131, I-124) have clinical utility (Table 2).[1-3,25-28] Following ingestion iodide is rapidly absorbed from the upper gastrointestinal tract and equilibrates with the extracellular water space. Several organs and tissues have the capacity to actively concentrate iodide from the extracellular water. These include the choroid plexus, nasopharynx, salivary glands, gastric mucosa, female breast (particularly when lactating), sweat glands, and thyroid gland.[1-3,26] Only the thyroid has the enzymatic mechanisms for the organification of iodide and the synthesis, storage, and release of thyroid hormones. A considerable fraction of absorbed

TABLE 2b

Physical Properties, Doses, and Dosimetry of Radiopharmaceuticals Used for Thyroid Studies

Radiopharmaceuticals	T$_{1/2}$ (Physical)	Photon Energies (keV)	Usual Dose	Route of Administration	Adult Absorbed Radiation Doses (cGy) Thyroid[a]	Adult Absorbed Radiation Doses (cGy) Whole Body	Remarks
Radioiodines of Current Clinical Utility							
I-123	13.3 h	159	200–400 μCi (for thyroid imaging) .2–10 μCi (for whole body imaging)	Oral	3.0–6.0 30–150	0.01–0.02 0.1–0.5	Cyclotron produced. Near-ideal radioisotope for imaging the thyroid. Decay by isomeric transition yields excellent radiation dosimetry. T$_{1/2}$ somewhat short for delayed whole body surveys. Permits performance of SPECT.
I-124	4.2 days	511,[b] 603	100–300 μCi	Oral	90–270	0.08	Cyclotron produced. Positron emitter requires PET. Unfavorable dosimetry makes its use justifiable only as part of radiation dosimetry prior to 131-I therapy.
I-125	60 days	28–35	50 μCi	Oral	52.0	0.17	Very low suboptimal photon energy. Long half-life only useful for prolonged turnover studies. Has been used for uptake studies but obsolete except for autoradiography of surgical specimens, intraoperative probe, and other special investigations.
I-131	8.1 days	364	5–10 μCi (uptake) 25–50 μCi (imaging) 2–5 mCi, occasionally as much as 10 mCi (postthyroidectomy whole body surveys)	Oral	8.0–160 75–150 3000.0–7500.0	0.03–0.05 0.22–0.44 8.8–22.0	High photon suboptimal for imaging. Suboptimal decay scheme with many beta particles makes ideal 131-I for therapy rather than imaging except for whole body postthyroidectomy surveys.
Radioiodines of Historical Interest							
I-211	2.1 h	2225, 5319	—	Oral	—	—	Has been used for uptake measurements.

(continued)

TABLE 2b (continued)
Physical Properties, Doses, and Dosimetry of Radiopharmaceuticals Used for Thyroid Studies

Radiopharmaceuticals	$T_{1/2}$ (Physical)	Photon Energies (keV)	Usual Dose	Route of Administration	Adult Absorbed Radiation Doses (cGy) Thyroid[a]	Whole Body	Remarks
I-126	13.3 days	666, 388	—	Oral	—	—	Has been used for uptake measurements.
I-128	25 min	433	—	Oral	—	—	First used in 1938 for uptake measurements.
I-129	16×10^6 years	39	—	Oral	—	—	Has been used for long-term animal studies.
I-130	12.5 h	536, 739, 668	—	Oral	—	—	Has been used for uptake measurements.
I-132	2.3 h	600, 760, 1410	25–50 µCi	Oral	40.0	0.05	Generator produced. Has been used for uptake measurements.
Tc-99m-O$_4$	6 h	140	5–15 mCi	Intravenous	1.0[a]	0.06	Generator produced. Decay by isomeric transition. Photon ideal for imaging. Excellent radiation dosimetry. Most widely used radiopharmaceutical for thyroid imaging.
Tc-99m DMSA-V	6 h	140	2–5 mCi	Intravenous	0.008–0.02	0.02–0.06	For imaging of medullary thyroid cancer.
Tc-99m MIBI	6 h	140	2–10 mCi	Intravenous	0.04–0.23	0.03–0.16	Distributes in proportion to blood flow. For evaluation of vascularity of thyroid nodules. May be used to locate metastatic medullary or other thyroid cancers.
I-131 MIBG	8.1 days	364	0.5–10.0 mCi	Intravenous	17.5–35	0.05–0.1	May locate a minority of primary and metastatic medullary thyroid cancers. High sensitivity for locating pheochromocytoma in the MEN 2 syndromes.

I-123 MIBG	13.3 h	159	2.0–10.0 mCi	Intravenous	4.4–22	0.04–0.2	May locate a minority of primary and metastatic medullary thyroid cancers. High sensitivity for locating pheochromocytoma in the MEN 2 syndromes. Better dosimetry and imaging properties than 131-I MIBG
Tl-201	3.0 days	68–82	1.0–3.0 mCi	Intravenous	0.9–2.8	0.21–0.62	Distributes in proportion to blood flow and taken up by viable cellular lesions. Has been used to characterize the vascularity of thyroid nodules and may be used to locate metastatic medullary and other thyroid cancers.
Ga-67	78.3 h	93, 185, 300	3.0–10.0 mCi	Intravenous	0.6–21	0.7–2.3	Nonspecific tumor- and inflammation-seeking radiopharmaceutical. Has been used to characterize thyroid nodules and to stage lymphoma.
In-111 Octreoscan	67.3 h	171, 245	3.0–6.0 mCi	Intravenous	0.74–1.49	1.3–2.6	High sensitivity for the location of many neuroendocrine tumors including medullary thyroid carcinoma and pheochromocytomas in the MEN 2 syndrome.
Am-241	458 years	60 (28 keV characteristic x-ray of 127-I emitted)	—	External irradiation only	0.06	Negligible	*In vivo* x-ray fluorescence of I-127 present in the thyroid. Requires solid-state detector rectilinear scanner used to quantify the total and regional iodine content of thyroid tissue and lesions.

a   For euthyroid patients; higher in hyperthyroid patients.
b   Annihilation photon from β+ decay.

iodide is excreted via the urine. Some thyroid hormone and its metabolites are excreted by the liver into the bile and thence into the gut. These factors must all be taken into account in the interpretation of radioiodine scintigraphy, particularly whole body scans, and contamination with urine, saliva, nasal mucus, sweat, and milk may all lead to artifacts which may be mistaken for disease.[1-3,26,29] Within the normal thyroid radioiodine is uniformly distributed and depicts the shape of the gland. The target-to-background ratio of thyroid tissue to adjacent soft tissues and salivary glands is high.[1-3,26] Pathology may be revealed by an abnormal location of the gland or generalized increased or decreased uptake of radioiodine (in general associated with increased and decreased thyroid function, respectively). Focal areas of decreased tracer uptake may be seen in the area of cysts, necrosis, and benign or malignant neoplasms, whereas focal areas of increased tracer uptake, usually associated with reduced uptake in adjacent normal tissues, result from metabolically active hyperfunctioning lesions that are always benign.[1-3,26,27,30]

The essential characteristics of the various radioiodines used for thyroid studies currently and in the past are listed in Table 2.[1] Unsatisfactory half-lives (too short with I-130 and I-132 and too long with I-125) and/or unsatisfactory photon energies or excessive particulate emissions (e.g., I-125) mean that only I-123 and I-131 are in widespread clinical[1-3,26-28,31-33] use, and I-124 is used in specialized centers for positron emission tomographic (PET) studies.[34,35] The near-ideal photon energy and favorable radiation dosimetry of I-123 make this the optimal thyroid imaging radiopharmaceutical.[1,27,31,32] The short (13-h) half-life and high cost are, however, something of a drawback. The longer lived I-131 (8 days) remains the principal tracer for the performance of postthyroidectomy whole body surveys for residual thyroid tissue and metastatic disease in thyroid cancer patients because it permits imaging 24–72 h after administration.[36,37] When the thyroid itself is imaged, this is usually 6–24 h after tracer administration.[1-3,26] The high radiation dosimetry of I-131 is not a major disadvantage if the majority of the patients studied go on to therapy with very large doses of I-131.[1-3,26,28,33] The very factors that make I-131 suboptimal for diagnostic imaging make it the standard therapeutic radionuclide for thyroid disease.[2,3,26,28,33]

Pertechnetate (Tc-99m-TcO₄)

The radionuclide Tc-99m is the metastable 6-h half-life radioisotope of Tc-99. For thyroid imaging Tc-99m is used in the form of the pertechnetate anion, which is derived, without further processing, by simple elution of the molybdenum-99 (Mo-99) generator with sterile normal saline.[1,38] The isomeric transition of Tc-99m to Tc-99 occurs with the emission of a 140-keV photon and thus Tc-99m has excellent radiation dosimetric properties.[2,3,26,31,38-40] As a small monovalent anion, it is transported by the same ion channel as iodide in many of the same tissues, including the thyroid gland, salivary glands, gastric mucosa, and choroid plexus. It is readily cleared by the kidney and to a lesser extent via the gut. Unlike iodide, once the pertechnetate is concentrated within the thyroid cell it is not further metabolized to technetium-labeled thyroid hormone analogs.[2,3,26,27,31,39,40] The thyroid is usually scanned 20 min after the intravenous injection of 1–10 mCi because only the initial uptake mechanism is traced. Anterior, both anterior oblique and occasionally lateral, views are obtained with and without radioactive markers on the chin, thyroid cartilage, and suprasternal notch. The patient should take a swallow of water immediately before imaging or the radioactivity in swallowed saliva may be confused with a pyramidal lobe.[1] The Tc-99m thyroid scan provides an *in vivo* map of trapping function within the gland.[1,39] Under certain conditions, thyroid tissue may manifest intact anion trapping function that is dissociated from the later steps of thyroid hormonogenesis.[27,31,39] Under these conditions the gland as a whole or a focal lesion within the gland may show a discordance between normal or increased pertechnetate uptake and decreased radioiodine retention.[2,3,26,31,39,41] The whole gland is affected by congenital inborn errors of iodide organification or by acquired factors such as antithyroid drugs or some cases

TABLE 3
Agents Interfering with Thyroid Imaging and Uptake Measurement

Agents	Recommended Withdrawal Interval
Competing anions: Br^-, ClO^-_4, SCN^-, $SeCN^-$, ReO^-_4	1–2 weeks
Sodium nitroprusside	1 week
Antithyroid drugs: propylthiouracil, methimazole	1 week
Nonsteroidal antiinflammatory drugs: salicylates, phenylbutazone	1–2 weeks
Iodine and inorganic iodides: expectorants and multivitamins	
Lugol's solution, saturated solution of potassium iodide (SSKI)	2 weeks
Kelp	2 weeks
Glucocorticoids	1 week
Natural or synthetic thyroid hormones	
Triiodothyronine (T_3)	2 weeks
Thyroid extract	4–6 weeks
Thyroglobulin	4–6 weeks
Thyroxine (T_4)	4–6 weeks
T_3/T_4 combinations	4–6 weeks
Topical iodophor skin preparations	1–9 months
Radiographic contrast media	
Water soluble intravenous (angiography, IVP, CT)	1–2 months
Intravenous cholecystographic agents	1–2 months
Oral cholecystographic agents	6–9 months
Iodinated oils for bronchography	6–12 months
Iodinated oils for myelography	2–10 years
Water soluble myelographic contrasts	6–12 months
Amiodirone	3–12 months

of Hashimoto's thyroiditis (see Table 3). Focal discordance may be seen in a minority of thyroid neoplasms including some carcinomas.[2,3,26,31,39]

Thallium Chloride (Tl-201)

Tl-201, when administered intravenously, is taken up by viable cellular tissues by the same energy-dependent ion exchange mechanism that takes up potassium and extrudes sodium. Because this mechanism is highly efficient, the tissue uptake of Tl-201 is proportional to blood flow.[42-45] Thus, Tl-201 scintigraphy has been used to characterize those thyroid nodules that are cellular and vascular (and thus possibly malignant) from those that are avascular and acellular (and thus probably benign).[43-47] The other utility of Tl-201 scintigraphy has been for the whole body survey of thyroid cancer patients.[43,44,48,49] Although Tl-201 uptake by metastases increases somewhat after thyroid hormone withdrawal and the consequent elevation of TSH, it is nevertheless possible to scan patients while on thyroid hormone. This is an advantage in patients who tolerate hypothyroidism poorly. Tl-201 scintigraphy may also be useful to depict the sites and extent of metastatic thyroid cancer in patients when serum thyroglobulin indicates the presence of disease but where I-131 scintigraphy is negative.[43,44,46,48] This phenomenon presumably results from a dissociation between thyroglobulin synthesis and iodide uptake and organification. Tl-201 may also have utility in depicting medullary carcinoma of the thyroid (MCT), which is a highly vascular neuroendocrine tumor that does not metabolize radioiodine.[2,42,50]

Sestamibi (Tc-99m MIBI)

This organic complex is labeled with the nearly optimal radionuclide Tc-99m and is rapidly cleared from the blood in proportion to blood flow. Thus, it has been used in a similar fashion to Tl-201 for the characterization of thyroid nodules, the whole body survey of thyroid cancer patients with lesions that are not iodide avid including dedifferentiated papillary cancer,

Hürthle cell cancer, and MCT.[2,51] As with Tl-201, patients may be scanned without withdrawal from thyroid hormone. The more favorable photon energy, half-life, and decay scheme of Tc-99m permits the administration of doses as high as 10 mCi Tc-99m MIBI versus 1–3 mCi Tl-201 and thus provides superior image quality and probably greater sensitivity.[47,51]

Gallium (Ga-67) Citrate

This agent binds rapidly to transferrin and is taken up by a wide range of tumors and inflammatory and infectious lesions.[1,52,53] The mechanisms for this remain controversial but may include the overexpression of the ferritin gene by tumors, the presence of lactoferrin in inflammatory cells, and siderophores in bacteria.[1] All of these specialized proteins will bind gallium. Thyroid nodules that are hypofunctioning by Tc-99m or I-123 imaging have been characterized by Ga-67 uptake. Those that are most Ga-67 avid have a greater propensity to malignancy.[52] This technique is, however, less sensitive than Tl-201 scintigraphy (being only approximately 40%) and lacks specificity for malignant tumors because Ga-67 is also taken up by inflammatory lesions.[52] There is, however, a sensitivity of greater than 90% for anaplastic carcinoma and thyroid lymphoma. In the latter, Ga-67 scintigraphy may be clinically useful.[1,52,53] Radiolabeled bleomycin has also shown avidity for thyroid cancers.[54]

Octreoscan (In-111 Octreotide)

This is an octapeptide analog of the peptide hormone/neurotransmitter somatostatin that is linked to the radionuclide In-111 by the chelator diethylene triamine pentaacetic acid (DTPA).[55,56] Octreoscan thus permits the *in vivo* depiction of somatostatin receptors that are present on a wide range of neuroendocrine and other tissues and the tumors derived from them. Recent studies have shown Octreoscan to be taken up by both primary and metastatic MCT with greater sensitivity and specificity than most other available techniques.[55-57] In the case of the multiple endocrine neoplasia syndromes, type 2a and 2b, where MCT is associated with pheochromocytoma, these other neuroendocrine tumors are also depicted with high sensitivity.[55,56]

Metaiodobenzylguanidine (MIBG)

This radiopharmaceutical, labeled with I-131 or more satisfactorily with I-123, is actively concentrated by neuroendocrine tissues, especially the sympathomedullary system, by an active amine uptake system.[1,58,59] Once MIBG enters the cytoplasm it may be further stored within the intracytoplasmic neurosecretory storage vesicles. These systems are most highly expressed in the sympathomedullary tumors such as pheochromocytomas and paragangliomas, which are depicted with an approximately 90% sensitivity and nearly 100% specificity.[59,60] Many other tumors of the amine precursor uptake and decarboxylation (APUD) series also express the amine uptake mechanism, albeit to a lesser extent, and thus may also be imaged with MIBG. In contrast to the high sensitivity for pheochromocytomas, the sensitivity for MCT is significantly lower, having been reported at between 20 and 40%.[58-62] Therapy with large doses of I-131 MIBG has been attempted in a few patients manifesting intense tracer uptake. MIBG scintigraphy has a significant role in depicting the pheochromocytomas of the MEN 2a and 2b (multiple endocrine neoplasia) syndromes.[1,59,60,64]

Dimercaptosuccinic Acid (DMSA-V-Tc-99m)

This radiopharmaceutical in trivalent form is usually used to image the kidney, but when reconstituted in nonstandard fashion with the addition of sodium bicarbonate to render the reaction alkaline it is transformed to a pentavalent form (DMSA-V-Tc-99m).[1,60,65-68] This complex, by an as yet unknown mechanism, binds to a variety of tumors including MCT. The sensitivity of this procedure for detecting MCT is controversial and has been reported as being as high as 95%, whereas others have found much lower sensitivity.[60,62,65,66] It does appear to be more sensitive than MIBG scintigraphy. In the case of the MEN syndromes

DMSA-V-Tc-99m is not taken up by pheochromocytomas and in this setting would have a greater specificity for MCT.[60,65,66] Because DMSA-V complex will bind other transition metals, rhenium-156 has been suggested as a label for the therapy of metastatic MCT.[1,60,61]

Anti-CEA Monoclonal Antibodies

A large proportion of MCT tumors express carcinoembryonic antigen (CEA). A number of anti-CEA monoclonal antibodies have been labeled with a range of radionuclides, including I-131, In-111, and Tc-99m, primarily for the detection of metastatic colon cancer. In principle, these same radiopharmaceuticals may have a role in depicting metastatic MCT, although clinical experience remains extremely limited.[1,69,70]

Fluorodeoxyglucose (FDG-F-18)

The glucose analog fluorodeoxyglucose (FDG), when labeled with the positron-emitting radionuclide F-18, may be used to trace the two initial steps of tissue glucose metabolism[71]—glucose uptake and phosphorylation—after which FDG-F-18 is not further metabolized. Because most malignant tumors metabolize glucose by the inefficient glycolytic pathway they manifest striking FDG-F-18 uptake.[71] This has been used to locate and characterize a wide range of tumors but requires PET to image the two 511-keV annihilation photons derived from the positrons.[71] Although experience in thyroid cancer is limited, this tumor appears to behave similarly to other malignancies.[71] The clinical role of FDG-F-18 PET in thyroid cancer remains to be clarified but may include whole body survey for noniodine avid thyroid cancers, which might be performed without thyroid hormone withdrawal and as an objective means to predict the effects of chemo- or radiotherapy when treating thyroid cancer.[71] A further increment in thyroid tumor FDG-F-18 uptake may occur after thyroid hormone withdrawal.

NUCLEAR MEDICINE INSTRUMENTATION

Various devices can be used to depict spatially or quantify radiopharmaceuticals *in vivo* and will be briefly considered below, because an understanding of the broad principles of these techniques is useful in interpreting and understanding the strengths and weaknesses of the various nuclear medicine procedures.

The Rectilinear Scanner

This was the original nuclear medicine imaging device but is no longer manufactured in North America, nevertheless many of these instruments are still in service for thyroid imaging.[24] A multi-hole focusing collimator is interfaced to a scintillation crystal/photomultiplier detector. The device is mechanically moved to and fro across the region to be imaged and the point-by-point countrate depicted as a two-dimensional map by means of several types of output devices (e.g., on paper by means of black or multicolored typewriter ribbon and mechanical tapper, or on photographic film by means of small light sources with the photo-scanner). Advantages of this technique are that the focusing collimators provide highest resolution at depth and thus a form of laminar tomography; the images are life size; and it is easy to mark anatomical and other features such as palpable nodules.[1,24]

The Planar Gamma Camera

The Anger gamma camera is now the principal nuclear medicine imaging device.[1,24] A variety of collimators are used to form the image. The pinhole collimators have highest resolution but very low sensitivity and are widely utilized to image the thyroid.[1,32,72] An alternative is the multi-hole converging collimator, which can be used to project a small organ like the thyroid onto the large gamma camera detector.[32] Multiple parallel hole collimators are used for whole body tumor surveys.[32] The higher the photon energy, the thicker the collimator septa and the longer the bore of the channels must be.[32] The collimator projects the gamma rays from the patient onto a detector which consists of a large, thin sodium iodide crystal where the energy is deposited and within milliseconds reemitted as a flash of visible light. The light photons are detected by an array of photomultipliers the outputs of which are combined to derive the x and y coordinates of the light flash, which are then used to produce a visible spot of light on an oscilloscope which is permanently recorded on photographic film. The oscilloscope is only activated if the total energy deposited in the detector (as determined by pulse height analysis) is that of an unscattered gamma ray. The location and energy of the event recorded by the detector can also be digitized and stored in a nuclear medicine computer interfaced to the gamma camera.[1] This permits image processing including background subtraction, the use of various color tables, image smoothing, region of interest and quantification, and quantitative data display in the form of time/activity graphs.[1]

Nuclear Angiography

If a fairly large activity (mCi) of a radiopharmaceutical (e.g., I-123 or Tc-99m) is rapidly injected as a bolus, the rapid acquisition of a series of serial images at a fast frame rate (e.g., 1 to 3 per second) will produce a nuclear angiogram that gives an indication of the degree of vascularity of thyroid nodules.[1,73] This may be viewed as a series of images on film or played in cine mode by the computer. The method has not been widely employed because of the relatively low resolution due to the limited count rates. Lesions that are hypofunctional on thyroid scintigraphy and hypervascular on nuclear angiography are more likely to be neoplasms than lesions that are hypovascular, which are usually cysts or colloid nodules.[1,73]

Single-Photon Emission Computed Tomography (SPECT)

A number of tomographic techniques have been applied to thyroid scintigraphy.[74] These include various multiple pinhole techniques (e.g., the seven pinhole or coded aperture), which produce coronal tomographic sections,[74] and single or multihead rotating gamma camera SPECT, in which multiple gamma camera images are made at multiple projections as the camera(s) is rotated around the patient.[75] These projections of the radionuclide distribution in the patient are then reconstructed by computer backprojection to derive transaxial, coronal, sagittal, and oblique tomograms. Tomography permits higher resolution at depth than planar scintigraphy and also may give a better three-dimensional depiction of abnormalities.[1,75]

Positron Emission Tomography (PET)

When a positron is emitted by a radionuclide, it may travel a few millimeters and then interact with an electron. The two particles mutually annihilate each other and, in so doing, emit two 511-keV photons at 180° to each other. Suitable opposing detector systems utilizing either coincidence circuitry or time-of-flight technology, rather than mechanical collimation, are used to locate the annihilation events and thus to create a transverse tomogram (positron emission tomogram or PET image). The technique has the potential for great sensitivity and for absolute quantification.[1,34,35,71]

Many positron-emitting radionuclides are short lived, produced by accelerators such as cyclotrons and, as such, may be both expensive and limited in availability. PET applications in thyroid disease have been limited to date but include I-124 for imaging and absolute quantification for dosimetry in the therapy of hyperthyroidism and thyroid cancer.[34,35] Another application is the *in vivo* characterization of tumor glucose metabolism by means of FDG-F-18 (vide supra).[1,71]

X-Ray Fluorescence Imaging

The principle of x-ray fluorescence has been widely used *in vitro* for the nondestructive analysis of samples (e.g., trace element analysis). It has also been applied as an *in vivo* technique to map the distribution of stable nonradioactive I-127 in the thyroid gland and to quantify the total thyroidal iodine content.[1,76,78] The physical principle on which this technique is based is the photoelectric effect and the emission of characteristic x-rays.[1,76,77] Thus, when the iodine within the thyroid is irradiated with photons of suitable energy (e.g., ~60 keV), these are absorbed by the inner, K shell, electron, which is ejected from its orbit (binding energy 33.2 keV). When the orbit is refilled by an electron from the L shell, a characteristic x-ray of 28.5 keV is emitted, and this is sufficiently energetic to permit detection outside the neck. The most widely used radiation source for thyroid x-ray fluorescence has been a sealed radioactive source containing americium (Am-241), which, in addition to alpha particles, also emits a 59.6-keV photon.[1,76,77] With a 458-year half-life, source replacement and adjustment for radioactive decay is not required. A focusing collimator is used to direct the Am-241 photons onto a point within the thyroid and the device is then moved back and forth across the neck in a rectilinear fashion by a scanning device. The characteristic x-rays that are emitted are detected by a solid-state semiconductor detector (e.g., lithium-drifted silicon or high-purity germanium) which has excellent energy resolution and is able to distinguish the characteristic x-rays of iodine from scattered Am-241 photons.[76-78] The output of the detector is subjected to pulse high analysis and then mapped by a photorecorder as a semiquantitative scan. By the use of computer analysis of the detector output, the total or regional thyroidal iodine content can be estimated by comparison to a suitable iodine-containing standard phantom.[1,76-78] The iodine content of nodules can be used to predict the nature of thyroid nodules.[1,76,77,79]

This technique has provided an excellent research tool in thyroidology but has had limited clinical adoption because of the need for liquid nitrogen cooling of the detector, the expense, the need to license the Am-241 sources, and the lack of commercial interest.[1,76,77,79]

Thyroid Uptake Probes

Among the first devices used in clinical nuclear medicine were simple, nonimaging, directionally collimated detector devices.[1,24,80] Initially, insensitive Geiger counters were used but these have been replaced by highly sensitive sodium iodide detectors.[24] The photon emitted by the radionuclide is absorbed by the detector and its energy reemitted as visible light. This is detected and amplified by a photomultiplier tube, the output of which is subject to further amplification. The voltage of the output is proportional to the energy of the photon detected, and thus it is possible to use pulse height analysis to exclude scattered photons (that have lost some of their energy) and to distinguish between two or more radionuclides that may be present simultaneously.[1,24,80]

Some systems may include two probes, one for counting the neck and another for simultaneously counting a background area such as the thigh. Modern devices include electronic packages that rapidly calibrate the instrument and perform uptake measurements (vide infra). It is a tribute to the unique physiological data generated by the uptake probe that it remains after 50 years an essential tool in clinical thyroidology.[1,24,80]

Whole Body Counters

A number of highly sensitive radiation detectors can be used to quantify the total retained radionuclide in a patient.[1,24] These devices have maximal sensitivity (detection thresholds in the nanocurie range) but no spatial resolution. These devices include shielded rooms (6-in steel plate) containing multiple large-scintillation detector probes around the patient as well as shadow shield machines in which shielded detectors face each other and the patient is slid between them on a movable bed (this will also yield a longitudinal profile of radioactivity in the patient). These devices are large, heavy, and cumbersome, are not commercially available, and are used primarily in research.[24]

Clinical whole body counting is nevertheless possible using larger tracer doses (e.g., after 2–5 mCi I-131 doses for whole body thyroid cancer surveys) by examining the seated patient at a distance of 2 m from a standard thyroid uptake probe. Such measurements may be important in determining whole body radiation doses from therapeutic doses of I-131.[1,81,82]

NONIMAGING THYROID STUDIES

Quantitative measurements of tracer uptake by the thyroid are among the first clinical nuclear medicine studies and one which is in routine clinical use today.[1,24,25,80]

Radioiodine Uptake

The earliest studies used I-128 ($T_{1/2}$ 23 min) and insensitive Geiger counters as detectors.[1,24] Modern studies use I-131 or I-123 and sensitive directional scintillation crystal probes.[80] Current instrumentation permits the use of minute tracer doses of radioactive iodine, 3–10 µCi I-131 or 200–300 µCi I-123, which are administered orally.[80] Ideally, the patient's neck should be counted with an uptake probe before tracer administration to exclude interference from any previously administered radionuclides. The patient dose and a standard are counted in a suitable neck phantom, which is made of plastic and approximates the size and attenuation of an average neck. At least 10,000 counts are required to give a counting standard deviation of less than 1%. The patient dose is administered and the count rate over the patient's thyroid determined at standard time intervals (e.g., 4, 6, 12, 24, or 48 h).[80] For most purposes, the 24-h uptake is utilized.[80] In addition to the thyroid counts obtained over the neck, it is necessary to correct for nonthyroidal background activity, which may be determined by counting over the patient's thigh, or by counting over the neck with and without a heavy lead shield over the thyroid. The effects of radioactive decay are compensated for by measuring the count rate of the phantom at the time of patient measurement.[80] The percent thyroid uptake is then calculated as

$$\% \text{ uptake } (\tau) = \frac{\text{Thyroid cpm } (\tau) - \text{Thigh cpm } (\tau)}{\text{Standard cpm } (\tau)} \times \frac{\text{Standard cpm } (0)}{\text{Patient cpm } (0)} \times 100 \quad [8.1]$$

or

$$\% \text{ uptake } (\tau) = \frac{\text{Unshielded cpm } (\tau) - \text{Shielded cpm } (\tau)}{\text{Unshielded cpm } (\tau)} \times \frac{\text{Standard cpm } (0)}{\text{Patient dose cpm } (0)} \times 100$$

$$[8.2]$$

The percent thyroid uptake is highly dependent on the dietary iodine intake, which varies greatly with geographical location.[80] The 24-h radioiodine uptake in North America today is between 5 and 30%, whereas in Graves' disease, values are typically 50–70%.[80,83,84] A small subset of thyrotoxic patients have such rapid radioiodine turnover that the 24-h uptake may be deceptively low and the highest uptakes are achieved at 6–12 hours.[80,83,84] The 24-h uptakes are somewhat inconvenient because they require two different visits to the nuclear medicine laboratory and, for many purposes, early radioiodine uptake measurements may suffice (e.g., at 4 or 6 h)—normal range at 6 h being 2–20%.[80,83] If the plasma inorganic iodide concentration is known, the absolute thyroidal iodide uptake rate can be calculated. Many factors including diet, drugs, and diseases must be taken into account when interpreting thyroid uptake measurements (Table 3).[80,83,85] Although the diagnosis of hyperthyroidism is no longer made by radioiodine uptake, its etiologies may be classified by this technique and those amenable to I-131 therapy determined.[83-86] Many I-131 therapy dosage schemes utilize the radioiodine uptake in their calculations.[83-85] Radioiodine uptake measurements performed on medically treated hyperthyroid patients (after a brief period of drug withdrawal) have been utilized to predict which patients will enter prolonged remission (normalized uptake) and those who will relapse (elevated uptake).[85]

Thyroid Technetium Pertechnetate (Tc-99m-O$_4$) Uptake Studies

Because Tc-99m-O4 is trapped but not organified within the thyroid, maximal uptake is achieved within 20 min of administration.[38-40] Except in those states where anion trapping and thyroid hormonogenesis are dissociated, the 20-min pertechnetate uptake may serve as a useful approximation of radioiodine uptake, although the absolute values are considerably lower.[31,38-40,86] In euthyroid patients, the 20-min Tc-99m-O$_4$ uptake is between 0.5 and 5%, and in thyrotoxic patients this may rise to as high as 25%. Uptake measurements may be performed with the probe system in a fashion analogous to radioiodine uptake or combined with gamma camera scintigraphy with thyroidal and background region of interest analysis.[86] A useful semiquantitative estimation of thyroid uptake may be obtained by comparing thyroid to salivary gland Tc-99m-O4 uptake at the time of thyroid scintigraphy.[40,86] With normal uptake, the intensity of the thyroid is equal or slightly greater than the salivary glands and visible blood background is present. With low uptake the thyroid is less intense than salivary glands and blood background is more intense than normal, whereas with high uptake the thyroid is much more intense than salivary glands and blood background activity is not visualized.[40,86]

Pharmacological Interventions

In the past, thyroid uptake measurements with and without various pharmacological interventions played a major role in the diagnosis of hyper- and hypothyroidism. Although simpler and more sensitive biochemical tests have replaced these interventional studies, they are worth reviewing for their graphic depiction of the pathophysiology and controlling feedback loops of the hypothalamic-pituitary-thyroidal axis.[2,80]

The Perchlorate Discharge Test

The perchlorate ion, like the pertechnetate ion, is trapped in thyroid tissue but not organified.[80] If administered in pharmacological quantities perchlorate will compete with iodine for thyroidal trapping.[80] This has been exploited to detect defects of iodide organification when 1 g of potassium perchlorate is administered (children 3 mg/kg body weight) 2 h after the radioiodine dose.[80] In normal subjects there is no change in the count rate over the thyroid before and after perchlorate administration, but in a positive test the count rate falls by at least 10% in conditions of congenital inborn errors of organification or acquired diseases such as Hashimoto's thyroiditis.[80] This test remains useful in determining the etiology of goitrous hypothyroidism in children and families, particularly where associated with deafness (Pendred's syndrome).[80]

The Triiodothyronine (T$_3$) Suppression Test

A graphic demonstration of the sensitive feedback loop controlling thyroid function is shown by the normal T$_3$ suppression test.[80] After determining a baseline radioiodine uptake the patient is treated with T$_3$ 100 mg daily for 7 days, following which the radioiodine uptake is again determined and will be documented to have fallen by at least 50%. A failure of the radioiodine uptake to suppress is striking proof of autonomous function due to a non-TSH stimulatory factor (e.g., stimulatory immunoglobulins in Graves' disease) or primary tissue autonomy (e.g., hyperfunctioning foci within multinodular goiters and hyperfunctioning adenomas).[80] Thyroid uptake measurements or I-123 or pertechnetate thyroid scintigraphy performed while a patient is taking suppressive or replacement doses of thyroxine may be used to establish whether glandular autonomy is present and thus the danger of iatrogenic thyrotoxicosis.[86] Autonomous thyroid tissue may be present under conditions of overall euthyroidism or hyperthyroidism depending on the degree of hormonogenesis.[80]

The TSH Stimulation Test

Before the availability of sensitive and specific serum TSH measurements, primary hypothyroidism could be distinguished from secondary hypothyroidism by measuring the thyroid uptake before and after 3 days of daily bovine TSH administration (10 IU intramuscularly).[80] In normal individuals and in secondary hypothyroidism radioiodine uptake increases by at least 15%, whereas there is no response in primary hypothyroidism.[80] A further elegant demonstration of thyroid pathophysiology occurs when TSH is administered to a patient with a hyperfunctioning thyroid nodule in which excessive secretion of thyroxine suppresses endogenous TSH and results in suppression of surrounding normal thyroid tissue.[80] In this case, the exogenous bovine TSH can be shown by scintigraphy to stimulate function and thus tracer uptake into the suppressed normal tissue. Bovine TSH was found to be allergenic and is no longer commercially available; however, biosynthetic recombinant human TSH is currently undergoing trials and will soon be available.[80,87] The greatest potential utility for human biosynthetic TSH lies not with these stimulation tests but as a means to perform whole body I-131 metastatic surveys in thyroid cancer patients without the need to withdraw thyroxine therapy (vide infra).[87]

PARATHYROID SCINTIGRAPHY

Parathyroid scintigraphy presents a number of unique challenges. The lesions being sought are small, very often less than 1 g, and they lie in an area with many large vascular structures and in close proximity to the highly vascular thyroid gland.[2,17,21]

Radiopharmaceuticals

A large number of radiotracers, including Tl-201 and MIBI-Tc-99m, have been examined for parathyroid scintigraphy but none are specific and even the best are suboptimal.[2,12,13,88-91]

Historical Background

Tracers that have been used with limited success in the past include cyanocobalomin (Co-57), which was the first investigated; selenomethionine (Se-75), a tracer of protein synthesis; and toluidine blue labeled with I-131 or subsequently with I-123 because it had been observed that intravenous toluidine blue stains the parathyroid glands *in vivo*.[2,88] There are also reports of gallium-67 locating parathyroid adenomas. All these agents suffered from poor radiation dosimetry, which limits the administered dose, which in turn limits the sensitivity and specificity of the methods. Attempts to stimulate parathyroid hormone (PTH) synthesis by infusion of EDTA (ethylene diamine tetraacetic acid) prior to Se-75 administration only slightly increased sensitivity.[2] Subsequent scintigraphic approaches to parathyroid imaging have depended on the nonspecific depiction of the highly vascular and cellular nature of parathyroid tissue by means of nonspecific blood flow tracers including Cs-131, Tl-201, and MIBI-Tc-99m.[2,92]

Thallium-Pertechnetate (Tl-201-Tc-99m) Subtraction Scintigraphy

There were a number of reports of the depiction of parathyroid adenomas by Tl-201 dating back to the 1970s.[2,92] The adjacent thyroid gland is also a highly vascular and cellular organ and thus it is difficult to distinguish the parathyroid tissue which often lies contiguous with the thyroid. This problem can be mitigated by subtracting a thyroid-specific radiopharmaceutical image from the nonspecific blood flow image by the use of computerized manipulation of digitized images. Many variations of the thallium-pertechnetate subtraction protocol have been advocated.[2,12,13,91,93,94] Initial studies utilized high-resolution, low-sensitivity pinhole collimation, which is now frequently replaced by converging or parallel hole collimation. There has been much debate about which tracer should be administered first. If the lower photon energy Tl-201 (80 keV) is injected first, there will be no interference with scattered photons from the higher energy Tc-99m (140 keV).[91] However, the patient must then be kept immobilized for at least 20 min after acquisition of the Tl-201 image to allow for sufficient Tc-99m uptake to permit thyroid imaging, which increases the risk of artifact due to patient movement. Conversely, although the period of immobilization is shorter when Tc-99m-O_4 is administered first, the scatter from Tc-99m photons into the Tl-201 energy window must be subtracted and compensated for prior to the administration of Tl-201.[2,12,91,93] Doses of Tl-201 between 1 and 5 mCi and Tc-99m-O_4 of 2–10 mCi in various combinations have been advocated.[2,12,40,91] A typical imaging sequence will display the Tl-201 and Tc-99m images acquired with the appropriate energy windows and the Tc-99m image on the Tl-201 window if the Tl-201 is administered after the Tc-99m.[91] In addition, a series of subtraction images (Tc-99m from Tl-201) are displayed, usually in 10% decrements between 0 and 100%.[2,12,91,93,94]

Sestamibi-Pertechnetate (MIBI-Tc-99m-Tc-99m-O$_4$) Subtraction Scintigraphy

The same principles have been applied using the Tc-99m-labeled blood flow agent MIBI-Tc-99m.[2,12,89,90] Because there is no difference in the photon energy between this agent and the Tc-99m-O$_4$ thyroid subtraction agent, the procedure is dependent on the relative size of the doses administered (e.g., 1–2 mCi Tc-99m-O$_4$ followed by 10 mCi MIBI-Tc-99m). In fact, the high-photon flux made possible by the large doses of MIBI-Tc-99m will frequently permit the depiction of parathyroid lesions without any subtraction.[2,12,89,90] Furthermore, the different kinetics of MIBI-Tc-99m retention in parathyroid and thyroid tissue may be exploited by comparing immediate postinjection with the 2 to 4 h delayed images because parathyroid lesions retain MIBI-Tc-99m longer than the thyroid.[2,89,95]

Other Subtraction Protocols

These are based on the same principles as the techniques already described but utilize I-123 as the thyroid-specific tracer, which is subtracted from the Tl-201 or Tc-99m-MIBI images. Thyroid subtraction with Tc-99m-O$_4$ has been applied to Se-75 imaging with little additional advantage.[2]

Limitations of Subtraction Scintigraphic Techniques

It can be seen from the protocols outlined above that successful thyroid subtraction depends on there being a fixed relationship between thyroidal uptake of the blood flow tracer (e.g., Tl-201 or MIBI-Tc-99m) and the thyroid specific (e.g., Tc-99m-O$_4$ or I-123). This holds true in normal and diffusely hyperplastic thyroid glands, but in the case of a number of pathologies, there may be a discordance. The most problematic lesion is the solitary thyroid nodule that is "cold" on thyroid scintigraphy but is also vascular. Similar areas within multinodular goiters may also pose this problem. Thus the value of parathyroid subtraction scintigraphy is markedly degraded in the presence of nodular thyroid disease.[2,92,93,96] Patient movement is a major source of artifact and every effort should be made to immobilize the patient between the acquisition of the blood flow and thyroid images. Radioactive surface markers may be placed on the chin and sternoclavicular joints to detect patient movement and, if the particular computer software permits, to realign the images.[2,92,93]

Bone Scan

The increased metabolic turnover in the skeleton in hyperparathyroidism can be depicted by the standard Tc-99m-disphosphonate nuclear medicine bone scan.[97-100] Patterns observed include diffuse increased skeletal uptake, particularly in the skull, ribs, and clavicles; focal increased uptake at the sites of brown tumors which may mimic tumor metastases; focal increased uptake at the site of pathological fractures; and uptake at sites of heterotopic calcification, including the lungs, kidneys, and stomach.[101]

The whole body retention of bone scan tracer can be determined by whole body counting, and this has been used as an index of overall skeletal turnover in metabolic bone diseases.

Thyroid Ultrasound

While early attempts to study the thyroid date back to the 1970s, early bistable and static scanner technology has been completely replaced by high-frequency (7.5–10.0 MHz), high-resolution, real-time devices.[1,14,42,102-107] The technique requires no preparation, there is no exposure to ionizing radiation, and there are no known side effects. The resolution for cysts is as small as 2 mm and for solid lesions 2–5 mm, and real-time facility permits the evaluation of pulsatile vascular structures and movement on swallowing.[1,14,102-104,107-110] The sonograms are intrinsically tomographic and are obtained in the axial, longitudinal (parasaggital), and oblique (along the axis of the thyroid lobes) planes. The patient is examined supine with the neck well extended, and swallowing may be needed to bring the lower poles of the thyroid into view.[1,14,102-104,106] Extensive retrosternal goiters cannot be fully evaluated due to the inadequate sonographic window. Fine-needle aspiration biopsy can be performed under real-time ultrasound guidance. This may be especially useful for lesions that are difficult to palpate easily and is essential for the biopsy of impalpable lesions.[1,14,104,107,111-116]

Color Doppler scanning has also been recently employed and may provide information on the vascularity of the gland as a whole or of focal lesions within the gland.[117,118]

With aging, the echogenicity of the gland increases and intraglandular fibrous septa are visualized. Small anechoic foci of colloid accumulation and echogenic vascular calcifications are also very common and may be difficult to distinguish from clinically significant pathology.[1,102,103,109,119,120]

PARATHYROID ULTRASOUND

To adequately depict parathyroid lesions by sonography it is essential to use high-resolution instrumentation (e.g., a 10-MHz transducer with a stand-off pad).[2,12-14,102,103] To explore the deeper regions of the neck it may be useful to change to a 7.5-MHz transducer.[2,11,12,102] After exploring the thyroid gland carefully the search is extended to the accessible part of the superior mediastinum (including studies while swallowing) and then to the regions of the hyoid bone and the neurovascular bundles. The normal parathyroid glands are seldom depicted by ultrasound, but enlarged glands are oval, hypoechoic solid structures which may arise at any site to which the gland may migrate.[2,11-14,93,102,103] The enlarged vasculature leading to the gland may also be visualized. Some have advocated the fine-needle aspiration of lesions suspected to be parathyroid enlargements. The aspirates are subjected to both cytology and assay of PTH and thus parathyroid lesions may be distinguished from thyroid lesions.[121]

RADIOGRAPHY

Conventional radiography has a limited but nevertheless significant role in the evaluation of the thyroid and parathyroid glands and the effects of glandular dysfunction. Evaluation of compression or deviation of the esophagus and trachea and evidence for significant extension of a goiter into the mediastinum are important factors to be weighed in deciding on surgical intervention.[1]

CHEST X-RAY AND PLANE RADIOGRAPHY

Generally the soft-tissue attenuation of thyroid lesions provides limited contrast with surrounding soft tissues. Some lesions, however, particularly papillary carcinoma, may manifest characteristic calcifications.[1] The effect of thyroid enlargements on the trachea is readily evaluated on the posterior-anterior and lateral chest x-rays. The thoracic inlet view may be especially valuable. Both tracheal compression and deviation are detected.[1] Substernal goiter extending into the superior mediastinum may also be depicted by mediastinal widening, effacement of normal contrast lines, and distortion or deviation of the trachea.[1] Rarely, goiters may extend into the posterior mediastinum in close proximity to the esophagus. The functional significance of tracheal compression may be estimated by calculation of the cross-sectional area of the lumen from measurements in two planes or better by performance of flow-volume loop spirometry.[1]

Careful serial chest radiography is essential in the management of thyroid cancer patients.[1-3,26,28] This also requires careful comparison of the chest X-ray and scintigraphic studies. Superior mediastinal and hilar lymphadenopathy may be demonstrated, and most important is the evaluation of the pulmonary parenchyma. The size and extent of pulmonary metastatic foci (and the relationship to I-131 uptake) are the most important factors in the prognosis of metastatic papillary thyroid cancer.[2,3,26,28,122] Deposits occur most often in the lower lung fields and may vary from barely perceptible miliary nodules through an obvious noduloreticular pattern to frank macronodules.[2,3,26,28,122] Very small lesions may be demonstrated by laminography or chest CT even if the face of an entirely normal chest x-ray is clear and shows no lesions (vide infra).

LAMINOGRAPHY

Thoracic laminography or poly-tomography is performed by simultaneously moving the x-ray source and the film so as to blur out the planes above and below the plane of interest. This provides better contrast and sensitivity than planar radiography but has in large measure been replaced by CT and MRI.[1]

BARIUM CONTRAST ESOPHAGOGRAPHY

By the ingestion of barium or other contrast media, compression, impression, or displacement of the esophagus can be well delineated. It is important for the examination to be performed in at least two planes. The images may be studied on image-intensified fluoroscopy with "spot" images recorded on film and/or as cine contrast esophagography.[1] Occasionally, larger parathyroid adenomas may cause a small focal indentation of the barium column.[1]

XERORADIOGRAPHY

In this technique, the x-ray image is formed on a charged xeroradiographic plate rather than a standard x-ray film. The charge is lost in proportion to the radiation exposure and the plate is then developed by its ability to attract a finely divided carbon powder, which can in turn be transferred to a paper substrate to which it can be permanently fixed by baking.[1,123] Xeroradiography has the advantage of intrinsic edge enhancement, which is especially effective in depicting small foci of calcification and thus it has been mainly utilized for mammography.[1,123] Because many papillary thyroid carcinomas may have foci of calcification or psammoma bodies, this technique has been advocated for the characterization of thyroid nodules.[1,123] Nevertheless, this approach has not been widely employed. When combined with 131-I scintigraphy, sensitivity of 75% and specificity of 85% has been reported.[1,123]

IMAGING THERMOGRAPHY

Techniques to map the pattern of skin surface temperature, which may reflect the degree of vascularity of deeper tissue structures, have been used in conjunction with thyroid scintigraphy to characterize thyroid nodules.[1,124] In the clinical setting of a scintigraphically hypofunctioning nodule, lesions that are thermographically warm are more likely to be neoplastic and thermographically cold lesions are often cysts or colloid nodules. The technique requires the examination of the patient in a controlled temperature environment and lacks both specificity and sensitivity.[1,124] There are reports of large parathyroid adenomas (which are highly vascular) being imaged by thermography.

ANGIOGRAPHY

The thyroid and associated parathyroid glands are highly vascular organs fed by multiple arteries. These can be visualized by the injection of radioopaque iodinated radiographic contrast media. The images can be observed directly on image-intensified fluoroscopy and/or recorded on film.[1,125] The images may be digitized and the pre- and postcontrast images subtracted from each other to yield images of the vessels in isolation. Direct intraarterial injection of contrast, which is an invasive and difficult procedure, may be avoided in digital venous arteriography in which a bolus of contrast is injected into the venous circulation and followed until it opacifies the arteries.[1,125] The inevitable dilution of the contrast results in images of lower quality but these may often suffice. The relatively large doses of contrast agent often result in flushing, headache, and other minor side effects. Occasionally, serious allergies (including fatal anaphylaxis) may occur. Other rare but serious side effects are heart failure, arrhythmia, and renal failure. Modern nonionic contrast media, although more expensive, may be somewhat safer. Whenever patients with thyroid disorders are subjected to contrast-enhanced radiological procedures using iodinated media (arteriography, venography, intravenous urography, contrast-enhanced CT), this must be done only after careful consideration of the following factors: (1) the patient must not be a potential candidate for I-131 therapy (the large iodine load will preclude this for at least 4 to 6 weeks); and (2) in areas with low dietary iodine intake the large iodine load may precipitate thyrotoxicosis in goiterous patients (the Jod Basedow syndrome) (see Table 3).

Many thyroid and parathyroid neoplasms are highly vascular and manifest a characteristic capillary blush.[1,125,126] Malignant lesions may also demonstrate the typical features of abnormal tumor vascularity including tortuosity, luminal irregularity, and shunt vessels.[125,126] Although angiography has been used to characterize hypofunctioning thyroid nodules, the invasive nature of the procedure and the complex vascular anatomy has made thyroid angiography obsolete.[1,125,126] In contrast, angiography still has a role in location of parathyroid lesions when noninvasive techniques have failed or provide equivocal or contradictory results. The sensitivity in this setting may, however, be relatively low (30–70%).[2,93,126] In postoperative recurrent or persistent hyperparathyroidism interpretation must be tempered by the potential for error due to altered vascular anatomy. The techniques applied include nonselective arterial digital angiography, venous digital angiography, and selective anteriography.[2,126] The latter is particularly technically challenging and requires the highest order of arteriographic skill. All these procedures carry the usual risks of iodinated contrast administration such as allergic responses. In addition, the risk of nephrotoxicity is increased in hypercalcemic patients with impaired renal function. Although nonselective arterial digital angiography and venous digital angiography are less invasive than selective angiography, they are also less sensitive. On the other hand, the selective approach carries a small risk of stroke and spinal cord infarction. Patients who are poor surgical risks or who refuse surgery may be treated by selective arteriographic injection of occlusive emboli or sclerosants (e.g., ethanol).

VENOGRAPHY AND VENOUS SAMPLING

The parathyroid venous drainage is highly variable, particularly in the case of ectopic glands.[17,22] Prior surgery can completely alter normal routes and directions of venous flow, rendering interpretation of venous sampling potentially misleading. Nevertheless, it is in this very circumstance that accurate parathyroid localization is most desirable.[2,11,17,19,20] Selective retrograde filling of all the venous radicals that might drain normally and ectopically located parathyroids is undertaken to verify the location of the catheter tip, rather than to depict the glandular lesion itself (although this is sometimes achieved).[126] When the location of the catheter tip is verified, the contrast within the catheter is flushed by means of free venous flow to avoid sample dilution. Any excessive syringe suction is to be avoided because it may disturb venous flow patterns and give rise to misleading results. Meticulous documentation of the site of sampling is essential. After the venous samples have been assayed for PTH, the results should be tabulated against the sites of sampling, or better should be plotted on a diagram that depicts the individual venous anatomy of a particular patient. A further refinement that may be practiced is to assay simultaneously acquired arterial blood samples for PTH and plot the arteriovenous PTH differences rather than absolute venous PTH concentrations. Parathyroid venous sampling is a complex and difficult procedure that should be performed only by the most experienced of arteriographers and should be reserved for those cases in whom all the usual noninvasive approaches have been unrewarding.[126] In addition to the usual risks of intravascular contrast (vide supra), venography and venous sampling carry the risks of rupture or infarction of the adenoma if excessive injection pressure is used and of air embolus during sampling.

BONE RADIOGRAPHY

The classical skeletal radiographic signs of hyperparathyroidism are now seldom seen in modern industrial countries.[127] Full-blown ostitis fibrosa cystica with erosive brown tumors, pathological fractures, pseudofractures, marked generalized osteopenia, and deformity of the softened bones is now rare. Characteristic subtle subperiosteal resorption of bone in the lateral areas of the phalanges is more frequent and is best depicted on magnification radiographs of the hands. As the population ages and the number of patients with end-stage renal disease and on dialysis increases, so the effects of renal osteodystrophy are observed more often. These include osteopenia, Looser's zones, brown tumors, abnormal sclerosis, and so-called "rugger jersey spine."[127]

Diffuse osteopenia may be observed in patients with long-standing severe hyperthyroidism.[127] Advanced metastatic follicular thyroid cancer deposits are characteristically completely lytic on bone radiographs and may not excite a response on skeletal scintigraphy. The I-131 whole body survey remains the most sensitive modality for these tumors.[1-3,6,26,28]

BONE DENSITOMETRY

Although skeletal radiography is insensitive for the evaluation of diffuse bone mineral loss, accurate quantification is possible if a narrow beam of X-rays or gamma rays are passed through the patient and detected quantitatively by means of a scintillation detector–photomultiplier tube combination.[127,128,130] The detector and radiation source (x-ray tube or sealed radionuclide source) are moved to and fro across the patient to produce a quantitative rectilinear scan. Sites evaluated include the forearm (using a single-photon I-125 source or single-energy x-ray source) or the spine, proximal femur, and/or whole body (using a dual-photon Gd source or dual-energy x-ray source). The differential attenuation of the lower energy (~40 keV) and the higher energy (~100 keV) photons permits the attenuation of surrounding soft tissue to be separated from that of the bone and thus the accurate evaluation of deep lying bones such as spine and femur.[129,131,132] The bone mineral loss due to hyperparathyroidism and hyperthyroidism can be quantified and partial recovery demonstrated after successful cure. The degree of bone mineral loss may be used in deciding which elderly patients with mild hyperparathyroidism should be subjected to surgery and to evaluate the risks of suppressive thyroid hormone administration in patients with goiter and thyroid cancer.

RENAL RADIOGRAPHY

Plane radiography may reveal renal stones and/or nephrocalcinosis in patients with hyperparathyroidism. Renal ultrasound may similarly depict stones, calcifications, or dilation of the pelvicalyceal system due to obstruction. The intravenous urogram (IVU) may delineate obstructing stones not demonstrated by other means, but care should be exercised in patients with marked hypercalcemia and impaired renal function. Contrast-enhanced CT is often performed in place of planar IVU.

THYROID COMPUTED TOMOGRAPHY

X-ray computed tomography is performed by quantifying the attenuation of a beam of x-rays passed through the patient at multiple angles and then reconstructing a cross-sectional image by filtered backprojection.[1,133,134] The windowing of the display can be adjusted to emphasize soft tissue, lung, or bone features. High-attenuation iodinated contrast media can be ingested to delineate the esophagus and the gut or injected intravenously to better delineate vascular structures and the vascularity of various lesions. Iodinated contrast media must never be administered if there is even a remote possibility that I-131 therapy might be required (e.g., for thyroid cancer or hyperthyroidism) (vide supra)[1,107,133,134] (see Table 3).

Normal thyroid tissue has a significantly greater x-ray attenuation (40 to 60 HU) than other surrounding soft tissue structures (20 to 30 HU) due to the normal high iodine content of the thyroid gland (after intravenous contrast injection the attenuation increases by 25 HU). Movement or the presence of metal clips and sutures may give rise to streak or "starburst" artifacts which degrade the diagnostic quality of the procedure.[1,107,133,134]

Thyroid and parathyroid CT are performed with the neck well extended and perhaps with some gantry tilt (10–15°). Contiguous or interdigitated 5-mm sections are obtained from the level of the hyoid bone to the root of the aorta for the study of thyroid masses, substernal goiter, and recurrent thyroid cancer.[107,134,135] For suspected pulmonary metastasis thin sections (2 or 3 mm) are obtained every centimeter.[1,133] CT of the skull, orbits, and pituitary has a major role in the evaluation of Graves' ophthalmopathy to depict the proptosis, occular muscle, and soft tissue thickening, and for the depiction of pituitary lesions, but that lies outside the scope of this review.[1]

PARATHYROID COMPUTED TOMOGRAPHY

Normal sized parathyroid glands are seldom visualized.[12,16,93] The sensitivity for the detection of lesions is very much dependent on their size. Because of the vascularity of parathyroid tissue, lesions may be well depicted by bolus contrast injection followed by dynamic acquisition. The technique is especially valuable in locating retroclavicular, mediastinal, and retrosternal glands.[12,16,93] Usually, contiguous or interdigitated 5-mm sections from the level of the hyoid bone to the root of the aorta will suffice. In some recurrent or persistent cases, it may be useful to extend the examination from the skull base through the heart.

THYROID MAGNETIC RESONANCE IMAGING

MRI generates tomographic sections in any desired plane without exposure to ionizing radiation. The patient is placed in a very high magnetic field and then interrogated with a suitable radiofrequency signal.[1,136] This causes paramagnetic nuclei, of which protons are by far the most abundant, to align off axis and precess. When they return to normal orientation they do so by emitting a radiofrequency signal that can be detected and decoded. The strong magnetic field is supplemented by gradient fields so that the emitted signal encodes not only the proton density and chemical milieu but also the spatial coordinates.[1] Various radiofrequency pulses are used to perturb the aligned nuclei.[136-139] Two different relaxation times can be calculated—T_2 (spin-spin) and T_1 (spin-lattice)—and images weighted to each of these parameters can be produced. The major advantage of MRI is the excellent and varied soft tissue contrast. On T_1 weighted images fat appears bright, whereas on T_2 weighted images tissues with high water content appear brightest and fat darker. Flowing blood yields no signal and thus vascular structures have black lumens. The iron present in the hemoglobin and hemosiderin of hemorrhages yields an intense signal.[1,136,138] The initial hope that analysis of MRI parameters would reliably differentiate between benign and malignant lesions has not been entirely borne out.[1,136,138-143] The intravenous administration of the paramagnetic metal gadolinium in chelated form (Gd-EDTA) can be used to depict the vascularity and capillary permeability of a tissue. Unlike iodinated radiographic contrast media, Gd-EDTA is not known to alter thyroid function and, most importantly, does not decrease subsequent I-131 uptake.

Clinical thyroid MRI is performed with the patient positioning similar to that for CT. The use of surface coils usually provides the best images, and 5- to 7-mm sections are created in the transaxial, coronal, and saggital planes.[1,136,143] On T_1 weighted images normal thyroid has a signal equal to or slightly greater than the adjacent muscles and is homogenous.[136-139,141-143] On T_2 weighted images the thyroid is more intense than the muscles and is homogenous in younger patients, but with age, some normal inhomogeneity may develop.[136-139,141-143] The normal gland enhances intensely with Gd-EDTA administration.

PARATHYROID MAGNETIC RESONANCE IMAGING

As with CT, the normal parathyroid gland is not usually visualized.[15,93,142,144] In general, positioning and technical procedures are as for thyroid MRI (vide supra). EKG gating and respiratory phase encoding can be applied to minimize the effects of vascular flow and pulsation and respiratory movement. Enlarged glands are oval with the long axis cranio-caudal.[15,142,144] On T_1-weighted images the parathyroid enlargement appears isointense with the thyroid, whereas it is hyperintense with T_2-weighted sequences. Hyperplasia cannot be reliably distinguished from adenoma.[15,142,144] All types of lesions enhance intensely with Gd-EDTA administration.[15,93,144]

THYROID DISEASES

The medical imaging procedures already discussed have a significant role to play in the management of many diseases and these applications are discussed below with reference to the individual pathologies.

CONGENITAL ABNORMALITIES

Abnormalities of embryological development may lead to ectopic thyroid tissue in the tongue, above the hyoid bone, in the mediastinum, or elsewhere. Such ectopic locations are often associated with hypothyroidism (vide infra) or may present as mass lesions of uncertain origin.[22,145] Anatomically based techniques such as ultrasound (most often used), CT, or MRI may provide detailed data as to anatomical relations and may be diagnostic for lesions such as cystic hygroma, but many thyroid-derived masses are nonspecific.[14,102-104,106,107] In contrast, radionuclide studies that demonstrate intense uptake of Tc-99m-O_4 or I-123 are diagnostic of thyroid tissue[22,145] (Figure 1).

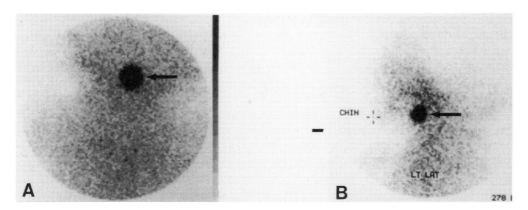

FIGURE 1. Tc-99m-O_4 scans (**A**, anterior; **B**, left lateral) in a hypothyroid patient with a lingual thyroid depicted as a single focus of tracer uptake in the base of the tongue (arrow).

Thyroglossal duct cysts present as midline neck masses. They frequently contain functioning thyroid tissue and may need removal for cosmetic reasons, infection, or very rarely for tumor.[22] Prior to cyst resection a thyroid scan should be performed to establish the location and site(s) of thyroid tissue (occasionally the tissue in the cyst is the only thyroid tissue present).[22,145] Hemiagenesis may occur and is well depicted by scintigraphy, but an ultrasound study may be needed to exclude a "cold" mass on the side of absent thyroid tissue.[22,102-104,106,107,145]

A very rare form of ectopic thyroid tissue can be found in ovarian teratomas. Such tissue may become hyperfunctional and autonomous, which leads to hyperthyroidism with suppressed radioiodine uptake over the thyroid in the neck (stroma ovarii). Even more rarely, malignant tumors may arise in stroma ovarii.

HYPOTHYROIDISM
Neonatal and Infant Hypothyroidism

All modern industrialized countries have introduced neonatal screening programs for the early detection of hypothyroidism.[145] Various programs use either free T_4 (thyroxine) or TSH as the primary test. By so doing, early treatment can be initiated and a vast burden of mental retardation, suffering, and cost prevented.[145] Once a diagnosis of hypothyroidism is made it is necessary to distinguish between those that are transient (e.g., antithyroid drugs taken by the mother or maternal TSH receptor-blocking antibodies) and those that are permanent. In the latter group it is important to separate those that are sporadic (e.g., agenesis, lingual [Figure 1], or other ectopic location) from those where the thyroid is in a normal location but in whom dyshormonogenesis is present, often due to an inherited error in the synthetic pathway.[145] The dyshomogeneses are inherited and thus subsequent pregnancies can also be affected. They can then be subject to intrauterine diagnosis (by ultrasound and intrauterine blood sampling) and even experimental treatment by the introduction of thyroid hormone into the amniotic fluid.[145] The perchlorate discharge test may be useful in definitely diagnosing hypothyroidism due to inherited dyshomogenesis (e.g., Pendred's syndrome) or acquired disorders (e.g., Hashimoto's thyroiditis).[80]

Hypothyroidism in Adults

Medical imaging has a limited role in adult hypothyroidism.[2,39,80] Although not required for diagnosis of hypothyroidism, the eitiology may be revealed in most cases by various combinations of thyroid scintigraphy (I-123 or Tc-99m-O_4) and ultrasound.[14,40,102-104] This may help define hypothyroidism associated with thyroiditis and multinodular goiter.[146,147] In goiterous hypothyroidism associated with acquired or inherited dyshomogenesis, the perchlorate discharge test may be positive.[80] Early in the natural history of such glands the goiter is a diffuse colloid process that may become multinodular over time. Very rarely CT or MRI might be needed to define a multinodular or intrathoracic goiter in patients who are hypothyroid (or hyperthyroid).[137,148,149]

HYPERTHYROIDISM
Diagnosis

Imaging procedures and nonimaging radionuclide studies have little role in the diagnosis of hyperthyroidism.[2,37,39,83,86,135,149] All primary hyperthyroidism has as a sine qua non suppressed TSH level which is the principal test for diagnosis.[83] Total or free T_4 and T_3 may further help to define the diagnosis and severity of the disease. In the very rare circumstance of TSH-secreting pituitary tumors, thyroid hormones and TSH are elevated and in such cases occasionally the radioiodine uptake and suppression tests may be useful.[83]

Differential Diagnosis

The correct classification of the type of hyperthyroidism may have an important role in the appropriate choice of management (Table 4).[2,83,86,150] Graves' disease may remit after a course of antithyroid drugs whereas toxic multinodular goiter and toxic solitary nodules do not. Forms of hyperthyroidism associated with increased radioiodine uptake can be treated by therapeutic doses of I-131, but those that are associated with low uptakes cannot (Table 4).[83,84,150,151] Some dosimetric schemes involve the administration of radioiodine and may utilize (1) radioiodine uptakes with I-131 or I-123, usually at 24 h but also in some approaches at 2, 4, 24, or 48 h, or even absolute measurements of iodine uptake using PET and I-124,[34,35,84] or (2) measurements of thyroid volume by clinical palpation or ultrasound.[84]

TABLE 4
Radioactive Iodine Uptake to Classify the Etiology of Thyrotoxicosis

A. Increased radioactive iodine uptake
  1. Graves' disease
  2. Toxic multinodular goiter (Plummer's disease)
  3. Solitary toxic nodule
  4. Trophoblastic tumors secreting chorionic gonadotropin
  5. Pituitary tumors secreting TSH
  6. Hypothalamic/pituitary thyroid hormone resistance
B. Reduced radioactive iodine uptake
  1. Subacute, granulomatous (DeQuervain's) thyroiditis
  2. Painless thyroiditis
  3. Hashimoto's thyroiditis
  4. Exogenous thyroid hormone ingestion (thyrotoxicosis factitia)
  5. Jod Basedow disease (thyrotoxicosis following iodide load)
  6. Ectopic thyroid tissue[a]
    a. mediastinal goiter
    b. metastatic well-differentiated thyroid carcinoma
    c. stroma ovarii

[a] Reduced radioactive iodine uptake in the neck; radioiodine uptake may be demonstrated at the site(s) of the ectopic tissue.

Separation of Graves' disease or toxic diffuse goiter from other forms of primary hyperthyroidism can be accomplished by careful physical examination that discloses an enlarged smooth occasionally firm thyroid and findings of ophthalmopathy and other manifestations of thyroid acropachy.[83,137,150] Often, even the most meticulous examinations will disclose only diffuse, and at times, not a striking amount of thyroid enlargement. Thyroid imaging with isotopes of iodine, either I-131 or I-123, or Tc-99m pertechnetate will portray the gland as diffusely and symmetrically enlarged[83,86,137,150,151] (Figures 2 and 3). Other forms of primary hyperthyroidism will be distinguished from Graves' disease by either patchy, but obviously increased, radiotracer uptake in toxic multinodular goiter or toxic nodule(s) with one (Plummer's disease) or more palpable nodules that avidly accumulate either radioiodine or Tc-99m pertechnetate with accompanying suppression of the remaining nonautonomous thyroid tissues[30,83,86,150,151] (Figures 4). Other forms of hyperthyroidism such as that from exogenous thyroid hormone administration or from hypothalamic-pituitary neoplasms, struma ovarii, or trophoblastic tissue secretion of human chorionic gonadotropin do not lend themselves to thyroid imaging per se because the etiology of the hyperthyroidism lies outside of the thyroid.[83,86,150]

THYROIDITIS

Thyroiditis syndromes are a heterogeneous group of disorders classified as acute suppurative, subacute, chronic, and fibrous (Riedels). Acute or suppurative thyroiditis is a rare condition associated with bacterial infection of the gland. Patients present with the abrupt onset of neck pain and clinical manifestations of systemic infection. Imaging of the gland will disclose focal, decreased area(s) of uptake that correspond to the affected areas of the gland. Gram stain and culture of materials aspirated from these regions will confirm the diagnosis of localized infection. Ga-67 may be positive in this condition.[52]

Subacute thyroiditis classically presents as a self-limited course of transient hyperthyroidism followed by either euthyroidism or hypothyroidism with a return to the euthyroid state over weeks to months.[146] The gland may be painful or painless (silent thyroiditis) to palpation.[146] Occasionally occurring in the immediate postpartum interval, thyroiditis can be mistaken for postpartum depression, especially if the patient presents in the hypothyroid

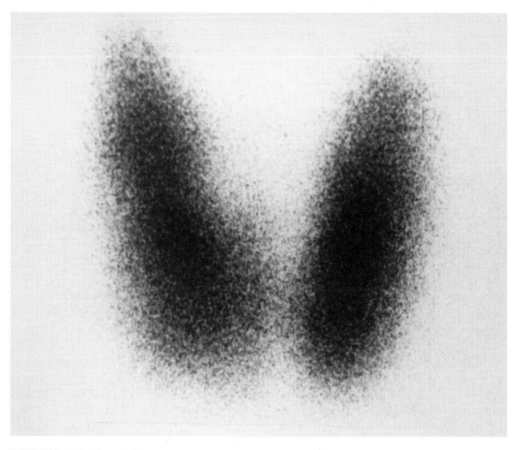

FIGURE 2. Mild Graves' disease. Tc-99m-O$_4$ scan shows a thyroid gland that is of normal configuration but shows somewhat increased diffuse tracer uptake and low background.

phase of the syndrome. The etiology of this thyroiditis is unknown but a causal relationship with antecedent viral illnesses has been made.[146] Thyroid inflammation results in the release of stored hormone and impaired accumulation of radioiodine leading to the important finding of a low (usually less than 1–2% at 24 h) radioiodine uptake in the setting of an elevated T$_4$ or T$_3$ and a suppressed TSH level.[27,38,39,40,42,86,146] Ultrasound may have a role in selected cases.[14,102-106,146,146a] The management of subacute thyroiditis is for the most part observation, but in some cases β-blockade to relieve symptoms of hyperthyroxinemia and corticosteroids to relieve pain may be used. It is not uncommon for patients to have more than one episode of thyroiditis.[10]

Chronic thyroiditis (Hashimoto's thyroiditis) typically presents as an asymptomatic thyroid enlargement more frequently observed in women than men. Chronic thyroiditis is usually seen in people who are in their 40s and 50s, but may occur in patients of any age. Antibodies against microsomal and/or thyroglobulin are usually detected, and the disease may be familial and/or associated with other autoimmune diseases including Graves' disease, diabetes mellitus, pernicious anemia, premature gonadal failure, vitiligo, and adrenal insufficiency. Lymphocytic and plasma cell infiltration with destruction of follicular elements of the thyroid is the pathologic hallmark of chronic thyroiditis. Thyroid dysfunction sufficient to cause frank hypothyroidism occurs in about 50% of patients, but hyperthyroidism is occasionally seen in patients with chronic thyroiditis ("Hashitoxicosis").

Thyroid scintigraphy typically depicts a gland with inhomogeneous distribution of radioiodine or technetium pertechnetate that can at times be focal.[2,27,31,38-41] Radioiodine uptake can be quite variable, ranging from high to normal or low depending on the stage of the

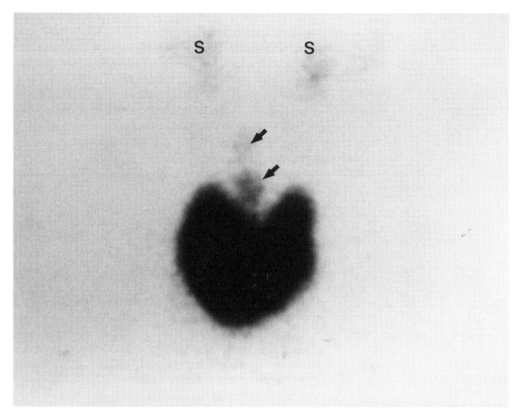

FIGURE 3. Severe Graves' disease. Tc-99m-O$_4$ scan shows intense uptake in a diffusely enlarged gland. There is uptake in a hypertrophic thyroglossal duct (arrows). Note the intensity of thyroid uptake relative to the normal salivary gland (S) and general background.

disease and the severity of lymphocytic infiltration.[80] As acquired organification defects may be seen in chronic thyroiditis, perchlorate discharge studies can be abnormal, but are more of a historical interest because these studies are infrequently performed in this clinical setting.[80] Diffuse enlargement and a number of nonspecific ultrasound patterns are observed.[14,103,104,106,107,110] Differentiation of chronic thyroiditis from primary lymphoma of the thyroid may be difficult, even with adequate cytology obtained at thyroid biopsy.[141]

In end-stage, hypothyroid chronic thyroiditis the thyroid may be completely destroyed with resultant very low radioiodine uptake and minimal thyroid visualization on scintigraphy.[80]

EUTHYROID DIFFUSE GOITER

Euthyroid or nontoxic goiter presents as a slowly enlarging gland usually over decades that is characterized by variable follicular size, colloidal content, cellular morphology, and iodine metabolism. Diffuse goiter may occur either as a sporadic event or in endemic form with epidemiologic patterns as a distinguishing factor separating these two entities. Diagnosis usually is not problematic with an enlarged gland in an otherwise asymptomatic patient usually with a family history of goiter.[4] Biochemical studies such as serum T$_4$ and TSH levels are normal.[2] Aside from clinical findings of a mass in the neck, other manifestations of thyroid disease are lacking.

Aside from simple, clinical examination and neck palpation, euthyroid diffuse goiter has no other distinguishing clinical features.[4] When the size of a gland is questioned a high-resolution ultrasound can be used to establish the presence of an enlarged thyroid and to distinguish a diffuse from nodular gland by ultrasound characteristics.[14,103,104,106,107,110] Ultra-

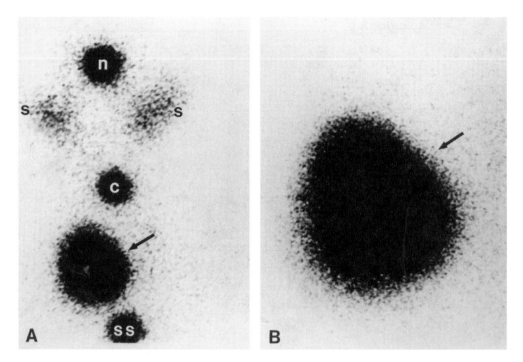

FIGURE 4. Toxic single nodule depicted by Tc-99m-O$_4$ scan. (**A**) Head and neck view showing intense tracer uptake in nodule (arrow) relative to normal salivary gland uptake (s). Radioactive markers on nose (n), chin (c), and suprasternal notch (ss). (**B**) Detailed view of toxic nodule (arrow). Note complete suppression of tracer uptake in adjacent normal thyroid tissue.

sonography is also useful in clinical circumstances where there is suspected compression of neck structures such as the trachea or esophagus.[14,103,104,106,107,110] Other anatomic imaging modalities such as chest x-rays, CT, and MRI have also been used to document thyroid compression of adjacent neck structures.[15,133-136,138,148,149] Barium swallow has proven useful in documenting esophageal compression, and pulmonary function studies of airflow (i.e., flow volume loops) may be able to quantify the functional significance of tracheal compression in patients presenting with either stridor or shortness of breath and an enlarged thyroid.

Scintigraphic studies with radioiodine or Tc-99m pertechnetate are useful to confirm the clinical findings of diffuse goiter.[2,27,31,38-41] Substernal extension of goiter is not an uncommon finding and may be identified on chest x-ray, CT, or MRI.[15,133,134,138,144,147-149] As a result of variable uptake of either radioiodine or Tc-99m pertechnetate, the substernal portion of the goiter may be depicted as functionally different than the cervical thyroid on scintigraphic studies.

MULTINODULAR EUTHYROID GOITER

Diffuse nodular enlargement of the thyroid is classically characterized as a multinodular gland in the absence of overt thyroid dysfunction. Palpation plays a major role in distinguishing this form of thyroid enlargement from euthyroid diffuse goiter.[4] The size of the gland and the presence of nodules can be readily ascertained from high-resolution ultrasound or scintigraphy with radioiodine or Tc99m pertechnetate[2,14,31,39,40,42,102-104,106,107,147] (Figure 5). Evaluation of patients with compression syndromes is identical to that used for the evaluation of diffuse thyroid goiter, with chest x-ray, CT, MRI, barium swallow, and pulmonary function studies (i.e., flow volume loops) (vide supra).[15,133,134,136,138,144,147-149]

The etiology of multinodular euthyroid goiter is felt to be the result of the same intrathyroidal goiterogenic processes that lead to diffuse colloid goiter, with functional variation of follicular elements leading to thyroid enlargement and nodule formation. Thus, diffuse

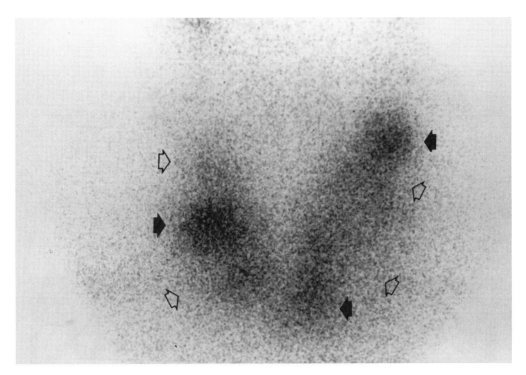

FIGURE 5. Euthyroid multinodular goiter depicted by Tc-99m-O$_4$ scan as multiple areas of increased tracer uptake (solid arrows) and areas of reduced tracer uptake (open arrows).

goiter may, in some instances, progress to a nodular form particularly in older patients. Growth-stimulating antibodies without resultant thyroid dysfunction has been evoked as a causative factor in the development of some diffuse and nodular goiters.

Although imaging plays only a limited role in most multinodular glands, scintigraphy or ultrasound can be used to assist in the prebiopsy identification of "clinically suspicious" nodules in these glands where fine-needle aspiration of dominant nodules or nodules enlarging under observation is undertaken.[1,2,7-10,111,152] Scintigraphy, CT, or MRI may be required to assess the full extent of substernal extension[15,40,44,102,103,134,135,144,147,149,151] (Figure 6).

SOLITARY AND DOMINANT NODULES

Imaging to characterize solitary or dominant nodules has largely been supplanted by needle biopsy in most clinical situations.[1,9,152-155] The presence of a solitary thyroid nodule in an otherwise impalpable normal gland or a dominant nodule in an enlarged or multinodular thyroid raises the question of thyroid malignancy.[4] Previously, scintigraphy was used to characterize the functional nature of thyroid nodules[1,9,151,153-155] (Table 5). Categorization into hot, warm, and cold nodules was used to guide further evaluation and therapy.[8,9] The classification of a suspect nodule as "cold" or nonfunctioning and not radioiodine-avid suggested that further evaluation was necessary to exclude malignancy (the risk being approximately 10%)[8,9,105,152,153,156] (Figures 7 and 8). A "hot" nodule (radioiodine-avid) virtually excludes malignancy but may evolve toward autonomous hyperfunction[8,30,88,135,153,156] (figures 4 and 9). Warm nodules are suspect but somewhat less so than those without apparent function (no accumulation of radioiodine). Other radioisotopes have been used to functionally characterize thyroid nodules. Although not organified, Tc-99m pertechnetate is accumulated by functioning thyroid tissues.[31,40] The absence of Tc-99m pertechnetate uptake by nodules is associated with a higher incidence of malignancy and has been used in this application to aid in the identification of potentially malignant nodules.[9,40,105,152,153] Conversely, technetium pertechnetate

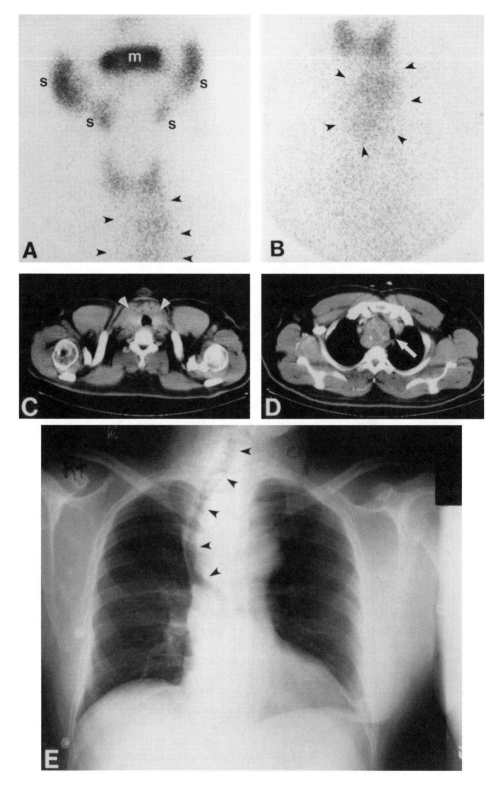

FIGURE 6.   Large substernal goiter. (**A** and **B**) Depiction by Tc-99m-O$_4$ scan: normal tracer uptake in salivary glands (s) and mouth (m). Large substernal goiter outlined by arrowheads. (**C** and **D**) Depiction by CT scan: the enlarged gland (white arrowheads) surrounds undisplaced cervical trachea (**C**) and large goiter (white arrow) displaces intrathoracic trachea (**D**). (**E**) Chest X-ray depicts marked tracheal deviation to the right (arrowheads).

uptake in a nodule may very rarely be misleading because some thyroid malignancies may accumulate technetium pertechnetate and image as "hot" or "warm" nodules.[31] The other major means of categorizing such nodules is ultrasonography, which can delineate solid from cystic lesions and find evidence of local invasiveness or lymph node enlargement.[102-107,109,112] Thallium-201 and Tc-99m MIBI have been used in addition to Tc-99m pertechnetate for the imaging of nodules.[2,44-47] These agents can be used to identify the vascularity of masses but provide no information concerning their functional status.[45] Gallium-67 citrate can also be used to characterize some thyroid nodules.[52] Lymphoma, metastases to the thyroid, and anaplastic thyroid carcinoma have all been imaged with radiogallium.[52] The use of CT or MRI is only occasionally required in the management of thyroid nodules.[135,141,149]

TABLE 5
Imaging Characteristics of Solitary Thyroid Nodules

	Possibly Malignant[a]	Probably Benign[a]
I-123 or Tc-99m-O$_4$	"Cold"[†]	"Hot" or "warm"[†]
Nuclear angiography	Vascular	Avascular
Tl-201	Positive[†]	Negative
Tc-99m MIBI scintigraphy	Positive[†]	Negative
Ga-67 scintigraphy	Positive	Negative
Thermography	Hot	
Xerography	Microcalcifications	No calcifications or laminar calcifications
Ultrasound	Obvious nodal metastases[†]	Thin-walled simple cyst[†]
	Ill-defined margins[†]	
	Solid mass[†]	
	Complex cyst	
CT	Obvious nodal metastases[†]	Thin-walled simple cyst[†]
	Ill-defined margins[†]	
	Solid mass[†]	
	Complex cyst	
MRI	Obvious nodal metastases[†]	Thin-walled simple cyst[†]
	Ill-defined margins[†]	
	Solid mass[†]	
	Complex cyst	

[a]   All tests lack both sensitivity and specificity; the most useful diagnostic features are indicated by [†].

THYROID CANCER

Thyroid cancer is classified into four major types: papillary, follicular, medullary, and anaplastic.[1-3,26] Papillary and follicular thyroid carcinoma arise from thyroid follicular cells and retain, to a variable degree, their ability to concentrate radioactive iodine, albeit to a lesser degree than normal thyroid tissues.[1-3,26] This radioiodine-concentrating ability may render such tumors amenable to effective therapy with I-131 after the removal of the bulk of primary tumor. Hürthle cell neoplasms are a subset of thyroid neoplasms that are characterized by abundant mitochondrial elements and have characteristic cytologic and pathologic characteristics.[1-3,26] Often presenting as a solitary nodule, these tumors can be benign or malignant. They frequently do not accumulate sufficient radioiodine for imaging or for attempts at therapy. Medullary cancer arises from the parafollicular or C cells of the thyroid, and does not concentrate radioiodine, but secretes calcitonin. Anaplastic carcinoma arises from follicular cells, but is so dedifferentiated that radioiodine accumulation for imaging or therapy with radioiodine does not occur.[1-3,26] In some instances a well-differentiated papillary or follicular cancer may dedifferentiate into an anaplastic cancer.[1-3,26]

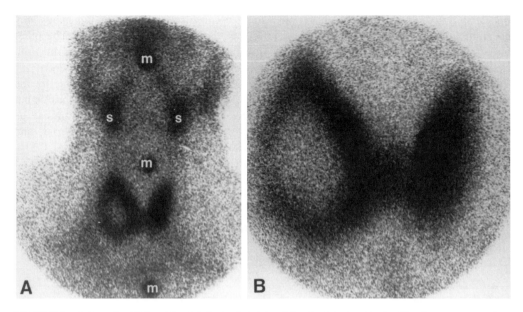

FIGURE 7.   Solitary "cold" thyroid nodule in the right lobe of the gland depicted by Tc-99m-O$_4$ scan. m = markers on nose, thyroid cartilage, and suprasternal notch; s = normal uptake in salivary glands. (**A**) head, neck, and upper chest; (**B**) detailed view.

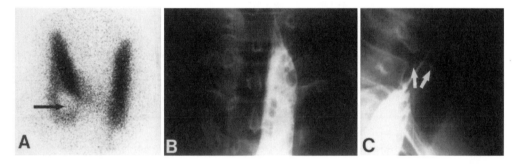

FIGURE 8.   Solitary thyroid nodule. (**A**) Depiction as a "cold" nodule by Tc-99m-O$_4$ scan (arrow). (**B**) Lateral displacement of barium-filled esophagus. (**C**) Thin rim of calcification (white arrows) in wall of a cyst due to organized hemorrhage.

Papillary Thyroid Cancer

Papillary thyroid cancer constitutes the majority of all thyroid neoplasms and comprises lesions that are "pure papillary" and those that demonstrate mixed papillary and follicular elements.[1-3,26] The degree of follicular differentiation and colloid formation varies considerably, but radioiodine concentrating ability may still be present in some neoplasms without detectable colloid formation. Papillary cancer is usually unifocal but presents as multicentric disease in about 25% of patients.[1-3,26] Papillary cancer may be divided into occult and clinical forms (intrathyroidal and extrathyroidal primaries) based on the size of the primary tumor. Neoplasms less than 1.0 cm in diameter are classified as occult because these are not usually detected on routine physical examination. Occult papillary thyroid cancer is seen at autopsy in up to 30% of patients without known thyroid disease. Very rarely, patients present with detectable metastases even with undetectable primary lesions.[1-3,26] The overall prognosis of lesions less than 1.0 cm is excellent and the term "occult" is used in this context to denote the clinical significance of these lesions.[1-3,26] Predictive factors that have been shown to affect prognosis in patients with papillary thyroid cancer are advanced age (>40 years), male sex,

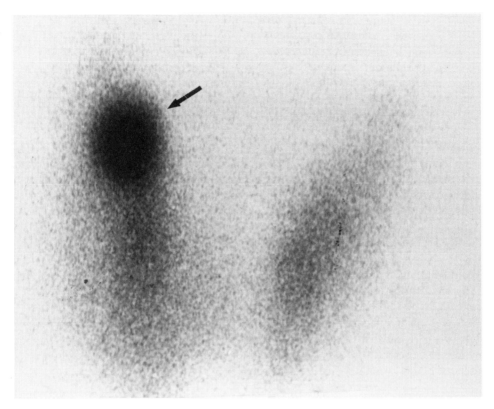

FIGURE 9. Tc-99m-O$_4$ scan of solitary "warm" nodule (arrow) in a euthyroid patient. Note tracer uptake in adjacent normal thyroid tissue is not completely suppressed.

tumor histologic grade, size of the primary lesion at initial diagnosis, regional invasion, local recurrence, and distant metastases.[1-3,26] Patients often present with local cervical lymph node metastases (approximately 1/3). These lymph node metastases do not appear to greatly influence survival, but do increase morbidity and the need for reoperation.[1-3,26] Metastases to lung or bone are relatively uncommon but are associated with higher mortality particularly when bone metastases are present.[1-3,26]

Follicular Thyroid Cancer

Pure follicular thyroid cancer represents up to 20% of all thyroid cancers and may be subdivided into encapsulated, minimally invasive or nonencapsulated and invasive.[1-3,26] Follicular cancer is usually unifocal and tends to occur in older patients who may have had long-standing goiters; the primary lesions are usually larger than papillary cancers at diagnosis. The major route of metastasis of follicular thyroid cancer is hematogenous with spread to bone and lung. The vast majority of these lesions show considerable avidity for radioactive iodine.[1-3,26]

Medullary Thyroid Cancer

Medullary cancer of the thyroid constitutes approximately 10% of all thyroid cancers.[1-3,26] MCT can be either sporadic or familial. Sporadic disease is characterized as unifocal tumors usually presenting as a solitary (usually large) thyroid mass. MCT metastasizes by both the hematogenous and lymphatic routes.[1-3,26] Metastasis may already be present in up to half of the patients at the time of initial diagnosis. Familial C-cell hyperplasia is a precursor of MCT, is present in both lobes, and allows differentiation of familial (e.g., associated with MEN 2a and 2b) from sporadic forms of the disease. The familial forms of MCT are usually bilateral and multifocal.[1-3,26] Familial MCT can be detected at an early stage of evolution by provocative testing using pentagastrin or calcium infusion. These same tests can also be used to detect early and occult metastatic MCT. Recently, gene mapping has been useful in identifying patients with the familial syndromes associated with medullary thyroid cancer. Because MCT is not derived from thyroid follicular cells this tumor is not radioactive iodine avid.[6] Many lesions can be demonstrated by nonspecific blood flow tracers (Tl-201 or Tc-99m MIBI)[11,42,43,50] or by MIBG,[58-62] Tc-99m DMSA-V,[2,51,60] or In-111-Octreotide.[54,55,74]

Anaplastic Thyroid Cancer

The highly malignant anaplastic thyroid cancers account for less than 5% of all thyroid cancers and are considered to be of dedifferentiated follicular origin.[1-3,26] They usually occur in older patients. A locally invasive and rapidly growing tumor, anaplastic thyroid cancer spreads late with regional metastases. Survival is very poor, usually measured in months. These malignancies do not concentrate radioactive iodine sufficient for diagnostic imaging or therapy,[2,3,26] but are often Ga-67 avid on scintigraphy.[1,52,53]

Thyroid Imaging

Thyroid imaging in suspected thyroid cancer is used to define the anatomy and functional status of a thyroid nodule (vide infra); detect early, occult, or minimal cancer in high risk patients (e.g., with a history of neck irradiation[3,26,157,158]); detect primary disease in a patient with known regional or distant thyroidal cancer metastases; detect thyroid cancer metastases (both regional or distant); assess suitability for radioactive iodine treatment; and monitor the therapeutic effects of radioiodine treatment(s).[2,3,26,28]

Preoperative Studies

Preoperative studies to evaluate patients with thyroid nodules have been discussed in a previous section. Radioiodine or Tc-99m pertechnetate have been used to characterize nodules prior to either biopsy or thyroidectomy.[2,3,9,26,31,36,38] A history of previous radiation exposure to the neck is important because functional imaging may predict malignancy in up to 40% of "cold" nodules in this clinical setting.[157,158] Distant metastases or regional involvement is usually not imaged scintigraphically in patients with known thyroid cancer while a significant mass of normal thyroid tissue remains in the neck.[1-3,26,39] Thus, in patients who present with thyroid nodules, nodes in the neck or disease demonstrable by palpation or anatomical imaging (e.g., CT or MRI), consideration of thyroid malignancy, radioiodine, or technetium pertechnetate may not offer sufficient specificity to distinguish thyroid from nonthyroid etiologies.[2,3,26,39,113-116]

Detection of Thyroid Cancer Metastases

Primary well-differentiated thyroid cancer and its metastases usually accumulate radio-iodine, but less avidly than normal thyroid tissue. In an effort to enhance radioiodine accumulation by both residual primary and metastatic thyroid cancer deposits, elevation of TSH is most useful.[1-3,26,28,122,159] Optimal preparation for the detection of metastatic thyroid cancer thus requires an initial subtotal or total thyroidectomy in order to remove the primary lesion and the major fraction of the normal functioning thyroid tissues. Usually, at an interval of approximately 6 weeks postsurgery is a time period sufficient to allow for the prolonged exposure to elevated levels of TSH and the imaging of potential thyroid cancer metastases[1-3,26,122,159] (Figures 10–13). An alternative to the 6-week protocol is to use 3 weeks of T_3 therapy which is discontinued 3 weeks prior to scanning. This is a welcome alternative for those patients who tolerate poorly the abrupt and prolonged removal of thyroid hormone.[1-3,26] TSH levels must be measured at the time of imaging to document adequate patient preparation, especially in those instances where there is no discernible radioiodine accumulation. Nonvisualization of metastatic disease in studies performed in the face of suboptimal

TSH elevation (<25–50 µIU/ml) must be interpreted with great caution.[2,3,26] Stimulation of radioiodine uptake with exogenous TSH (bovine and more recently recombinent human) or oral thyrotropin-releasing hormone has been proposed and may have clinical utility.[87] The general availability of human recombinant TSH (which is anticipated within 2 years) may obviate the problems inherent in the use of thyroid hormone withdrawal protocols.[87] The visualization of metastases may be further enhanced with low-iodine diets and diuretics or other drugs used to reduce circulating iodine levels.[2,3,26] The review of pathologic tissues with emphasis on the evaluation of colloid and thyroglobulin is critical to ensure that proper patient selection is maintained. Those tumors without radioiodine accumulation such as Hürthle cell neoplasms, anaplastic cancer, or MCT do not lend themselves to radioiodine imaging or therapy and should be excluded from this type of evaluation.[1-3,26]

The ideal dose of radioactive iodine to be used for postthyroidectomy imaging of well-differentiated thyroid cancer remains controversial.[2,3,26,36,122,159] It is evident that higher doses of radioiodine will allow imaging of a greater number of smaller metastatic foci (Figure 14), but higher initial radiation exposure from the diagnostic dose to neoplastic tissues may result in injury or "stunning" and thus render subsequent therapeutic doses of radioiodine less efficacious.[36,159,160] The finding of activity within the thyroid bed postthyroidectomy is not unusual because even the best of thyroid surgeons finds a true, total thyroidectomy difficult to perform without morbidity. Regional lymph node metastases and distant metastases can usually be identified as foci of 131-I uptake outside of the normal distribution of radioiodine (Figures 15–17). In situations where 24-h postadministration images are ambiguous, delayed images at 48 to 72 h may be helpful in further defining potential abnormal foci of radioiodine uptake.[2,3,26,28,36,37,122] Treatment plans are usually based upon finding metastatic disease and where metastases are located.[2,3,26,28,122,160] Conventional doses of 131-I for therapy of well-differentiated thyroid cancer typically range from 30 to 100 mCi for the ablation of normal thyroid tissues in the neck, 100 to 150 mCi for therapy of regional lymph node metastases and 150 to 250 mCi for remote metastases to lung, bone, and other sites[2,3,26,28,33,122,160] (Figures 14 and 18). An alternative approach is to individualize the dose on the basis of radiation dosimetry measurements.[2,3,26,28,81,82,122,160] Dosimetric evaluation of radioactive iodine therapy can be extremely useful in escalating doses to maximize therapy, particularly in patients with metastases to lung and bone where the conventional limits of I-131 doses are typically 200–250 mCi. Dosimetric measurements allow administration of much larger doses (300–600 mCi) without significant morbidity if the whole body and blood self-irradiation remain below 200 rads.[81,82] A small number of patients (particularly those with poor renal function and large I-131 avid tumor burdens) are administered smaller doses of I-131 than would be the case if standardized doses are used.[81,82] Pulmonary fibrosis can be avoided if the lung uptake of I-131 at 48 h is kept below 80 mCi.[3,26,28,81,82]

Posttherapy Images

Posttherapy images obtained after the therapeutic administration of I-131 (when residual I-131 radioactivity levels are <5mR/nR at 1 m of <30 mCi) take advantage of existing radioactive iodine accumulation. And in patients with known metastatic disease, they are most useful in further documenting delivery of radioiodine to metastatic deposits and provide more detailed images of regions of abnormal radioiodine accumulation.[1-3,26,28,29,82] Occasionally lesions are depicted that cannot be seen on the diagnostic tracer studies, thus identifying a greater extent of disease than that anticipated from smaller 2–5 mCi I-131 diagnostic images. This can be useful in subsequent therapy planning.[1-3,26,28,36,82]

Assessment of Therapeutic Effects of Treatment

Assessment of the therapeutic effects of prior I-131 treatment and monitoring for disease progression with scintigraphy have great value in managing patients with well-differentiated thyroid cancer[2,3,26,28,33] (Figure 18). In addition to clinical palpation of the neck to detect

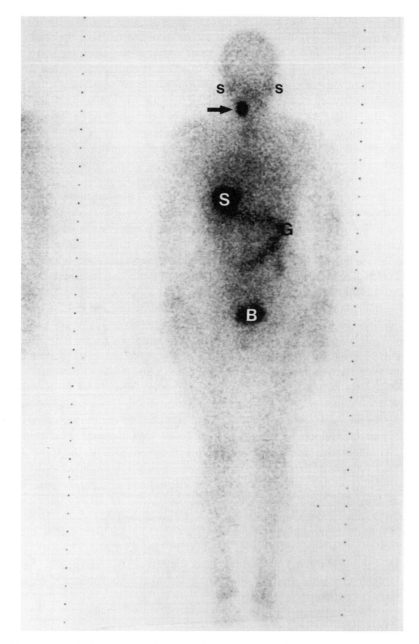

FIGURE 10. Whole body I-131 scan performed with 2 mCi 6 weeks following total thyroidectomy (posterior projection performed at 24 h). A small focus of I-131 uptake in the left thyroid bed (0.3% of administered dose) (arrow). Normal uptake is present in salivary gland (s), stomach (white S), and gut (G), and excretion via the bladder (B).

lymphadenopathy, many advocate the use of ultrasound to confirm and characterize palpable iodes and to detect impalpable lesions.[4,113-116] Although the intervals at which repeat diagnostic imaging are optimally performed remain controversial, regimens designed to evaluate patients at regular intervals are critical to proper management (these are typically once yearly initially and with longer intervals if preceding scans are negative).[2,3,26,28] Withdrawal of thyroid hormone for at least 6 weeks prior to imaging or using T_3 for 3 weeks with imaging performed 3 weeks later is essential to elevate the TSH.[3,26] Diagnostic image sequences will then demonstrate local and distant radioiodine-avid metastatic involvement if present. Thyroglobulin

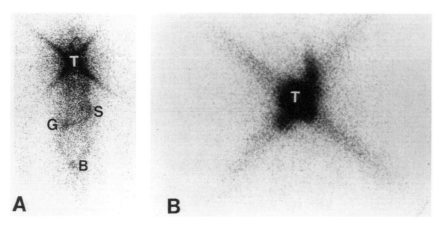

FIGURE 11. **(A)** Whole body I-131 scan performed with 2 mCi 6 weeks following attempted total thyroidectomy. Large intense focus of residual I-131 uptake in large remnant of thyroid tissue (T) (15% of administered dose). Septal penetration of photons from intense uptake makes detailed examination of neck and chest impossible. Normal I-131 uptake in stomach (S) and gut (G) and excretion via bladder (B). **(B)** Detailed view of neck again shows marked septal penetration from large thyroid bed remnant (T).

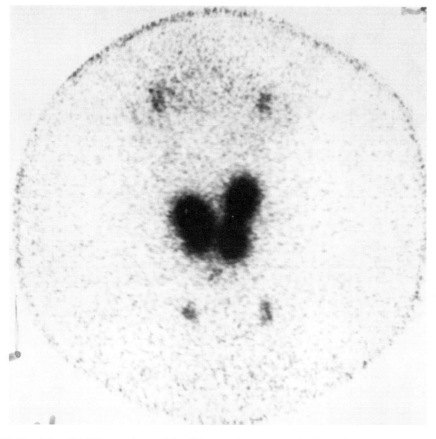

FIGURE 12. A 2-mCi I-131 scan after total thyroidectomy demonstrates significant thyroid bed activity. The 24-h radioiodine uptake was 6%. *(From Freitas, J.E., Gross, M.D., Ripley, S., and Shapiro, B., Semin. Nucl. Med., 15, 102, 1985. With permission.)*

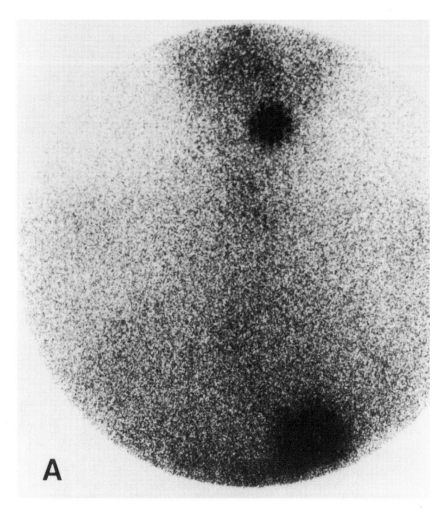

FIGURE 13.   I-131 thyroid scan performed 6 weeks after total thyroidectomy. The anterior view, which includes the lower face and chest (**A**), shows a midline focus of activity above the thyroid bed. A lateral view (**B**) demonstrates this focus of uptake in the region of the base of the tongue. *(From Sud, A.M. and Gross, M.D., Clin. Nucl. Med., 16, 894, 1991. With permission.)*

levels can be useful in following patients with well-differentiated thyroid cancer in much the same manner as radioiodine scans (measurements performed in the face of thyroid hormone treatment are, however, much less sensitive than those after T_4 withdrawal).[4,6] The presence of an increasing thyroglobulin level in a patient after thyroidectomy, I-131 ablation, and I-131 therapy is suspicious for recurrence or progression of disease and may be particularly useful in those patients where subsequent I-131 scans are truly negative.[2-6,26,28] The decision to treat a patient with rising thyroglobulins and a negative diagnostic I-131 scan is controversial.[5,5a,6] In patients whose neoplasms do not accumulate radioiodine, other radiotracers such as Tl-201 or Tc-99m sestamibi can be used to identify metastases (although the treatment options under these circumstances are limited).[4,44,48,61]

Medullary Thyroid Cancer

Often the first suspicion of medullary thyroid cancer (MCT) is after resection of a sporadic solitary nodule when the characteristic histology is observed.[1-3,26,161] This can be confirmed by the presence of calcitonin by immunohistochemistry. The evaluation of patients with suspected metastatic or familial carcinoma (MCT) generally begins with the evaluation of

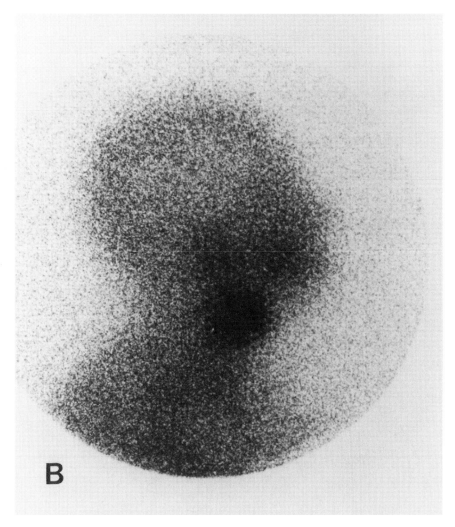

FIGURE 13 (continued).

basal and stimulated calcitonin levels. Pentagastrin, calcium, or the combination of penta-gastrin and calcium infusions have been used to assess patients with suspected sporadic and familial MCT.[3,26,161] Findings suggestive of MCT in the proper clinical setting should prompt biochemical evaluation for parathyroid adenoma, pheochromocytoma, and/or pheochromocy-toma (MEN 2a); mucosal neuromas; and thickened corneal nerves (MEN 2b or MEN 3) (Table 6).[3,26] Genetic mapping has recently been shown useful in identifying patients carrying the gene for MCT in multiple endocrine neoplasia syndromes (MEN 2a).

Nonspecific blood flow agents such as Tl-201 and Tc-99m sestamibi can be used to locate these highly vascular tumors[51,161] (Figure 19A). Scintigraphic imaging of medullary thyroid cancer has recently been expanded to include Tc-99m DMSA-V, a traditional renal tracer wherein the valence of technetium is changed from +7 to +5, allowing imaging of primary MCT and metastases.[60,62,65,66,68,162] Other radiotracers that have shown promise for localizing MCT are I-131 and I-123 MIBG[58,59,60,62-64,162] (Figures 19B and 20), and the recently intro-duced somatostatin analog Octreotide labeled with either I-123 or In-111 has been highly effective in imaging MCT.[55,56,59] Radiolabeled, anti-CEA antibody has also been used to localize MCT.[69,70]

Once detected, the most effective therapy for MCT is surgical extirpation of all thyroid tissues including obvious primary and local metastatic disease.[3,26] Because these neoplasms

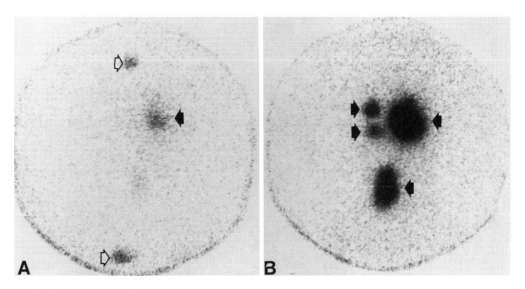

FIGURE 14.   (**A**) A 2-mCi I-131 scan after total thyroidectomy shows uptake in the thyroid bed (closed arrow). Markers are placed at the thyroid cartilage and sternal notch (open arrows). (**B**) A scan of the same patient 3 days after a 150-mCi dose of I-131. Note the increased uptake within the thyroid bed and the presence of paratracheal node activity (closed arrows) that was not appreciated on the 2-mCi I-131 scan. *(From Freitas, J.E., Gross, M.D., Ripley, S., and Shapiro B.,* Semin. Nucl. Med., *15, 102, 1985. With permission.)*

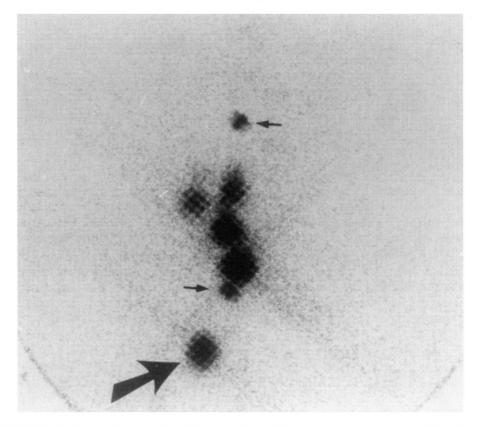

FIGURE 15.   I-131 thyroid scan performed 6 weeks after total thyroidectomy demonstrates a midline focus of activity below the thyroid notch (large arrow). The small arrows point to markers on the chin and the suprasternal notch. *(From Freitas, J.E., Gross, M.D., Ripley, S., and Shapiro B.,* Semin. Nucl. Med., *15, 102, 1985. With permission.)*

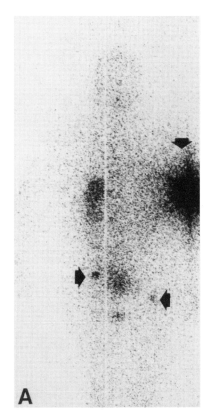
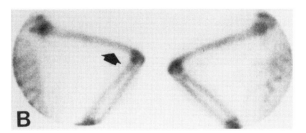

FIGURE 16. (**A**) A 2-mCi I-131 anterior body scan demonstrating metastatic involvement in the pelvis and humerus (closed arrows). (**B**) A Tc-99m MDP (methylene diphosphonate) bone scan demonstrates a subtle abnormality in the distal (left) humerus (arrow). *(From Freitas, J.E., Gross, M.D., Ripley, S., and Shapiro B.,* Semin. Nucl. Med., *15, 102, 1985. With permission.)*

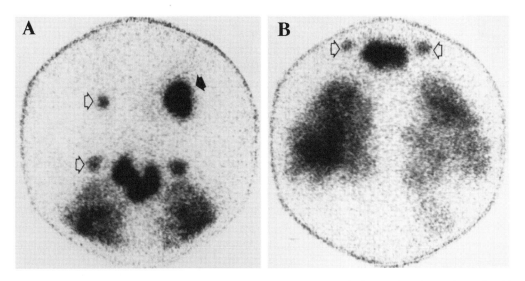

FIGURE 17. (**A**) A 2-mCi I-131 scan obtained 6 weeks after attempted surgical removal of a large primary thyroid carcinoma. Extensive metastases are noted in the neck (closed arrow) and in the lungs. (**B**) These areas of metastatic involvement image in spite of considerable thyroid bed activity from presumably remaining normal thyroid tissue. The open arrows identify radioactive markers. *(From Freitas, J.E., Gross, M.D., Ripley, S., and Shapiro B.,* Semin. Nucl. Med., *15, 102, 1985. With permission.)*

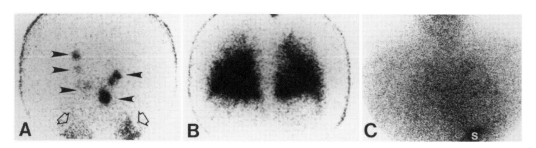

FIGURE 18. Well-differentiated thyroid cancer metastatic to cervical lymph nodes and lungs. (**A**) I-131 scan of neck and upper chest performed with 2 mCi 6 weeks after total thyroidectomy shows multiple foci in the neck (arrowheads) and in both pulmonary apices (open arrows). (**B**) I-131 scan of anterior chest with 2 mCi 6 weeks after total thyroidectomy showing intense diffuse uptake of tracer throughout the lungs. (**C**) I-131 scan of anterior chest with 2 mCi 1 year after therapy with 200 mCi I-131 shows only minimal residual abnormal tracer uptake throughout the lungs.

TABLE 6
Features of the Multiple Endocrine Neoplasia (MEN) Syndromes

MEN 1 (Wermer's Syndrome)
    Parathyroid hyperplasia
    Pituitary adenoma (functional or nonfunctional)
    Pancreatic islet cell tumors (often multiple)
MEN 2a (Sipple's Syndrome)
    C-cell hyperplasia—medullary thyroid cancer (MCT)
    Parathyroid hyperplasia
    Adrenomedullary hyperplasia—pheochromocytomas (often bilateral intraadrenal)
MEN 2b
    C-cell hyperplasia—medullary thyroid cancer (MCT)
    Adrenomedullary hyperplasia—pheochromocytomas (often bilateral intraadrenal)
    Ganglioneuromatosis of lips, tongue, eyelids, and gut
    Medullated corneal nerves
    Pseudomarfanoid body habitus

do not concentrate radioactive iodine, other therapies including systemic chemotherapy and external radiation therapy have been attempted but generally do not provide satisfactory therapeutic results.[3,26] More recently, I-131 MIBG has been studied in limited numbers of patients as a potential radiotherapeutic agent in the therapy of MCT.[60]

IMAGING OF PARATHYROID DISEASES

DIAGNOSIS

Before embarking on any attempts to locate the site(s) of parathyroid neoplasms or hyperplasia it is essential that a firm clinical and biochemical diagnosis of hyperparathyroidism be made (e.g., primary, secondary, tertiary, or associated with the MEN syndromes).[2,11,12,15,17,93] The hallmarks of primary hyperparathyroidism include elevated serum calcium, low serum inorganic phosphate, inappropriate elevation of PTH, hypercalciuria, and increased nephrogenous cAMP generation. It is essential that other causes of hypercalcemia be excluded, particularly before invasive and expensive procedures are performed. The vast majority of primary hyperparathyroid patients are now diagnosed at an asymptomatic or barely symptomatic stage by the widespread use of screening biochemical panels, all of which include a measurement of serum calcium.[2,17,18] A smaller proportion have renal stones, and hyperparathyroid bone disease is becoming increasingly rare[2] (Figure 21). The majority of cases (80–85%) of primary hyperparathyroidism are due to solitary parathyroid adenomas,

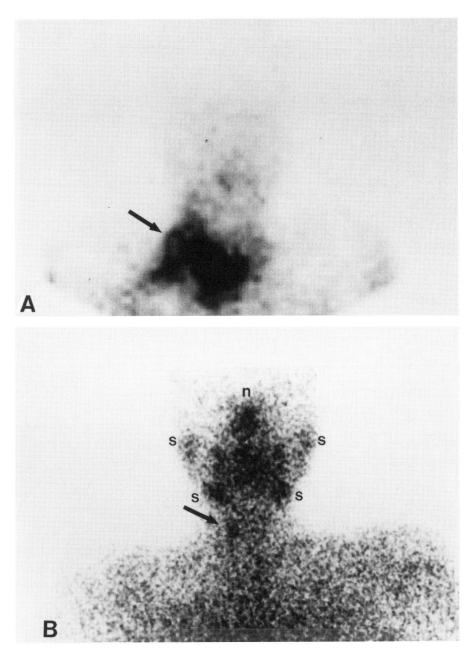

FIGURE 19. Primary and locally metastatic medullary thyroid carcinoma. (**A**) Tl-201 scan of anterior head and neck shows extensive intense abnormal uptake (arrow). (**B**) I-131 MIBG scan of anterior head and neck shows normal uptake in nasopharynx (n) and salivary glands (s). There is only minimal abnormal uptake in the right lobe of the thyroid (arrow).

15% are due to multigland hyperplasia (in which case the association with the MEN syndromes must be considered), and 1–2% are due to parathyroid carcinoma.[2,17,18]

The need for preoperative studies to locate parathyroid disease in all new patients is controversial.[2,17,18,92,93] Some experienced endocrine surgeons have success rates of 95% without localizing procedures, whereas others advocate preoperative localization in the belief that it may increase the rate of success and/or that it may shorten and simplify the operation. Few would disagree with the proposition that every effort should be made to successfully

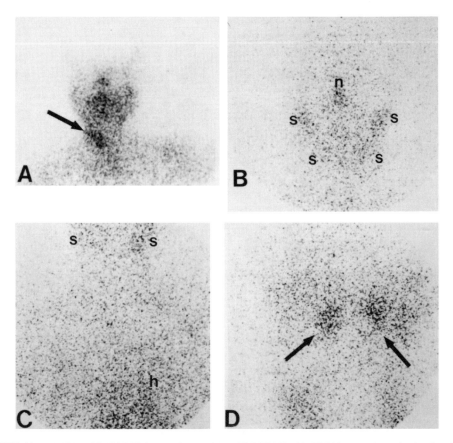

FIGURE 20. Tl-201 and I-131 MIBG scans in a patient with MEN 2b. (**A**) Tl-201 scan of anterior head and neck shows abnormal uptake in right thyroid (arrow). (**B**) I-131 MIBG scan of anterior head and neck and (**C**) anterior neck and chest shows normal uptake in nasopharynx (n), salivary glands (s), and heart (h). There is no abnormal uptake in the neck. (**D**) I-131 MIBG scan of posterior chest and abdomen shows abnormal increased adrenal uptake due to bilateral pheochromocytomas (arrows).

locate the lesion(s) responsible for recurrent or persistent hyperparathyroidism in patients who have undergone prior neck exploration, because repeated surgery becomes increasingly more difficult.[2,11,18-20] Nevertheless, it is in this setting that distortion of anatomy and post-surgical artifacts are most frequent and in which most localizing techniques may fail.

PARATHYROID ADENOMAS (NO PRIOR NECK EXPLORATION)

Solitary adenomas constitute at least 80% of the cause of primary hyperparathyroidism. The choice of localizing techniques is highly dependent on the technology and expertise available at any particular institution.[2,11-14,16,18,93,149]

In general, high-resolution, high-frequency ultrasound is the technique of first choice (sensitivity ranges from 44 to 92% with a specificity of ~95%).[2,12-16,93] The lesions being depicted are solid, hypoechoic, oval lesions with a craniocaudal orientation. If the lesion is only equivocally depicted on sonography or does not appear in the neck, subtraction scintigraphy (with Tl-201/Tc-99m-O_4 or MIBI-Tc-99m/Tc-99m-O_4) may be chosen next, particularly if the thyroid gland is free of nodules (sensitivity ranges from 44 to 86% with a specificity of 90–98%)[2,12,13,15,92,93] (Figure 22). CT or MRI might also be applied to confirm equivocal sonography and/or subtraction scintigraphy or to search for ectopic extracervical lesions.[2,58,96,149] MRI sensitivity ranges 57 to 100% with specificity of 88–97% and CT sensitivity ranges from 60 to 86% with a specificity of 92–95%.[15,16,144,149] There is little

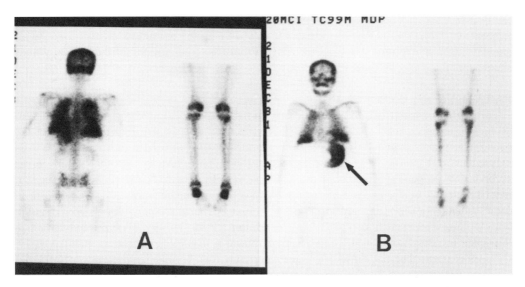

FIGURE 21. Whole body Tc-99m MDP (methylene disphosphonate) bone scan (**A** = anterior, **B** = posterior) in a patient with hypercalcemia due to primary hyperparathyroidism. There is increased tracer uptake in the skull, jaw, clavicles, and lower limbs characteristic of metabolic bone disease. In addition, there is intense abnormal uptake in the lungs and stomach (arrow) due to heterotopic calcification.

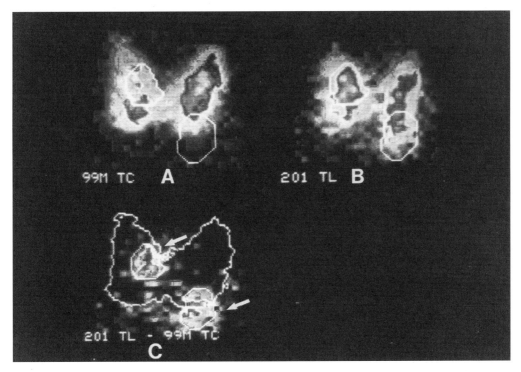

FIGURE 22. (**A**) Tc-99m-O4 thyroid scan with a left inferior pole adenoma outlined. (**B**) Tl-201 scan identifies two areas of increased tracer accumulation. (**C**) The subtraction image (**A** from **B**) localizes the two areas of parathyroid adenomas more clearly (arrows). *(From Ferlin, G., et al., J. Nucl. Med. Allied Sci., 25, 119, 1981. With permission.)*

justification under normal circumstances to resort to arteriography, venography, and venous sampling in patients with no prior neck surgery and in whom at least one noninvasive study is localizing.[2,15,93]

In about 5% of cases there may be more than one parathyroid adenoma present. Such cases are extremely difficult to distinguish from asymmetrical multigland hyperplasia and all glands should be explored and biopsied (only if there is actual atrophy of the normal glands should this diagnosis be made).[17,93]

PARATHYROID HYPERPLASIA

Multigland hyperplasia may be primary (associated with the MEN 1 or MEN 2a syndromes or as an isolated phenomenon) due to inherited defects affecting the growth of the parathyroid glands (and other neuroendocrine tissues).[2] Alternatively, parathyroid hyperplasia may occur in response to the hypocalcemia and hyperphosphatemia of renal failure in the secondary hyperparathyroidisms of renal osteodystrophy. Finally, even when the effects of renal failure are corrected by adequate dialysis or renal transplantation, the hyperplasia in some patients does not regress but rather autonomous hyperfunction continues with ongoing bone disease and even hypercalcemia, a condition termed tertiary hyperthyroidism.[2] It is important to recognize that although the hyperplasia is usually symmetrical, marked asymmetry may occur. The largest hyperplastic gland may then be misidentified as a parathyroid adenoma.[2] Hyperparathyroidism may persist or recur if an inadequate subtotal parathyroidectomy is performed, either because all the normally located glands are not identified or if ectopic and/or supernumerary glands are present.[20] To prevent this and to avoid the difficulties involved in repeated neck exploration some surgeons will intentionally perform a total parathyroidectomy and implant fragments of parathyroid tissue in the forearm or neck muscles (vide infra).[2] None of the anatomical or functional parathyroid localizing procedures are as sensitive for parathyroid hyperplasia as for adenoma because the hyperplastic glands are usually considerably smaller.[2,13-16,92,93,103] Sensitivity is typically 50–75% that for adenoma location.[15,149] During initial surgery a meticulous exploration to locate, identify, and biopsy all glands must be undertaken, exploring all the embryologically determined potential sites of gland location. The results of imaging studies may aid and speed this meticulous exploration but are not a substitute for it.[2,16]

PARATHYROID CARCINOMA

Fortunately this highly malignant tumor is rare (1–2% of primary hyperparathyroidism). It is characterized by very high serum calcium and PTH levels. There are no diagnostic features to unequivocally distinguish it from adenoma on any medical imaging modality. It should be suspected when the lesion is large (>2.5 cm), shows evidence of local invasion, or is accompanied by lymphadenopathy. Intense vascularity of the primary and metastatic foci may be demonstrated by the uptake of Tl-201 or MIBI-Tc-99m, contrast-enhanced CT or MRI, or angiography.[2,15]

PERSISTENT HYPERPARATHYROIDISM

When hypercalcemia and elevated PTH persists after surgical neck exploration whether or not the putative causative lesion(s) were resected, this situation suggests one of several possibilities, and it is essential to review the biochemistry most carefully to exclude other pathologies (e.g., sarcoid or hypocalciuric hypercalcemia) and to review the histology of all resected material.[2,11,18,19] If no parathyroid lesion has been resected then an ectopic adenoma is most probable (Figures 23–25). If one or more hyperplastic glands have been resected (and can be distinguished from an adenoma) then one or more residual hyperplastic glands are probably present and it is essential to consider supernumerary glands and ectopic sites as well as glands in the usual location which might have been missed.[2,11,15,19]

In these circumstances preoperative localizing procedures can be invaluable.[2,11,19,20] However, prior surgery may result in distortion of normal architecture, scarring, reactive lymphadenopathy, artifacts due to radioopaque or paramagnetic clips, altered vascularity, and abnormal patterns of venous drainage, which all serve to degrade both the sensitivity and

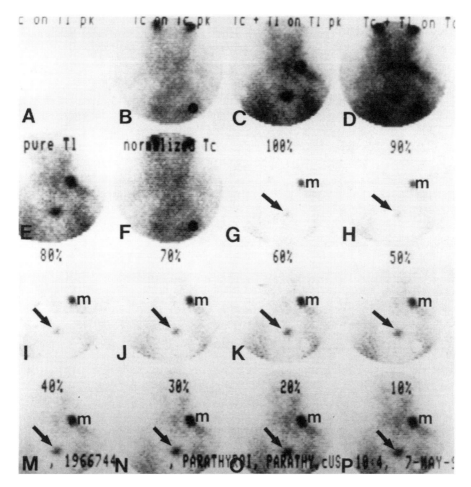

FIGURE 23. Prior negative neck exploration, ectopic mediastinal parathyroid adenoma. Tl-201/Tc-99-mO$_4$ subtraction scintigraphy. (**A**) Tc-99m imaged on the Tl-201 peak before Tc-99-mO$_4$ injection. (**B**) Tc-99m imaged on the Tc-99m peak. (**C**) Tc-99m + Tl-201 imaged on Tl-201 peak. (**D**) Tc-99m + Tl-201 imaged on Tc-99m peak. (**E**) "Pure Tl-201." (**F**) "Normalized Tc-99m." (**G–P**) Serial 10% subtraction of Tc-99m from Tl-201 from 100% to 10%. This shows abnormal uptake in the mediastinum (arrows). Note marker on left lateral neck (m).

specificity of all available techniques.[2,11,19] Nevertheless, the performance of one or more localizing studies is preferable to blind repeat neck and mediastinal exploration (e.g., ultrasound sensitivity 36–65%, CT sensitivity 46–55%, MRI sensitivity 50–91%).[15,149] Some believe that subtraction scintigraphy, which is not dependent on high-resolution anatomical depiction, is the best modality of first choice in this circumstance.[2,11,19] Reported sensitivity and specificity in this situation vary widely (sensitivity 26–70%).[2,11,19]

RECURRENT HYPERPARATHYROIDISM

Whereas in persistent hyperparathyroidism the biochemistry does not return to normal after neck exploration, in recurrent hyperparathyroidism there is a period of biochemical normality that may last weeks to years.[2,11,19,20] The issues are similar in the two conditions. The hormonal hypersecretion of an adenoma may be temporarily reduced by vascular injury during exploration, and when the adenoma recovers the hyperparathyroidism recurs. In the case of primary or secondary hyperplasia, a similar situation may occur when subtotal parathyroidectomy is performed or if there is ongoing further growth and hyperplasia in unexplored glands (e.g., ectopic and supernumerary glands).[2,11,19] The medical imaging procedures are as for persistent disease and indeed many publications do not distinguish between the two.[2,11,15,19]

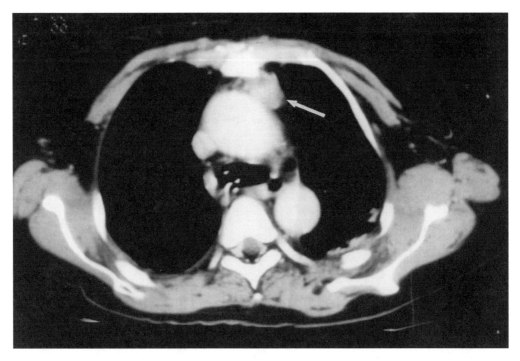

FIGURE 24. Prior negative neck exploration, ectopic parathyroid adenoma. CT scan shows soft tissue mass in the anterior mediastinum (arrow) corresponding to the abnormality on the Tl-201/ Tc-99-mO$_4$ subtraction study. The lesion proved to be a parathyroid adenoma.

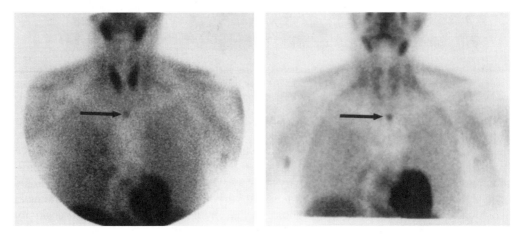

FIGURE 25. Prior negative neck exploration, ectopic parathyroid adenoma. Anterior neck-chest Tc-99m MIBI scintigraphy at 20 min (left) and 3 h (right) postinjection showing mediastinal parathyroid adenoma (arrow). Note that MIBI is better retained in the parathyroid adenoma than in the normal thyroid gland.

PARATHYROID REIMPLANTATION

The treatment of multigland hyperplasia requires the resection of the majority (typically 3½) of the glands. Insufficient resection may lead to relapse, and reexploration of the neck is technically difficult.[2,11,15,18-20] Thus, some surgeons implant fragments of parathyroid tissue in the forearm or sternocleidomastoid after total parathyroidectomy where these may be imaged using Tl-201 or Tc-99m MIBI.[2,15] In the case of forearm implants the PTH concentration in the draining superficial arm veins may be readily monitored.

CONCLUSION

The availability of multiple tests including high-resolution anatomic imaging provided by ultrasound, CT, and MRI, and functional mapping by scintigraphy provide a spectrum of tools to characterize abnormal anatomy and secretion of hormones by the thyroid and parathyroid. Each test affords different information that, when used judiciously, allows for not only complementary imaging analysis, but also accurate, timely, and cost-effective diagnosis and therapy.

ACKNOWLEDGMENTS

The authors wish to thank Ms. Joan Fogarty for help in the preparation of the manuscript. This work was supported in part by the following grants: NCI T32: CA09015 and NIH MO1 RR00042 to the Clinical Research Center at the University of Michigan.

REFERENCES

1. **Shulkin, B. L. and Shapiro, B.,** The role of imaging tests in the diagnosis of thyroid carcinoma, *Endocrinol. Metab. Clin. North Am.,* 19, 523, 1990.
2. **Freitas, J. E. and Freitas, A. E.,** Thyroid and parathyroid imaging, *Semin. Nucl. Med.,* 24, 234, 1994.
3. **Freitas, J. E., Gross, M. D., Ripley, S., and Shapiro, B.,** Radionuclide diagnosis and therapy of thyroid cancer: current status report, in *Freeman and Johnson's Radionuclide Imaging,* 3rd ed., Freeman, L. M., Ed., Grune & Stratton, New York, 1986, p. 1994.
4. **Christensen, S. B. and Tibblin, S.,** The reliability of the clinical examination of the thyroid gland, *Ann. Chir. Gynaecol. Fenn.,* 74, 151, 1985.
5. **Pacini F., Lippi, F., Formica, N., et al.,** Therapeutic doses of iodine-131 reveal undiagnosed metastases in thyroid cancer patients with detectable serum thyroglobulin levels, *J. Nucl. Med.,* 28, 1888, 1987.
5a. **Ozata, M., Suzuki, S., Miyamoto, T., Liu, R. T., Fierro-Renoy, F., and DeGroot, L. J.,** Serum thyroglobulin in the follow-up of patients with treated differentiated thyroid cancer, *J. Clin. Endocrinol. Metab.,* 79, 98, 1994.
6. **Schlumberger, M. and Tubiana, M.,** Serum Tg measurements and total body I-131 scans in the follow-up of thyroid cancer patients, in *Diagnostic Methods in Clinical Thyroidology,* Hamburger, J. I., Ed., Springer-Verlag, New York, 1989, 147.
7. **Caruso D. and Mazzaferri, E. L.,** Fine needle aspiration biopsy in the management of thyroid nodules, *Endocrinologist,* 1, 194, 1991.
8. **Blum, M.,** Imaging in the management of thyroid nodules: a personal perspective, *Thyroid Today,* 9(1), 1, 1986.
9. **Gharib H. and Goellner, J. R.,** Fine needle aspiration biopsy of the thyroid: an appraisal, *Ann. Intern. Med.,* 118, 282, 1993.
10. **Hamburger, J. I.,** Extensive personal experience: diagnosis of thyroid nodules by fine needle biopsy, *J. Clin. Endocrinol. Metab.,* 79, 335, 1994.
11. **Clark, O. H., Okerlund, M. D., Moss, A. A., et al.,** Localization studies in patients with persistent or recurrent hyperparathyroidism, *Surgery,* 98, 1983, 1985.
12. **Geatti, O., Shapiro, B., Orsolon, P. G., Proto, G., Guerra, U. P., Antonucci, F., and Gasparini, D.,** Localization of parathyroid enlargement: experience with 99mTc methoxyisobutylisonitrile and thallium 201 scintigraphy, ultrasound and computed tomography, *Eur. J. Nucl. Med.,* 21, 17, 1994.
13. **Gooding, G. A. W., Okerlund, M. D., Stark, D. D., and Clark, O. H.,** Parathyroid imaging: comparison of double-tracer (Tl-201, Tc-99m) scintigraphy and high-resolution US, *Radiology,* 161, 57, 1986.
14. **Gooding, G. A. W.,** Sonography of the thyroid and parathyroid, *Radiol. Clin. North Am.,* 31, 967, 1993.
15. **Milestone, B. N. and Gefter, W. B.,** Magnetic resonance imaging of parathyroid disorders, in *Imaging of the Thyroid and Parathyroid Glands: A Practical Guide,* Eisenberg, B., Ed., Churchill Livingstone, New York, 1991, 177.
16. **Stark, D. D., Clark, O. H., Gooding, G. A., and Moss, A. A.,** High-resolution ultrasonography and computed tomography of thyroid lesions in patients with hyperparathyroidism, *Surgery,* 94, 863, 1983.

17. **Thompson, N. M. W., Eckhauser, F. E., and Harkness, J. K.,** The anatomy of primary hyperparathyroidism, *Surgery,* 92, 814, 1982.

18. **Lafferty F. W. and Hubay, C. A.,** Primary hyperparathyroidism: a review of the long-term surgical and nonsurgical morbidities as a basis for a rational approach to treatment, *Arch. Intern. Med.,* 149, 789, 1989.

19. **Levin, K. E., Gooding, G. A. W., Okerlund, M. D., Higgins, C. B., Norman, D., Newton, T. H., Duh, Q. V., Arnaud, C. D., Siperstein, A. E., and Zeng, Q. H.,** Localizing studies in patients with persistent or recurrent hyperparathyroidism, *Surgery,* 102, 917, 1987.

20. **Brennan, M. F., Marx, S. J., and Doppman, J.,** Results of reoperation for persistent and recurrent hyperparathyroidism, *Ann. Surg.,* 194, 671, 1984.

21. **Som, P. M. and Bergeron, R. T.,** Normal anatomy of the neck, in *Head and Neck Imaging,* Som, P. M., Bergeron, R. T., Curtin, H. D., and Reede, D. L., Eds., C. V. Mosby, St. Louis, MO, 1991, 498.

22. **Som, P. M. and Bergeron, R. T.,** Congenital lesions of the neck, in *Head and Neck Imaging,* Som, P. M., Bergeron, R. T., Curtin, H. D., and Reede, D. L., Eds., C. V. Mosby, St. Louis, MO, 1991, 531.

23. **Akerstrom G., Malmaeus J., and Bergstrom R.,** Surgical anatomy of human parathyroid glands, *Surgery,* 95, 14, 1984.

24. **Brucer, M.,** *A Chronology of Nuclear Medicine,* Heritage Publications, St. Louis, MO, 1990, 223.

25. **Hamilton, J. G.,** The rates of absorption of the radioactive isotopes of sodium, potassium, chlorine, bromine and iodine in normal human subjects, *Am. J. Physiol.,* 124, 667, 1938.

26. **Freitas, J. E., Gross, M. D., Ripley, S., and Shapiro, B.,** Radionuclide diagnosis and therapy of thyroid cancer: current status report, *Semin. Nucl. Med.,* 15, 106, 1985.

27. **Kusic Z, Becker, D. V., Saenger, E. L., Paras, P., Gartside, P., Wessler, T., and Spaventi, S.,** Comparison of technetium-99m and iodine-123 imaging of thyroid nodules: correlation with pathologic findings, *J. Nucl. Med.,* 31, 393, 1990.

28. **Maxon, H. R., III and Smith, H. S.,** Radioiodine-131 in the diagnosis and treatment of metastatic well differentiated thyroid cancer, *Endocrinol. Metab. Clin. North Am.,* 19, 685, 1990.

29. **Greenler, D. P. and Klein, H. A.,** The scope of false-positive iodine-131 images for thyroid carcinoma, *Clin. Nucl. Med.,* 14, 111, 1989.

30. **Hamburger, J. I.,** Evolution of toxicity in solitary non-toxic autonomously functioning thyroid nodules, *J. Clin. Endocrinol. Metab.,* 50, 1089, 1980.

31. **Atkins, H. L., Klopper, J. F., Laubrerit, R. M., and Wolf, A. P.,** A comparison of technetium 99m and iodine 123 for thyroid imaging, *Am. J. Roentgenol. Radium Ther. Nucl. Med.,* 117, 195, 1973.

32. **McKeighen, R. E., Nuhllehner, G., and Moyer, R. A.,** Gamma camera collimator considerations for imaging ^{123}I, *J. Nucl. Med.,* 15, 328, 1974.

33. **Waxman, A., Ramanna, L., Chapman, N., Chapman, D., Brachman, M., Tanasescu, D., Berman, D., Catz, B., and Braunstein, G.,** Significance of 131-I scan dose in patients with thyroid cancer: determination of ablation: concise communication, *J. Nucl. Med.,* 22, 861, 1981.

34. **Frey, P., Townsend, D., Flattet, A., et al.,** Tomographic imaging of the human thyroid using 124-I, *J. Clin. Endocrinol. Metab.,* 63, 918, 1980.

35. **Lambrecht, R. M., Woodhouse, N., Phillips, R., Wolczak, D., Qureshi, A., Reyes, E. D., Graser, C., Al-Vanbawi, S., Al-Rabiah, A., Meyer, W., et al.,** Investigational study of 124-iodine with a positron camera, *Am. J. Physiol. Imaging,* 3, 197, 1988.

36. **Arnstein, N. B., Carey, J. E., Spaulding, S. A., and Sisson, J. C.,** Determination of iodine-131 diagnostic dose for imaging metastatic thyroid cancer, *J. Nucl. Med.,* 27, 1764, 1986.

37. **Bianchi, R., Iervasi, G., Matteucci, F., Turchi, S., Cazzuola F., Bellina, C. R., Boni, G., Molea, N., Ferdeghini, M., Toni, M. G., and Mariani, G.,** Chromatographic identification in serum of endogenously radioiodinated thyroid hormones after iodine 131 whole-body scintigraphy in the follow up of patients with differentiated thyroid carcinoma, *J. Nucl. Med.,* 34, 2032, 1993.

38. **Sodee, D. B.,** The study of thyroid physiology utilizing intravenous sodium pertechnetate, *J. Nucl. Med.,* 7, 564, 1966.

39. **Dos Remedioas, L. V., Weber, P. M., and Jasko, I. A.,** Thyroid scintiphotography in 1000 patients: rational use of 99mTc and 131-I compounds, *J. Nucl. Med.,* 12, 673, 1971.

40. **Andros, G., Harper, P. V., Lathrop K. A., et al.,** Pertechnetate 99m localization in man with applications to thyroid scanning and the study of thyroid physiology, *J. Clin. Endocrinol. Metab.,* 25, 2067, 1985.

41. **Shambaugh, G. E., III, Quinn, J. L., Oyasu, R., and Freinkel, N.,** Disparate thyroid imaging: combined studies with sodium pertechnetate Tc-99m and radioactive iodine, *J. Am. Med. Assoc.,* 228, 866, 1974.

42. **Arnstein, N. B., Juni, J. E., Sisson, J. C., Lloyd, R. V., and Thompson, N. W.,** Recurrent medullary carcinoma of the thyroid demonstrated by thallium-201 scintigraphy, *J. Nucl. Med.,* 27, 1564, 1986.

43. **Brendel, A. J., Guyot, M., Jeandot, R., Lefort, G., and Manciet, G.,** Thallium-201 imaging in the follow up of differentiated thyroid carcinoma, *J. Nucl. Med.,* 29, 1515, 1988.

44. **Nemec, J., Zamrazil, V., Pohunková, D., Rohling, S., and Holub, V.,** The rational use of ^{201}Tl scintigraphy in the evaluation of differentiated thyroid cancer, *Eur. J. Nucl. Med.,* 9, 261, 1984.

45. **Pavoni, P. and Mango, L.,** Clinical evaluation of [201]thallium chloride scan for thyroid nodule, *Eur. J. Nucl. Med.,* 6, 47, 1981.

46. **Henze, E., Roth, J., Boerer, H., and Adam, W. E.,** Diagnostic value of early and delayed ^{201}Tl thyroid scintigraphy in the evaluation of cold nodules for malignancy, *Eur. J. Nucl. Med.,* 11, 413, 1986.

47. **Ochi, H., Sawa, H., Fukuda, T., Inoue, Y., Nakajima, H., Masuda, Y., Okamura, T., Onoyoma, Y., Sugano, S., Ohkita, H., Tei, Y., Kamino, K., and Kabayashi, Y.,** [201]Thallium-chloride thyroid scintigraphy to evaluate benign and/or malignant nodules, *Cancer,* 50, 236, 1982.

48. **Piers, D. A., Sluiter, W. J., Willemse, P. H. B., and Doorenbas, H.,** Scintigraphy with ^{201}Tl for detection of thyroid cancer metastases, *Eur. J. Nucl. Med.,* 7, 515, 1982.

49. **Hoefnagel, C. A., Delprat, C. C., Marcuse, H. R., and deVijlder, J. J.,** Role of [201]thallium total body scintigraphy in follow-up of thyroid carcinoma, *J. Nucl. Med.,* 27, 1854, 1986.

50. **Talpos, C. B., Jackson, C. E., Froelich, J. W., Kambouris, A. A., Block, M. A., and Tashyian, A. H., Jr.,** Localization of residual medullary thyroid cancer by thallium/technetium scintigraphy, *Surgery,* 98, 1189, 1985.

51. **O'Driscoll, C. M., Baker, F., Casey, M. J., and Duffy, G. J.,** Localization of recurrent medullary thyroid carcinoma with technetium-99m-methoxyisobutylnitrile scintigraphy: a case report, *J. Nucl. Med.,,* 32, 2281, 1991.

52. **Beckerman, C., Hoffer, P. B., and Bitran, J. D.,** The role of gallium-67 in the clinical evaluation of cancer, *Semin. Nucl. Med.*, 14, 296, 1984.

53. **Pinsky, S. M. and Henkin, R. E.,** Gallium-67 tumor scanning, *Semin. Nucl. Med.*, 6(4), 397, 1976.

54. **Mori, T., Hamamoto, K. and Morita, R.,** Clinical evaluation of ^{99m}Tc-bleomycin scintigraphy for diagnosis of thyroid cancer, *J. Nucl. Med.,* 15, 518, 1974.

55. **Dörr, U., Frank-Raue, K., Raue, F., Soutter-Bihl, M. L., Guzman, G., Buhr, H. J., and Bihl, H.,** The potential value of somatostatin receptor scintigraphy in medullary thyroid carcinoma, *Nucl. Med. Commun.*, 14, 439, 1993.

56. **Kweekeboom, D. J., Reubi, J. C., Lamberts, S. W. J., Bruining, H. A., Mulder, A. H., Oei, H. Y., and Krenning, E. P.,** In vivo somatostatin receptor imaging in medullary thyroid carcinoma, *J. Clin. Endocrinol. Metab.,* 76, 1413, 1993.

57. **Waddington, W. A., Kettle, A. G., Heddle, R. M., and Coakley, A. J.,** Intra-operative localization of recurrent medullary carcinoma of the thyroid using indium-111 pentetreotide and a nuclear surgical probe, *Eur. J. Nucl. Med.,* 21, 363, 1994.

58. **Endo, K., Shiomi, K., Kasagi, K., Konishi, J., Torizuka, K., Nakao, K., and Tanimura, H.,** Imaging of medullary thyroid cancer with ^{131}I-MIBG, *Lancet,* 2, 233, 1984.

59. **Von Moll, L., McEwan, A. J., Shapiro, B., Sisson, J. C., Gross, M. D., Lloyd, R., Beals, E., Beierwaltes, W. H., and Thompson N. W.,** Iodine-131-MIBG scintigraphy of neuroendocrine tumors other than pheochromocytoma and neuroblastoma, *J. Nucl. Med.,* 28(6), 979, 1987.

60. **Clarke, S. E. M., Lazarus, C. R., Wraight, P., et al.,** Pentavalent (99mTc) DMSA, (131-I) MIBG, and (99mTc) MDP—an evaluation of three imaging techniques in patients with medullary carcinoma of the thyroid, *J. Nucl. Med.,* 29, 33, 1988.

61. **Hoefnagel, C. A., Delprat, C. C., Zanin, D., van der and Shoot, J. B.,** New radionuclide tracers for the diagnosis and therapy of medullary thyroid carcinoma, *Clin. Nucl. Med.*, 13, 159, 1988.

62. **Hilditch, T. E., Connell, J. M. C., Elliot, A. T., Murray, T., Reed, N. S.,** Poor results with 99m-technetium [V] DMS and 131-iodine MIBG in the imaging of medullary thyroid carcinoma, *J. Nucl. Med.,* 27, 1150, 1986.

63. **Courtis, G., Talbot, J. W., Kable, G., et al,** Uptake of ^{131}I-MIBG by medullary carcinoma of thyroid in familial cases, *Eur. J. Nucl. Med.,* 12, 77, 1986.

64. **Perdrisot, B., Rohmer, V., Lejeune, J. J., Bigorgne, J. C., and Jallet, P.,** Thyroid uptake of MIBG in Sipple's syndrome, *Eur. J. Nucl. Med.,* 14, 37, 1988.

65. **Ramamoorthy, N., Shetye, S. V., Pandey, P. M., Mani, R. S., Patel, M. C., Patel, R. B., Ramanathon, P., Krishna, B. A., and Sharma, S. M.,** Preparation and evaluation of [99m]Tc (V)-DMSA complex: studies in medullary carcinoma of the thyroid, *Eur. J. Nucl. Med.,* 12, 623, 1987.

66. **Patel, M. C., Patel, R. B., Ramanathan, P., Ramamoorthy, N., Krishna, B. A., Sharma, S. M.,** Clinical evaluation of [99m]Tc [V]-dimercaptosuccinic acid (DMSA) for imaging medullary carcinoma of thyroid and its metastasis, *Eur. J. Nucl. Med.,* 13, 507, 1988.

67. **Ohta, H., Yamamoto, K., Endo, K., Mori, T., Hamanaka, D., Shimazu, A., Ikekubo, K., Makimoto, K., Iida, Y., Konishi, J., et al.,** A new imaging agent for medullary carcinoma of the thyroid, *J. Nucl. Med.,* 25, 323, 1984.

68. **Endo, K., Ohta, H., Torizuka, K., et al.,** [99m]Technetium (V)-DMSA in the imaging of medullary thyroid carcinoma, *J. Nucl. Med.,* 28, 252, 1987.

69. **Edington, H. D., Watson, C. G., Levine, G., Tauxe, W. N., Vousem, S. A., Unger, M., and Kowal, C. D.,** Radioimmuno-imaging of metastatic medullary carcinoma of the thyroid gland using an indium-111 labeled monoclonal antibody to CEA, *Surgery,* 104, 1004, 1988.

70. **Reiners, C., Eilles, C., Spiegel, W., et al.,** Immunoscintigraphy in medullary thyroid cancer using a 123-I or 111-In-labeled monoclonal anti-CEA antibody fragment, *Nucl. Med.,* 25, 227, 1986.

71. **Hawkins, R. A., Choi, Y., Huang, S. C., Messa, C., Hoh, C. K., and Phelps, M. E.,** Quantitating tumor glucose metabolism with FDG and PET, *J. Nucl. Med.,* 33, 339, 1992.

72. **McKitrick, W. L., Park, H. M., and Kosegi, J. E.,** Parallax error in pinhole thyroid scintigraphy: a critical consideration in the evaluation of substernal goiters, *J. Nucl. Med.,* 26, 418, 1985.

73. **Lee, V. W., Almass, N. W., Shapiro, J. H., and Angtuaco, E.,** Radionuclide angiography for assessment of hyperthyroidism, *Radiology,* 142, 237, 1982.

74. **Koral, K. F., Freitas, J. E., Rogers, W. L., et al.,** Thyroid scintigraphy with time-coded aperture, *J. Nucl. Med.,* 20, 345, 1979.

75. **Chen, J. J. S., LaFrance, N. D., Allo, M. D., Cooper, D. S., and Ladenson, P. W.,** Single photon emission computed tomography of the thyroid, *J. Clin. Endocrinol. Metab.,* 66, 1240, 1988.

76. **Thrall, J. H., Burman, K. D., Gillin, M. T., Corcoran, R. J., Johnson, M. C., and Wartofsky, L.,** Solitary autonomous thyroid nodules: comparison of fluorescent and pertechnetate imaging, *J. Nucl. Med.,* 18(11), 1064, 1977.

77. **Patton, J. A. and Sandler, M. P.,** X-ray fluorescent scanning in thyroid imaging, in *Thyroid and Parathyroid Imaging,* Sandler, M. P., Patton, J. A., and Partain, C. L., Eds., Appleton-Century-Crofts, Norwalk, CT, 1986, 247.

78. **Jonckheer, M. H. and Deconinck, F.,** X-ray fluorescence determination of stable iodine in the thyroid: a review, *Acta Clin. Belg.,* 37, 92, 1982.

79. **Patton, J. A., Sandler, M. P., and Partain, C. L.,** Prediction of benignancy of the solitary "cold" thyroid nodule by fluorescent scanning, *J. Nucl. Med.,* 26, 461, 1985.

80. **Powers, T. A.,** Radioiodine thyroid uptake measurement, in *Thyroid and Parathyroid Imaging,* Sandler, M. P., Patton, J. A., and Partain, C. L., Eds., Appleton-Century-Crofts, Norwalk, CT, 1986, 179.

81. **Leeper, R.,** Controversies in the treatment of thyroid carcinoma: the New York Memorial Hospital approach, *Thyroid Today,* 4, 1, 1982.

82. **Leeper, R. D. and Shimaoka, K.,** Treatment of metastatic thyroid cancer, *J. Clin. Endocrinol. Metab.,* 9, 383, 1980.

83. **Klein, I., Becker, D. V., and Levey, G. S.,** Treatment of hyperthyroid disease, *Ann. Intern. Med.,* 121, 281, 1994.

84. **Shapiro, B.,** Optimization of radioiodine therapy of thyrotoxicosis: What have we learned after 50 years?, *J. Nucl. Med.,* 34, 1638, 1993.

85. **Hayes, A. A., Akre, C. M., and Gorman, C. A.,** 131-Iodine treatment of Graves' disease using modified early 131-iodine uptake measurements in therapy dose calculations, *J. Nucl. Med.,* 31, 519, 1990.

86. **Fogelman I., Cooke, S. G., and Maisey, M. N.,** The role of thyroid scanning in hyperthyroidism, *Eur. J. Nucl. Med.,* 22, 397, 1986.

87. **Meier, C. A., Braverman, L. S., Ebner, S. A., Veronikis, I., Daniels, G. H., Ross, D. S., Deraska, D. J., Davies, T. F., Valentine, M., and DeGroot, L. J.,** Diagnostic use of recombinant human thyrotropin in patients with thyroid carcinoma (phase I/II study), *J. Clin. Endocrinol. Metab.,* 78, 188, 1994.

88. **Blower, P. J., Kettle, A. G., O'Doherty, M. J., Collins, R. E. C., and Coakley, A. J.,** 123 I-methylene blue: an unsatisfactory parathyroid imaging agent, *Nucl. Med. Commun.,* 13, 522, 1992.

89. **Coakley, A. J., Kettle, A. G., Wells, C. P., et al.,** Tc-99m sestamibi—A new agent for parathyroid imaging, *Nucl. Med. Commun.,* 10, 791, 1984.

90. **O'Doherty, M. J., Kettle, A. G., Wells, P., Collins, R. E., and Coakley, A. J.,** Parathyroid imaging with technetium 99m-sestamibi: pre-operative localization and tissue uptake studies, *J. Nucl. Med.,* 33, 313, 1992.

91. **Sandrock, D., Dunham, R. G., and Neumann, R. D.,** Simultaneous dual energy acquisition for ^{201}Tl/99-Tc-m parathyroid subtraction scintigraphy: physical and physiological considerations, *Nucl. Med. Commun.,* 11, 503, 1990.

92. **Ferlin, G., Borsato, N., Camerani, M., Conte, N., and Zotti, D.,** New perspectives in localizing enlarged parathyroids by technetium-thallium subtraction scan, *J. Nucl. Med.,* 24, 438, 1983.

93. **Erdman, W. A., Breslau, N. A., Weintreb, J. C., Weatherall, P., Setiawan, H., Harrell, R., and Snyder, W.,** Non-invasive localization of parathyroid adenomas: a comparison of x-ray computerized tomography, ultrasound, scintigraphy, and MRI, *Magn. Reson. Imaging,* 7, 187, 1989.

94. **Fogelman, I., McKillop, J. H., Bessent, R. G., Boyle, I. T., Gray, H. W., Gunn, I., and Hutchinson, J. S.,** Successful localization of parathyroid adenomata by thallium-201 and technetium-99 subtraction scintigraphy: description of a new technique, *Eur. J. Nucl. Med.,* 9, 545, 1984.

95. **Taillefer, R., Boucher, Y., Potvin, C., and Lambert, R.,** Detection and localization of parathyroid adenomas in patients with hyperparathyroidism using a single radionuclide imaging procedure with technetium 99m-sestamibi (double phase study), *J. Nucl. Med.,* 33, 1801, 1992.

96. **Geatti, O., Proto, G., Mazzolini, A., Shapiro, B., Orsolon, P. G., and Guerra, U. P.,** Concurrent Plummer's Disease and parathyroid adenoma: diagnostic and therapeutic approaches to a difficult clinical problem, *Clin. Nucl. Med.,* 19, 508, 1994.

97. **Holder, L. E.,** Clinical radionuclide bone imaging, *Radiology,* 176, 607, 1990.

98. **Holmes, R. A.,** [99mTc] pyrophosphate in demonstrating bone disease of parathyroid dysfunction, *J. Nucl. Med.,* 19, 330, 1978.

99. **Lutwak, L., Singer, F. R., and Urist, M. R.,** Current concepts of bone metabolism, *Ann. Intern. Med.,* 80, 630, 1974.

100. **Ram, P. C. and Fordham, E. W.,** An historical survey of bone scanning, *Semin. Nucl. Med.,* 9, 190, 1979.

101. **Fogelman, I., Bessent, R. G., Turner, J. G., Citrin, D. L., Boyle, I. T., and Greig, W. R.,** The use of whole-body retention of 99mTc disphosphonate in the diagnosis of metabolic bone disease, *J. Nucl. Med.,* 19, 270, 1978.

102. **Austin, C. W.,** Ultrasound evaluation of thyroid and parathyroid disease, *Semin. Ultrasound,* 4, 250, 1982.

103. **Butch, R. J., Simeone, J. F., and Mueller, T. R.,** Thyroid and parathyroid ultrasonography, *Radiol. Clin. North Am.,* 23, 57, 1985.

104. **Fleischer, A. C.,** Thyroid sonography, in *Thyroid and Parathyroid Imaging,* Sandler, M. P., Patton, J. A., and Partain, C. L., Eds., Appleton-Century-Crofts, Norwalk, CT, 1986, 275.

105. **Solbiati, L., Volterrani, L., Rizzatto, G., Bazzocchi, M., Busilacci, P., Candiani, F., Ferrari, F., Giuseppetti, G., Maresca, G., Mirk, P., et al.,** The thyroid gland with low uptake lesions: evaluations by ultrasound, *Radiology,* 155, 187, 1985.

106. **Simeone, J. F., Daniels, G. H., Mueller, P. R., Maloof, F., van Sonnenbrg, E., Hall, D. A., O'Connell, R. S., Ferrucci, J. T., Jr., and Wittenberg, J.,** High-resolution real-time sonography of the thyroid, *Radiology,* 145, 431, 1982.

107. **Radecki, P. D., Arger, P. H., Arenson, R. L., Jennings, A. S., Coleman, B. G., Mintz, M. C., and Kressel, H. V.,** Thyroid imaging: comparison of high-resolution of real-time ultrasound and computed tomography, *Radiology,* 153, 145, 1984.

108. **Propper, R. A., Skolnick, M. L., Weinstein, B. J., et al.,** The nonspecificity of the thyroid halo sign, *J. Clin. Ultrasound,* 8, 129, 1980.

109. **Katz, J. F., Kane, R. A., and Reyes, J.,** Thyroid nodules: sonographic-pathologic correlation, *Radiology,* 151, 741, 1984.

110. **Hassani, S. N. and Bard, R. L.,** Evaluation of solid thyroid neoplasms by gray-scale and real-time ultrasonography: the "halo" sign, *Ultrasound Med.,* 4, 323, 1977.

111. **Eftekhari, F. and Peuchot, M.,** Thyroid metastases: combined role of ultrasonography and fine needle aspiration biopsy, *J. Clin. Ultrasound,* 17, 657, 1989.

112. **Jones, A. J., Aitman, T. J., Edmonds, C. J., Burke, M., Hudson, E., and Tellez, M.,** Comparison of fine needle aspiration cytology, radioisotopic and ultrasound scanning in the management of thyroid nodules, *Postgrad. Med. J.,* 66, 914, 1990.

113. **Rubaltelli, L., Proto, E., Salmaso, R., Bortoletto, P., Candiani, F., and Cagol, P.,** Sonography of abnormal lymph nodes in vitro: correlation of sonographic and histologic findings, *Am. J. Roentgenol.,* 155, 1241, 1990.

114. **Simeone, J. F., Daniels, G. H., Hall, D. A., McCarthy, K., Kopans, D. B., Butch, R. J., Mueller, P. R., Stark, D. D., and Ferrucci, J. T., Jr.,** Sonography in the follow-up of 100 patients with thyroid carcinoma, *Am. J. Roentgenol.,* 148, 45, 1987.

115. **Sutton, R. T., Reading, C. C., Charboneau, J. W., James, E. M., Grant, C. S., and Hay, I. D.,** US-guided biopsy of neck masses in postoperative management of patients with thyroid cancer, *Radiology,* 168, 769, 1988.

116. **Vassallo, P., Wernecke, K., Roos, N., et al.,** Differentiation of benign from malignant superficial lymphadenopathy: the role of high-resolution US, *Radiology,* 183, 215, 1991.

117. **Fobbe, F., Finke, R., Reichenstein, E., Schieusener, W., and Wolf, K. J.,** Appearance of thyroid diseases using colour-coded duplex sonography, Eur. J. Radiol., 9, 29, 1989.

118. **Ralls, P. W., Mayekawa, S., and Lee, K.,** Color-flow doppler sonography in Graves disease: "thyroid inferno," *Am. J. Radiol.,* 150, 781, 1988.

119. **Carroll, B. A.,** Asymptomatic thyroid nodules: incidental sonographic detection, *Am. J. Roentgenol.,* 138, 499, 1982.

120. **Brander, A., Viikinkoski, P., Nickels, J., and Kivisaar, L.,** Thyroid gland: US screening in a random adult population, *Radiology,* 181, 683, 1991.

121. **Doppman, J. L., Krudy, A. G., Marx, S. J., Saxe, A., Schneider, P., Norton, J. A., Spiegel, A. M., Downs, R. W., Schaaf, M., Brennan, M. E., Schneider, A. B., and Aurbach, G. D.,** Aspiration of enlarged parathyroid glands for parathyroid hormone assay, *Radiology,* 148, 31, 1983.

122. **Schlumberger, M., Tubiana, M., DeVathaire, F., Hill, C., Gardet, P., Travagli, J. P., Fragu, P., Lumbroso, J., Caillou, B., and Parmenter, C.,** Long-term results of treatment of 283 patients with lung and bone metastases from differentiated thyroid carcinoma, *J. Clin. Endocrinol. Metab.,* 63, 960, 1986.

123. **Kasai, N. and Tsuva, A.,** Xeroradiography of the thyroid, *Radiology,* 141, 439, 1981.

124. **Samuels, B. I.,** Thermography: a valuable tool in the detection of thyroid disease, *Radiology,* 102, 53, 1972.

125. **Zachrisson, B. F.,** Thyroid angiography, *Acta Radiol. (Suppl),* 350, 1, 1976.

126. **Brennan, M. F., Doppman, J. L., Krudy, A. G., Marx, S. J., Spiegel, A. M., and Aurbach, G. D.,** Assessment of techniques for preoperative parathyroid gland localization in patients undergoing reoperation for hyperparathyroidism, *Surgery,* 91, 6, 1982.

127. **Genant, H. K., Vogler, J. B., and Block, J. E.,** Radiology of osteoporosis, in *Osteoporosis Etiology, Diagnosis and Management,* Riggs, B. L. and Melton, L. J., III, Eds., Raven Press, New York, 1988.

128. **Robinson, R. G.,** Dual-photon absorptiometry in clinical practice, *J. Nucl. Med.,* 31, 1781, 1990.

129. **Wahner, H. W., Dunn, W. L., Mazess, R. B., Towsley, M., Lindsay, R., Markhard, L., and Dempster, D.,** Dual photon (153-Gd) absorptiometry of bone, *Radiology,* 156, 203, 1985.

130. **Ott, S. M., Kilcoyne, R. G., and Chestnut, C. H., III,** Ability of four different techniques of measuring bone mass to diagnose vertebral fractures in postmenopausal women, *J. Bone Min. Res.,* 2, 201, 1987.

131. **Wahner, H. W., Dunn, W. L., Brown, M. L., Marin, R. L., and Riggs, B. L.,** Comparison of dual-energy x-ray absorptiometry and dual photon absorptiometry for bone mineral measurements of the lumbar spine, *Mayo Clin. Proc.,* 63, 1075, 1988.

132. **Heymsfield, S. B., Wang J, Heshka, S., Kehayias, J. J., and Pierson, R. N.,** Dual-photon absorptiometry: comparison of bone mineral and soft tissue mass measurements in vivo with established methods, *Am. J. Clin. Nutr.,* 49, 1283, 1989.

133. **Vette, J. K.,** Computed tomography of the thyroid gland, *Acta Endocrinol. (Suppl.),* 268, 1, 1985.

134. **Silverman, P. M., Newman, G. E., and Korobkin, M.,** Computed tomography in the evaluation of thyroid disease, *Am. J. Roentgenol.,* 142(5), 897, 1984.

135. **Bashist, B., Ellis, K., and Gold, R. P.,** Computed tomography of intrathoracic goiters, *Am. J. Roentgenol.,* 140(3), 455, 1983.

136. **Gefter, W. B., Spritzer, C. E., Eisenberg, B., LiVolsi, V. A., Axel, L., Velchik, M., Alavi A., Schenck, J., and Kressel, H. V.,** Thyroid imaging with high-field-strength surface-coil MR, *Radiology,* 164(2), 483, 1987.

137. **Charkes, N. D., Maurer, A. H., Siegel, J. A., Radecki, P. D., and Malmud, L. S.,** MR imaging in thyroid disorders, correlation of signal intensity with Graves disease activity, *Radiology,* 164(2), 491, 1987.

138. **Mountz, J. M., Glazer, G. M., Dmuchowski, C., and Sisson, J. C.,** MR imaging of the thyroid: comparison with scintigraphy in the normal and diseased gland, *J. Comput. Assisted Tomogr.,* 11, 612, 1987.

139. **Noma, S., Kanaoka, M., Minami, S., Sagoh, T., Yamashita, K., Nishimuro, K., Togashi, Itoh, K., Fujisawa, I., Nakano, V., et al.,** Thyroid masses: MR imaging and pathologic correlation, *Radiology,* 168(3), 759, 1988.

140. **Auffermann, W., Clark, O. H., Thurnher, S., Galante, M., and Higgins, C. B.,** Recurrent thyroid carcinoma: characteristics on MR images, *Radiology,* 168(3), 753, 1988.

141. **Takashima, S., Ikezoe, J., Morimoto, S., Harada, K., Kozuka, T., and Matsuzuka, F.,** MR imaging of primary thyroid lymphoma, *J. Comput. Assisted Tomogr.,* 13(3), 517, 1989.

142. **Rafto, E. S. and Gefter, W. B.,** MRI of the upper aerodigestive tract and neck, *Radiol. Clin. North Am.,* 26(3), 547, 1988.

143. **Higgins, C. B., McNamara, M. T., Fisher, M. R., et al.,** MR imaging of the thyroid, *Am. J. Roentgenol.,* 147, 1255, 1986.

144. **Kang, Y. S., Rosen, K., and Clark, O. H., et al.,** Localization of abnormal parathyroid glands of the mediastinum with MR imaging, *Radiology,* 189, 137, 1993.

145. **Fisher, D. A.,** Clinical review 19: management of congenital hypothyroidism, *J. Clin. Endocrinol. Metab.,* 72, 523, 1991.

146. **Benker, G., Olbricht, T. H., Windeck, R., Wagner, R., Albers, H., Lederbagen, S., Hoff, H. G., and Reinwein, D.,** The sonographic and functional sequelae of De Quervain's subacute thyroiditis: long term follow-up, *Acta Endocrinol. (Copenhagen),* 117, 435, 1988.

146a. **Tokuda, Y., Kasagi, K., Iida Y., Yamamoto, K., Hatabu, H., Hidaka, A., Konishi, J., and Ishii, Y.,** Sonography of subacute thyroiditis: changes in the findings during the course of the disease, *J. Clin. Ultrasound,* 18, 21, 1990.

147. **Park, H. M., Carver, R. D., Siddiqui, A. R., Elisei, R., Anelli, S., Ciccarelli, C., and Pinchera, A.,** Efficacy of thyroid scintigraphy in the diagnosis of intrathoracic goiter, *Am. J. Roentgenol.,* 148, 527, 1987.

148. **Glazer, G. M., Axel, L., and Moss, A. A.,** CT diagnosis of mediastinal thyroid, *Am. J. Roentgenol.,* 138, 495, 1982.

149. **Higgins, C. B. and Auffermann, W.,** MR imaging of thyroid and parathyroid glands: a review of current status, *Am. J. Roentgenol.,* 151(6), 1095, 1988.

150. **Ripley, S. D., Freitas, J. E., and Nagle, C. E.,** Is thyroid scintigraphy necessary before 131I therapy for hyperthyroidism: concise communication, *J. Nucl. Med.,* 25, 664, 1984.

151. **Goldstein, R. and Hart, I. R.,** Follow up of solitary autonomous thyroid nodules treated with I131, *N. Engl. J. Med.,* 309, 1473, 1983.

152. **Sisson, J. C., Bartold, S. P., and Bartold, S. L.,** The dilemma of the solitary thyroid nodule: resolution through decision analysis, *Semin. Nucl. Med.,* 8, 59, 1978.

153. **Van Herle, A. J., Rich, P., Ljung, B.-M. E., et al.,** The thyroid nodule, *Ann. Intern. Med.,* 96, 221, 1982.

154. **Ridgway, E. C.,** Clinical review 30: clinician's evaluation of a solitary thyroid nodule, *J. Clin. Endocrinol. Metab.,* 74, 231, 1992.

155. **Ross, D. S.,** Evaluation of the thyroid nodule, *J. Nucl. Med.,* 32, 2181, 1991.

156. **Molitch, M. E., Beck, J. R., Dreisman, M., Gottlieb, J. E., and Pauker, S. G.,** The cold thyroid nodule: an analysis of diagnostic and therapeutic options, *Endocr. Rev.,* 5, 185, 1984.

157. **Refetoff S., Harrison J., Karanfilski, B. T., Kaplan, E. L., DeGroot, L. J., and Beckerman, C.,** Continuing occurrence of thyroid carcinoma after irradiation to the neck in infancy and childhood, *N. Engl. J. Med.,* 292, 171, 1975.

158. **Schneider, A. B.,** Radiation-induced thyroid tumors, *Endocrinol. Metab. Clin. North Am.,* 19, 495, 1990.

159. **Coakley, A. J., Page, C. J., and Croft, B.,** Scanning dose and detection of thyroid metastases, *J. Nucl. Med.,* 21, 803, 1980.

160. **Bushnell, D. L., Boles, M. A., Kaufman, G. E., Wodas, M. A., and Barnes, W. E.,** Complications, sequela and dosimetry of iodine-131 therapy for thyroid carcinoma, *J. Nuc. Med.,* 33, 2214, 1992.

161. **Cabezas, R. C., Berena, L., Estorch, M., Carrio, I., and Garcia-Ameijeiras, A.,** Localization of metastases from medullary thyroid carcinoma using different methods, *Henry Ford Hosp. Med. J.,* 37, 169, 1989.

162. **Guerra, U. P., Pizzocaro, C., Terzi, A., et al.,** New tracers for the imaging of the medullary thyroid carcinoma, *Nucl. Med. Commun.,* 10, 285, 1989.

Chapter 9

GRAVES' OPHTHALMOPATHY:
THE ROLE OF CYTOKINES IN PATHOGENESIS

Rebecca S. Bahn

CONTENTS

INTRODUCTION

The clinical triad of goiter, rapid heart rate, and eye disease was first described in the early 19th century.[1,2] This form of hyperthyroidism is commonly called Graves' disease, and the associated eye condition is referred to as Graves' ophthalmopathy (GO), thyroid ophthalmopathy, or endocrine ophthalmopathy. Symptoms described by patients with GO include a "gritty" sensation in the eyes, sensitivity to light, increased tearing, double vision, blurring of vision, and a feeling of pressure behind the eyes.[3] Findings on physical examination include extraocular muscle dysfunction, proptosis (forward protrusion of the eyes), periorbital and eyelid edema, conjunctival chemosis (swelling) and injection (redness), lid lag and retraction (or "stare"), and exposure keratitis (corneal injury due to dryness) (Figure 1). Most patients experience only the minor congestive signs of GO (chemosis, injection, lid edema), which generally improve within several months' time without treatment. In a minority of patients, however, the disease progresses and one or more of the components (proptosis, extraocular muscle dysfunction, periorbital edema) become severe and symptomatic for several years' time. In rare instances, patients develop optic neuropathy with decreased visual acuity, dulling of color perception, visual field defects, and, rarely, blindness.[3] Pretibial dermopathy, a diffuse or nodular thickening of the skin that generally occurs on the anterior lower leg, is a rare

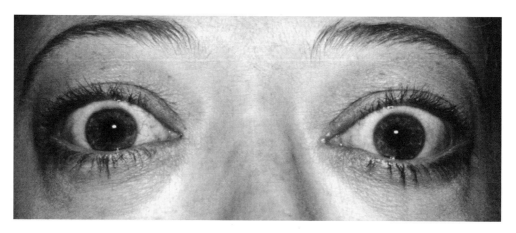

FIGURE 1. Hyperthyroid patient with Graves' ophthalmopathy. Clinical signs include periorbital edema, proptosis, and lid retraction.

condition that is occasionally seen in patients with GO (Figure 2). These skin changes occur rarely on other parts of the body, often following local trauma.[4]

ASSOCIATION WITH HYPERTHYROIDISM

GO is clinically evident in 25 to 50% of patients with Graves' hyperthyroidism and pretibial dermopathy is diagnosed in a small percentage of patients with GO.[4] However, subtle ocular and dermal involvement can be demonstrated in the vast majority of patients with Graves' disease when sensitive techniques are used.[5,6] Conversely, although approximately 10% of patients with GO do not have hyperthyroidism, the majority of these patients have laboratory evidence of thyroid autoimmune disease, including the presence of antibodies directed against the thyroid-stimulating hormone (TSH) receptor or thyroid peroxidase.[7] Regardless of whether GO or hyperthyroidism occurs first, the other manifestation occurs in 85% of patients within 18 months.[8]

The target cell involved in Graves' hyperthyroidism is the thyroid follicular cell. The TSH receptor is the specific autoantigen against which the autoimmune response is directed.[9] Stimulation of TSH receptors on thyroid follicular cells by circulating autoantibodies in Graves' disease results in unregulated and excessive production of thyroid hormones. Although still a matter of some controversy, the fibroblast in the orbit and pretibial skin is thought to be the target cell involved in GO and pretibial dermopathy.[10,11] Because of the close clinical association between Graves' hyperthyroidism, GO, and pretibial dermopathy, it is reasonable to suspect that a single pathogenic mechanism involving a common antigen may be responsible for all three conditions. The demonstration of RNA encoding the TSH receptor in human fibroblasts[12] and orbital tissue specimens[13] allows for the possibility that the TSH receptor is that common autoantigen. It has been suggested that an autoimmune reaction against TSH receptors on fibroblasts throughout the body occurs in Graves' disease.[11] That the clinically apparent connective tissue manifestations are generally limited to the orbit and pretibial skin may be explained by the known phenotypic differences between fibroblasts from various anatomic sites with regard to their biosynthetic capabilities and sensitivity to stimuli.[14-17]

PATHOLOGY

The clinical symptoms and signs of GO can be explained mechanically by an increase in the volume of retroocular tissue within the bony orbit. Histologic examination of this tissue

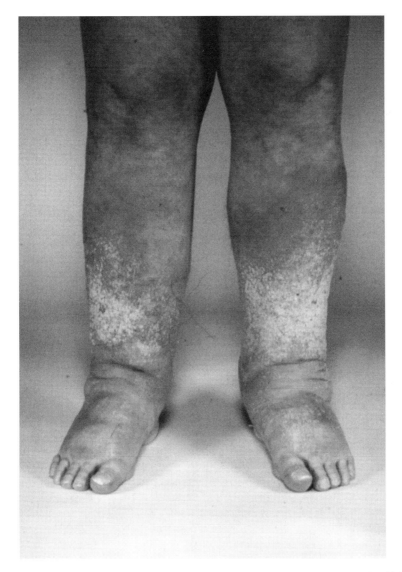

FIGURE 2.   Patient with severe pretibial dermopathy. Marked swelling of lower legs and feet with thickened, scaly skin is apparent.

reveals an accumulation of glycosaminoglycans (GAG) within the connective tissue components of the extraocular muscles and orbital fat.[18] GAG are hydrophilic macromolecules that are produced by orbital fibroblasts.[4] Orbital GAG accumulation results in an enlargement of the extraocular muscles and their surrounding fatty connective tissues.[19] Swelling of the extraocular muscles at the apex of the orbit can cause a compressive optic neuropathy. Proptosis, a forward displacement of the globe, serves to decompress the enlarged, edematous tissues contained within the orbit. Extraocular muscle dysfunction results from an accumulation of GAG and edema in the endomysial connective tissues investing the extraocular muscle fibers. The muscle fibers themselves are intact[20,21] but are widely separated by increased amounts of connective tissue and hydrophilic extracellular matrix components. In late stages of the disease, the extraocular muscles can become fibrotic and atrophic as a result of chronic compression of the muscle fibers.[22] Chemosis and periorbital edema are caused by intraorbital inflammation and decreased venous drainage from the orbit due to compression of orbital lymphatics.

In addition to tissue edema and an accumulation of GAG, an infiltration of inflammatory cells is characteristically seen in orbital tissues from patients with GO.[19,23] A prominent diffuse infiltration of lymphocytes, as well as some aggregates, has been demonstrated in the eye muscle interstitial connective tissue and in the connective tissue remote from the extraocular muscles in the posterior orbit. The majority of these cells are T-lymphocytes (CD2+/CD3+), the minority being B-lymphocytes (Leu26+). Both helper/inducer (CD4+) and suppressor/cytotoxic (CD8+) T-lymphocytes are present, with a slight predominance of the latter. Immunoreactivity for interferon-γ (IFN-γ), tumor necrosis factor-α (TNF-α), and interleukin-1α (IL-1α) can be shown both in the cytoplasm of infiltrating mononuclear cells and in adjacent connective tissue.[23] The presence of cytokines in close spatial relationship to the cellular infiltrate suggests that these cytokines are derived from the activated mononuclear cells, or from the neighboring connective tissue cells that may be stimulated by mononuclear cell-derived factors.

CYTOKINES: BACKGROUND

Cytokines are produced by a variety of different cell types and act on nearly every tissue and organ system in the body. IL-1 and TNF, cytokines known to be present in affected orbital connective tissues in GO,[23] are highly proinflammatory factors. They act in a synergistic fashion to stimulate the release of other inflammatory cytokines and secondary mediators of inflammation such as platelet-activating factor and prostaglandins.[24] TNF (α and β forms) is produced mainly by monocytes and stimulated lymphocytes. This cytokine enhances the cytolytic activity of natural killer cells, perhaps mediating tumor regression through this mechanism.[25] The IL-1 family consists of three structurally related polypeptides, IL-1α, IL-1β, and IL-1 receptor antagonist. IL-1 (α and β) can induce fever, anorexia, and hypotension. In addition, this cytokine has host-defense properties including stimulation of the growth and differentiation of T- and B-lymphocytes. The IL-1 receptor antagonist binds to IL-1 receptors but has no intrinsic stimulatory activity.[26] Elevated serum levels of IL-1 are found in individuals with various autoimmune or inflammatory diseases including rheumatoid arthritis, inflammatory bowel disease, and insulin-dependent diabetes mellitus.[27] IFN-γ is another cytokine present in affected connective tissues in GO.[23] This cytokine is produced by macrophages and T-lymphocytes. IFN-γ is a potent activator of tumor-killing macrophages, induces HLA (human leukocyte antigen) class I and class II expression in target tissues and plays an important role in B cell differentiation and immunoglobulin secretion.[28]

In general, the initiating event in an autoimmune disease is an abnormal response to infection, toxins, environmental factors, foreign antigens, or trauma. The host response to the abnormal immune process initially includes the synthesis of cytokines, which then contribute to the T-cell response, propagation of the disease process, and further production of cytokines. Cytokines have been shown to have "effector" functions in the pathogenesis of some autoimmune diseases.[25] In insulin-dependent type I diabetes mellitus, IL-1 has a role in the selective destruction of beta cells during insulitis.[29] In the BB rat model for type I diabetes mellitus, blocking the binding of IL-1 with the IL-1 receptor antagonist delays the onset of diabetes.[25] In GO, instead of causing destruction of ocular connective tissue, IL-1 and IFN-γ stimulate orbital fibroblasts to produce excessive quantities of GAG.[14,30] The accumulation of GAG and edema in the orbital tissues is primarily responsible for the development of the clinical signs and symptoms of the disease. In addition, particular cytokines stimulate the expression of immunomodulatory proteins on orbital fibroblasts[11] and thus aid in the propagation of the disease (see below).

EFFECTS OF CYTOKINES ON FIBROBLASTS

GLYCOSAMINOGLYCAN SYNTHESIS AND CELL PROLIFERATION

In a cell culture system of fibroblasts derived from patients with GO and pretibial dermopathy,[31] IFN-γ stimulates GAG production in fibroblasts from orbital connective tissue but not in fibroblasts from pretibial or abdominal skin.[14] In contrast, IL-1α and transforming growth factor-β (TGF-β) stimulate GAG accumulation equally in fibroblasts from extraocular perimysial connective tissue, abdominal skin, pretibial skin, and orbital connective tissue.[30] The known presence of IFN-γ and IL-1α in affected tissues in GO[23] and pretibial dermopathy offers an explanation for the excessive accumulation of GAG in these tissues. In addition, the selective stimulation of orbital fibroblast GAG production by IFN-γ suggests that fibroblasts from this site may be especially susceptible to immunologic pertubation of their biosynthetic capabilities.

Another effect of cytokines relevant to GO is the ability of particular cytokines to stimulate the proliferation of orbital fibroblasts.[32] Significant stimulation of proliferation of orbital fibroblasts from patients with GO was observed with IL-1α, IL-4, insulin-like growth factor I (IGF-I), and TGF-β, but not with IL-2 or IL-6. These former cytokines may be important in the development of the extraocular muscle fibrosis seen in late stages of GO.

EXPRESSION OF HUMAN LEUKOCYTE ANTIGENS

The human leukocyte antigen termed DR (HLA-DR) is expressed on cells that are capable of presenting antigens to CD4+ lymphocytes. HLA-DR is normally present on activated T cells, monocytes, B cells, macrophages, and endothelial cells. In the setting of an autoimmune disorder, HLA-DR can be expressed on other cells that do not generally express this antigen, such as thyrocytes.[33,34] In frozen biopsy specimens of orbital tissues from patients with severe GO, marked HLA-DR immunoreactivity can be detected in orbital fibroblasts including those forming the endomysial connective tissue that separates and surrounds the extraocular muscle fibers.[35] No HLA-DR reactivity is apparent on the extraocular muscle cells themselves or in orbital connective tissue obtained from normal individuals. Cultured orbital, pretibial, and abdominal fibroblasts from patients with Graves' disease or normal individuals do not express HLA-DR spontaneously. However, as is the case with many cell types, treatment *in vitro* of fibroblasts with IFN-γ results in induction of HLA-DR expression.[17] Of particular significance is that HLA-DR expression induced by IFN-γ in orbital and pretibial fibroblasts from patients with GO and pretibial dermopathy is greater in magnitude than that expressed in abdominal fibroblasts from the same patients. These results suggest that orbital and pretibial fibroblasts may be particularly susceptible to involvement in the autoimmune process.

EXPRESSION OF HEAT SHOCK PROTEINS

Heat shock proteins (HSPs) are highly conserved proteins that are synthesized in increased quantities in cells that are under the influence of stressful stimuli. These proteins act to maintain cellular homeostasis during stress and possess roles in the intracellular processing, membrane anchoring, and presentation of antigens. These latter functions of HSPs are important in the local modulation of the immune response.[36] The inducible HSP-72, a protein not constitutively expressed in human fibroblasts, has been detected in cultured orbital and pretibial fibroblasts from patients with severe GO and pretibial dermopathy, even after several cell passages.[37] This protein is not detectable in abdominal skin fibroblasts from the same patients nor in fibroblasts derived from the orbit or skin of normal individuals. The expression of HSP-72 is significantly enhanced following treatment with IFN-γ or TNF-α in orbital fibroblasts from patients with GO, but not in normal orbital fibroblasts.[37] Treatment with IL-1 (α and β), IL-6, and TGF-β stimulates HSP-72 expression in both normal and GO patients' orbital fibroblasts. These findings suggest that particular cytokines may aid in the propagation of the autoimmune response in the orbit by stimulating the expression of these immuno-modulatory proteins on orbital fibroblasts.

EXPRESSION OF INTERCELLULAR ADHESION MOLECULES

Adhesion molecules are important receptors for a variety of interactions between immuno-competent cells, connective tissue cells, and extracellular matrix.[38] In GO, strong immuno-reactivity for intercellular adhesion molecule-1 (ICAM-1) is present in the endomysial connective tissue that surrounds the extraocular muscle fibers and throughout the fatty connective tissue in the posterior orbit.[35] ICAM-1 cannot be demonstrated in normal orbital connective tissue. However, its expression is induced *in vitro* in normal orbital fibroblasts and in fibroblasts from patients with GO following treatment with IL-1α, TNF-α, or IFN-γ.[39]

TREATMENT OF GRAVES' OPHTHALMOPATHY

CURRENT STRATEGIES

There is currently no way to prevent GO, and the condition is usually treated only when symptoms become substantial or when vision is affected. Patients with only mildly symptomatic disease are not treated because of the risks inherent in each therapeutic option and because those patients most likely to progress to severe disease cannot be identified. Corticosteroids and orbital radiotherapy are most effective for the inflammatory symptoms and signs of the disease such as periorbital edema and ocular discomfort.[3] These two treatments may inhibit the production of cytokines by activated mononuclear cells and orbital fibroblasts. Transantral orbital decompression surgery, in which a portion of the bony orbit is excised, is considered when proptosis is substantial or when vision is acutely threatened.[3] This procedure decompresses the orbit by allowing some of the retroorbital tissue to prolapse into the maxillary sinus. Orbital decompression surgery is frequently followed by extraocular muscle recession surgery to correct diplopia.

FUTURE APPROACHES

The clinical expressions of GO result most directly from an increased volume of orbital connective tissues due to accumulation of GAG and edema. The excessive production of GAG by orbital connective tissue fibroblasts is likely stimulated by cytokines, including IL-1 and IFN-γ, known to be present in affected orbital tissues. Therefore, agents that either directly or indirectly inhibit the production or activity of particular cytokines might prove to be useful in the treatment of GO.

Specific blockade of the orbital fibroblast IL-1 receptor *in vitro* and *in vivo* is possible using the naturally occurring IL-1 receptor antagonist.[40] This antagonist is structurally related to IL-1, is produced by the same cells, and binds to cellular IL-1 receptors without activating them.[41] The administration of IL-1 receptor antagonist to animals reduces the severity of inflammatory disorders including streptococcal cell wall-induced arthritis in rats, and immune-complex-induced inflammatory bowel disease in rabbits.[26] In a phase I clinical trial in normal individuals, plasma concentrations of IL-1 receptor antagonist as high as 25–30 μg/ml caused no symptoms or changes in vital signs and did not alter white blood cell counts or routine biochemical parameters.[42] Thus, at least in short-term administration, the IL-1 receptor antagonist appears to be safe for human administration.

Soluble IL-1 receptors, produced by recombinant techniques or found naturally occurring in body fluids, specifically bind IL-1 and prevent its binding to cell receptors. Administration of soluble IL-1 receptor to rats with autoimmune encephalomyelitis reduces the severity of the paralysis and delays the onset of neurologic disease.[26] Early studies in humans suggest that soluble IL-1 can be administered safely; currently phase II clinical trials are underway.[27] In a similar fashion, soluble TNF receptors bind TNF and prevent its binding to cell surface

TABLE 1
Effector Functions of Cytokines in Graves' Ophthalmopathy

Cytokines Potentially Involved	Effector Functions	Resulting Pathology	Clinical Sequelae
IFN-γ IL-1α TGF-β	Stimulation of orbital fibroblast glycosaminoglycan production[14,30]	Enlarged and edematous extraocular muscles and connective tissue compartment	Proptosis Chemosis Periorbital edema Early extraocular muscle dysfunction Pain Optic neuropathy
IL-1α IL-4 IGF-1 TGF-β	Stimulation of fibroblast proliferation[32]	Fibrosis of extraocular muscles	Late diplopia
IFN-γ TNF-α	Induction of HLA-DR antigens on fibroblasts[17]	Continued presentation of antigen to immune system	Disease propagation
IL-1α TNF-α IFN-γ	Stimulation of fibroblast ICAM-I expression[39]	Recruitment of lymphocytes into the orbit	Disease propagation Inflammation Pain
IFN-γ TNF-α IL-1 IL-6 TGF-β	Induction of HSP-72 expression on fibroblasts[37]	Enhanced antigen processing and presentation	Disease propagation

IFN-γ, interferon-γ; IL-1α, interleukin-1; TGF-β, transforming growth factor-β; IGF-1, insulin-like growth factor-1; TNF-α, tumor necrosis factor-α; HLA-DR, human leukocyte antigen-DR; ICAM-I, intercellular adhesion molecule-1; HSP-72, heat shock protein-72.

receptors. Blocking TNF receptors, at least for short periods, appears to be safe in humans. Because synergistic actions of IL-1 and TNF are likely important in the pathophysiologic events of infectious or inflammatory diseases, blocking either cytokine can be expected to reduce the severity of the disease process.[24]

SUMMARY

Circulating T cells in Graves' disease, directed against an antigen on thyroid follicular cells, may recognize this same antigen on orbital and pretibial fibroblasts and consequently infiltrate the orbit and pretibial skin. The TSH receptor is a likely candidate for this common antigen because it is known to be present on both fibroblasts and thyroid follicular cells. Interaction between activated T cells and their target antigen on fibroblasts would result in release of cytokines into the surrounding tissues. IFN-γ, IL-1α, and TNF-β are known to be present in affected tissues in GO and pretibial dermopathy and may play a major role as disease "effectors" (Table 1). These cytokines are capable of stimulating the expression of immunomodulatory proteins (HSP-72, ICAM-I, and HLA-DR) in orbital and pretibial fibroblasts. These proteins would be instrumental in perpetuating the autoimmune response in the orbital and dermal connective tissues. Further, particular cytokines (IFN-γ, IL-1α, TGF-β, IGF-I) stimulate fibroblast GAG production and proliferation, resulting in an accumulation of GAG, edema, and fibrosis in the connective tissues. This resulting increase in connective tissue volume and fibrotic restriction of extraocular muscle movement leads to the clinical manifestations of GO. A similar process occurring in the pretibial connective tissues results in the nodular or diffuse skin thickening characteristic of pretibial dermopathy. The apparent clinical limitation of the connective tissue manifestations of Graves' disease to the orbit and pretibial skin may be due to local mechanical features, as well as to phenotypic differences known to exist between fibroblasts from various sites. However, it is likely that subclinical or subtle connective tissue involvement in Graves' disease is more widespread.

Cytokines are an important effector link in GO between the autoimmune process and the connective tissue manifestations of the disease. Interactions between particular cytokines and fibroblasts in the orbit and skin, resulting in alterations of particular fibroblast biosynthetic and immunologic properties, appear to be important in the development and propagation of the orbital and dermal pathology. Future therapy for GO and pretibial dermopathy may be aimed at blocking the production, receptor binding, or activity of these cytokines.

REFERENCES

1. **Graves, R. J.,** Clinical lectures, Lecture XII (1835), *Med. Classics,* 5, 25, 1940.
2. **Von Basedow, C.,** Exophthalmos durch hypertrophie des zengewebes in der augenhohle, *Wochschr. Ges. Aeilk.,* 13, 197, 1840.
3. **Bahn, R. S., Garrity, J. A., and Gorman, C. A.,** Diagnosis and management of Graves' ophthalmopathy, *J. Clin. Endocrinol. Metab.,* 71, 559, 1990.
4. **Smith, T. J., Bahn, R. S., and Gorman, C. A.,** Connective tissue, glycosaminoglycans, and diseases of the thyroid, *Endocr. Rev.,* 10, 366, 1989.
5. **Werner, S., Coleman, D. J., and Franzen, L. A.,** Ultrasonic evidence of a consistent orbital involvement in Graves' disease, *N. Engl. J. Med.,* 29, 1447, 1974.
6. **Wortsman, J., Dietrich, J., Traycoff, R. B., and Stone, S.,** Preradial myxedema in thyroid disease, *Arch. Dermatol.,* 117, 635, 1981.
7. **Salvi, M., Zhang, Z.-G., Haegert, D., et al.,** Patients with endocrine ophthalmopathy not associated with overt thyroid disease have multiple thyroid immunological abnormalities, *J. Clin. Endocrinol. Metab.,* 70, 89, 1990.
8. **Marcocci, C., Bartalena, L., Bogazzi, F. M., and Pinchera, A.,** Studies on the occurrence of ophthalmopathy in Graves disease, *Acta Endocrinol.,* 120, 473, 1989.
9. **McKenzie, J. M., Zakarija, M., and Sato, A.,** Humoral immunity in Graves' disease, *J. Clin. Endocrinol. Metab.,* 7, 31, 1978.
10. **Weetman, A. P.,** Thyroid-associated eye disease: pathophysiology, *Lancet,* 338, 25, 1991.
11. **Bahn, R. S. and Heufelder, A. E.,** Mechanisms of disease: pathogenesis of Graves' ophthalmopathy, *N. Engl. J. Med.,* 329, 1468, 1993.
12. **Heufelder, A. E., Dutton, C. M., Sarkar, G., Donovan, K. A., and Bahn, R. S.,** Detection of TSH receptor RNA in cultured fibroblasts from patients with Graves' ophthalmopathy and pretibial dermopathy, *Thyroid,* 3, 297, 1993.
13. **Feliciello, A., Porcellini, A., Ciullo, I., Bonavolonta, G., Avvedimento, V. E., and Fenzi, G. F.,** Expression of thyrotropin-receptor mRNA in healthy and Graves' disease retro-orbital tissue, *Lancet,* 342, 337, 1993.
14. **Smith, T. J., Bahn, R. S., Gorman, C. A., and Cheavens, M.,** Stimulation of glycosaminoglycan accumulation by interferon gamma in cultured retro-ocular fibroblasts, *J. Clin. Endocrinol. Metab.,* 72, 1162, 1991.
15. **Smith, T. J., Bahn, R. S., and Gorman, C. A.,** Hormonal regulation of hyaluronate synthesis in cultured human fibroblasts: evidence for differences between retro-ocular and dermal fibroblasts, *J. Clin. Endocrinol. Metab.,* 69, 1019, 1989.
16. **Imai, Y., Odajima, R., Inoue, Y., Shishiba, Y.,** Effect of growth factors on hyaluronan and proteoglycan synthesis by retroocular tissue fibroblasts of Graves' ophthalmopathy in culture, *Acta Endocrinol.,* 126, 541, 1992.
17. **Heufelder, A. E., Smith, T. J., Gorman, C. A., and Bahn, R. S.,** Increased induction of HLA-DR by interferon gamma in cultured fibroblasts derived from patients with Graves' ophthalmopathy and pretibial dermopathy, *J. Clin. Endocrinol. Metab.,* 73, 307, 1991.
18. **Campbell, R. J.,** Pathology of Graves' ophthalmopathy, in *The Eye and Orbit in Thyroid Disease,* Gorman, C. A., Waller, R. A., and Dyer, J. A., Eds., Raven Press, New York, 1984, 25.

19. **Weetman, A. P., Cohen, S., Gatter, K. C., Fells, P., and Shine, B.,** Immunohistochemical analysis of the retrobulbar tissues in Graves' ophthalmopathy, *Clin. Exp. Immunol.,* 75, 222, 1989.

20. **Hufnagel, T. J., Hickey, W. J., Cobbs, W. H., Jacobiec, F. A., Iwamoto, T., and Eagle, R. C.,** Immuno-histochemical and ultrastructural studies on the exenterated orbital tissues of a patient with Graves' disease, *Ophthalmopathy,* 91, 1411, 1987.

21. **Tallstedt, L. and Norberg, R.,** Immunohistochemical staining of normal and Graves' extraocular muscle, *Invest. Ophthalmol. Vis. Sci.,* 29, 175, 1988.

22. **Weetman, A. P.,** Thyroid-associated ophthalmopathy, *Autoimmunity,* 12, 215, 1992.

23. **Heufelder, A. E. and Bahn, R. S.,** Detection and localization of cytokine immunoreactivity in retroocular connective tissue in Graves' ophthalmopathy, *Eur. J. Clin. Invest.,* 23, 10, 1993.

24. **Okusawa, S., Gelfand, G. A., Ikejima, T., Connolly, R. J., and Dinarello, C. A.,** Interleukin-1 induces a shock-like state in rabbits: synergism with tumor necrosis factor and the effect of cyclooxygenase inhibition, *J. Clin. Invest.,* 81, 1162, 1988.

25. **Dinarello, C. A.,** inflammatory cytokines: interleukin-1 and tumor necrosis factor as effector molecules in autoimmune diseases, *Curr. Opin. Immunol.,* 4, 941, 1991.

26. **Dinarello, C. A.,** Interleukin-1 and interleukin-1 antagonism, *Blood,* 77, 1627, 1991.

27. **Dinarello, C. A. and Wolff, S. M.,** The role of interleukin-1 in disease, *N. Engl. J. Med.,* 328, 106, 1993.

28. **Becker, S.,** Interferons as modulators of human monocyte-macrophage differentiation. I. Interferon-γ in-creases HLA-DR expression and inhibits phagocytosis of zymosan, *J. Immunol.,* 132, 1249, 1984.

29. **Bendtzen, K., Mandrup-Poulsen, T., Nerup, J., Nielsen, J. H., Dinarello, C. A., and Svenson, M.,** Cytotoxicity of human pI 7 interleukin-1 for pancreatic islets of Langerhans, *Science,* 232, 1545, 1986.

30. **Korducki, J. M., Loftus, S. J., and Bahn, R. S.,** Stimulation of glycosaminoglycan production in cultured human retroocular fibroblasts, *Invest. Ophthalmol. Vis. Sci.,* 33, 2037, 1992.

31. **Bahn, R. S., Gorman, C. A., Woloschak, G. E., et al.,** Human retroocular fibroblasts *in vivo*: a model for the study of Graves' ophthalmopathy, *J. Clin. Endocrinol. Metab.,* 65, 665, 1987.

32. **Heufelder, A. E. and Bahn, R. S.,** Modulation of orbital fibroblast proliferation by cytokines and glucocor-ticoid receptor agonists, *Invest. Ophthalmol. Vis. Sci.,* 35, 120, 1994.

33. **Bottazzo, G., Pujol-Borrell, R., and Hanafusa, T.,** Role of aberrant HLA-DR expression and antigen presentation in induction of endocrine autoimmunity, *Lancet,* 2, 1115, 1983.

34. **Davies, T. and Piccinini, L.,** Intrathyroidal MHC class II antigen expression and thyroid autoimmunity, *Endocrinol. Metab. Clin. North Am.,* 16, 247, 1987.

35. **Heufelder, A. E. and Bahn, R. S.,** Elevated expression in situ of selectin and immunoglobulin superfamily type adhesion molecules in retroocular connective tissue from patients with Graves' ophthalmopathy, *Clin. Exp. Immunol.,* 91, 381, 1993.

36. **Kaufmann, S. H. E.,** Heat shock proteins and the immune response, *Immunol. Today,* 11, 129, 1990.

37. **Heufelder, A. E., Wenzel, B. E., Gorman, C. A., and Bahn, R. S.,** Detection, cellular localization and modulation of heat shock proteins in cultured fibroblasts from patients with extrathyroidal manifestations of Graves' disease, *J. Clin. Endocrinol. Metab.,* 73, 739, 1991.

38. **Shimizu, Y. and Shaw, S.,** Lymphocyte interaction with extracellular matrix, *FASEB J.,* 5, 2292, 1991.

39. **Heufelder, A. E. and Bahn, R. S.,** Graves' immunoglobulins and cytokines stimulate the expression of intercellular adhesion molecule-1 (ICAM-1) in cultured Graves' orbital fibroblasts, *Eur. J. Clin. Invest.,* 22, 529, 1992.

40. **Tan, G. H., Dutton, C. M., and Bahn, R. S.,** Interleukin-1 (IL-1) receptor antagonist and soluble IL-1 receptor inhibit IL-1-induced glycosaminoglycan production in cultured human orbital fibroblasts from patients with Graves' ophthalmopathy, *J. Clin. Endocrinol. Metab.,* 81, 449, 1996.

41. **Arend, W. P.,** Interleukin-1 receptor antagonist: a new member of the interleukin-1 family, *J. Clin. Invest.,* 88, 1445, 1991.

42. **Granowitz, E. V., Porat, R., and Mier, J. W.,** Pharmacokinetics, safety, and immunomodulatory effects of human recombinant interleukin-1 receptor antagonist in healthy humans, *Cytokine,* 4, 353, 1992.

Chapter 10

THE ENDOCRINE PANCREAS

Monica E. Doerr and John B. Buse

CONTENTS

INTRODUCTION

The pancreas is a retroperitoneal organ whose function is critical in the digestion of food and the metabolic regulation of fuels. The mature organ consists primarily of acinar exocrine tissue which produces digestive juices—predominantly bicarbonate and enzymes. The acinar production of bicarbonate and the release of its watery alkaline fluid through the pancreatic duct into the first portion of the duodenum is regulated through complex hormonal and physiochemical mechanisms. This bicarbonate-rich fluid neutralizes stomach acid to allow the action of pancreatic enzymes. Pancreatic amylase completes the digestion of ingested starches to disaccharides, a process begun in the mouth by salivary amylase; the absorption of monosaccharides through specific transporters occurs after action of disaccharidases on the microvilli of intestinal luminal cells. The breakdown of proteins to amino acids begins in the stomach with the action of pepsin. In a process akin to carbohydrate digestion, protein hydrolysis is mediated in large part by trypsin, chymotrypsin, and other endo- and ectopeptidases secreted from the pancreas, with intracellular and extracellular dipeptidases completing the process in the intestinal lining. Fat digestion begins in the intestine where bile salts allow for interaction of pancreatic lipase and co-lipase with dietary triglycerides resulting in their cleavage to fatty acids and monoglycerides, which are absorbed from the surface of intestinal cells by diffusion. Failure of the exocrine function of the pancreas is evidenced by weight loss, malnutrition, and diarrhea as a consequence of the malabsorption of nutrients; this generally occurs as a result of obstruction of the pancreatic ducts by stones or chronic inflammation.

The focus of this chapter is on the endocrine actions of cells within the pancreas, which are contained within dispersed clusters termed islets of Langerhans. The islets comprise approximately 1–2% of the total pancreatic mass. These islets are complex mini-organs with specialized blood supply, autonomic innervation, and complex microcirculation. Of the endocrine cells within the islet, approximately 70–80% are the insulin-producing β cells, 5% somatostatin-producing δ cells, and 10–15% either glucagon-producing α cells or pancreatic-polypeptide producing PP cells. A variety of other hormone products are secreted in very small amounts from these and other rare cell types within islets.

A critical problem for essentially all multicellular organisms is that basal energy needs are constant and increase in response to stress and activity while fuel intake is intermittent. The concerted action of the endocrine hormones of the pancreas produce the efficient deposition of carbohydrates, amino acids, and fats in the postabsorptive state and their regulated release from stores in the interdigestive period. In the pages that follow, we will consider the ontogeny of the pancreatic islet and then individually discuss the secretion and action of the major islet hormones. Although the absorptive consequences of exocrine pancreatic dysfunction can generally be effectively managed with dietary interventions and replacement of pancreatic enzymes, pancreatic endocrine dysfunction is accompanied by severe metabolic consequences such as diabetes mellitus and hypoglycemia and may be at the root of disorders of lipid metabolism, blood pressure regulation, and atherosclerosis.

ISLET ONTOGENY

In the development of the pancreas, two outpocketings of the primitive duodenal endoderm form. The first, so-called dorsal bud, develops opposite the bile duct and gives rise to the body and tail of the pancreas. It receives its vascular supply from the celiac trunk and contains mainly glucagon-rich islets essentially devoid of pancreatic polypeptide-secreting cells. The second, ventral bud develops adjacent to the bile duct and rotates around the gut fusing with the dorsal bud and largely becomes the head of the pancreas. This portion of the pancreas is generally supplied from the superior mesenteric artery and contains few if any glucagon-producing cells. These buds develop as branching ductal epithelium with both endocrine and exocrine tissue subsequently differentiating. Genes for islet hormones are transcribed before true bud development and prior to the genes for exocrine enzymes. It is unknown whether exocrine and islet cells derive from different progenitor cells. Furthermore, the precise stimuli and regulators of islet cell differentiation are largely unknown. In ontogeny, glucagon gene expression occurs first, followed by insulin expression, somatostatin expression, and finally pancreatic polypeptide expression. In transplantable tumor lines, cells have been shown to sequentially contain glucagon, then glucagon and insulin, followed by insulin or glucagon alone, with a later transition to insulin plus somatostatin or pancreatic polypeptide. The molecular regulation of islet cell development and differentiations is just beginning to be understood through the techniques of molecular biology.[1,2]

Whereas, in general, islet mass as a percentage of the total pancreas decreases with age—accounting for 20% of pancreatic mass in newborns, 7.5% in preadolescents, and 1% in adults—the process of pancreatic and islet differentiation seems to occur throughout life. In the normal adult pancreas, rare ductal epithelial cells immunostain for islet hormones.

There is proliferation of ductal epithelium with subsequent differentiation into mature ductal epithelium, acinar tissue, and islets. This process of new islet formation is accelerated in recent onset insulin-dependent diabetes and severe liver disease as well as by a variety of experimental conditions. Evidence from a variety of experimental approaches suggest that transforming growth factor-α (TGF-α), epidermal growth factor (EGF), insulin-like growth factor (IGF), and TGF-β may play a role in neo-islet formation. Because transient expression in fetal islets of gastrin, secretin, and thyrotropin-releasing hormone (TRH) has been observed, involvement of these hormones in islet replication has been postulated. Finally, a factor has been partially purified from cellophane wrapped pancreas that has islet trophic effects. Obviously, further understanding of these processes could lend important therapeutic strategies in disease involving islet dysfunction.[3]

ISLET ARCHITECTURE

As mentioned above, the islet can be viewed as a mini-organ with very special organization of its cellular components.[1] It seems to have a capsule consisting of a single layer of fibroblasts with deposited collagen. Insulin-producing β cells form the core of the islet. There is a mantle of non-β cells one to three cells thick. In humans, the glucagon-secreting α cells form a layer at the periphery of the core with the somatostatin-secreting δ cells being the most peripheral cells within the surrounding mantle. Occasional human islets display characteristics that suggest that larger islets may actually exist as compound islets of several mantle-core subunits or lobules.

The islet has a specialized capillary blood supply. Each islet is vascularized by one to three arterioles which penetrate to the core of the islet through breaches in the mantle. In the core, the capillaries are fenestrated and therefore highly permeable. The capillary network passes along the inside of the mantle before penetrating the mantle and draining into collecting venules. The endocrine cells seem to be aligned along vascular structures. Polyhedral β cells generally have two vascular borders with one face opposed to an "arterial" capillary and another face opposed to a "venous" capillary generally in a draining sinusoidal pattern. Adjacent β cells are joined by calcium-dependent and calcium-independent cell adhesion molecules as well as desmosomes with canalicular spaces formed where three or more β cells adjoin. It is believed that glucose uptake and "sensing" as well as a significant portion of insulin secretion occurs into these canaliculi where bulk flow of interstitial fluid occurs from the arterial to the venous side of the capillary web.

Blood flow to the islet is prodigious, with the islet receiving approximately 20-fold per unit volume the blood flow of the exocrine pancreas. Furthermore, islet blood flow is regulated, possibly by vasoactive intestinal polypeptide (VIP) and increases with increased levels of circulating glucose.

The pancreas is innervated by the sympathetic nervous system through the celiac ganglion and by the parasympathetic nervous system through the vagus nerve. Cholinergic, adrenergic, and peptidergic neurons are present and have a variety of known and suspected actions on individual endocrine cell types. There are ganglia within the pancreas that contain parasympathetic neurons as well as cell bodies that seem to express peptidergic nerve products. These peptidergic neurons may mediate intra-islet coordination and the "pacemaker" function which is hypothesized to drive the pulsatile release of insulin; their nerve fibers follow the vascular supply and terminate in the pericapillary space, just within the capillary basement membrane, and on the surface of individual endocrine cells.

Through the vascular arrangement of the islet with a perfusion pattern in which β cells are perfused first with their effluent then reaching the α cell and finally the δ cell, a hierarchy of intra-islet endocrine mechanisms is established; this results in insulin playing a dominant role in islet hormonal regulation. Insulin secretion (released proximally in the islet microcirculation) inhibits both α- and δ-cell glucagon and somatostatin production. The increase in glucagon that occurs in the absence of insulin results in a massive increase in δ-cell somatostatin secretion.[4] Other pharmacologic and physiologic actions of glucagon and soma-tostatin on insulin secretion may be mediated through the peri-islet interstitial space, which theoretically could allow for islet hormones as well as neurotransmitters to exert paracrine effects. Intracellular electrical communication as well as the passage of small molecules has been shown to occur within islets through tight junctions. In fact, some have suggested that individual islets should be thought of as an endocrine syncytium, and these connections may account for the observation that *in vitro* individual islets tend to secrete insulin in a coordinated fashion, with islets having various threshold levels of glucose at which insulin release tends to occur.

Finally, it is very likely that islet hormones, particularly somatostatin and pancreatic polypeptide, play a central role in the regulation of acinar pancreatic function. The venules that pass from the islet form an insulo-acinar (islet-acinar) portal system, with islet hormones apparently regulating both acinar tissue development as well as the production and release of various components of pancreatic digestive juice.

INSULIN

INTRODUCTION

Insulin is the predominant hormone produced within the islets of Langerhans. Insulin secretion is the dominant regulator of metabolism in the fed state; its secretion is maintained at basal levels during the fasted state. The net effect of its secretion is twofold: (1) the clearance of glucose from the circulation and (2) the inhibition of the breakdown of fuel storage forms (protein, fat, and glycogen). Thus, it results in the net deposition of fuels in all tissues. Diabetes is the disease state that results from inadequate insulin action and is characterized by high levels of glucose as well as relatively unrestrained mobilization of amino acids, fatty acids, and glycogen from muscle and fat. Diabetes in its more severe forms has been termed starvation in the face of plenty because this imbalance results in progressive weight loss despite adequate and often increased food intake.

The human insulin gene is located on the short arm of chromosome 11 adjacent to the IGF-II gene. The amino acid sequence of insulin across species is highly conserved and allowed for the clinical use of porcine (1 amino acid different from human insulin) and bovine insulin (3 amino acid differences) in the treatment of diabetes prior to the availability of recombinant human insulin. There has been considerable controversy as to whether insulin is expressed in cells other than pancreatic β cells. If there is extrapancreatic insulin production, expression is at low levels and physiologic effects have not been demonstrated. Glucose is the major regulator of all steps of insulin production and secretion. In insulinoma cell lines, there is a threefold increase in insulin gene transcriptional rate as early as 10 min after incubation in a high glucose containing medium. Glucose effects on proported transcriptional regulators seem to require metabolism of glucose because they can be blocked by inhibitors of glucose phosphorylation (the first step in glucose metabolism). These effects are specific and cannot be demonstrated with fructose, pyruvate, or nonmetabolizable analogues of glucose. Tremendous progress has been made in our understanding regarding the details of the insulin gene's transcriptional regulation. This could have significant impact in the therapy of diabetes as well as the creation by molecular engineering of insulin-secreting cell lines useful in therapeutic transplantation.[5]

INSULIN BIOSYNTHESIS AND RELEASE

Insulin is secreted as an α-, β-heterodimer joined by two disulfide bridges and was the first protein whose amino acid sequence was determined. Subsequently, insulin was the first protein for which a precursor protein was demonstrated. Through intracellular proteolysis the precursor is converted to a fully biologically active hormone. Its translation is regulated primarily by glucose and cyclic AMP but also is regulated by amino acids, nucleosides, and other sugars. The nascent insulin molecule is translated as a preproinsulin with an approximately 23-amino acid leader sequence at the amino terminus of the eventual β-chain. Preproinsulin is then cleaved after entry into the rough endoplasmic reticulum (RER) to form proinsulin, generally before translation is complete. Proinsulin is sorted through the Golgi apparatus and condenses with at least six other soluble proteins in association with clathrin-coated membranes. Vesicles subsequently bud off from the Golgi. Within these granules, a low pH and high calcium concentration develop, which allows for proinsulin conversion to insulin in a multistep process that occurs in association with clathrin uncoating of the vesicle. This is accomplished by cleaving out from within the proinsulin molecule a connecting peptide termed C-peptide, producing the insulin α-, β-heterodimer. The α-chain and the β-chain C-peptide junctions are preferentially cleaved and trimmed by different enzymes. In different species this process results in various intermediate forms of intact and split proinsulin which can be found in the circulation in minute quantities. Besides the highly regulated transport mechanism found in secretory cells such as the β cell, through which most insulin is secreted, there is a constitutive pathway. This pathway is a default pathway present in all cells. In the β cell, insulin conversion is less efficient in the constitutive pathway. In β-cell stress as is seen in early diabetes or in insulinoma tumor cells, higher levels of circulating proinsulin and split proinsulin molecule are seen. These result from less efficient proinsulin conversion within the granule or from a greater proportion of insulin being secreted through the unregulated pathway. Though considerable advances in our understanding of granule formation and insulin processing have been made in the last decade, many of the specifics remain to be elucidated.[6,7]

Other protein constituents of the secretory granule besides insulin, C-peptide, and processing enzymes include β-granin (a conversion product of chromogrannin A), pancreastatin, and islet amyloid polypeptide (IAPP). The biologic function of these molecules is uncertain, although intense interest surrounds their potential roles in the pathophysiology of diabetes. Whereas no function of isolated C-peptide other than in the folding of the proinsulin molecule could be demonstrated in initial studies, recent interest has turned to the potential role of the absence of C-peptide in the development of complications of insulin-dependent diabetes and in the development of insulin resistance.[8] Pancreastatin reportedly inhibits insulin release.[9] IAPP is found in insoluble amyloid deposits within islets in non–insulin-dependent diabetes mellitus (NIDDM) as well as within insulinomas. Some have postulated that IAPP may play a role in the insulin secretory defect and/or peripheral insulin resistance observed in diabetes, but compelling evidence for both is lacking.[10]

As the secretory granule matures, insulin crystallizes into hexamers coordinated around zinc divalent cations, which produces the dense granule observed with electron microscopy. Insulin is stored in such dense granules until released or degraded. The process of insulin release involves exocytosis or fusion of secretory vesicles with the plasma membrane, resulting in the discharge of insulin and other granule components into the extracellular space. Granule transport throughout the cell from the RER to the Golgi and from the Golgi to the cell surface is energy dependent, highly regulated, and requires a variety of cytoskeletal, membrane, and other cytoplasmic proteins. A small guanosine triphosphate (GTP)-binding protein, Rab3A, seems to play a critical role in the process of regulated insulin exocytosis. It is thought to mediate exocytosis through interaction of an effector domain with two membrane-associated proteins that are released into the cytoplasm in concert with exocytosis.[11] Further work on the regulation of granule processing and membrane fusion is one of the most promising avenues for identifying novel targets for drug development and the potential molecular defects in insulin secretion present in diabetes.

REGULATION OF SECRETION

Glucose is, by far, the most important physiologic regulator of insulin secretion. However, insulin secretion in response to glucose is modulated by many factors including amino acids, other sugars, fatty acids, ketone bodies, hormones, and drugs. Studies on insulin secretion can and have been performed in isolated β cells, isolated islets, and perfused pancreases, as well as in whole organisms stimulated with either oral or intravenous secretagogues. Each model provides slightly different insights. Many volumes have been written on the regulation and regulators of insulin secretion and here we will touch on the highlights, particularly of *in vivo* insulin secretion. *In vivo* insulin secretion generally cannot be measured directly but only inferred because of clearance of insulin by the liver. Because C-peptide is secreted in equimolar concentrations with insulin from the β cell and is not subject to first-pass metabolism in the liver, insulin secretory rates can be determined after determining C-peptide kinetics by measuring the C-peptide in blood.

Normally, as one contemplates eating a meal, sights and smells stimulate vagal efferents whose cholinergic influence seems to heighten the insulin response to glucose stimuli.[12] Oral ingestion of sugars, fats, and proteins results in greater insulin responses than the same nutrients administered intravenously. This effect, known as the incretin effect, seems to be mediated by a series of gut hormones and has led to the concept of an entero-insular (gut-islet) axis in the regulation of metabolism. The most important of these gut hormones in the regulation of insulin metabolism are glucagon-like peptide 1 (GLP-1), cholecystokinin (CCK), and glucose-dependent insulinotropic peptide (also known as gastric inhibitory peptide, or GIP). At least GLP-1 is under development as a potential therapeutic agent in diabetes.[13,14]

In response to a constant-rate intravenous infusion of glucose, insulin is secreted in a biphasic pattern with an initial surge of insulin secretion (peak in a matter of minutes) and a subsequent second phase that is proportional to the glucose level attained and lasting for a few hours. The mechanisms that account for this biphasic pattern are uncertain and may reflect either transient intracellular signals, a readily releasable pool of preformed vesicles, and/or heterogeneity in the responses of different β cells or different islets. A variety of other carbohydrate molecules have been shown to either stimulate directly or potentiate insulin secretion. The amino acids leucine, arginine, and lysine are potent insulin secretagogues and their effects are potentiated by glucose. Acutely, lipids seem to have minimal effects on insulin secretion *in vivo*, although *in vitro* there appear to be a variety of responses in which fatty acid chain length and degree of unsaturation are important. Approximately 50% of insulin secretion during any 24 h period is related to basal insulin requirements, and the remainder is secreted in response to meals. In both basal and stimulated secretion, insulin is secreted at a basal rate with superimposed large pulses (20–600% increase) at a frequency of 1.5 to 2 h, with the pulse amplitude largely determined by the glucose concentration. Superimposed on these ultradian rhythms are rapid oscillations, with a frequency of 8 to 16 min, that are not clearly related to glucose concentration. These pulses are barely measurable in the peripheral circulation but are larger in the portal circulation. The physiologic significance of these oscillations is unknown, although pulsatile insulin delivery seems to be more effective pharmacologically than continuous insulin delivery. Finally, there are circadian rhythms in insulin secretion, with greater insulin responses in the morning than in the evening associated with an increase in glucose concentration, suggesting a decrease in the glucose responsiveness of the β cell to insulin.[15-17]

Over the last several years, tremendous advances have been made in our understanding of the molecular physiology of insulin secretion. When β cells are exposed to glucose, glucose enters the cells through a specific high-capacity low-affinity facilitative glucose transporter molecule termed GLUT-2, which is structurally similar to the higher affinity transporters expressed in other tissues. Because of these affinity differences, glucose will enter the β cell well at relatively high levels of circulating glucose and less well than other tissues at lower glucose concentrations. Thus other tissues, particularly the brain, are able to obtain glucose in the fasting state while glucose-mediated insulin secretion is abrogated.

Glucose metabolism is critical for all effects of glucose on insulin secretion. Glucose metabolism occurs almost exclusively through the glycolytic pathway within the islet. The rate-limiting step of glucose metabolism within β cells is phosphorylation, which is catalyzed by two enzyme systems, a high-affinity hexokinase that is active at low glucose concentrations but severely inhibited by its product (glucose-6-phosphate), and a low-affinity enzyme termed glucokinase. Glucokinase activity over the physiologic range of glucose concentration exactly parallels insulin secretion, suggesting that glucokinase is the glucose sensor of the β cell. It is believed that stimulus secretion coupling is mediated by transmembrane electrical changes that occur in response to glucose metabolism. Glucose metabolism is classically believed to be coupled to insulin metabolism through alterations in cytosolic ATP/ADP ratios which result in closure of ATP-sensitive potassium channels expressed on the surface of the β cell. This closure results in depolarization of the cell. When a certain threshold is reached voltage dependent calcium channels open, allowing calcium to enter cells. Intracellular calcium results in activation of Ca^{2+}-calmodulin-dependent protein kinase, which is thought to result in a phosphorylation cascade. The net result of this cascade is granule fusion with the plasma membrane and insulin release. Voltage- and calcium-dependent potassium channels are subsequently activated and the membrane is repolarized. This is an extremely simplified explanation of what seems to be occurring. Molecular techniques have resulted in the identification of at least 20 ion channels within islets. The effects of various neurotransmitters and hormones on insulin secretion seem to be mediated through the cyclic AMP-protein kinase C pathway as well as the phosphoinositide-protein kinase A pathway, both of which can amplify glucose-mediated signals as regards intracellular calcium. The three kinase systems discussed are known to have at least 20 identified endogenous substrates for phosphorylation.[18,19] Further unveiling the complexity of intracellular fuel metabolism and stimulus secretion coupling will require many years of continued effort by large numbers of investigators in different disciplines.

INSULIN ACTION

Insulin binds on a specific cell surface receptor on most cells. The insulin receptor has endogenous tyrosine kinase activity, and insulin action is thought to be mediated by an extensively studied but still fairly poorly understood cascade of phosphorylation.[20] The vast majority of glucose clearance from the circulation in response to insulin occurs into muscle, with a smaller fraction taken up by adipocytes. This effect is mediated by the so-called insulin regulated facilitative glucose transporter, or GLUT4. In the absence of insulin, GLUT4 is not present on the cell surface but within a pool of intracellular vesicles. In the presence of insulin, these vesicles rapidly translocate to the cell surface and fuse with the plasma membrane, resulting in a dramatic increase in glucose transport capacity. Because glucose is rapidly phosphorylated intracellularly, there is a net flux of glucose across the membrane as it enters by facilitated diffusion down its concentration gradient. Insulin also results in the dephosphorylation and activation of glycogen synthase, resulting in a stimulation of glycogen synthesis. Simultaneously, glycogenolysis is inhibited by the action of a phosphatase to inhibit phosphorylase b kinase. Insulin promotes protein synthesis. In adipose tissue, glucose uptake is stimulated through the actions of insulin on adipose GLUT4. Hormone-sensitive lipase within the adipocyte is inhibited, resulting in a decrease in the mobilization of triglycerides from the intracellular lipid droplet. Simultaneously, the synthesis and activity of lipoprotein lipase, a secreted product of the adipocyte and myocyte, is increased. This results in accelerated clearance of fatty acids and glycerol from absorbed dietary chylomicrons as well as VLDL primarily into muscle and fat. The rate-limiting step of triglyceride formation (α-glycerol phosphate acyltransferase) is likewise activated through a phosphorylation event in the presence of insulin. In the liver, glucose uptake is mediated by the same low-affinity transporter (GLUT2) as is employed in the β cell and is not regulated by insulin. However, glucose uptake increases in the fed state as a result of higher portal glucose concentrations and blood flow. High levels of insulin (and concomitant low levels of glucagon) result in stimulation of glycogen synthase and inhibition of glycogen phosphorylase. This combination thus tilts the balance of hepatic glucose metabolism toward glycogen deposition. In general, very low levels of insulin secretion, as would occur many hours after a meal, are associated with a disinhibition of glucagon secretion and a reversal of the effects listed above.[21]

INSULIN-DEPENDENT DIABETES MELLITUS

IDDM is the form of diabetes usually found in children and young adults and is characterized generally by leanness, insulin deficiency, and an absolute requirement for insulin treatment to maintain life. This form of diabetes seems to be the result of a specific autoimmune attack in which the β cells are specifically destroyed. The disease has both genetic and environmental influences highlighted by the fact that approximately 2% of fraternal twins will share the trait while approximately 30% of identical twins are concordant for the condition. The genes responsible for IDDM are largely unknown. The single largest genetic effect is encoded within the major histocompatibility complex (MHC) on the short arm of chromosome 6 in linkage disequilibrium with the class II molecules of the region (HLA-DQ in particular). There seems to be at least two diabetogenic loci within the MHC that can synergize in conferring diabetes risk. Other genetic influence is linked to the human insulin gene, although the nature of this gene's influence is completely unknown. However, because of the known higher prevalence of diabetes among the children of diabetic men than women and the known effect of genomic imprinting on the nearby IGF-II locus, it has been speculated that this locus may explain the difference in transmission of diabetes risk from mothers and fathers. Several other genetic loci have been postulated.[22-24]

What results in the conversion of genetically determined risk to ongoing islet destruction is unknown, but several mechanisms are hypothesized. One compelling recent strand of evidence in the triggering of islet autoimmunity links a shared amino acid sequence. This sequence is homologous between a suspected islet pathogen (Coxsackie virus B4), an islet cell surface protein (ICA-69) that is expressed in the presence of γ-interferon (produced in response to inflammation such as viral infection), and bovine serum albumin, a major protein constituent of cows' milk. It has been shown in some but not all populations that early exposure of infants to cows' milk in the form of infant formulas is associated with an increased risk of IDDM. This raises the possibility that cows' milk exposure while the gut immune system is immature and relatively leaky to peptides results in an immunization to a peptide that alternatively could be encountered with a common viral exposure (Coxsackie B4). Later, any viral exposure or low-level inflammation of islets would result in the expression of the similar peptide on the surface of islets in the form of ICA-69, thus creating a potential target for immunologic destruction. Further interest in this mechanism has been raised by the demonstration that diabetes can be prevented in an animal model by immunizing weanlings with this putative peptide.[22,25]

Once the autoimmune process is started, circulating antibodies to a variety of islet proteins and glycolipids are found in the circulation, which can be useful for determining the prediabetic state. The exact mechanisms of immune destruction are unknown, and considerable controversy exists as to whether the β cell is specifically destroyed through a lymphocyte-mediated cellular destruction ("kiss of death") or through its exquisite sensitivity to certain cytokines and oxidative damage. Strategies to predict who will develop IDDM and when they are in place have produced a variety of intervention trials that are underway to try to prevent IDDM in children and adults at high risk.[22]

Because patients with IDDM are absolutely deficient in insulin, they require injected insulin to live. In the absence of injected insulin, the combination of essentially nonexistent insulin levels and inappropriately elevated glucagon levels (as a result of the release of normal β-cell inhibition of glucagon secretion) results in unrestrained lipolysis and increased hepatic glucose production. Increased production and decreased clearance of ketone bodies as breakdown products of fatty acid metabolism also occur. This produces severe hyperglycemia or high blood sugar and ketone accumulation, which cause dehydration and severe acidosis. The resulting diabetic ketoacidosis may progress rapidly, causing death as a result of cardiovascular collapse.[26]

NON–INSULIN-DEPENDENT DIABETES MELLITUS

NIDDM is loosely used to refer to a spectrum of disorders characterized generally by elevations of fasting blood glucose usually occurring in adults. Pathophysiologically, many diverse mechanisms are operative and our understanding of these has advanced fairly rapidly over the past decade. Most patients with NIDDM are obese and middle-aged. Age, sedentary lifestyle, and obesity are risk factors for diabetes, and most seem to be associated with "insulin resistance." This term is used to convey the notion that in some individuals the tissues, particularly muscle and liver, are relatively resistant to the actions of insulin. Normally, this can be overcome by the β cell compensating through increased insulin secretion. This clearly occurs in the majority of people with obesity, old age, and a sedentary lifestyle who do not develop diabetes. However, in people genetically predisposed to the development of diabetes, complete compensation for insulin resistance with increased insulin production fails. Then, although the absolute levels of insulin in the circulation may be significantly higher than in a thin, young, active insulin-sensitive subject, diabetes ensues. Hyperglycemia develops because of increased hepatic glucose production (a dysfunctional process when the fasting blood glucose is already high) and decreased glucose clearance into muscle. This dysregulation of glucose metabolism results from inadequate insulin action in the liver and muscle. The mechanisms by which insulin resistance is produced are completely unknown, although abundant hypotheses exist. Obesity is the most common cause of insulin resistance in Western society and can be reduced by caloric restriction and exercise. Drugs are under investigation that lessen insulin resistance both in muscle and in liver, although their mechanisms of action are unclear.

The role of insulin secretory defects has been more controversial but more clearly established in the last few years. Most interesting has been the discovery that a significant proportion of patients with an autosomal dominant form of NIDDM termed maturity onset diabetes of youth, or MODY, have mutations in the glucokinase gene. Glucokinase is the putative glucose sensor that catalyzes the rate-limiting step in islet glucose metabolism. As would be expected, patients carrying these mutations have a mild form of disease because their levels of the normal allele are only 50% reduced. It has been well established that glucokinase gene transcription is regulated by glucose. Therefore, there is almost complete compensation for the inactive mutant enzyme by the normal allele as glucose levels increase marginally. Another as yet unknown mutation linked to the adenosine deaminase locus produces a form of MODY with another insulin secretory defect. A third genetic form of NIDDM has been discovered in association with various mutations in the mitochondrial genome (exclusively inherited from one's mother). Several mitochondrial mutations are associated with defects in insulin secretion; they are variable in their phenotype, generally involving a variety of organ systems, with the diabetes usually being relatively mild.[26-28]

Careful study of patients with mild forms of diabetes has demonstrated defects in almost all aspects of glucose metabolism discussed above. In early diabetes, before the blood glucose is significantly elevated, there is decreased expression of the islet glucose transport molecule, GLUT2, both in humans and in animal models. This in effect blinds the β cell to circulating glucose levels. However, the β cell maintains its sensitivity to amino acids as a secretagogue. Therefore, it is suggested that patients with NIDDM consume meals consisting of mixed protein and carbohydrate. The first phase of insulin secretion seems to be specifically lost. Therefore, consuming carbohydrates, which are more difficult to digest (high in fiber), can be associated with an improvement in glucose levels. A new therapy is aimed at improving the coupling of intestinal carbohydrate absorption and the delayed pancreatic insulin secretion.

Several glucosidase inhibitors have been developed that inhibit disaccharidase activity in the proximal intestine, shifting carbohydrate absorption distally and thereby allowing the pancreas more time to respond with insulin secretion. The pulsatility of insulin secretion is lost in early diabetes and even in the metabolically normal relatives of patients with NIDDM. This suggests a fundamental change in either islet glucose metabolism or the electrical regulation of stimulus secretion coupling that precedes the development of NIDDM. These and other aspects of insulin secretion are areas of intense exploration aimed at providing better screening for patient risk of developing diabetes as well as directing new targets for drug development.[26,28]

INSULINOMA

Insulin-producing adenomas of the pancreas, although the most common endocrine pancreatic tumors, are quite rare and are characterized by hypoglycemia. A discussion of hypoglycemia follows in the section on glucagon and, therefore, we will make only a few points as they relate to the discussion above. These tumors are almost always solitary, although they can occur as part of the multiple endocrine neoplasia type 1 (MEN 1) syndrome. Because the insulin secretion within these tumors can remain fairly regulated, it is often quite difficult to make the diagnosis. These tumors can produce hypoglycemia after a meal because of increased insulin secretion from a large mass of β cells. However, they classically produce fasting hypoglycemia as a result of modestly increased insulin secretion and thereby decreased glucagon secretion between meals. Generally, the ratio of proinsulin to insulin is somewhat elevated, reflecting the fact that more of the secretion is occurring through relatively unregulated mechanisms. Hypoglycemia produced from insulinomas must be distinguished from factitious hypoglycemia. This can generally be accomplished by simultaneous measurements of serum glucose, insulin, and C-peptide along with antibodies to insulin and serum sulfonylurea levels. If the hypoglycemia were caused by surreptitious insulin administration, the glucose level would be low, while the insulin level would be very high and the C-peptide low. C-peptide is not contained within commercial insulin preparations, and the hypoglycemia would have suppressed endogenous insulin secretion. Sulfonylureas are medications that enhance glucose-stimulated insulin secretion by activating the ATP-dependent potassium channel and can cause hypoglycemia. In such cases, the glucose would be low while insulin and C-peptide would be high. Serum and urine toxicology studies would reveal the presence of sulfonylurea medication. Insulin antibodies rarely are produced by myeloma tumors and in other cases are the consequence of injection of insulin. When they cause hypoglycemia, these are high-capacity but usually low-affinity antibodies. As such they can cause binding of insulin after meals as insulin concentrations become quite high; later, as insulin levels fall, insulin will be released from the immunologic complex and can produce hypoglycemia. In such a condition, the circulating insulin levels will generally be extremely high, the C-peptide level relatively low, and the antibody assay for insulin binding will be high. Other tumors, particularly hepatobiliary tumors, can produce high levels of free IGF-I, which can produce hypoglycemia, but these patients are almost always affected by a clinically advanced malignancy. The insulin and C-peptide levels are low because insulin production is not part of the pathophysiology in these non-islet cell tumors.[29,30]

Generally, the appropriate treatment for insulinomas is surgical removal. Occasionally the tumors are malignant or the patient is too ill to undergo surgery. In such cases, specific therapy can be targeted to molecules important in the insulin secretory pathway. Diazoxide is a drug with a well-established record of ameliorating hypoglycemia in the setting of insulinoma. It is a specific activator of the ATP-dependent potassium channel and as such keeps the insulin-producing cell hyperpolarized and resistant to depolarization. Calcium channel blockers have been used but less frequently produce significant benefits. Rare tumors have been treated with somatostatin analogues with variable results.[29,30]

GLUCAGON

INTRODUCTION

Glucagon is a single-chain polypeptide that is synthesized by the α cells of the pancreas from a 160-amino acid preprohormone. It is also produced in intestinal cells where alternative hormone products such as GLP-1 are produced. The gene for glucagon is located on chromosome 2 in humans. The end result of its various physiologic actions is the raising of serum glucose levels. As opposed to insulin, which acts throughout the body, glucagon has only one target organ outside of the pancreas—the liver. Its specific actions include the stimulation of glycogenolysis and gluconeogenesis, as well as the production of ketone bodies from fatty acid precursors. Although glucagon differs from insulin in that it is catabolic, they both exert their effects in two distinct ways. First, they rapidly induce changes in the catalytic properties of critical enzymes by either phosphorylation or dephosphorylation, usually within minutes to hours. Over hours to days, the actual synthesis of these enzymes is up-regulated. Glucagon is one of many peptide hormones that utilizes the adenylate cyclase and cyclic AMP second messenger system. Glucagon binds to a membrane receptor in hepatocytes, thereby increasing cyclic AMP levels through a Gs-protein linked intermediate. When glucagon levels are high relative to those of insulin, glucose-6-phosphatase, fructose-1,6-bisphosphatase, and phosphoenolpyruvate carboxykinase are all induced, resulting in increased glucose production.

REGULATION OF SECRETION

The production and secretion of glucagon is affected by a great number of substances in addition to glucose. Although hypoglycemia is perhaps the most obvious stimulant, amino acids, other hormones, and the autonomic nervous system all play important roles in modulating glucagon levels. Each of these, in the appropriate physiologic context, will be reviewed. The role of glucagon in the prevention of and recovery from hypoglycemia will be discussed separately in the following section.

It is clearly established that glucose inhibits the release of glucagon from α cells. The threshold for this inhibition is 2–3 mM, which is below that associated with stimulation of insulin release. Glucose metabolism in the α cell is only around 15–20% of that found in the β cell; furthermore, glucose uptake into purified α cells is not stimulated by insulin. It should be noted that glucose-induced inhibition of glucagon is effectively counteracted by inhibitors of cellular glucose metabolism. Anoxia, which is a powerful inhibitor of metabolism, actually stimulates glucagon release, regardless of glucose concentration.[31] The role of β receptors and their agonists in glucagon secretion from isolated islets of Langerhans has been studied. A selective β$_2$ adrenoreceptor agonist was found to raise cyclic AMP levels and stimulate glucagon secretion from rat islets, and this effect was specific for islet α cells.[32] As reflected in the previous discussion on insulin, in the past, the pancreatic α cell was thought to be a prototypical insulin-sensitive cell. Careful studies on purified α cells have shown, however, that there are less than 400 insulin receptors per α cell. This receptor density is 50- to 500-fold lower than that found in classical insulin-sensitive cells. Furthermore, insulin itself has no effect on α-cell electrical activity or glucagon release.[31] Islet cell studies have also established the presence of γ-aminobutyric acid (GABA)-activated Cl– channels, which are subject to desensitization after prolonged exposure to GABA. Through this mechanism, β cells may be able to suppress glucagon release by production of GABA in response to elevated glucose levels. It would then follow that glucagon secretion will increase whenever β-cell function is impaired. This represents one potential explanation for the observation that patients with diabetes often have inappropriate excess secretion of glucagon, despite their hyperglycemia.[31]

In terms of the regulation of glucagon secretion, recurrent hypoglycemia has a somewhat paradoxical effect, even in the absence of diabetes. When healthy rats experienced iatrogenic insulin-induced hypoglycemia repeatedly over a 4-week period, their glucagon response to this stimulus decreased by 84% compared to controls. After a 3- to 4-week recovery period, the glucagon response recovered somewhat, but it remained significantly less than the untreated control. This effect was found to be very specific for hypoglycemia. When arginine was given to stimulate glucagon release in the same animals, the response was completely normal. This demonstrated that the secretory reserves of the α cells and adrenal medulla were intact, and the defects caused by recurrent hypoglycemia were not due to depletion of glucagon itself.[33]

Amino acids affect glucagon release to varying degrees. Alanine causes a swift and dramatic rise in glucagon concentrations, as do glycine and serine. The other neutral amino acids (Asn, Thr, Met, Phe, and Gln) also increase glucagon levels but not to the same degree. Among the basic amino acids, arginine is a more effective stimulant than lysine or histidine. Leucine is the only amino acid that has been shown to significantly decrease the plasma glucagon level. It must be pointed out that most amino acids also stimulate insulin secretion. One possible explanation for this effect on glucagon is that certain amino acids are potent glycogenic precursors. When these particular amino acids (such as alanine and glycine) are present, the increase in glucagon secretion relative to that of insulin would favor efficient glucose production via gluconeogenesis.[34] When comparing the effects of an intravenous infusion of 21 amino acids with oral consumption of a protein-rich meal, the stimulation of both insulin and glucagon release is nearly identical. This is true only when the amino acid mixture is prepared so as to accurately imitate the pattern of plasma amino acid elevations seen after eating a typical protein-rich meal.[35]

Certain medical conditions, such as cirrhosis and hyperthyroidism, are associated with decreased glycogen stores. These patients have significantly higher glucagon and insulin levels than healthy adults, despite having normal glucose concentrations. These same patients have markedly blunted glucose responses to intravenous glucagon after an overnight fast. Because it is known that hepatectomized animals have markedly elevated glucagon levels chronically, it can be postulated that glucagon release may depend on glycogen stores in the liver. This is supported by the fact that in healthy adults during a prolonged fast, glucagon significantly increases only after 48 to 72 h, which is correlated with the complete exhaustion of glycogen stores. Furthermore, plasma glucagon levels are at their lowest when glycogen content is at its peak, as in the immediate postabsorptive period. If starvation continues for more than 72 h, plasma glucagon increases progressively, regardless of the lack of any significant change in glucose or insulin levels. These special situations may represent a breakdown of the classic feedback between glucose levels and glucagon secretion.[36]

The autonomic nervous system plays an important role, which has been increasingly recognized in the past decade, in the regulation of pancreatic endocrine function. Three separate yet interrelated autonomic inputs affect the pancreas and thereby glucagon secretion: (1) adrenal medullary epinephrine, (2) pancreatic parasympathetic nerves, and (3) pancreatic sympathetic nerves. When the sympathoadrenal system is activated, preganglionic sympathetic nerves discharge; the impulses travel to the adrenal medulla via the splanchnic nerves, which synapse on the postganglionic epinephrine-secreting adrenal chromaffin cells. Epinephrine, which reaches the pancreas through the systemic circulation, inhibits insulin while stimulating the release of glucagon. The islets contain approximately ten times higher levels of choline acetyltransferase than adjacent exocrine tissue, which clearly suggests extensive cholinergic innervation.[37] Furthermore, it has been shown that electrical activation of the vagus nerve stimulates the secretion of both glucagon and insulin. Exogenous VIP or gastrin-releasing peptide (GRP) both closely mimic the effect of the parasympathetic nervous system on the islet cells. Recent studies have suggested that preganglionic sympathetic fibers enter the pancreas directly and innervate sympathetic ganglia within the pancreatic parenchyma. In fact, sympathetic nerve terminals have been found in close proximity to islet cells. When these nerves are activated, glucagon release is also stimulated. Central pathways may also be involved, but their role is less clear. Electrical stimulation of the lateral hypothalamus causes insulin and glucagon levels to rise.[37]

In summary, it is clear that the regulation of glucagon secretion involves multiple mechanisms. In addition to familiar stimuli such as hypoglycemia (except as noted above), amino acids, glucocorticoids, and other hormones can influence its release. The autonomic nervous system can play a significant role, especially in settings of stress. Both somatostatin (discussed later in this chapter) and high serum levels of fatty acids inhibit the release of glucagon, as can GABA and β antagonists.

ROLE IN HYPOGLYCEMIA

Adequate plasma glucose levels are vital to the normal functioning of the human brain, which has very limited glucose storage capacity and requires weeks to convert to efficient metabolism of alternative fuels such as ketone bodies. It is interesting to note that there is only one hormone responsible for lowering glucose levels, but several mechanisms are in place to prevent and correct hypoglycemia. There is a predictable sequence of responses to decreasing glucose levels, which starts with an inhibition of insulin secretion, followed by increasing glucagon, epinephrine, and growth hormone secretion. This is followed by an increase in cortisol production; followed by neurogenic symptoms (tachycardia, sweating), neuroglycopenic symptoms, and then overt cognitive dysfunction, with some changes in brain autoregulation of blood flow occurring subsequently. If the hypoglycemia is not corrected, severe cases can lead to seizures, coma, and death.[38] The glycemic threshold for glucagon release is about 68 mg/dl, which is almost exactly the glucose concentration corresponding to a significant drop in cerebral metabolism.

Among the counterregulatory factors that protect against hypoglycemia, glucagon has a central and critical role. In the setting of acute or transient hypoglycemia, glucagon is responsible for approximately 40% of recovery. Selective glucagon deficiency has been shown to cause lower glucose concentrations, but it does not lead to overt hypoglycemia even after a 3-day fast or moderate exercise. However, if hyperinsulinemia is experimentally induced while simultaneously blocking glucagon release, severe hypoglycemia ensues. It should be noted that hypoglycemia virtually never occurs when the secretion and actions of both insulin and glucagon are normal.[38] Studies performed to evaluate the counterregulatory mechanisms at work during periods of moderate prolonged hypoglycemia, as would be seen in insulin treated diabetics or patients with insulinomas, demonstrate the vital role of glucagon. When incremental increases in glucagon are prevented by somatostatin, lower glucose production rates were seen, and glucose infusions were necessary to prevent severe hypoglycemia. These same studies provide evidence that the long-held belief that epinephrine can completely compensate for glucagon deficiency may be incorrect. In healthy adults, lack of adequate glucagon response led to decreases in plasma glucose to as low as 38 mg/dl despite increasing levels of epinephrine.[39] It must be noted that patients with IDDM typically lose the normal production of glucagon for counterregulation after only a few years of the disease and therefore (as discussed in the previous section) are at high risk for hypoglycemic complications.[33]

Epinephrine is the other counterregulatory hormone of key importance. The contribution of adrenal activation toward correction of hypoglycemia increases with the severity of the stimulus. It turns out that the plasma glucose nadir rather than the change in level or even the rate of change is the major determinant of the peak epinephrine response.[37] Physiologic increases in epinephrine that occur in response to hypoglycemia lead to both sustained increases in hepatic glucose production and suppression of peripheral glucose utilization.[39] These mechanisms are mediated through both α- and β-adrenergic receptors. In addition, mobilization of certain fatty acids has been found to be an indirect effect of elevated epinephrine levels, and these fatty acids further enhance glucose production while limiting utilization.[38] Although epinephrine deficiency (as would be seen after bilateral adrenalectomy or experimentally caused by both α and β blockade) does not impair glucose recovery from hypoglycemia if glucagon secretion is normal, the absence of both inevitably leads to severe hypoglycemia.

Although both the sympathoadrenal and parasympathetic portions of the autonomic nervous system contribute to hypoglycemic responses, there are a few distinctions between their roles. First, pancreatic parasympathetic nerves are activated at less severe levels of glucopenia than required for epinephrine release from the adrenal medulla. Surgical procedures such as vagotomy or pyloric transection, which disrupt parasympathetic pathways, abolish parasympathetic responses to hypoglycemia. The hormones cortisol and growth hormone are also involved in counterregulation of hypoglycemia, but to a lesser degree than glucagon or epinephrine. Neither cortisol nor growth hormone is activated to a significant degree in transient hypoglycemia, but they do contribute to recovery in the setting of prolonged hypoglycemia. They act by further stimulating hepatic glucose production and also by helping to suppress glucose utilization by peripheral tissues.[38] It should be emphasized that neither of these hormones plays a critical role in correcting hypoglycemia, even when prolonged, if glucagon and epinephrine responses are intact. This has been shown by experiments that carefully isolated the relative contributions of all four major counterregulatory substances.[39]

GLUCAGONOMA

The glucagonoma syndrome is extremely rare, with approximately 100 cases reported in the literature. The mean age at diagnosis is 55, yet many patients have a long history of symptoms that suggest the tumor's presence for 5 to 10 years. The associated clinical features include weight loss, mild diabetes, depression, and anemia. Other conditions that are more specific for glucagonoma are painful tongue enlargement and ulcers at the angles of the mouth as well as a characteristic red, migratory, oozing rash. This rash is thought to be associated with zinc deficiency and low levels of amino acids. A less common but potentially fatal complication of glucagonoma results from blood clots forming in large veins within the body in about 30% of patients. Diagnosis is easily accomplished with modern assays, in which the upper limit of normal for glucagon levels is 20 pmol/L. The cutoff for diagnosis is generally set at 50 pmol/L or higher. Other conditions that can lead to elevated glucagon levels are renal failure, hepatic failure, prolonged hypoglycemia, and severe stress. Current treatment options include surgical removal, which is the treatment of choice when technically possible. Alternative therapies in selected cases include hepatic artery embolization and chemotherapy with either streptozotocin or octreotide, a long-acting somatostatin analog.[40]

SOMATOSTATIN

Somatostatin is a 14-amino acid peptide with a disulfide ring which was first isolated from ovine hypothalamus in 1973. It was later discovered that most of the total body stores of somatostatin are located in the digestive tract, with 65% contained in the gut and approximately 5% within the pancreas. It is found in δ cells at the periphery of the islets.[41] The two biologically active forms, SOM-14 and SOM-28, are both derived from a 116-amino acid preprosomatostatin encoded on the long arm of chromosome 3. SOM-14 is the predominant form in the pancreas.[42]

PHYSIOLOGIC ACTIONS AND REGULATION

Pancreatic and gut somatostatin inhibit the release of numerous other hormones and peptides. These include insulin and glucagon within the pancreas as well as gastrin, secretin, motilin, and VIP from other portions of the digestive system. The release of somatostatin inhibits gastric acid secretion, gastric emptying, gastrointestinal blood flow, and absorption of nutrients from the intestinal lumen. A specific example of this is the effect on absorption of triglycerides. Low levels have been found to contribute to the postprandial rise in triglycerides while intravenous infusions attenuate the peak value of serum triglycerides after meals. Somatostatin also decreases pancreatic exocrine function by lowering enzyme and bicarbonate secretion from the pancreas.[43] The large number of inhibitory effects of somatostatin is mainly due to the broad distribution of its receptors across different cell types. Binding studies with radioactively labeled somatostatin have revealed receptors on G cells and parietal cells within the stomach and on δ cells themselves. This finding strongly suggests a negative feedback of somatostatin on its own biosynthesis and secretion. Binding sites have also been found on other pancreatic islet cells as well as exocrine pancreatic cells. Four structurally related somatostatin receptors ranging from 369 to 428 amino acids have been isolated and cloned since 1992.[41] They are members of the G-protein-linked family of receptors, something this group has in common with the glucagon receptor. Pancreatic α cells contain a higher proportion of SOM-14 binding sites, which explains the fact that the 14-amino acid form is more potent than the 28-amino acid form at inhibiting glucagon release. This distribution is reversed in the β cell, and consequently the 28-amino acid form is more effective at suppressing insulin release.[44] Within the cell, somatostatin activates the inhibitory G protein, which in turn inhibits adenylate cyclase activity and lowers cAMP levels. Direct effects on calcium channels have also been reported. An additional mechanism is protein dephosphorylation, as somatostatin has been found to increase phosphoprotein phosphatase activity in the digestive system.[43]

Plasma concentrations of somatostatin under basal conditions range from 5 to 30 pmol/L. Meals containing fat and protein typically increase this value to 10 to 50 pmol/L, yet it must be noted that because there is a 30–45% transhepatic gradient for somatostatin, much of it released into the portal vein is metabolized prior to reaching the peripheral circulation. SOM-28 is metabolized more slowly than SOM-14 and therefore may be more important as a hormonal mediator. Somatostatin secretion is also stimulated by a number of other peptides and hormones, including GRP, gastrin itself, CCK, secretin, glucagon, and VIP. Because all of these peptides also inhibit gastric acid secretion, somatostatin may represent the common inhibitory mediator for hormonal and nervous system effectors. Among all of the aforementioned secretagogues, CCK and gastrin are relatively weak.[41]

THERAPEUTIC USES

It has been extremely difficult to distinguish between the physiological and pharmacological actions of somatostatin. The reasons for this include its widespread distribution, the fact that it does not necessarily act by release into the general circulation, and the lack of specific antagonists to its actions. Furthermore, because the circulating half-life of somatostatin is less than 3 min, a longer acting analog was developed for therapeutic applications. This analog, originally known as SMS 201-995, is now widely known as octreotide. Compared to somatostatin, octreotide is a much more potent inhibitor of secretion and has a half-life of 1 to 2 h. It cannot be absorbed orally and therefore must be administered by subcutaneous injections three times a day or via a continuous infusion pump.

The most effective applications for octreotide involve the treatment of gastrointestinal or pancreatic neuroendocrine tumors. These types of tumors are extremely rare and most are slow growing. This category of tumor includes insulinomas, carcinoids, glucagonomas, gastrinomas, and vasoactive intestinal peptidomas. Surgical removal, whenever possible, is the best treatment option for these tumors. When complete cure cannot be accomplished surgically, octreotide is effective at lowering levels of the secreted hormone or peptide and can produce marked improvements in related symptoms. For example, vasoactive intestinal peptidomas are characterized by profuse watery diarrhea of the secretory type. Octreotide inhibits secretion of VIP and also reduces intestinal secretion directly, thereby effectively controlling the diarrhea. It is also helpful with the flushing, wheezing, and diarrhea associated with overproduction of 5-hydroxytryptamine in the carcinoid syndrome. However, octreotide has not produced long-term reductions in the size of these tumors, and therefore, must be considered primarily as a palliative agent at this time. Although octreotide has been shown to inhibit gastric, pancreatic, and colonic cancer cell lines *in vitro* and *in vivo*, phase II studies demonstrated no benefit from its use in patients with these types of metastatic cancer.

There are several other disease settings in which octreotide has definite or potential therapeutic uses. One of these is in the treatment of diabetes. In this case, its benefit would be associated with lowering growth hormone and IGF-I levels, rather than controlling serum glucose concentration. These two hormones are thought to be involved in the vascular proliferation that underlies both diabetic retinopathy and nephropathy. Another promising application for octreotide is in the treatment of bleeding esophageal varices in patients with cirrhosis. Octreotide reduces portal pressure and hepatic blood flow and has been shown to be of equal efficacy to vasopressin in randomized trials. Furthermore, octreotide is less costly and has fewer side effects than vasopressin, which can cause coronary artery spasm. Many types of diarrhea respond to octreotide therapy, such as those associated with short bowel syndrome, ileostomy, diabetes with autonomic neuropathy, and medullary thyroid carcinoma. Although somatostatin is thought to be a major regulator of pancreatic exocrine function, a clear role of octreotide in the treatment of acute or chronic pancreatitis has not been established. The use of octreotide is relatively safe, with complications mainly limited to gallstone formation, steatorrhea, and transient diarrhea.[41]

SOMATOSTATINOMAS

Like glucagonomas, these neuroendocrine tumors are extremely rare. They occur both in the pancreas and in the intestine with roughly equal incidence. The mean age at diagnosis is about 50, and there is a slight (1.5:1) female preponderance. The pancreatic tumors are metastatic in 85–90% of cases, whereas the intestinal tumors are metastatic in only about 50% of cases. The liver is the organ most frequently involved in metastatic spread. Clinical features include gallbladder disease, weight loss, and glucose abnormalities. In patients with pancreatic somatostatinomas, diabetes is present in 60–70%; however, less than 20% of intestinal tumors are associated with hyperglycemia. When evaluated in these patients, hypochlorhydria is also found but rarely produces clinical symptoms. When metastases are present, prognosis is extremely poor. Furthermore, these tumors do not respond to chemotherapy to any significant extent; therefore, complete surgical excision is the only chance for a cure.[38]

PANCREATIC POLYPEPTIDE

Pancreatic polypeptide is secreted as a 36-amino acid peptide from the PP cells within the islet as well as from cells scattered throughout the exocrine pancreas and in the gut. Pancreatic polypeptide seems to inhibit gallbladder contraction, pancreatic enzyme production, and gastric acid secretion. However, its effects in these regards are weak and of unclear physiologic significance. Pancreatic polypeptide seems to be largely released in response to cholinergic innervation in response to meals, and hypoglycemia and high serum levels are attained. Pancreatic polypeptide-secreting tumors are associated with no metabolic or other abnormalities except for occasional rash and diarrhea.[45]

REFERENCES

1. **Bonner-Weir, S. and Smith, F. E.,** Islet of Langerhans: morphology and its implications, in *Joslin's Diabetes Mellitus*, 13th ed., Kahn, C. R. and Weir, G. C., Eds., Lea & Febiger, Philadelphia, 1994, chap. 2.

2. **Rudnick, A., Ling, T.-Y., Odagiri, H., Rutter, W. J., and German, M. S.,** Pancreatic beta cells express a diverse set of homeobox gene, *Proc. Nat. Acad. Sci., U.S.A.,* 91, 12203, 1994.

3. **Bonner-Weir, S. and Smith, F. E.,** Islet cell growth and the growth factors involved, *Trends Endocrinol. Metab.,* 5, 60, 1994.

4. **Stagner, J. I. and Samols, E.,** The vascular order of islet cellular perfusion in the human pancreas, *Diabetes*, 41, 93, 1992.

5. **Melloul, D. and Cerasi, E.,** Transcription of the insulin gene: towards defining the glucose-sensitive cis-element and trans-acting factors, *Diabetologia*, 37(Suppl. 2), 3, 1994.

6. **Hutton, J. C.,** Insulin secretory granule biogenesis and the proinsulin-processing endopeptidases, *Diabetologia*, 37(Suppl. 2), 48, 1994.

7. **Halban, P. A.,** Proinsulin processing in the regulated and the constitutive secretory pathway, *Diabetologia*, 37(Suppl. 2), 65, 1994.

8. **Wahren, J., Johansson, B.-L., and Wallberg-Henriksson, H.,** Does C-peptide have a physiological role?, *Diabetologia*, 37(Suppl. 2), 99, 1994.

9. **Ahren, B., Lindskog, S., Tatemoto, K., and Efendic, S.,** Pancreastatin inhibits insulin secretion and stimulates glucagon secretion in mice, *Diabetes*, 37, 281, 1988.

10. **Bennet, W. M., Smith, D. M., and Bloom, S. R.,** Islet amyloid polypeptide: Does it play a pathophysiological role in the development of diabetes? *Diabetic Med.*, 11, 825, 1994.

11. **Olszewski, S., Deeney, J. T., Schuppin, G. T., Williams, K. P., Corkey, B. E., and Rhodes, C. J.,** Rab3A effector domain peptides induce insulin exocytosis via a specific interaction with a cytosolic protein doublet, *J. Biol. Chem.*, 269, 27987, 1994.

12. **Bruce, D. G., Storlein, L. H., Furler, S. M., and Chrisholm, D. J.,** Cephalic phase metabolic responses in normal weight adults, *Metabolism*, 36, 721, 1987.

13. **Gutniack, M. C., Orskov, C., Holst, J. J., Ahren, B., and Efendic, S.,** Antidiabetogenic effect of glucagon-like peptide-1 (7-36) amide in normal subjects and patients with diabetes mellitus, *N. Engl. J. Med.*, 326, 1316, 1992.

14. **Wang, Z. L., Wang, R. M., Owji, A. A., Smith, D. M., Ghatei, M. A., and Bloom, S. R.,** Glucagon-like peptide-1 is a physiologic incretin in rat, *J. Clin. Invest.*, 93, 2263, 1995.

15. **Pipeleers, D., Kiekens, R., Ling, Z., Wilikens, A., and Schuit, F.,** Physiologic relevance of heterogeneity in the pancreatic beta-cell population, *Diabetologia*, 37 (Suppl. 2), 57, 1994.

16. **O'Meara, N. M. and Polonsky, K. S.,** Insulin secretion in vivo, in *Joslin's Diabetes Mellitus*, 13th ed., Kahn, C. R. and Weir, G. C., Eds., Lea & Febiger, Philadelphia, 1994, chap. 5.

17. **Opara, E. C., Garfinkel, M., Hubbard, V. S., Burch, W. M., and Akwari, O. E.,** Effect of fatty acids on insulin release: role of chain length and degree of unsaturation, *Am. J. Physiol.*, 266, E635, 1994.

18. **Henquin, J.-C.,** Cell biology of insulin secretion, in *Joslin's Diabetes Mellitus*, 13th ed., Kahn, C. R. and Weir, G. C., Eds., Lea & Febiger, Philadelphia, 1994, chap. 4.

19. **Howell, S. L., Jones, P. M., and Persaud, S. J.,** Regulation of insulin secretion: the role of second messengers, *Diabetologia*, 37(Suppl. 2), 30, 1994.

20. **Quon, M. J., Butte, A. J., and Taylor, S. I.,** Insulin signal transduction pathways, *Trends Endocrinol. Metab.*, 5, 369, 1994,

21. **Chipkin, S. R., Kelly, K. L., and Ruderman, N. B.,** Hormone-fuel interrelationships: fed state, starvation and diabetes mellitus, in *Joslin's Diabetes Mellitus*, 13th ed., Kahn, C. R. and Weir, G. C., Eds., Lea & Febiger, Philadelphia, 1994, chap. 6.

22. **Atkinson, M. A. and Maclaren, N. K.,** The pathogenesis of insulin-dependent diabetes mellitus, *N. Engl. J. Med.*, 331, 1428, 1994.

23. **Davies, J. L., Kawaguchi, Y., Bennett, S. T., Copeman, J. B., Cordell, H. J., Pritchard, L. E., Reed, P. W., Gough, S. C., Jenkins, S. C., Palmer, S. M., Balfour, K. M., Rowe, B. R., Farrall, M., Barnett, A. H., Baln, S. C., and Todd, J. A.,** A genome-wide search for human type 1 diabetes susceptibility genes, *Nature*, 371, 130, 1994.

24. **Bennett, S. T., Lucasses, A. M., Bough, S. C. L., Powell, E. E., Undelien, D. E., Pritchard, L. E., Merriman, M. E., Kawaguchi, Y., Dronsfield, M. J., Pociot, F., Nerup, J., Bouzekri, N., Cambon-Thomsen, A., Ronningen, K. S., Barnett, A. H., Bain, S. C., and Todd, J. A.,** Susceptibility to human type 1 diabetes at *IDDM2* is determined by tandem repeat variation at the insulin gene minisatellite locus, *Nat. Genet.*, 9, 284, 1995.

25. **Akerblom, H. K., Savilahti, E., Saukkonen, T. T., Paganus, A., Virtanen, S. M., Teramo, K., Knip, M., Ilonen, J., Reijonen, H., Karjalainen, J., Vaarala, O., and Reunanen, A.,** The case for elimination of cow's milk in early infancy in the prevention of type 1 diabetes: the Finnish experience, *Diabetes/Metab. Rev.*, 9, 269, 1993.

26. **Foster D.,** Diabetes mellitus, in *Harrison's Principles of Internal Medicine*, 13th ed., Isselbacher, K. J., Braunwald, E., Wealson, J. D., Martin, J. B., Fauci, A. S., and Kasper, D. L., Eds., McGraw-Hill, New York, 1994, chap. 337, pp. 1979, 2000.

27. **Alcolado, J. C., Majid, A., Brockington, M., Sweeney, M. G., Morgan, R., Rees, A., Harding, A. E., and Barnett, A. H.,** Mitochondrial gene defects in patients with NIDDM, *Diabetologia*, 37, 372, 1994.

28. **Beck-Nielsen, H. and Groop, L. C.,** Metabolic and genetic characterization of prediabetic states. Sequence of events leading to non-insulin-dependent diabetes mellitus, *J. Clin. Invest.*, 94, 1714, 1994.

29. **Service, F. J., McMahon, M. M., O'Brien, P. C., and Ballard, D. J.,** Functioning insulinoma—incidence, recurrence, and long-term survival of patients: a 60-year study, *Mayo Clin. Proc.,* 66, 711, 1991.

30. **Polonsky, K. S.,** A practical approach to fasting hypoglycemia, *N. Engl. J. Med.,* 326, 1020, 1992.

31. **Rorsman, P., Ashcroft, F. M., and Bergren, P.-O.,** Regulation of glucagon release from pancreatic A-cells, *Biochem. Pharmacol.,* 41, 1783, 1991.

32. **Lacey, R. J., Berrow, N. S., Scarpello, J. H. B., and Morgan, N. G.,** Selective stimulation of glucagon secretion by beta-2 adrenoceptors in isolated islets of Langerhans of the rat, *Br. J. Pharmacol.,* 103, 1824, 1991.

33. **Powell, A. M., Sherwin, R. S. and Shulman, G. I.,** Impaired hormonal responses to hypoglycemia in spontaneously diabetic and recurrently hypoglycemic rats, *J. Clin. Invest.,* 92, 2667, 1993.

34. **Kuhara, T., Ikeda, S., Ohneda, A., and Sasaki, Y.,** Effects of intravenous infusion of 17 amino acids on the secretion of GH, glucagon, and insulin in sheep, *Am. J. Physiol.,* 260, E21, 1991.

35. **Schmid, R., Schulte-Frohlinde, E., Schusdziarra, V., Neubauer, J., Stegmann, M., Maier, V., and Classen, M.,** Contribution of postprandial amino acid levels to stimulation of insulin, glucagon, and pancreatic polypeptide in humans, *Pancreas,* 7, 698, 1991.

36. **Kabadi, U. M.,** Is hepatic glycogen content a regulator of glucagon secretion?, *Metabolism,* 41, 113, 1992.

37. **Havel, P. J. and Taborsky, G. J.,** The contribution of the autonomic nervous system to changes of glucagon and insulin secretion during hypoglycemic stress, *Endocr. Rev.,* 10, 332, 1989.

38. **Cryer, P. E.,** Glucose counterregulation: prevention and correction of hypoglycemia in humans, *Am. J. Physiol.,* 264, E149, 1993.

39. **DeFeo, P., Perriello, G., Torlone, E., Fanelli, C., Ventura, M. M., Santeusanio, F., Brunetti, P., Gerich, J., and Bolli, G. B.,** Evidence against important catecholamine compensation for absent glucagon counterregulation, *Am. J. Physiol.,* 260, E203, 1991.

40. **Bloom, S. R. and Polak, J. M.,** Glucagonoma syndrome, *Am. J. Med.,* 82, 25, 1987.

41. **Shulkes, A.,** Somatostatin: physiology and clinical applications, *Balliere's Clin. Endocrinol. Metab.,* 8, 215, 1994.

42. **Rabbani, S. H. and Patel, Y. C.,** Peptides derived by processing of rat prosomatostatin near the aminoterminus: characterization, tissue distribution, and release, *Endocrinology,* 126, 2054, 1990.

43. **Patel, Y. C. and Tannebaum, G. S.,** Somatostatin: basic and clinical aspects, *Metabolism,* 39, 1, 1990.

44. **Rens-Domiano, S. and Reisine, T.,** Biochemical and functional properties of somatostatin receptors, *J. Neurochem.,* 58, 1987, 1992.

45. **Vinik, A. I., Strodel, W. E., Eckhauser, F. E., Moattari, A. R., and Lloyd, R.,** Somatostatinomas, PPomas, neurotensinomas, *Semin. Oncol.,* 14, 263, 1987.

Chapter 11

GENETICS OF ENDOCRINE DISORDERS AND DIABETES MELLITUS

Bess Adkins Marshall and Abby Solomon Hollander

CONTENTS

0-8493-9429-5/96/$0.00+$.50
© 1996 by CRC Press, Inc.

INTRODUCTION

The advent of molecular genetics techniques has led to an explosion in information regarding the molecular basis and genetics of disease. Any review of the topic rapidly becomes outdated in light of this rapid advancement of knowledge. Nevertheless, this chapter attempts to review the genetic aspects of some of the endocrinologic disorders about which much is known. In the case of diabetes mellitus, the tremendous amount of work that has been published has not yet revealed the molecular genetic basis of either of the common types of diabetes, but many possibilities have been examined and either ruled out or found to be important in a subset of disease. Because of the mass of data available, this chapter necessarily neglects some disorders. However, those relatively common disorders about which much is known and those with particularly interesting etiologies are included in detail.

GENETICS OF GROWTH HORMONE

INTRODUCTION

Human growth is a complex physiologic phenomenon. Growth is influenced and controlled by a multitude of genetic and environmental factors. Growth hormone (GH) is a peptide that has an important role in linear growth. GH is secreted from the pituitary under the positive regulation of the hypothalamic factor growth hormone releasing factor (GRF) and the negative regulation of the hypothalamic factor somatostatin. After release from the pituitary, GH must bind to its receptor on the surface of target cells to exert biologic effects.[1] GH produces a variety of growth-promoting effects on tissues both directly, via binding to its receptor, and indirectly, through the insulin-like growth factors or somatomedins. In children, abnormalities of growth hormone production or action result in a clinical picture of GH deficiency or pituitary dwarfism.

Newborns with growth hormone deficiency usually have normal length and weight. They may present with hypoglycemia or prolonged hyperbilirubinemia.[2] Boys will often have a micropenis.[3] In children with GH deficiency, the facial bones develop slowly, leading to protrusion of the frontal bones and poor development of the bridge of the nose. Tooth eruption is delayed. The hair is thin and the nail growth is poor. The voice is often high-pitched. The linear growth is retarded, and the child will often appear mildly obese and cherubic.[2] These features can be corrected via therapy with recombinant human growth hormone (hGH). The discovery of the GH gene locus on human chromosome 17 made possible the development of recombinant hGH. In the last several years, much has been elucidated about the control of GH gene expression. The remainder of this section will focus on growth hormone gene expression, its regulation by transcription factors, and clinical examples of abnormalities of these processes.

THE GH GENE

Five related genes on the long arm of chromosome 17 comprise the GH/placental lactogen (PL) gene cluster. Two of these genes code for two GH isohormones, two code for PL, and the fifth codes for a PL pseudogene or PL-related protein.[4] The two GH genes are hGH-N (normal) and hGH-V (variant), and they are highly homologous. They differ in only 13 of 191 amino acids, and the differences are dispersed throughout the polypeptide chain.[5] The hGH-N gene is expressed in the pituitary, and the hGH-V gene is expressed primarily in placenta.[6] Recombinant hGH utilizes the sequence of the hGH-N gene after splicing at the transition between intron B and exon 3. The resulting mRNA codes for the most abundant form of pituitary GH with a molecular weight of 22 kDa.[7]

Deletion of the hGH-N gene results in a syndrome termed GH deficiency type IA.[8] This abnormality is transmitted by an autosomal recessive mode. Affected infants have a birth length that is slightly below average but significantly shorter than siblings. They will initially show a good response to exogenous GH therapy, but subsequently develop resistance to the treatment due to the production of neutralizing antibodies to GH. Affected individuals have a very short final adult height.

GH deficiency type IB is also transmitted in an autosomal recessive pattern. In this syndrome, there is no known abnormality of the GH gene, and small quantities of GH can be measured in the serum. Affected individuals do not produce meaningful levels of antibodies during treatment with exogenous GH, and response to therapy is generally good.[2] Two other forms of genetically transmitted GH deficiency have been described.[9] Type II GH deficiency is clinically similar to type IB but is transmitted in an autosomal dominant fashion. Type III GH deficiency also has no definable defect in the GH gene, and there is no propensity to produce neutralizing antibodies. This syndrome is transmitted in an X-linked mode. In each of these syndromes, the deficiency is restricted to GH.[9]

TRANSCRIPTION FACTORS IN GH GENE EXPRESSION

The promoter region of the GH gene regulates somatotroph-specific expression of GH. Transcription factors interact with the promoter to control gene expression. There are four main categories of transcription factors that interact with the GH gene promoter:[10] Pit-l or GHF-1; CTF/NF-1, USF/MCTF, SP1; inhibitory factors; and GCR, TR, RAR, RXR. Pit-1 (GHF-1) is a POU domain transcription factor expressed only in pituitary somatotrophs, lactotrophs, and thyrotrophs. The POU domain is a novel DNA-binding motif which appears to exert critical developmental actions. It is absolutely necessary for GH gene transcription *in vivo*.[11] Much has been elucidated regarding expression of this factor, and it will be discussed in greater detail. The transcription factors CTF/NF-1, USF/MCTF, and SPl are ubiquitous sequence-specific factors, and they are required for high-level activity of the GH promoter in pituitary cells. They do not activate the GH gene in nonpituitary cells.[10,12] Inhibitory factors include inhibitory proteins that bind to silencer elements, such as silencer 1.[13] The inhibitory elements do not overlap with the stimulatory elements, so the mechanism does not appear to involve hindering access to positive regulators. The silencer proteins appear to attenuate GH gene expression.[10] GCR, TR, RAR, and RXR are hormone-activated nuclear receptors. Their function in the context of the GH promoter is thought to involve opening of the GH chromatin structure to allow access for GHF-1 and other factors.[10]

GHF-1, which is also known as Pit-l or GC1, is a pituitary-specific factor that has been found to bind to two *cis*-acting elements within the GH promoter.[14] The gene and protein have been sequenced in humans and rodents. At the amino acid level, there is 96% identity between the human and mouse sequences, and at the DNA level, identity is 90%, indicating a high level of conservation of structure and function.[10] GHF-1 is a member of the POU domain family of transcriptional regulators. The POU-domain proteins have important developmental and transcriptional functions. During development of the fetal mouse, the detectability of GHF-1 protein accumulation coincides with the earliest time that GH transcription is evident, indicating that GHF-1 plays a role in pituitary cell differentiation.[15] A zinc finger protein involved in GHF-1 activation of the GH promoter has recently been described.[16] This protein, called Zn-15, binds to a sequence of GH called the GH-Z box. The binding of Zn-15 to GH appears to be critical for GHF-1-dependent GH expression.

A model for the expression and action of GHF-1 has been proposed.[10] GHF-1 accumulation is believed to activate the GRF receptor (GRFR) gene.[10] The expression of GRFR, in turn, allows the developing somatotrophs to respond to GRF. GRF stimulation leads to production of cAMP responding element binding protein (CREB), a stimulatory protein that binds to the GHF-1 promoter. An autoregulatory loop is thereby established, with permanent activation of GHF-1.

Several factors that regulate GH production do so through their effects on GHF-1 expression. Factors that increase the intracellular cAMP in the somatotroph will increase GHF-1 expression, whereas those that decrease intracellular cAMP will attenuate GHF-1. When GRF binds to its receptor on the somatotroph, it causes an increase in intracellular cAMP.[17] GRFR is known to belong to the family of G_s-linked cell surface receptors.[18] Somatostatin, however, has the opposite effect on intracellular cAMP and is a negative regulator of GH secretion. Somatostatin binds to a receptor that belongs to the family of G_i-linked cell surface receptors.[18] Activin is a hormone synthesized in the pituitary gonadotrophs. It is known to stimulate follicle-stimulating hormone (FSH) secretion, but also acts as a negative regulator of GH. Activin binds to the distal GHF-1 binding site and reduces binding of GHF-1 to its recognition elements. Because activin down-regulates GH through a different mechanism than somatostatin, their suppressive effects are additive.[19]

DEFECTS OF GHF-1: DWARF MOUSE MODELS AND HUMAN HOMOLOGUES

The Snell dwarf mouse and the Jackson dwarf mouse are two mutant mouse strains that have defects in the GHF-1 gene. Both strains exhibit anterior pituitary hypoplasia, and they produce no detectable GH, prolactin (PRL), or thyroid-stimulating hormone (TSH).[20] The Jackson dwarf mouse has a gross rearrangement of the GHF-1 gene. The GHF-1 gene in the Snell dwarf mouse contains a single point mutation which substitutes cysteine for an invariant tryptophan in the homeodomain. This results in a GHF-1 protein that is very deficient in DNA binding. The Snell dwarf mouse has very little detectable pituitary GHF-1 mRNA or protein.[21] The Snell and Jackson strains produce mice that have very little transcription of GHF-1, and this results in absence of the pituitary cell populations (somatotrophs, lactotrophs, thyrotrophs) that would usually express GHF-1.[20] GRFR expression is absent in the Snell dwarf mouse. This indicates that GHF-1 is necessary for the appearance of GRFR.[22]

Human homologues to the dwarf mouse phenotype have been described. Patients with severe mental and growth retardation have been shown to have combined deficiencies of GH, PRL, and TSH. One such patient was found to be homozygous for a nonsense mutation in the GHF-1 gene that resulted in the production of a GHF-1 variant lacking the entire POU homeodomain.[23] Other patients with this constellation of pituitary hormone deficiencies have been shown to be homozygous for mutations in the POU_s region. These mutations result in defects in DNA binding to GHF-1.[24] Two patients with combined pituitary hormone deficiencies have been studied who are heterozygous for separate point mutations in the GHF-1 gene.[25] The dominant nature of these two point mutations suggest that GHF-1 functions as a dimer. As more is known about the regulators of pituitary development and function, it will be possible to more clearly define the genetic etiology of many more cases of GH deficiency.

REFERENCES

1. **Daughaday, W.H.,** Growth hormone: normal synthesis, secretion, control, and mechanisms of action, in *Endocrinology*, DeGroot, L.J., Ed., W. B. Saunders, Philadelphia, 1989, 318.

2. **Kaplan, S.A.,** Growth and growth hormone, in *Clinical Pediatric Endocrinology*, Kaplan, S.A., Ed., W. B. Saunders, Philadelphia, 1990, 1.

3. **Herber, S.M. and Milner, R.D.G.,** Growth hormone deficiency presenting under age 2 years, *Arch. Dis. Child.,* 59, 557, 1984.

4. **Parks, J.S.,** Molecular biology of growth hormone, *Acta Paediatr. Scand.* (Suppl.), 349, 127, 1989.

5. **Seeberg, P.H.,** The human growth hormone gene family: nucleotide sequences show recent divergence and predict a new polypeptide hormone, *DNA,* 1, 239, 1982.

6. **Frankenne, F., Renier-Delrue, F., Scippo, M.L., Martial, J., and Henner, G.,** Expression of the growth hormone variant gene in human placenta, *J. Clin. Endocrinol. Metab.,* 64, 635, 1987.

7. **Baumann, G.,** Growth hormone heterogeneity: genes, isohormones, variants, and binding proteins, *Endocr. Rev.,* 12, 124, 1991.

8. **Illig, R., Prader, A., Fernandez, A., et al.,** Hereditary prenatal growth hormone deficiency with increased tendency to growth hormone antibody formation ("a-type" of isolated growth hormone deficiency), *Acta Paediatr. Scand.,* 60, 607, 1971.

9. **Phillips, J.A.,** Genetic diagnosis: differentiating growth disorders, *Hosp. Pract.,* 20, 85, 1985.

10. **Theill, L.E. and Karin, M.,** Transcriptional control of GH expression and anterior pituitary development, *Endocr. Rev.,* 14, 670, 1993.

11. **Castrillo, J.-L., Theill, L.E., and Karin, M.,** Function of the homeodomain protein GHF-1 in pituitary cell proliferation, *Science,* 253, 197, 1991.

12. **LeMaigre, F.P., Courtois, S.J., Durviaux, S.M., Egan, C.J., LaFontaine, D.A., and Rousseau, G.G.,** Analysis of cis- and trans-acting elements in the hormone-sensitive human somatotropin gene promoter, *J. Steroid Biochem.,* 34, 19, 1989.

13. **Roy, R.J., Gosselin, P., Anzivino, M.J., Moore, D.D., and Guerin, S.L.,** Binding of a nuclear protein to the rat growth hormone silencer element, *Nucleic Acids Res.,* 20, 401, 1992.

14. **West, B.L., Cantanzaro, D.F., Mello, S.H., Cattini, P.A., Baxter, J.D., and Reudelhuber, T.L.,** Interaction of a tissue-specific factor with an essential rat growth hormone gene promoter element, *Mol. Cell. Biol.,* 7, 1193, 1987.

15. **Dolle, P., Castrillo, J.-L., Theill, L.E., Deernick, T., Ellisman, M., and Karin, M.,** Expression of the GHF-1 protein in mouse pituitaries correlates both temporally and spatially with the onset of growth hormone gene activity, *Cell,* 60, 809, 1990

16. **Lipkin, S.M., Naar, A.M., Kalla, K.A., Sack, R.A., and Rosenfeld, M.G.,** Identification of a novel zinc finger protein binding a conserved element critical for pit-1-dependent growth hormone gene expression, *Genes Dev.,* 7, 1674, 1993.

17. **Seifert, H., Perrin, M., Rivier, J., and Vale, W.,** Binding sites for growth hormone releasing factor on rat anterior pituitary cells, *Nature,* 313, 487, 1985.

18. **Bilezikjian, L.M. and Vale, W.,** Stimulation of adenosine 3'-5'-monophosphate production by growth hormone-releasing factor and its inhibition by somatostatin in anterior pituitary cells *in vitro, Endocrinology,* 113, 1726, 1983.

19. **Struthers, R.S., Gaddy-Kurten, D., and Vale, W.W.,** Activin inhibits binding of transcription factor pit-1 to the growth hormone promoter, *Proc. Natl. Acad. Sci. U.S.A.,* 89, 11451, 1992.

20. **Wilson, D.B. and Wyatt, D.P.,** Ultrastructural immunocytochemistry of somatotrophs and mammotrophs in embryos of the dwarf mutant mouse, *Anat. Rec.,* 215, 282, 1986.

21. **Li, S., Crenshaw, E.B., III, Rawson, E.J., Simmons, D.M., Swanson, L.W., and Rosenfeld, M.G.,** Dwarf locus mutants lacking three pituitary cell types result from mutation in the POU-domain gene pit-l, *Nature,* 347, 528, 1990.

22. **Lin, C., Lin, S.-C., Chang, C.-P., and Rosenfeld, M.G.,** Pit-l-dependent expression of the receptor for growth hormone releasing factor mediates pituitary cell growth, *Nature,* 360, 765, 1992.

23. **Tatsumi, K., Miyai, K., Notomi, T., Kaibe, K., Amino, N., Mizono, Y., and Kohono, H.,** Cretinism with combined hormone deficiency caused by a mutation in the pit-1 gene, *Nat. Genet.,* 1, 56, 1992.

24. **Pfaffle, R.W., DiMattia, G.E., Parks, I.S., Brown, M.R., Wit, J.M., Jansen, M., Van der Nat, H., Van den Brande, J.L., Rosenfeld, M.G., and Ingraham, H.A.,** Mutation of the POU-specific domain of pit-l without pituitary hypoplasia, *Science,* 257, 1118, 1992.

25. **Ohta, K., Nobukuni, Y., Mitsubchi, H., Fujimoto, S., Matsuo, N., Inagaki, H., Endo, F., and Matsuda, I.,** Mutations in the pit-1 gene in children with combined pituitary hormone deficiency, *Biochem. Biophys. Res. Commun.,* 189, 851, 1992.

GENETICS OF 21-HYDROXYLASE DEFICIENCY

INTRODUCTION

Congenital adrenal hyperplasia (CAH) is a disorder characterized by a deficiency of one of the adrenal enzymes required for cortisol biosynthesis. Cortisol deficiency leads to hypersecretion of adrenocorticotropic hormone (ACTH), resulting in adrenal hyperplasia. The most common etiology of this disorder is deficiency of 21-hydroxylase, the enzyme required to convert 17-hydroxyprogesterone to 11-deoxycortisol. This enzyme deficiency accounts for approximately 90–95% of all cases of CAH.[1] 21-Hydroxylase deficiency is a common inborn error of metabolism, occurring in about 1 in 15,000 births as an autosomal recessive disorder.[2] The genetic basis of this disease has been thoroughly studied. The clinical variants of 21-hydroxylase deficiency, localization of the gene, known mutations, and progress in prenatal diagnosis and treatment will be discussed.

CLINICAL VARIANTS OF 21-HYDROXYLASE DEFICIENCY

21-Hydroxylase deficiency exists as two "classical" variants and one "nonclassical" variant. The classical variants are divided into "salt-wasting" (SW) and "simple virilizing" (SV) forms. The nonclassical variant is also referred to as "late onset" or "cryptic." These variants are distinguishable based on their clinical presentations, and there is evidence that their genetic bases differ.[3]

The clinical distinction between the SW and SV forms of 21-hydroxylase deficiency can be made based on the patient's ability to produce aldosterone. Aldosterone biosynthesis requires 21-hydroxylase. The SV form of the disorder occurs in individuals who have only a partial deficiency of 21-hydroxylase. In both SW and SV disease, there will be high circulating levels of 17-hydroxyprogesterone. In large amounts, this precursor produces a salt-losing tendency. This effect in turn causes increased plasma renin activity, which will stimulate aldosterone production.[4] Patients with SV disease will produce enough aldosterone to maintain a normal serum sodium, whereas those with SW disease will develop salt-losing crises. It appears, however, that a continuum of severity of salt-losing tendency exists, and that all patients with classical 21-hydroxylase deficiency have some degree of salt-losing tendency.[5]

Female newborns with both SW and SV forms of 21-hydroxylase deficiency will present with masculinization of the external genitalia. *In utero*, elevated levels of 17-hydroxyprogesterone in these fetuses give rise to high levels of androstenedione. This androgen is not biologically active, but approximately 10% will be converted to testosterone in peripheral tissues.[5] The testosterone will be converted to dihydrotestosterone, which is responsible for the virilization of the genitalia. A typical female infant with classical 21-hydroxylase deficiency will exhibit clitoromegaly, enlarged labia which may be rugated, posterior fusion of the labia, and a perineal urogenital sinus. On occasion, the degree of virilization is so marked that the infant is presumed to be male.[5] These infants often require clitoroplasty or more extensive reconstructive surgery. Male newborns with classical 21-hydroxylase deficiency have normal sexual differentiation. Those with SW disease will usually present with a salt-losing crisis in the first several weeks of life. Males with SV disease may present with rapid growth, advanced skeletal development, and premature adrenarche.

Nonclassical (NC) 21-hydroxylase deficiency is much more common than the classical forms, affecting approximately 1 in 1000 of the general Caucasian population.[6] Individuals with NC disease are asymptomatic at birth and usually develop signs of androgen excess during childhood or soon after puberty. Affected males may present with severe acne or premature adrenarche, but they may be difficult to detect on a clinical basis. Females may additionally present with hirsutism or oligomenorrhea. NC 21-hydroxylase is felt to account for 1–2% of hyperandrogenism in women.[7] NC 21-hydroxylase deficiency is diagnosed by measuring elevated 17-hydroxyprogesterone levels produced in response to stimulation with ACTH.

Therapy for all forms of 21-hydroxylase deficiency involves the use of glucocorticoid to suppress pituitary ACTH production. Doses must be carefully monitored, especially during childhood, to avoid Cushingoid effects of overreplacement or rapid skeletal development due to underreplacement. Individuals with SW disease require mineralocorticoid replacement, and infants will also require sodium supplementation to the diet.

LOCALIZATION OF THE 21-HYDROXYLASE GENES

The discovery of the locus for the 21-hydroxylase genes involved some degree of serendipity. In 1977, Levine and Dupont did HLA (human leukocyte antigen) typing of their patients with 21-hydroxylase deficiency and the patients' families. They discovered that 21-hydroxylase deficiency was closely linked to the HLA haplotype.[8,9] Further studies showed that 21-hydroxylase deficiency cosegregated with gene products of MHC (major histocompatibility complex) classes I, II, and III. It was then concluded that the genes for 21-hydroxylase deficiency were located on the short arm of chromosome 6.[5,10]

Subsequent localization and characterization of the 21-hydroxylase genes was made possible after the enzyme was isolated in 1980 by Kominami and colleagues.[11] The 21-hydroxylase enzyme was established to be a cytochrome P-450 termed P-450c21.[5] The human P-450c21 has 494 amino acids. White and colleagues[12] purified bovine P-450c21 and generated an antibody to it. They were able to isolate the bovine adrenal mRNA that coded for P-450c21 through an *in vitro* translation reaction screened with the antibody. Reverse transcription was then used to produce cDNA. Bovine cDNA was used as a probe to isolate human P-450c21 from a fetal adrenal cDNA library.[12]

The genes for P-450c21 are located between the genes for HLA-B and HLA-DR (Figure 1). The locus contains an active gene (CYP21 or CYP21B) and a pseudogene (CYP21P or CYP21A). They are about 30 kb apart, adjacent to and alternating with the C4B and C4A genes, which encode the fourth component of serum complement.[13] The nucleotide sequences for CYP21B and CYP21A are 98% identical in the coding sequences and 96% identical in the intron sequences.[12] CYP21A contains nine deleterious mutations.[14] The specific mutations that have been found in 21-hydroxylase deficiency and their clinical expression will be discussed.

MOLECULAR GENOTYPES IN 21-HYDROXYLASE DEFICIENCY

Early investigations into the genetic differences between the various forms of 21-hydroxylase deficiency utilized HLA typing. In 1985, Holler and colleagues[3] studied 114 patients with classical disease and 13 patients with NC disease. They found overrepresentation of HLA-B14 in NC cases, of HLA-Bw47 in all forms, especially SW, and of HLA-B5(w51) in SV cases. In studying patients' family members, they found that the SV form of the disease is dominant over the SW form.[3]

Recently, much more detailed genetic analyses of the precise mutations in the CYP21B gene responsible for 21-hydroxylase deficiency have been carried out using techniques such as Southern blot analysis, allele-specific hybridization following DNA amplification by the polymerase chain reaction (PCR), and PCR single-strand conformation polymorphism. A summary of the mutations that have been described appears in Table 1. The most common mutations found have been point mutations. Several of these result in the conversion of the CYP21B to the pseudogene, CYP21A. Another common mutation is a deletion in the CYP21B gene that results in no gene product.[14-16]

In 1992, Speiser and colleagues[15] examined the correlation between the severity of various mutations and the clinical expression of disease. They found, for the most part, that the severity of the mutation predicted the severity of disease with respect to the degree of virilization or the degree of elevation of 17-hydroxyprogesterone. This correlation did not hold with respect to the tendency for salt loss. They found that aldosterone synthesis and sodium homeostasis showed great variability, even between genetically identical siblings or

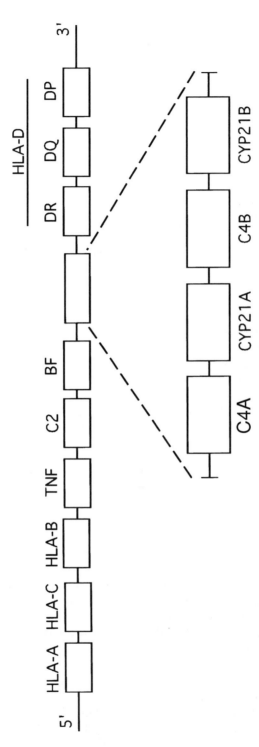

FIGURE 1. Map of the short arm of human chromosome 6 showing the MHC region and the location of the structural gene (CYP21B) and the pseudogene (CYP21A) for 21-hydroxylase.

TABLE 1
Mutations Causing 21-Hydroxylase Deficiency

Clinical Phenotype	Mutation		References
Salt-wasting	Intron 2:	A to C or G	14,16
	Exon 4:	Ile to Asn	15
	Exon 6:	Ile to Asp	21
		Val to Glu	21
		Met to Lys	21
	Exon 7:	Val to Leu	15
	Exon 8:	Gln to term	14
		Arg to Trp	14
	Deletion:	CYP21B	15–17
	Deletion:	CYP21A	17
Simple virilizing	Intron 2:	A to C or G	14
	Exon 1:	Pro to Leu	15
	Exon 4:	Ile to Asn	14,15
	Exon 8:	Gln to term	15
		Arg to Trp	15
	Deletion:	CYP21B	14,15
	Deletion:	CYP21A	17
Nonclassical	Exon 1:	Pro to Leu	15
	Exon 4:	Ile to Asn	14,15

in the same individual over time. They concluded that the factors that control salt balance in these patients are remote from the 21-hydroxylase gene.

The frequency of the mutations responsible for 21-hydroxylase deficiency depends on the population studied. Tajima and colleagues,[14] studying patients in Japan, found only 10% of the mutations resulted in a deletion, while the remainder involved point mutations. Strumberg and colleagues[17] looked at patients in Germany with SW disease and found 25% with deletion mutations, 25% with point mutations, and nearly 50% whose haplotype was not informative. Manfras and colleagues[16] studied patients in Pittsburgh who were of European origin. They found point mutations of intron 2 in 32.4% and deletion mutations in 23.5%. Koppens and colleagues[18] studied families in the Netherlands and found 12% had point mutations resulting in the conversion of CYP21B to CYP21A and 23% had deletion mutations.

Most patients with mutations in the CYP21B gene are homozygotes for a specific mutation or compound heterozygotes. In some, however, a mutation is found on only one allele.[14] Additionally, pedigree analysis has revealed patients with *de novo* mutations on both the maternally and paternally derived chromosomes.[14] This finding can explain the existence of affected and unaffected HLA-identical siblings.[19] The improved techniques currently available for genetic analysis of the CYP21B gene is making possible earlier and more accurate prenatal diagnosis of 21-hydroxylase deficiency.

PRENATAL DIAGNOSIS AND TREATMENT
OF 21-HYDROXYLASE DEFICIENCY

Because 21-hydroxylase deficiency is an autosomal recessive disorder, the possibility of prenatal diagnosis in subsequent pregnancies is of interest to parents with one affected child. It has been shown that treatment of the mother with glucocorticoids during pregnancy can prevent virilization in affected female infants.[20-22] For this reason, accurate prenatal diagnosis at the earliest possible time in gestation has become an important concern in the management of families with 21-hydroxylase deficiency.

The earliest method of prenatal diagnosis of 21-hydroxylase deficiency, reported in 1975, was the detection of elevated hormone levels in the amniotic fluid during the second trimester. Affected pregnancies have elevated levels of 17-hydroxyprogesterone, androstenedione, and testosterone.[21] This method may not be accurate for SV or NC disease, however.[23]

After the association between 21-hydroxylase deficiency and the HLA locus was established, HLA typing was found to be another indirect method of prenatal diagnosis.[24] This method requires prior HLA typing of the parents and the proband. HLA typing may be done during the first trimester, using chorionic villus tissue, and will detect any of the clinical forms of 21-hydroxylase deficiency. A pitfall of this method occurs when the parents have shared HLA antigens, which can make the HLA typing inconclusive. The HLA typing can produce inaccurate results when an intra-HLA recombination event occurs, and this has been reported to happen in approximately 1% of cases.[21]

The most accurate way to establish prenatal diagnosis of 21-hydroxylase deficiency is to do molecular genetic studies on amniotic or chorionic villus samples. Extracted DNA can be evaluated by Southern blot analysis.[20,21] Mutations in the 21-hydroxylase gene can be detected using polynucleotide probes designed to detect mutations in CYP21B. Through the use of PCR, amplified DNA can be obtained from very small samples.[22] Although the reports of direct molecular genetic testing to establish prenatal diagnosis of 21-hydroxylase deficiency contain small numbers of patients, the results are uniformly accurate.[20-22]

Prenatal treatment of 21-hydroxylase deficiency has shown variable success, usually based on how early in pregnancy the treatment begins. When therapy is started before 10 weeks gestation, virilization of an affected female fetus can usually be prevented or minimized.[20-22] There have been reports of virilization of infants where treatment was started early but was interrupted for several days to perform confirmatory amniotic fluid studies.[20] Currently, treatment is not interrupted unless it is shown to be unnecessary. The typical treatment of the mother is with dexamethasone, 0.5 mg every 8 h or 0.5 mg every 12 h.[21] This dose is usually well tolerated, although mothers have complained of increased weight gain, edema, mood fluctuations, and striae.[21] It is desirable, therefore, to establish prenatal diagnosis as early as possible during pregnancy, to avoid unneeded treatment. When chromosomal studies are done, prenatal treatment can be halted if the sex of the fetus is determined to be male. Parents of infants who have little to no virilization following prenatal treatment tend to be very satisfied with the outcome.[21] The ability of prenatal treatment to prevent or minimize virilization of females with classical 21-hydroxylase deficiency avoids the need for plastic surgery in these infants, an important advantage.

REFERENCES

1. **White, P.C., New, M.I., and Dupont, B.,** Congenital adrenal hyperplasia, *New Engl. J. Med.,* 316, 1519, 1987.
2. **Pang, S., Wallace, M.A., Hofman, L., Thuline, M.C., Dorche, C., Lyon, I.C.T., Dobbind, R.H., Kling, S., Fujieda, K., and Suwa, S.,** Worldwide experience in newborn screening for classical congenital adrenal hyperplasia due to 21-hydroxylase deficiency, *Pediatrics,* 81, 866, 1988.
3. **Holler, W., Scholz, S., Knorr, D., Bidlingmaier, F., Keller, E., and Albert, E.D.,** Genetic differences between the salt-wasting, simple virilizing, and nonclassical types of congenital adrenal hyperplasia, *J. Clin. Endocrinol. Metab.,* 60, 757, 1985.
4. **Kowarski, A., Finkelstein, J.W., Spaulding, J.S., et al.,** Aldosterone secretion rate in congenital adrenal hyperplasia: a discussion of the theories on the pathogenesis of the salt-losing form of the syndrome, *J. Clin. Invest.,* 44, 1505, 1965.
5. **Migeon, C.J. and Donohue, P.A.,** Congenital adrenal hyperplasia caused by 21-hydroxylase deficiency: its molecular basis and its remaining therapeutic problems, *Endocrinol. Metab. Clin. North Am.,* 20(2), 277, 1991.

6. **Speiser, P.W., Dupont, B., Rubenstin, P., et al.,** High frequency of nonclassical steroid 21-hydroxylase deficiency, *Am. J. Hum. Genet.,* 37, 650, 1985.

7. **Kuttenn, F., Couillin, P., Girard, F., et al.,** Late onset adrenal hyperplasia in hirsutism, *N. Engl. J. Med.,* 313, 224, 1985.

8. **Dupont, B., Oberfield, S.E., Smithwick, E.M., et al.,** Close genetic linkage between HLA and congenital adrenal hyperplasia (21-hydroxylase deficiencey), *Lancet,* 2, 1309, 1977.

9. **Levine, L.S., Zachmann, M., New, M.I., et al.,** Genetic mapping of the 21-hydroxylase gene within the HLA linkage group, *N. Engl. J. Med.,* 299, 911, 1978.

10. **O'Neill, G.J., Dupont, B., Pollack, M.S., et al.,** Complement C4 allotypes in congenital adrenal hyperplasia due to 21-hydroxylase deficiency: further evidence for different allelic variants at the 21-hydroxylase locus, *Clin. Immunol. Immunopathol.,* 23, 312, 1982.

11. **Kominami, S., Ochi, H., Kobayashi, Y., et al.,** Studies on the steroid hydroxylation system in adrenal cortex microsomes: purification and characterization of cytochrome p-450 specific for steroid c-21 hydroxylation, *J. Biol. Chem.,* 255, 3386, 1980.

12. **White, P.C., New, M.I., and Dupont, B.,** Structure of human steroid 21-hydroxylase genes, *Proc. Natl. Acad. Sci. U.S.A.,* 83, 5111, 1986.

13. **White, P.C. and New, M.I.,** Genetic basis of endocrine disease 2: congenital adrenal hyperplasia due to 21-hydroxylase deficiency, *J. Clin. Endocrinol. Metab.,* 74(1), 6, 1992.

14. **Tajima, T., Fujieda, K., Nakayama, K., and Fujii-Kuriyama, Y.,** Molecular analysis of patient and carrier genes with congenital steroid 21-hydroxylase deficiency by using polymerase chain reaction and single strand conformation polymorphism, *J. Clin. Invest.,* 92, 2182, 1993.

15. **Speiser, P.W., Dupont, J., Zhu, D., Serrat, J., Buegeleisen, M., Tusie-Luna, M.-T., Lesser, M., New, M.I., and White, P.C.,** Disease expression and molecular genotype in congenital adrenal hyperplasia due to 21-hydroxylase deficiency, *J. Clin. Invest.,* 90, 584, 1992.

16. **Manfras, B.J., Swinyard, M., Rudert, W.A., Ball, E.J., Lee, P.A., Kuhnl, P., Trucco, M., and Bohm, B.,** Altered CYP21B genes in HLA-haplotypes associated with congenital adrenal hyperplasia (cah): a family study, *Hum. Genet.,* 92, 33, 1993.

17. **Strumberg, D., Hauffa, B.P., and Grosse-Wilde, H.,** Molecular detection of genetic defects in congenital adrenal hyperplasia due to 21-hydroxylase deficiency: a study of 27 families, *Eur. J. Pediatr.,* 151, 821, 1992.

18. **Koppens, P.F.J., Hoogenboezem, T., Halley, D.J.J., Barendse, C.A.M., Oostenbrink, A.J., and Degenhart, H.J.,** Family studies of the steroid 21-hydroxylase and complement C4 genes define 11 haplotypes in classical congenital adrenal hyperplasia in the Netherlands, *Eur. J. Pediatr.,* 151, 885, 1992.

19. **Tajima, T., Fujieda, K., and Fujii-Kuriyama, Y.,** De novo mutation causes steroid 21-hydroxylase deficiency in one family of HLA-identical affected and unaffected siblings, *J. Clin. Endocrinol. Metab.,* 77, 86, 1993.

20. **Speiser, P.W., Laforgia, N., Kato, K., Pareira, J., et al.,** First trimester prenatal treatment and molecular genetic diagnosis of congenital adrenal hyperplasia (21-hydroxylase deficiency), *J. Clin. Endocrinol. Metab.,* 70, 838, 1990.

21. **Forest, M.G., David, M., and Morel, Y.,** Prenatal diagnosis and treatment of 21-hydroxylase deficiency, *J. Steroid Biochem. Mol. Biol.,* 45(1-3), 75, 1993.

22. **Rumsby, G., Honour, J.W., and Rodeck, C.,** Prenatal diagnosis of congenital adrenal hyperplasia by direct detection of mutations in the steroid 21-hydroxylase gene, *Clin. Endocrinol.,* 38, 421, 1993.

23. **Pang, S., Pollack, M.S., Loo, M., Green, O., et al.,** Pitfalls of prenatal diagnosis of 21-hydroxylase deficiency congenital adrenal hyperplasia, *J. Clin. Endocrinol. Metab.,* 61, 89, 1985.

24. **Pollack, M.S., Levine, L.S., Pang, S., Owens, R.P., Nitowsky, H.M., Maurer, D., New, M.I., Duchon, M., Merkatz, I.R., Sahs, G., and Dupont, B.,** Prenatal diagnosis of congenital adrenal hyperplasia (21-hydroxylase deficiency) by HLA typing, *Lancet,* i, 1107, 1979.

GENETICS OF PSEUDOHYPOPARATHYROIDISM

CLINICAL AND BIOCHEMICAL ASPECTS
OF PSEUDOHYPOPARATHYROIDISM

Pseudohypoparathyroidism (PHP) is a clinical problem characterized by resistance to parathyroid hormone (PTH) resulting in hypocalcemia and hyperphosphatemia. Patients with PHP do not increase serum calcium, urine phosphate, or urinary cAMP following parenteral administration of PTH.[1] There are several types of PHP, designated PHP-Ia, PHP-Ib, and PHP-II. PHP-Ia, the most common form of PHP, consists of renal resistance to PTH and a phenotype known as Albright's hereditary osteodystrophy (AHO). This phenotype was first described by Albright et al.[2] in 1942. The features include short stature, round facies, obesity, brachymetaphalangia, other skeletal abnormalities, and subcutaneous ossifications. Additionally, individuals with PHP-Ia have reduced activity of the α subunit of G_s, a G protein that stimulates adenylate cyclase.[3,4] A more detailed discussion of G_s will follow. Patients with PHP-Ia usually present with problems related to PTH resistance, but they often have subclinical resistance to other hormones whose actions are mediated by cAMP, such as gonadotropins and thyroid hormone. Patients with PHP-Ib have resistance to PTH, but their cells do not have reduced αG_s activity.[1] They rarely have the AHO phenotype.[5] PHP-II refers to patients who have normal urinary cAMP in response to PTH, but have a defective phosphaturic response.[6] The genetic basis of PHP-II is not known.[1]

AHO may exist without PTH resistance. This is termed pseudopseudohypoparathyroidism (PPHP). PPHP occurs in kindreds along with PHP-Ia, and affected individuals have reduced αG_s activity.[7] AHO is transmitted as an autosomal dominant disorder.[2]

MUTATIONS OF αG_S IN PHP

The G proteins are a family of proteins that couple cell-surface receptors for a variety of extracellular signals to enzymes or ion channels, resulting in the generation of an intracellular second messenger.[8] In the inactive state, G proteins are heterotrimers consisting of α, β, and γ subunits. The α subunits bind guanine nucleotide, and the β and γ subunits form stable noncovalent heterodimers that are tightly associated with cell membranes. The inactive G protein has an α subunit associated with a β-γ complex and has GDP bound to the guanine nucleotide binding site. Activation of a G protein may occur when a ligand binds to its receptor. GTP is exchanged for GDP on the α subunit, and the α subunit dissociates form the β-γ complex. The free GTP-bound α subunit then dirctly interacts with and modulates its appropriate effector.[8]

There have been at least 16 mammalian α subunit genes described, and they are grouped into categories based on amino acid sequence[9] or function.[8] The α_s family functions to stimulate adenylyl cyclase. Its gene spans approximately 20 kb and contains 13 exons and 12 introns. It has been localized to human chromosome 20ql2-ql3.2.[10] The α_s subunit is deficient in individuals with AHO. There is a reduction of approximately 50% in the amount of functional αG_s in patients with AHO, whether they have PHP or PPHP.[11] In most patients, this is associated with a 50% decrease in the amounts of steady state αG_s mRNA[11] and protein.[12]

Several specific mutations in αG_s have been described in kindreds with AHO.[7,13] Patten et al.[13] evaluated the αG_s sequence from the erythrocytes of a woman with PPHP and her son with PHP. They found a mutation in exon 1, an A-to-G substitution at the +1 position. This mutation converts methionine to valine, resulting in blockage of the initiation of translation. Weinstein et al.[7] studied two kindreds with AHO. The first consisted of a woman with PPHP, four daughters with PHP, and a grandson with PHP. DNA analysis revealed a G-to-C substitution at the splice junction bordering the 3' end of exon 10. The second kindred involved a woman with PPHP and her daughter with PHP. DNA analysis of these individuals revealed a single base deletion in exon 10. The αG_s deletions in AHO appear to be very heterogeneous, however. Lin et al.[14] studied 24 unrelated patients with PHP-Ia, and none had the mutations described by Patten or Weinstein.

GENETIC TRANSMISSION OF PHP-Ia AND PPHP

The mode of inheritance of PHP-Ia (AHO plus hormone resistance) and PPHP (AHO without hormone resistance) is considered to be autosomal dominant.[2,15] What remains unclear is why, in affected kindreds, some members have PHP and others have PPHP. It is believed that PHP-Ia represents full expression of the defective gene, whereas PPHP represents its partial expression. Many reported kindreds have an excess of affected females. This was initially thought to represent sex-linked dominant inheritance, but it was later suggested that the mode of transmission was autosomal dominant with sex modification of expression.[15] Davies and Hughes[16] recently reviewed 31 reports of AHO in two or more generations. They found full expression of the gene (PHP) in maternally transmitted cases and partial expression of the gene (PPHP) in paternally transmitted cases. They concluded that genomic imprinting is likely to be involved in the expression of PHP. Schuster et al.,[17] however, recently studied a family with AHO that showed paternal as well as maternal transmission of PHP. Future studies will be needed to clarify the role of genomic imprinting in the expression of PHP.

REFERENCES

1. **van Dop, C.,** Pseudohypoparathyroidism: clinical and molecular aspects, *Semin. Nephrol.,* 9(2), 168, 1989.
2. **Albright, F., Burnett, C.H., Smith, P.H., et al.,** Pseudo-hypoparathyroidism—an example of 'Seabright-Bantam syndrome'—report of three cases, *Endocrinology,* 30, 922, 1942.
3. **Farfel, Z., Brickman, A.S., Kaslow, H.R., et al.,** Defect of receptor-cyclase coupling protein in pseudohypoparathyroidism, *N. Engl. J. Med.,* 303, 237, 1980.
4. **Levine, M.A., Downs, R.W., Jr., Singer, M., et al.,** Deficient activity of guanine nucleotide regulatory proteins in erythrocytes from patients with pseudohypoparathyroidism, *Biochem. Biophys. Res. Commun.,* 94, 1319, 1980.
5. **Farfel, Z. and Bourne, H.R.,** Pseudohypoparathyroidism: mutation affecting adenylate cyclase, *Miner. Electrolyte Metab.,* 8, 227, 1982.
6. **Drezner, M., Neelon, F.A., and Lebovitz, H.E.,** Pseudohypoparathyroidism type II: a possible defect in the reception of the cyclic AMP signal, *N. Engl. J. Med.,* 289, 1056, 1973.
7. **Weinstein, L.S., Gejman, P.V., Friedman, E., et al.,** Mutations of the G_s α-subunit gene in Albright hereditary osteodystrophy detected by denaturing gradient gel electrophoresis, *Proc. Natl. Acad. Sci. U.S.A.,* 87, 8287, 1990.
8. **Weinstein, L.S. and Shenker, A.,** G protein mutations in human disease, *Clin. Biochem.,* 26, 333, 1993.
9. **Simon, M.I., Strathmann, M.P., and Gautam, N.,** Diversity of G proteins in signal transduction, *Science,* 252, 802, 1991.
10. **Gopal Rao, V.V.N., Schnittger, S., and Hansmann, I.,** G protein $G_s\alpha$ (GNAS1), the probable candidate gene for Albright hereditary osteodystrophy, is assigned to human chromosome 20ql2-ql3.2, *Genomics,* 10, 257, 1991.
11. **Levine, M.A., Ahn, T.G., Klupt, S.F., et al.,** Genetic deficiency of the alpha subunit of the guanine nucleotide-binding protein G_s as the molecular basis for Albright hereditary osteodystrophy, *Proc. Natl. Acad. Sci. U.S.A.,* 85, 617, 1988.
12. **Patten, J.L. and Levine, M.A.,** Immunochemical analysis of the α-subunit of the stimulatory G-protein of adenylyl cyclase in patients with Albright hereditary osteodystrophy, *J. Clin. Endocrinol. Metab.,* 71, 1208, 1990.
13. **Patten, J.L., Johns, D.R., Valle, D., et al.,** Mutation in the gene encoding the stimulatory G protein of adenylate cyclase in Albright's hereditary osteodystrophy, *N. Engl. J. Med.,* 322, 1412, 1990.
14. **Lin, C.K., Hakakha, M.J., Nakamoto, J.M., et al.,** Prevalence of three mutations in the $G_s\alpha$ gene among 24 families with pseudohypoparathyroidism type Ia, *Biochem. Biophys. Res. Commun.,* 189(1), 343, 1992.
15. **Fitch, N.,** Albright's hereditary osteodystrophy: a review, *Am. J. Med. Genet.,* 11, 11, 1982.
16. **Davies, S.J. and Hughes, H.E.,** Imprinting in Albright's hereditary osteodystrophy, *J. Med. Genet.,* 30, 101, 1993.
17. **Schuster, V., Kress, W., and Kruse, K.,** Paternal and maternal transmission of pseudohypoparathyroidism type Ia in a family with Albright hereditary osteodystrophy: no evidence of genomic imprinting, *J. Med. Genet.,* 31, 84, 1994.

GENETICS OF KALLMANN SYNDROME

INTRODUCTION

Kallmann syndrome is characterized by anosmia and hypogonadotropic hypogonadism. Familial Kallmann syndrome can be transmitted in an X-linked, autosomal recessive, or autosomal dominant fashion.[1-6] The X-linked form of the syndrome is the most common, and the gene responsible for this form of the syndrome has been identified. The gene appears to be necessary for proper migration of the cells of the olfactory placode.

The association between the sense of smell and hypogonadism is due to the common embryologic site of origin of the neurons of the olfactory bulb and LHRH (luteinizing hormone-releasing hormone) producing cells.[7] The neurons secreting LHRH originate embryologically in the olfactory placode[8] then migrate with the nervus terminalis into the septal-preoptic and hypothalamic regions.[9] A defect in migration appears to be the cause of X-linked Kallmann syndrome.

THE GENE OF X-LINKED KALLMANN SYNDROME

The X-linked Kallmann gene was mapped to chromosome Xp22.3 by linkage and deletion studies.[10,11] A gene from this region was cloned and found to code for a 679-amino acid extracellular protein with homology with cell adhesion molecules and serine protease inhibitors.[7,12] The protein, called KALIG-1 (Kallmann syndrome interval gene 1)[7] or ADMLX (adhesion molecule-like from the X-chromosome),[12] is deleted or defective[13,14] in patients with Kallmann syndrome.[7] The mRNA from the KALIG-1 gene is found in fetal brain, muscle, kidney, liver, and intestine.[7] The presence of the mRNA in these tissues may explain the association of Kallmann syndrome with renal aplasia and hypoplasia, synkinesia, and nystagmus.

REFERENCES

1. **Sparkes, R.S., Simpson, R.W., and Paulsen, C.A.,** Familial hypogonadotropic hypogonadism with anosmia, *Arch. Int. Med.,* 121, 534, 1968.
2. **Santen, R.J. and Paulsen, C.A.,** Hypogonadotropic eunuchoidism. I. Clinical study of the mode of inheritance, *J. Clin. Endocrinol. Metab.,* 36, 47, 1972.
3. **White, B.J., Rogol, A.D., Brown, K.S., Lieblich, J.M., and Rosen, S.W.,** The syndrome of anosmia with hypogonadotropic hypogonadism: a genetic study of 18 new families and a review, *Am. J. Med. Genet.,* 15, 417, 1983.
4. **Chaussain, J.L., Toublanc, J.E., Feingold, J., Naud, C., Vassal, J., and Job, J.C.,** Mode of inheritance in familial cases of primary gonadotropic deficiency, *Horm. Res.,* 29, 202, 1988.
5. **Merriam, G.R., Beitins, I.Z., and Bode, H.H.,** Father-to-son transmission of hypogonadism with anosmia, *Am. J. Dis. Child.,* 131, 1216, 1977.
6. **Kallmann, F.J., Schoenfeld, W.A., and Barrera, S.E.,** The genetic aspects of primary eunuchoidism, *Am. J. Ment. Defic.,* 48, 203, 1944.
7. **Franco, B., Guioli, S., Pragliola, A., Incerti, B., Bardoni, B., Tonlorenzi, R., Carrozzo, R., Maestrini, E., Pieretti, M., Taillon-Miller, P., Brown, C.J., Willard, H.F., Lawrence, C., Persico, M.G., Camerino, G., and Ballabio, A.,** A gene deleted in Kallmann's syndrome shares homology with neural cell adhesion and axonal path-finding molecules, *Nature,* 353, 529, 1991.
8. **Wray, S., Grant, P., and Gainer, H.,** Evidence that cells expressing luteinizing hormone-releasing hormone mRNA in the mouse are derived from progenitor cells in the olfactory placode, *Proc. Natl. Acad. Sci. U.S.A.,* 86, 8132, 1989.
9. **Schwanzel-Fukada, M. and Pfaff, D.W.,** Origin of luteinizing hormone-releasing hormone neurons, *Nature,* 338, 161, 1989.
10. **Ballabio, A., Bardoni, B., Guioli, S., Basler, E., and Camerino, G.,** Two families of low-copy number repeats are interspersed on Xp22.3: implications for the high frequency of deletions in this region, *Genomics,* 8, 263, 1990.

11. **Petit, C., Levilliers, J., and Weissenbach, J.,** Long-range restriction map of the terminal part of the short arm of the human X chromosome, *Proc. Natl. Acad. Sci. U.S.A.,* 87, 3680, 1990.
12. **Legouis, R., Hardelin, J.-P., Levilliers, J., Claverie, J.-M., Compain, S., Wunderle, V., Millasseau, P., Le Paslier, D., Cohen, D., Caterina, D., Bougueleret, L., Delemarre-Van de Waal, H., Lutfalla, G., Weissenbach, J., and Petit, C.,** The candidate gene for the X-linked Kallmann syndrome encodes a protein related to adhesion molecules, *Cell,* 67, 423, 1991.
13. **Bick, D., Franco, B., Sherins, R.J., Heye, B., Pike, L., Crawford, J., Maddalena, A., Incerti, B., Pragliola, A., Meitinger, T., and Ballabio, A.,** Brief report: intragenic deletion of the KALIG-1 gene in Kallmann's syndrome, *N. Engl. J. Med.,* 326, 1752, 1992.
14. **Hardelin, J.-P., Levilliers, J., Del Castillo, I., Cohen-Salmon, M., Legouis, R., Blanchard, S., Compain, S., Bouloux, P., Kirk, J., Moraine, C., Chaussain, J.-L., Weissenbach, J., and Petit, C.,** X chromosome-linked Kallmann syndrome: stop mutations validate the candidate gene, *Proc. Natl. Acad. Sci. U.S.A.,* 89, 8190, 1992.

GENETICS OF MULTIPLE ENDOCRINE NEOPLASIA

INTRODUCTION

The two types of multiple endocrine neoplasia (MEN) have separate clinical presentations and different genetic associations, as described below.

PROPOSED MEN1 GENES

MEN1 patients manifest tumors of the anterior pituitary, the parathyroid glands, and the pancreatic islets. Adrenocortical and thyroid tumors are occasionally associated with the syndrome.[1] The disorder is inherited in an autosomal dominant manner. The MEN1 gene has been mapped to chromosome 11q13 by linkage analysis.[2] Two recent papers propose two different genes in the area of the chromosome linked to the syndrome. The first proposes a gene termed ZFM1 (for zinc finger gene in the MEN1 locus). The nucleotide sequence of the clone predicts a gene containing 14 exons and 623 amino acids, part of which appears to be a metal-binding domain (zinc finger motif), which is seen in nucleic acid-binding proteins. The putative protein has some similarity to the Wilms' tumor gene product and the early growth response 2 protein.[3] The other proposed gene is nearby on chromosome 11q13 and was located using deletion mapping of parathyroid tumors. This gene codes for a previously described protein, phospholipase C β3 (PLC β3), which, based on the activity of similar proteins, may be involved in signal transduction, intracellular calcium regulation, or activation of protein kinase C, which are in turn involved in cell growth and differentiation.[4] There are no studies to date showing specific defects in either of these genes that cosegregate with MEN1 syndrome in affected families, so it is not yet clear which, if either, of these genes is responsible for the syndrome.

THE MEN2 GENE

The gene responsible for MEN2 is more clearly defined. MEN2 is an autosomal dominant disorder. The more common form, MEN2A, is characterized by tumors of the thyroid C cells (medullary thyroid carcinoma, or MTC), pheochromocytoma, and parathyroid adenoma or hyperplasia.[1] The less common form, MEN2B, differs in that the syndrome includes a Marfanoid habitus and hyperplasia of the intestinal autonomic ganglia. In familial MTC, MTC alone is inherited in an autosomal dominant fashion.

The genes for these disorders map to chromosome 10q11. Mutations in a single gene in the chromosome 10q11 region[5,6] have been positively linked to MEN2A, MEN2B, familial MTC, and Hirschsprung's disease, characterized by absence of intestinal autonomic ganglia in contrast to the hyperplasia of the ganglia sometimes seen in MEN2B.[7-12] This gene is the RET protooncogene in the family of receptor tyrosine kinases. The gene contains 17 exons over 22 kb[7] and encodes a protein that contains an extracellular domain, a transmembrane region, and an intracellular tyrosine kinase domain capable of autophosphorylation.[13] The normal function of the RET protooncogene is not known.

Interestingly, the mutations for each disease associated with the RET protooncogene are found in specific locations of the protein. The mutations found in MEN2A patients are missense mutations of five cysteine residues found near the plasma membrane in the extracellular domain of the molecule.[7,11,14] In most cases of MEN2A, it is the cysteine at position 634 that is mutated,[8,10,15] whereas mutations of the other four cysteines are more commonly found in familial MTC.[15] When cysteine 634 is changed to arginine, the family is more likely to manifest hyperparathyroidism as part of their MEN syndrome.[12,15] This specific amino acid change appears to be specific for this subtype of MEN2A, because it occurs in unrelated families who have differing polymorphisms of nearby genetic markers.[12]

In MEN2B, the mutation is a missense mutation changing methionine 918 to threonine in the intracellular tyrosine kinase region.[9] Hirschsprung's disease is most commonly associated with large deletions or truncations that would be expected to inactivate the protein.

Ponder[13] speculates that the MEN and familial MTC mutations cause constitutive activation or an increase in activity of the RET protooncogene protein, thereby allowing them to act in a dominant fashion. The Hirschsprung's disease mutations would cause inactivation, which has physiological significance, causing defects in the autonomic ganglia of the intestine in transgenic mice even in the heterozygous state.[13]

REFERENCES

1. **Larsson, C. and Nordenskjold, M.,** Multiple endocrine neoplasia, *Cancer Surv.,* 9, 703, 1990.
2. **Larsson, C., Skogseid, B., Oberg, K., Nakamura, Y., and Nordenskjold, M.,** Multiple endocrine neoplasia type 1 maps to chromosome 11 and is lost in insulinoma, *Nature,* 332, 85, 1988.
3. **Toda, T., Iida, A., Miwa, T., Nakamura, Y., and Imai, T.,** Isolation and characterization of a novel gene encoding nuclear protein at a locus (D11S636) tightly linked to multiple endocrine neoplasia type 1 (MEN1), *Hum. Mol. Genet.,* 3, 465, 1994.
4. **Weber, G., Friedman, E., Grimmond, S., Hayward, N.K., Phelan, C., Skogseid, B., Gobl, A., Zedenius, J., Sandelin, K., Teh, B.T., Carson, E., White, I., Oberg, K., Shepherd, J., Nordenskjold, M., and Larsson, C.,** The phospholipase c beta3 gene located in the MEN1 region shows loss of expression in endocrine tumours, *Hum. Mol. Genet.,* 3, 1775, 1994.
5. **Gardner, E., Papi, L., Easton, D.F., Cummings, T., Jackson, C.E., Kaplan, M., Love, D.R., Mole, S.E., Moore, J.K., Mulligan, L.M., Norum, R.A., Ponder, M.A., Reichlin, S., Stall, G., Telenius, H., Telenius-Berg, M., Tunnacliffe, A., and Ponder, B.A.J.,** Genetic linkage studies map the multiple endocrine neoplasia type 2 loci to a small interval on chromosome 10q11.2, *Hum. Mol. Genet.,* 2, 241, 1993.
6. **Mole, S.E., Mulligan, L.M., Healey, C.S., Ponder, B.A.J., and Tunnacliffe, A.,** Localisation of the gene for multiple endocrine neoplasia type 2A to a 480 KB region in chromosome band 10q11.2, *Hum. Mol. Genet.,* 3, 247, 1993.
7. **Donis-Keller, H., Dou, S., Chi, D., Carlson, K.M., Toshima, K., Lairmore, T.C., Howe, J.R., Moley, J.F., Goodfellow, P., and Wells, S.A., Jr.,** Mutations in the RET proto-oncogene are associated with MEN2A and FMTC, *Hum. Mol. Genet.,* 2, 851, 1993.
8. **Mulligan, L.M., Kwok, J.B.J., Healey, C.S., Elsdon, M.J., Eng, C., Gardner, E., Love, D.R., Mole, S.E., Moore, J.K., Papi, L., Ponder, M.A., Telenius, H., Tunnacliffe, A., and Ponder, B.A.J.,** Germ-line mutations of the RET proto-oncogene in multiple endocrine neoplasia type 2A, *Nature,* 363, 458, 1993.
9. **Eng, C., Smith, D.P., Mulligan, L.M., Nagai, M.A., Healey, C.S., Ponder, M.A., Gardner, E., Scheumann, G.F.W., Jackson, C.E., Tunnacliffe, A., and Ponder, B.A.J.,** Point mutation within the tyrosine kinase domain of the RET proto-oncogene in multiple endocrine neoplasia type 2B and related sporadic tumours, *Hum. Mol. Genet.,* 3, 237, 1994.
10. **Mulligan, L.M., Eng, C., Healey, C.S., Ponder, M.A., Feldman, G.L., Li, P., Jackson, C.E., and Ponder, B.A.J.,** A de novo mutation of the RET proto-oncogene in a patient with MEN2A, *Hum. Mol. Genet.,* 3, 1007, 1994.

11. **Quadro, L.L.P., Salvatore, D., Carlomagno, F., Del Prete, M., Numziata, V., Colantuoni, V., Di Giovanni, G., Brandi, M.L., Mannelli, M., Gheri, M., Verga, U., Libroia, A., Berger, N., Fusco, A., Grieco, M., and Santoro, M.,** Frequent RET protooncogene mutation in multiple endocrine neoplasia type 2A, *J. Clin. Endocrinol. Metab.,* 79, 590, 1994.
12. **Gardner, E., Mulligan, L.M., Eng, C., Healey, C.S., Kwok, J.B.J., Ponder, M.A., and Ponder, B.A.J.,** Haplotype analysis of MEN 2 mutations, *Hum. Mol. Genet.,* 3, 1771, 1994.
13. **Ponder, B.A.J.,** The gene causing multiple endocrine neoplasia type 2 (MEN2), *Ann. Med.,* 26, 199, 1994.
14. **Xue, F., Yu, H., Maurer, L.H., Memoli, V.A., Nutile-McMenemy, N., Schuster, M.K., Bowden, D.W., Mao, J.-I., and Noll, W.W.,** Germline RET mutations in MEN 2A and FMTC and their detection by simple DNA diagnostic tests, *Hum. Mol. Genet.,* 3, 635, 1994.
15. **Mulligan, L.M., Eng, C., Healey, C.S., Clayton, D., Kwok, J.B.J., Gardner, E., Ponder, M.A., Frilling, A., Jackson, C.E., Lehnert, H., Neumann, H.P.H., Thibodeau, S.N., and Ponder, B.A.J.,** Specific mutations of the RET proto-oncogene are related to disease phenotype in MEN2A and FMTC, *Nat. Genet.,* 6, 70, 1994.

GENETICS OF TYPE I DIABETES MELLITUS

INTRODUCTION

Type I insulin-dependent diabetes mellitus (IDDM) is characterized by progressive autoimmune destruction of the pancreatic β cells resulting in insulin deficiency. The etiology of IDDM clearly involves contributions from both genetic and environmental factors. The most convincing evidence of this is data from twin studies, which have shown as much as 55% concordance of IDDM in identical twins,[1] indicating a significant, but not absolute, genetic etiology. The environmental factors that lead to or prevent the appearance of IDDM in genetically predisposed individuals are unknown. Two genetic susceptibility loci are currently under intense scrutiny, one on chromosome 6 and the other on chromosome 11 near the insulin gene. The first genes found to be associated with susceptibility to IDDM were alleles of MHC class I genes of chromosome 6.[2-4] Despite much investigation, the mechanism by which the gene products of these genes may cause IDDM is not yet known.

HLA ASSOCIATIONS

The earliest associations of IDDM susceptibility were with the class I MHC alleles B8 and B15.[2-4] Further work has shown more significant associations with certain class II MHC alleles. The MHC class I antigens (HLA-A, -B, and -C) contain a cytoplasmic domain, a transmembrane domain, and three extracellular domains. Two of the extracelelar domains combine to form a groove in which an antigen-derived peptide is held for presentation to T-cell receptors of cytotoxic (CD8+) T-lymphocytes. MHC class I antigens are found on the surface of all nucleated cells. The MHC class II antigens are composed of an α and a β chain, each encoded by a separate gene in the DP, DQ, or DR region of the MHC. The two chains form a structure analagous to the class I molecule, with an antigen-presenting groove composed of parts of both chains. The class II antigens are expressed on the surface of macrophages, B lymphocytes, T helper lymphocytes, monocytes, and some epithelial cells. When a foreign antigen is endocytosed by an antigen-presenting cell, the foreign antigen is partially degraded and presented on the surface of the antigen-presenting cell in the antigen binding groove of an MHC molecule. The MHC class II molecule with the foreign antigen then associates with a T-cell receptor of T helper (CD4+) lymphocytes, triggering the immune response to the foreign antigen.

The particular HLA antigens associated with susceptibility or resistance to IDDM vary somewhat from one population to another. The DR3 allele is found to be associated with IDDM susceptibility in Caucasian,[5,6] Chinese,[7] and Finnish[8] populations. HLA-DR4 is a susceptibility allele in Caucasian,[5,6] Finnish,[8] and Japanese[9,10] populations. DR9 is associated with susceptibility in Japanese IDDM.[9,10] The DR2 allele is considered protective from IDDM in Caucasians[5,6] and Japanese.[9,10] The presence of aspartate at position 57 of the DQ α chain is usually associated with resistance to IDDM, and the presence of an arginine at position 52 of the DQ β chain is associated with susceptibility to IDDM in Japanese[9,11] and Caucasian[12,13] populations.

The associations become more complex when the particular combination of class II alleles in a given subject is taken into account. Studies suggest that heterozygosity for DR3 and DR4 in Caucasians[14] or DR3 and DRw9 in Chinese[7] may confer particular susceptibility, while another suggests that the combination of an α chain containing an arginine at position 52 and a β chain without an aspartate at position 57 is crucial for IDDM susceptibility.[13] A large study, the WHO Multinational Project for Childhood Diabetes, or the DIAMOND project, has been initiated that will help address the question of whether population differences in diabetes susceptibility genes correlate with the observed differences in the rates of IDDM in different populations.[15] It may be that comparison of the DNA sequence of the various alleles of the MHC region in different populations will reveal the basis for the population-based differences in MHC susceptibility genes.

The mechanism by which certain HLA types predispose to the development of IDDM is not clear. One proposed explanation for the various associations, presented by Nepom,[16] suggests that the affinity of an individual's various MHC molecules for diabetogenic peptides determines that subject's risk of developing diabetes—the peptide-affinity model. Nepom[16] proposed that certain MHC gene products confer susceptibility. Those gene products coexist in the endosome with the other MHC gene products expressed in that person and there they compete for binding of diabetogenic antigen peptides. The immune response resulting in diabetes would occur when the susceptibility MHC gene product bound the diabetogenic peptide. The risk of the susceptibility MHC molecule binding the diabetogenic peptide would be determined by the relative affinity of the peptide for all of the MHC molecules present. The susceptibility molecules could be homodimers or heterodimers. This would explain the protective effect of some haplotypes and the apparent synergistic effect of others. The nature of the diabetogenic peptides is unknown. At the amino acid level, it is believed that the two residues associated with diabetes susceptibility (Asp57 of the β chain and Arg52 of the α chain of the MHC class II molecule) are located in the antigen binding groove and that they are therefore in an ideal location to affect antigen binding or presentation.[13] Further work is needed to clarify the molecular basis of diabetes susceptibility due to the MHC genes.

CHROMOSOME 11 SUSCEPTIBILITY LOCUS

The insulin gene is found on the short arm of chromosome 11.[17,18] A region of DNA 363 base pairs 5′ of the insulin mRNA start site has been found to be associated with IDDM.[19,20] This region is a polymorphic locus of varying size that had been previously found to be associated with NIDDM.[16,18] Another region of chromosome 11, the c-Ha-*ras*-protooncogene (HRAS1), which is independent of the 5′ flanking region of the insulin gene, is associated with IDDM in some families.[21] As with the MHC susceptibility genes, the molecular mechanism by which these regions are related to IDDM is not known.

SUMMARY

Although it is clear that genetic and environmental factors influence the susceptibility to IDDM, the mechanism for their action is not known. The genes of the MHC region appear to be most strongly linked to development of IDDM. Likewise, genes in the vicinity of the insulin gene itself, although not including the insulin mRNA-coding region, are linked to IDDM. The specific region or gene product of this locus that predisposes to diabetes has not yet been determined. It is possible that more than one genetic locus is involved in the pathogenesis of IDDM, and these loci may or may not interact with one another and with various environmental factors.

REFERENCES

1. **Barnett, A.H., Eff, C., Leslie, R.D.G., and Pyke, D.A.,** Diabetes in identical twins: a study of 200 pairs, *Diabetologia,* 20, 87, 1981.
2. **Singal, D.P. and Blajchman, M.A.,** Histocompatibility (HL-A) antigens, lymphocytotoxic antibodies and tissue antibodies in patients with diabetes mellitus, *Diabetes,* 22, 429, 1972.
3. **Nerup, J., Platz, P., Andersen, O.O., Christy, M., Lyngsoe, J., Poulsen, J.E., Ryder, L.P., Nielsen, L.S., Thomsen, M., and Svejgaard, A.,** HL-A antigens and diabetes mellitus, *Lancet,* 864, 1974.
4. **Cudworth, A.G. and Woodrow, J.C.,** HL-A system and diabetes mellitus, *Diabetes,* 24, 345, 1975.
5. **Wolf, E., Spencer, K.M., and Cudworth, A.G.,** The genetic susceptibility to Type 1 (insulin-dependent) diabetes: analysis of the HLA-DR association, *Diabetologia,* 24, 224, 1983.
6. **Sachs, J.A., Cudworth, A.G., Jaraquemada, D., Gorsuch, A.N., and Festenstein, H.,** Type 1 diabetes and the HLA-D locus, *Diabetologia,* 18, 41, 1980.
7. **Hawkins, B.R., Lam, K.S.L., Ma, J.T.C., Low, L.C.K., Cheung, P.T., Serjeantson, S.W., and Yeung, R.T.T.,** Strong association of HLA-DR3/DRw9 heterozygosity with early-onset insulin-dependent diabetes mellitus in Chinese, *Diabetes,* 36, 1297, 1987.
8. **Tuomilehto-Wolf, E., Tuomilehto, J., Cepaitis, Z., Lounamaa, R., and Group, D.S.,** New susceptibility haplotype for type I diabetes, *Lancet,* Aug 5, 299, 1989.
9. **Maruyama, T., Shimada, A., Kasuga, A., Kasatani, T., Ozawa, Y., Ishii, M., Takei, I., Suzuki, Y., Kobayashi, A., Takeda, S., Matsubara, K., and Saruta, T.,** Analysis of MHC Class II antigens in Japanese IDDM by a novel HLA-typing method, hybridization protection assay, *Diabetes Res. Clin. Practice,* 23, 77, 1994.
10. **Ito, M., Taminato, M., Kamura, H., Yoneda, M., Morishima, Y., Takasuki, K., Itatsu, T., and Saito, H.,** Association of HLA-DR phenotypes and T-lymphocyte-receptor b-chain-region RFLP with IDDM in Japanese, *Diabetes,* 37, 1633, 1988.
11. **Awata, T., Kuzuya, T., Matsuda, A., et al.,** High frequency of aspartic acid at position 57 of HLA-DQ beta-chain in Japanese IDDM patients and non-diabetic subjects, *Diabetes,* 39, 266, 1990.
12. **Todd, J.A., Bell, J.I., and McDevitt, H.O.,** HLA-DQb gene contributes to susceptibility and resistance to insulin-dependent diabetes mellitus, *Nature (London),* 329, 599, 1987.
13. **Khalil, I., d'Auriol, L., Gobet, M., Morin, L., Lepage, V., Deschamps, I., Park, M.S., Degos, L., Galibert, F., and Hors, J.,** A combination of HLA-DQb Asp57-negative and HLA DQa Arg52 confers susceptibility to insulin-dependent diabetes mellitus, *J. Clin. Invest.,* 85, 1315, 1990.
14. **Rotter, J.I., Anderson, C.E., Rubin, R., Congleton, J.E., Terasaki, P.I., and Rimoin, D.L.,** HLA genotypic study of insulin-dependent diabetes: the excess of DR3/DR4 heterozygotes allows rejection of the recessive hypothesis, *Diabetes,* 32, 169, 1983.
15. **Group, W.P.,** WHO multinational project for childhood diabetes, *Diabetes Care,* 13, 1062, 1990.
16. **Nepom, G.T.,** A unified hypothesis for the complex genetics of HLA associations with IDDM, *Diabetes,* 39, 1153, 1990.
17. **Owerbach, D., Bell, G.I., Rutter, W.J., Brown, J.A., and Shows, T.B.,** The insulin gene is located on the short arm of chromosome 11 in humans, *Diabetes,* 30, 267, 1981.
18. **Harper, M.E., Ullrich, A., and Saunders, G.F.,** Localization of the human insulin gene to the distal end of the short arm of chromosome 11, *Proc. Natl. Acad. Sci. U.S.A.,* 78, 4458, 1981.
19. **Bell, G.I., Horita, S., and Karam, J.H.,** A polymorphic locus near the human insulin gene is associated with insulin-dependent diabetes mellitus, *Diabetes,* 33, 176, 1984.
20. **Hitman, G.A., Tarn, A.C., Winter, R.M., Drummond, V., Williams, L.G., Jowett, N.I., Bottazzo, G.F., and Galton, D.J.,** Type 1 (insulin-dependent) diabetes and a highly variable locus close to the insulin gene on chromosome 11, *Diabetologia,* 28, 218, 1985.
21. **Owerbach, D., Gunn, S., and Gabbay, K.H.,** Multigenic basis for type 1 diabetes: association of HRAS1 polymorphism with HLA-DR3, DQw2/DR4,DQw8, *Diabetes,* 39, 1504, 1990.

GENETICS OF THE SYNDROMES OF INSULIN RESISTANCE AND TYPE II DIABETES MELLITUS

INTRODUCTION

Type II (non–insulin-dependent) diabetes mellitus, or NIDDM, is characterized by hyperglycemia due to insulin resistance and relative insulin deficiency. Family studies indicate as much as 90% concordance for NIDDM in monozygotic twins, indicating a significant genetic contribution to the etiology of NIDDM.[1] However, some patients with NIDDM have two unaffected parents.[2] Patients with NIDDM are twice as likely to have an affected mother than father,[3,4] suggesting either an *in utero* influence or maternal inheritance. Population and family studies of typical NIDDM are complicated by the late onset of the disease, the heterogeneity of the disease, and the potential uncertainty of differentiating IDDM, NIDDM, and other syndromes of insulin resistance. The disease is likely polygenic in origin.

Several genes have been found to be associated with various subtypes of insulin-resistant diabetes, such as maturity onset diabetes of youth or Type A severe insulin resistance syndrome, which have typical Mendelian inheritance patterns. None has yet been definitively linked to typical NIDDM. Candidate genes that have been proposed include genes of the MHC region, the insulin gene, the insulin receptor gene, the gene for insulin receptor substrate 1 (IRS-1), the glycogen synthase gene, the Glut4 or Glut2 glucose transporter genes, the adenosine deaminase gene, mitochondrial transfer RNA genes, and the glucokinase gene. Some of these genes have been found to be the causative genes in some rare syndromes of insulin resistance, as discussed below. Others have been proposed as susceptibility genes for NIDDM.

GENES OF THE MHC REGION

Many studies have shown associations between the MHC region and IDDM (see IDDM section of this chapter), but some have also reported associations with NIDDM. In Finland, which has the highest incidence of IDDM and a substantial incidence of NIDDM, the same HLA haplotypes that are associated with IDDM are also associated with NIDDM.[5] In a population in Minnesota (predominantly of Northern European ancestry), Rich and colleagues[6] found an increased frequency of HLA-DR4 in both IDDM and NIDDM patients. As with IDDM, the mechanism by which genes of the MHC region may cause NIDDM is undetermined.

INSULIN GENE

Some studies have found an association between NIDDM and the insulin gene. Particular restriction-fragment-length polymorphisms in the 5′ flanking region of the insulin gene have been associated with NIDDM in some populations but not others.[7,12] An abnormally high ratio of proinsulin to insulin has been reported in patients with NIDDM.[13,15] However, in six American Pima Indians, a group in which an elevated proinsulin:insulin ratio has been reported,[15] and in Micronesian Nauruans, another group with a high incidence of NIDDM, the insulin gene sequence has been found to be normal.[16] One study looked for a particular silent mutation of the coding region of the insulin gene in over 200 NIDDM patients and found only one mutation.[17] Overall, the insulin gene itself appears to be a minor contributor to typical NIDDM.

A few cases of mutations that alter the structure of the insulin molecule have been reported[18-21] in patients with diabetes mellitus and hyperinsulinemia. The abnormal insulins have been given the names insulin Chicago, Los Angeles, and Wakayama, denoting the cities where the patients were found. These patients respond normally to exogenously administered insulin and represent a rare subtype of diabetes mellitus.

In addition, a few families have been found in which a mutation in the insulin gene prevents cleavage of proinsulin to insulin and causes familial hyperproinsulinemia.[22-24] These patients have elevated immunoreactive insulin measurable in their serum, but the majority is proinsulin rather than insulin. They are normoglycemic or mildly hyperglycemic.

INSULIN RECEPTOR GENE

The human insulin receptor gene is located on chromosome 19, is >120 kb long,[25,26] and contains 22 exons. Exon 11 may or may not be included in the mature mRNA of the receptor, depending on alternative splicing of the receptor mRNA.[27] There is some tissue specificity in expression of the alternative forms.[28] The insulin receptor mRNA in liver is primarily that containing exon 11, whereas other tissues contain both types.[28] The insulin receptor gene product is a single-precursor 1382-amino acid polypeptide that is cleaved into the α and β subunits and a 27-amino acid signal peptide. The protein undergoes posttranslational glycosylation and fatty acylation (reviewed by Taylor et al.[29]). The insulin receptor is a tetramer protein consisting of two extracellular α subunits and two membrane-spanning β subunits joined by disulfide bonds.[30,31] The α subunits form the insulin binding domain[32] and the β subunits form the intracellular tyrosine kinase domain.[33] Binding of insulin to the receptor elicits autophosphorylation of multiple tyrosine residues and activation of tyrosine kinase activity.[34-36] After activation of the receptor, various substrates are phosphorylated, including IRS-1.[37,38] The insulin receptor is an attractive candidate for defects leading to insulin resistance.

A relatively large number of defects have been described in the insulin receptor gene in patients with three rare syndromes: the syndrome of Type A severe insulin resistance, characterized by marked hyperinsulinemia and insulin resistance, acanthosis nigricans, and hyperandrogenism of ovarian origin;[39] leprechaunism, characterized by severe primordial dwarfism, hyperinsulinism, and fasting hypoglycemia;[40] and Rabson-Mendenhall syndrome, characterized by insulin resistance, abnormal dentition, and thickened nails.[41] Some of these mutations are outlined in Table 2. In many cases defects in the binding of insulin,[42-46] the kinase activity of the receptor,[43,47-55] mRNA abundance,[56,57] or the posttranslational processing or trafficking of the receptor[43,45,58-60] have been found in these mutant receptors. One mutation appeared to cause constitutive activation of receptor autophosphorylation, kinase activity, and glucose transport.[61] Some of the mutations act in a "dominant-negative" fashion, causing severe insulin resistance in the heterozygous state despite the presence of a normal receptor allele.[49,51,52,55] One functionally silent mutation,[62,63] Val[985] to Met, has been found in patients with Type A insulin resistance, NIDDM, and in normal subjects.[62-65] It is not clear why defects in the receptor present with varying clinical syndromes. Insulin receptor defects appear thus far to be the cause of all cases of leprechaunism and the Rabson-Mendenhall syndrome, both of which are extremely rare. However, insulin receptor defects may be only a minor cause of the more common Type A severe insulin resistance syndrome. In a study of 22 women with this syndrome, only one had a detectable defect in the insulin receptor.[64]

All the data available to date suggest that defects in the insulin receptor are not a major cause of insulin resistance in NIDDM. The cDNA and the amino acid sequences of the insulin receptor in Pima Indians and others with NIDDM were normal in those examined thus far.[66,67] Linkage studies have shown weak or no association of the insulin receptor gene with NIDDM[12,68-73] or its subtype, maturity onset diabetes of the young (MODY).[68,74] The reported mutations in the insulin receptor gene in patients with NIDDM include one found to be functionally silent and 1 found in one of 30 NIDDM patients, the functional importance of which is not known.[65] Although the possible polygenic and heterogeneous nature of NIDDM may reduce the sensitivity of linkage studies, thus far there does not appear to be good evidence that insulin receptor gene mutations are a common cause of insulin resistance in NIDDM.

INSULIN RECEPTOR SUBSTRATE-1 GENE

IRS-1 was the first described substrate for the insulin receptor tyrosine kinase.[37,38] It is a cytoplasmic protein of between 165 and 185 kDa that is phosphorylated by the activated insulin receptor at multiple sites. An analysis of polymorphisms of the IRS-1 showed polymorphisms at two sites, glycine[972] to arginine and alanine[513] to proline, were more common in NIDDM patients than controls in a subset of white subjects.[81] The functional significance of the amino acid changes is not yet known. IRS-1 was not linked to MODY in a recent study of 15 MODY families.[82] Further studies will be needed to conclude whether IRS-1 gene defects are important in the genetics of NIDDM.

TABLE 2
Mutations in the Insulin Receptor Gene Associated with Clinical Syndromes

Syndrome and Associated Insulin Receptor Defects	References
Type A Insulin Resistance	
1. Heterozygous for mutant receptor lacking receptor kinase domain	49
2. Heterozygous for missense mutation Gly[1008] to Val	48
3. Heterozygous for missense mutation Trp[1200] to Ser	52, 75
4. Homozygous for missense mutation Phe[382] to Val	60
5. Heterozygous for missense mutation Ala[1134] to Thr	51
6. Compound heterozygote for mutations—nonsense: termination at codon 133 and missense Asn462 to Ser	56
7. Compound heterozygote for a deletion of the 14th exon and termination at codon 867 and an unknown mutation of the other allele	76
8. Compound heterozygote for mutations—missense: Arg[981] to Gln and nonsense: termination at codon 988	54
9. Heterozygous for missense mutation Arg[1174] to Gln	55, 64
10. Heterozygous for missense mutation Pro[1178] to Leu	77
11. Heterozygous for missense mutation Arg[1351] to Gln	77
12. Heterozygous for missense mutation Arg[1131] to Gln	47
13. Heterozygous for deletion of exon 3 with frameshift leading to chain termination after exon 2	78
Leprechaunism	
1. Compound heterozygote for mutations—missense: Lys[460] to Glu and nonsense: termination at codon 671 (patient Leprechaun/Ark-1)	44
2. Homozygous missense mutation Leu[233] to Pro (patient Leprechaun/Geldermalsen)	43, 50
3. Homozygous missense mutation His[209] to Arg (patient Leprechaun/Winnipeg)	56
4. Compound heterozygote for mutations—nonsense: termination at codon 897 and *cis*-acting mutation: decreasing transcription from other allele (patient Leprechaun/Minn-1)	57
5. Compound heterozygote for mutations—missense: Val[28] to Ala and missense: Gly[366] to Arg (patient Leprechaun/Verona-1)	79
6. Homozygous missense mutation Trp[412] to Ser	58
7. Homozygous missense mutation Ile[119] to Met	80
8. Homozygous missense mutation Arg[86] to Pro (patient Leprechaun/Atl-1)	61
Rabson-Mendenhall Syndrome	
1. Homozygous (?) point mutation, prevents cleavage of proreceptor to α and β subunits	59
2. Compound heterozygote for mutations—nonsense: termination at codon 1000 and missense: Asn[15] to Lys	45, 56
3. Compound heterozygote for mutations—missense: Ser[323] to Leu and nonsense with truncation prior to transmembrane domain	46
4. Homozygous for missense mutation Ser[323] to Leu	77
NIDDM	
1. Heterozygote for missense mutation Lys[1068] to Glu	65
2. Heterozygote for missense mutation Val[985] to Met (mutation not functionally active, also present in nondiabetics)	62, 63, 65

GLUCOSE TRANSPORTER GENES

Three of the facilitative glucose transporters have been considered possible candidates in the etiology of diabetes mellitus, including Glut1, Glut2, and Glut4. Glut1 is found in many tissues and is believed to be responsible for basal transport in those tissues. The Glut1 gene is on chromosome 1p. Glut2, on chromosome 3q, is a high-K_m transporter found primarily in the liver and in pancreatic β cell, where it is thought to contribute to the glucose sensing mechanism responsible for glucose-responsive insulin secretion. Glut4, on chromosome 17p, is the insulin regulatable glucose transporter, found primarily in muscle and adipose tissue (see Mueckler[83] for a review of transporters).

Studies looking for an association of Glut1 and Glut4 with diabetes mellitus using restriction length polymorphisms have shown weak associations. In an Italian population and in Northern European and Southern European populations, an XbaI restriction length polymorphism was found more commonly in NIDDM patients than controls.[84,85] A subsequent sib-pair analysis and studies of a West Indian population and a Caucasian population showed only a weak or no association with NIDDM.[86-88] No cases of a defective Glut1 transporter have been described in cases of diabetes.

Studies of Glut4 have shown no associations with NIDDM. In one study a missense mutation (Val[383] to Ile) was found in one diabetic patient, but the mutation is a conservative one that would not be likely to cause defective transport activity.[89] A study of a silent polymorphism at codon 130 of Glut4 showed no association with NIDDM in a Welsh population,[63] and another study of a KpnI polymorphism showed no associations with NIDDM in African Americans.[90] Thus, despite the prominent position of Glut4 as the insulin-responsive transporter, no defects in this protein appear to be responsible for insulin resistance in NIDDM.

There is some evidence for a minor role of Glut2 in the etiology of diabetes. A missense mutation (Val[197] to Ile) that destroys the transport activity of Glut2[91] has been identified in 1 of 48 patients with gestational diabetes.[92] Studies have shown a possible association between a restriction length polymorphism of Glut2 and NIDDM in a British and a Caucasian population.[88,93] But, polymorphism analyses in NIDDM patients from populations of Pima Indians,[94] African Americans,[90] British Caucasians,[95] and MODY patients from French,[96] Danish,[97] and British[97] families show no association of the Glut2 gene with diabetes. Based on all the available data, it appears that Glut2 has a minor role, if any, in the susceptibility to NIDDM or MODY.

GLUCOKINASE GENE

Glucokinase (type IV hexokinase) catalyzes the first step of glucose metabolism, phosphorylation to glucose-6-phosphate, in the β cell and the liver. The enzyme belongs to a family of hexokinases (type I–IV) but has a higher K_m for glucose (5 mM vs. 20–130 μM) and is not inhibited by glucose-6-phosphate, as are the other three hexokinases. The glucokinase gene is on chromosome 7 and contains two different first exons and promoters. One of these is utilized exclusively in β-cell glucokinase and the other in hepatocyte glucokinase (see Magnuson[98] for review). It has been proposed that glucokinase, perhaps in combination with the high-K_m glucose transporter (GLUT2), acts as the "glucose sensor" in the pancreas.[99]

Glucokinase was first found to be associated with insulin resistance in 1992 when close linkage of the glucokinase locus to MODY was found in a study of families affected by MODY.[96,100] Several defects in the glucokinase gene have been found in affected members of families with MODY linked to the glucokinase gene. These include patients who are heterozygous for nonsense mutations,[101,102] missense mutations,[101,103,104] and deletions.[101,105] Functional studies of MODY patients in families linked to the glucokinase gene have an elevated threshold for insulin secretion from the β cell, as one would predict based on a decrease in glucokinase activity if glucokinase is indeed part of the regulatory mechanism for insulin secretion.[106,107]

Although most glucokinase mutations have been found in patients with MODY, a few have been described in families with typical late-onset NIDDM. One such family carried a nonsense mutation,[108] another a missense mutation.[103] Likewise, nonsense and missense mutations in glucokinase have been identified in patients with gestational diabetes who have a family history of diabetes.[109]

Studies of the activity of the glucokinase enzyme carrying missense mutations associated with diabetes show that most of the mutations affect the K_m and/or the V_{max} of the enzyme.[110] Glucokinase defects cause disease in an autosomal dominant fashion because even relatively small decreases in glucokinase activity affect insulin secretion. The mutations are found in exons 5, 7, and 8. Exons 7 and 8 are believed to form most of the surface of the glucose binding and catalytic cleft of the enzyme, while exon 5 is in an area believed to undergo a conformational change on glucose binding.[110]

Although a large number of glucokinase mutations have been found and associated with diabetes mellitus, some populations show minor linkage or no linkage of the glucokinase gene. Associations have been found in French MODY families,[96] British MODY,[100] Americans with gestational diabetes,[109] South Indians with NIDDM,[111] Japanese with MODY,[112] and elderly Finnish men with glucose intolerance,[113] but not in Japanese with NIDDM,[114] North-western Italians with NIDDM,[115] or French with NIDDM.[116] Additionally, defects of gluco-kinase are not found in all cases of MODY. One study found that 44% of French MODY patients do not have a detectable glucokinase mutation.[116]

There is ample evidence that glucokinase defects contribute strongly to the etiology of MODY and in a minor way to the etiology of NIDDM and gestational diabetes. In addition, the mechanism by which these defects cause diabetes is evident.

GLYCOGEN SYNTHASE AND TYPE 1 PROTEIN PHOSPHATASE GENES

Defective insulin-stimulated glycogen storage has been found in NIDDM,[117] so the enzymes involved in glycogen synthesis are possible candidates for defects in NIDDM. Glycogen synthase catalyzes the addition of uridine diphosphate glucose (UDP glucose) to glycogen, an important step in the nonoxidative pathway of glucose metabolism. The glycogen synthase gene is found on chromosome 19.[118,119] A restriction fragment length polymorphism, called XbaI RFLP A_2, in the glycogen synthase gene was found to be associated with NIDDM in a Finnish population.[118] The patients with this polymorphism had a higher likelihood of hypertension than NIDDM patients without the polymorphism.[118] The association of this polymorphism and NIDDM was not found in a French population,[120] a Japanese population,[121] or a Swedish population.[122] However, an association with the alternative allele, XbaI RFLP A_1 allele, was found in the French subjects.[120] Additionally, a simple tandem repeat polymor-phism in the synthase gene was associated with NIDDM in a different group of Japanese NIDDM patients.[123] The glycogen synthase locus was not linked to MODY in a study of 15 MODY families.[82] Further studies are needed, but it appears there may be a real association with the glycogen synthase gene and NIDDM.

Protein phosphatase type 1, found in skeletal muscle, is activated by insulin and in turn activates glycogen synthase by catalyzing the change from the inactive phosphorylated D form of glycogen synthase to the active, dephosphorylated I form.[124] A recent paper found a missense mutation in 1 of 30 NIDDM patients studied,[125] providing preliminary evidence of a possible association.

MITOCHONDRIAL GENES

The maternal effect noted in the inheritance patterns of NIDDM suggests a role for mitochondrial genes in NIDDM susceptibility.[4] Mitochondrial DNA carried the genes for the enzymes of oxidative phosphorylation and for the 2 ribosomal and 22 transfer RNA necessary for mitochondrial protein synthesis.[126] The mitochondria are inherited exclusively from the mother. Several defects in mitochondrial genes have been reported in association with sub-types of diabetes. A mutation in the leucine transfer RNA (tRNA[leu(UUR)]), which has been found frequently in patients with the syndrome of mitochondrial myopathy, encephalopathy, lactic acidosis, and stroke (MELAS syndrome), has also been found in the families of patients with maternally transmitted late-onset diabetes and nerve deafness.[127-132] One study estimates that mutation accounts for more than 1% of maternally inherited diabetes in Japan.[131] The diabetic patients with the mutation tended to require insulin despite the absence of islet cell antibodies. There also was a lower incidence of obesity and a younger age of onset than NIDDM patients without the mutation.[129] Some of the patients with the mutation had relatives with MELAS syndrome, but the patients themselves did not manifest MELAS syndrome, possibly because a smaller percentage of their mitochondrial DNA carried the mutation than in patients with MELAS and possibly because the MELAS patients carried another contrib-uting defect.[128] A 10.4-kb deletion on mitochondrial DNA has been associated with a similar subtype of maternally transmitted diabetes and nerve deafness.[133] A mutation in the mitochondrial lysine transfer RNA has been described in a family with maternally transmitted diabetes, deafness, and myoclonic epilepsy with ragged red fibers (MERRF).[134] Mitochondrial DNA mutations have been found in patients with Wolfram syndrome (also known as DIDMOAD for diabetes insipidus, diabetes mellitus, optic atrophy, and deafness).[135] In summary, mitochondrial DNA mutations are responsible for diabetes in certain subtypes of diabetes. These patients may not be initially recognized as having one of these subtypes because the diabetes may precede the appearance of the deafness or other manifestations of disease.[129]

ADENOSINE DEAMINASE LOCUS/CHROMOSOME 20

A locus on chromosome 20 in or near the adenosine deaminase (ADA) gene locus cosegregates with MODY in some families.[136,137] These families do not show linkage between MODY and the glucokinase gene. The chromosome 20 locus was not associated with MODY in a study of Japanese families[112] or in a study of two pedigrees, one from Denmark and another from Britain which was subsequently found to show a linkage of the glucokinase gene.[97] A study of 15 French MODY families did not reveal a linkage between the ADA locus and MODY.[82] Although the linkage to the chromosome 20 locus is strong in those families in which it has been found, it has been found in few families. Therefore, this locus may be a less common cause of MODY than defects in glucokinase. The chromosome 20 gene product that is defective is not yet known.

Ras ASSOCIATED WITH DIABETES (Rad)

A recent study used "subtraction cloning" to screen skeletal muscle mRNA from normal and NIDDM subjects and found a novel protein overexpressed almost ninefold in the NIDDM patients.[138] The protein is a 29-kDa protein that has similarity with the Ras-guanosine triphosphatase (GTPase) superfamily. The function of the protein and the degree of its linkage with NIDDM or other forms of diabetes are not yet known.

REFERENCES

1. **Barnett, A.H., Eff, C., Leslie, R.D.G., and Pyke, D.A.,** Diabetes in identical twins: a study of 200 pairs, *Diabetologia,* 20, 87, 1981.
2. **Cook, J.T.E., Hattersley, A.T., Levy, J.C., Patel, P., Wainscot, J.S., Hockaday, T.D.R., and Turner, R.C.,** Distribution of type II diabetes in nuclear families, *Diabetes,* 42, 106, 1993.
3. **Thomas, F., Balkau, B., Vauzelle-Kervroedan, F., Papoz, L., and Group TC-I-ZS,** Maternal effect and familial aggregation in NIDDM: the CODIAB Study, *Diabetes,* 43, 63, 1994.
4. **Alcolado, J.C. and Alcolado, R.,** Importance of maternal history of non-insulin dependent diabetic patients, *Br. Med. J.,* 302, 1178, 1991.
5. **Tuomilehto-Wolf, E., Tuomilehto, J., Hitman, G.A., Nissinen, A., Stengard, J., Pekkanen, J., Kivinen, P., Kaarsalo, E., and Karvonen, M.J.,** Genetic susceptibility to non-insulin dependent diabetes mellitus and glucose intolerance are located in HLA region, *Br. Med. J.,* 307, 155, 1993.
6. **Rich, S.S., French, L.R., Sprafka, J.M., Clements, J.P., and Goetz, F.C.,** HLA-associated susceptibility to type 2 (non-insulin-dependent) diabetes mellitus: the Wadena City Health Study, *Diabetologia,* 36, 234, 1993.
7. **Owerbach, D. and Nerup, J.,** Restriction fragment length polymorphism of the insulin gene in diabetes mellitus, *Diabetes,* 31, 275, 1982.
8. **Rotwein, P.S., Chirgwin, J., Province, M., Knowler, W.C., Pettitt, D.J., Cordell, B., Goodman, H.M., and Permutt, M.A.,** Polymorphism in the 5′ flanking region of the human insulin gene: a genetic marker for non-insulin dependent diabetes mellitus, *N. Engl. J. Med.,* 308, 65, 1983.
9. **Knowler, W.C., Pettitt, D.J., Vasquez, B., Rotwein, P.S., Andreone, T.L., and Permutt, M.A.,** Polymorphism in the 5′ flanking region of the human insulin gene, *J. Clin. Invest.,* 74, 2129, 1984.

10. **Elbein, S., Rotwein, P., Permutt, M.A., Bell, G.I., Sanz, N., and Karam, J.H.,** Lack of association of the polymorphic locus in the 5′-flanking region of the human insulin gene and diabetes in American Blacks, *Diabetes,* 34, 433, 1988.

11. **Elbein, S.C., Corsetti, L., Goldgar, D., Skolnick, M., and Permutt, M.A.,** Insulin gene in familial NIDDM: lack of linkage in Utah Mormon pedigrees, *Diabetes,* 37, 569, 1988.

12. **Cox, N.J., Epstein, P.A., and Spielman, R.S.,** Linkage studies on NIDDM and the insulin and insulin-receptor genes, *Diabetes,* 38, 653, 1989.

13. **Ward, W.K., LaCava, E.C., Paquette, T.L., Beard, J.C., Wallum, B.J., and Porte, D., Jr.,** Disproportionate elevation of immunoreactive proinsulin in type 2 (non-insulin-dependent) diabetes mellitus and in experimental insulin resistance, *Diabetologia,* 30, 698, 1987.

14. **Temple, R.C., Carrington, C.A., Luzio, S.D., Owens, D.R., Schneider, A.E., Sobey, W.J., and Hales, C.N.,** Insulin deficiency in non-insulin-dependent diabetes, *Lancet,* 1 (8633), 1989.

15. **Saad, M.F., Kahn, S.E., Nelson, R.G., Pettitt, D.J., Knowler, W.C., Schwartz, M.W., Kowalyk, S., Bennett, P.H., and Porte, D., Jr.,** Disproportionately elevated proinsulin in Pima Indians with non-insulin dependent diabetes mellitus, *J. Clin. Endocrinol. Metab.,* 70, 1247, 1990.

16. **Raben, N., Barbetti, F., Cama, A., Lesniak, M.A., Lillioja, S., Zimmet, P., Serjeantson, S.W., Taylor, S., and Roth, J.,** Normal coding sequence of insulin gene in Pima Indians and Nauruans, two groups with highest prevalence of type II diabetes, *Diabetes,* 40, 118, 1991.

17. **Sanz, N., Karam, J.H., Horita, S., and Bell, G.I.,** Prevalence of insulin-gene mutations in non-insulin-dependent diabetes mellitus, *N. Engl. J. Med.,* 314, 1322, 1986.

18. **Tager, H., Given, B., Baldwin, D., Mako, M., Markese, J., Rubenstein, A., Olefsky, J., Kobayashi, M., Kolterman, O., and Poucher, R.,** A structurally abnormal insulin causing human diabetes, *Nature,* 281, 122, 1979.

19. **Shoelson, S., Haneda, M., Blix, P., Nanjo, A., Sanke, T., Inouye, K., Steiner, D., Rubenstein, A., and Tager, H.,** Three mutant insulins in man, *Nature,* 302, 540, 1983.

20. **Kwok, S.C.M., Steiner, D.F., Rubenstein, A.H., and Tager, H.S.,** Identification of a point mutation in the human insulin gene giving rise to a structurally abnormal insulin (Insulin Chicago), *Diabetes,* 32, 872, 1983.

21. **Sakura, H., Ywamoto, Y., Sakamoto, Y., Kuzuya, T., and Hirata, H.,** Structurally abnormal insulin in a diabetic patient: characterization of a mutant insulin A3 (Val-Leu) isolated from the pancreas, *J. Clin. Invest.,* 78, 1666, 1986.

22. **Shibasaki, Y., Kawakami, T., Kanazawa, Y., Akanuma, Y., and Takaku, F.,** Posttranslational cleavage of proinsulin is blocked by a point mutation in familial hyperinsulinemia, *J. Clin. Invest.,* 76, 378, 1985.

23. **Barbetti, F., Raben, N., Kadowaki, T., Cama, A., Accili, D., Gabbay, K., Merenich, J.A., Taylor, S., and Roth, J.,** Two unrelated patients with familial hyperproinsulinemia due to a mutation substituting histidine for arginine at position 65 in the proinsulin molecule: identification of the mutation by direct sequencing of genomic deoxyribonucleic acid amplified by polymerase chain reaction, *J. Clin. Endocrinol. Metab.,* 71, 164, 1990.

24. **Chan, S.J., Seino, S., Gruppuso, P.A., Schwartz, R., and Steiner, D.F.,** A mutation in the A chain coding region is associated with impaired proinsulin conversion in a family with hyperproinsulinemia, *Proc. Natl. Acad. Sci. U.S.A.,* 84, 2194, 1987.

25. **Yang-Feng, T.L., Franke, U., and Ullrich, A.,** Gene for human insulin receptor: localization to site on chromosome 19 involved in pre-B-cell leukemia, *Science,* 228, 728, 1985.

26. **Seino, S., Seino, M., Nishi, S., and Bell, G.I.,** Structure of the human insulin receptor gene and characterization of its promoter, *Proc. Natl. Acad. Sci. U.S.A.,* 86, 114, 1989.

27. **Seino, S. and Bell, G.I.,** Alternative splicing of human insulin receptor messenger RNA, *Biochem. Biophys. Res. Commun.,* 159, 312, 1989.

28. **Moller, D.E., Yokata, A.C., Caro, J.F., and Flier, J.S.,** Tissue-specific expression of two alternatively spliced insulin receptor mRNAs in man, *Mol. Endocrinol.,* 3, 1263, 1989.

29. **Taylor, S.I., Kadowaki, T., Kadowaki, H., Accili, D., Cama, A., and McKeon, C.,** Mutations in insulin-receptor gene in insulin-resistant patients, *Diabetes Care,* 13, 257, 1990.

30. **Ullrich, A., Bell, J.R., Chen, E.Y., Herrera, R., Petruzzelli, L.M., Dull, T.J., Gray, A., Coussens, L., Liao, Y.C., Tsubokawa, M., Mason, A., Seburg, P., Grunfeld, C., Rosen, O.M., and Ramachandran, J.,** Human insulin receptor and its relationship to the tyrosine kinase family of oncogenes, *Nature,* 313, 756, 1985.

31. **Ebina, Y., Ellis, L., Jarnagin, K., Edery, M., Graf, L., Clauser, E., Ou, J.H., Masiarz, F., Kan, Y.W., Goldfine, I.D., Roth, R.A., and Rutter, W.J.,** The human insulin receptor cDNA: the structural basis for hormone-activated transmembrane signaling, *Cell,* 40, 747, 1985.

32. **DeMeyts, P., Gu, J.L., Shymko, R.M., Kaplan, B.E., Bell, G.I., and Whittaker, J.,** Identification of a ligand-binding region of the human insulin receptor encoded by the second exon of the gene, *Mol. Endocrinol.,* 4, 409, 1990.

33. **Kasuga, M., Fujita-Yamaguchi, Y., Blithe, D.L., and Kahn, C.R.,** Tyrosine-specific protein kinase activity is associated with the purified insulin receptor, *Proc. Natl. Acad. Sci. U.S.A.,* 80, 2137, 1983.

34. **Kasuga, M., Karlsson, F.A., and Kahn, C.R.,** Insulin stimulates the phosphorylation of the 95,000-dalton subunit of its own receptor, *Science,* 215, 185, 1982.

35. **Rees-Jones, R.W. and Taylor, S.I.,** An endogenous substrate for the insulin receptor-associated tyrosine kinase, *J. Biol. Chem.,* 260, 4461, 1985.

36. **White, M.F., Maron, R., and Kahn, C.R.,** Insulin rapidly stimulates tyrosine phosphorylation of a Mr-185,000 protein in intact cells, *Nature,* 318, 183, 1985.

37. **Rothenberg, P., Lane, W.S., Karasik, A., Backer, J., White, M.F., and Kahn, C.R.,** Purification and partial sequence of pp185, the major cellular substrate of the insulin receptor tyrosine kinase, *J. Biol. Chem.,* 266, 8302, 1991.

38. **Sun, X.J., Rothenberg, P., Kahn, C.R., Backer, J.M., Araki, E., Wilden, P.A., Cahill, D.A., Goldstein, B.J., and White, M.F.,** Structure of the insulin receptor substrate IRS-1 defines a unique signal transduction protein, *Nature,* 352, 73, 1991.

39. **Kahn, C.R., Flier, J.S., Bar, R.S., Archer, J.A., Gorden, P., Martin, N.M., and Roth, J.,** The syndromes of insulin resistance and acanthosis nigricans: insulin receptor disorders in man, *N. Engl. J. Med.,* 294, 739, 1976.

40. **Rosenberg, A.M., Haworth, J.C., DeGroot, G.W., Trevanen, C.L., and Rechler, M.M.,** A case of leprechaunism with severe hyperinsulinemia, *Am. J. Dis. Child.,* 134, 170, 1980.

41. **West, R.J., Lloyd, J.K., and Turner, W.M.L.,** Familial insulin-resistant diabetes multiple somatic anomalies, and pineal hyperplasia, *Arch. Dis. Child.,* 50, 703, 1975.

42. **Taouis, M., Levy-Toledano, R., Roach, P., Taylor, S.I., and Gorden, P.,** Structural basis by which a recessive mutation in the alpha-subunit of the insulin receptor affects insulin binding, *J. Biol. Chem.,* 269, 14912, 1994.

43. **Maassen, J.A., van der Vorm, E.R., van der Zon, G.C.M., Klinkhamer, M.P., Krans, H.M.J., and Moller, W.,** A leucine to proline mutation at position 233 in the insulin receptor inhibits cleavage of the proreceptor and transport to the cell surface, *Biochemistry,* 30, 10778, 1991.

44. **Kadowaki, T., Bevins, C.L., Cama, A., Ojamaa, K., Marcus-Samuels, B., Kadowaki, H., Beitz, L., McKeon, C., and Taylor, S.,** Two mutant alleles of the insulin receptor gene in a patient with extreme insulin resistance, *Science,* 240, 787, 1988.

45. **Kadowaki, T., Kadowaki, H., Accili, D., and Taylor, S.,** Substitution of lysine for asparagine at position 15 in the alpha-subunit of the human insulin receptor: a mutation that impairs transport of receptors to the cell surface and decreases the affinity of insulin binding, *J. Biol. Chem.,* 265, 19143, 1990.

46. **Roach, P., Zick, Y., Formisano, P., Accili, D., Taylor, S., and Gorden, P.,** A novel human insulin receptor gene mutation uniquely inhibits insulin binding without impairing posttranslational processing, *Diabetes,* 43, 1096, 1994.

47. **Kishimoto, M., Hashiramoto, M., Yonezawa, K., Shii, K., Kazumi, T., and Kasuga, M.,** Substitution of glutamine for arginine 1131: a newly identified mutation in the catalytic loop of the tyrosine kinase domain of the human insulin receptor, *J. Biol. Chem.,* 269, 11349, 1994.

48. **Odawara, M., Kadowaki, T., Yamamoto, R., Shibasaki, Y., Tobe, K., Accili, D., Bevins, C., Mikami, Y., Matsuura, N., Akanuma, Y., Takaku, F., Taylor, S., and Kasuga, M.,** Human diabetes associated with a mutation in the tyrosine kinase domain of the insulin receptor, *Science,* 245, 66, 1989.

49. **Taira, M., Hashimoto, N., Shimada, F., Suzuki, Y., Kanatsuka, A., Nakamura, F., Ebina, Y., Tatibana, M., Makino, H., and Yoshida, S.,** Human diabetes associated with a deletion of the tyrosine kinase domain of the insulin receptor, *Science,* 245, 63, 1989.

50. **Klinkhamer, M.P., Groen, N.A., van der Zon, G.C.M., Lindhout, D., Sandkuyl, L.A., Krans, H.M.J., Moller, W., and Maassen, J.A.,** A leucine-to-proline mutation in the insulin receptor in a family with insulin resistance, *EMBO J.,* 8, 2503, 1989.

51. **Moller, D.E., Yokota, A., White, M.F., Pazianos, A.G., and Flier, J.S.,** A naturally occurring mutation of insulin receptor alanine 1134 impairs tyrosine kinase function and is associated with dominantly inherited insulin resistance, *J. Biol. Chem.,* 265, 14979, 1990.

52. **Moller, D.E., Yokota, A., Ginsberg-Fellner, F., and Flier, J.,** Functional properties of a naturally occurring Trp1200 to Ser1200 mutation of the insulin receptor, *Mol. Endocrinol.,* 4, 1183, 1990.

53. **Haft, C.R. and Taylor, S.I.,** Deletion of 343 amino acids from the carboxyl terminus of the beta-subunit of the insulin receptor inhibits insulin signaling, *Biochemistry,* 33, 9143, 1994.

54. **Kusari, J., Takata, Y., Hatada, E., Freidenberg, G., Kolterman, O., and Olefsky, J.M.,** Insulin resistance and diabetes due to different mutation in the tyrosine kinase domain of both insulin receptor gene alleles, *J. Biol. Chem.,* 266, 5260, 1991.

55. **Moritz, W., Froesch, E.R., and Boni-Schnetzler, M.,** Functional properties of a heterozygous mutation (Arg1174 to Gln) in the tyrosine kinase domain of the insulin receptor from a type A insulin resistant patient, *FEBS Lett.,* 351, 276, 1994.

56. **Kadowaki, T., Kadowaki, H., Rechler, M.M., Serrano-Rios, M., Roth, J., Gordon, P., and Taylor, S.,** Five mutant alleles of the insulin receptor gene in patients with genetic forms of insulin resistance, *J. Clin. Invest.,* 86, 254, 1990.

57. **Kadowaki, T., Kadowaki, H., and Taylor, S.,** A nonsense mutation causing decreased levels of insulin receptor mRNA: detection by a simplified technique for direct sequencing of genomic DNA amplified by the polymerase chain reaction, *Proc. Natl. Acad. Sci. U.S.A.,* 87, 658, 1990.

58. van der Vorm, E.R., Kuipers, A., Kielkopf-Renner, S., Krans, H.M.J., Moller, W., and Maassen, J.A., A mutation in the insulin receptor that impairs prorecptor processing but not insulin binding, *J. Biol. Chem.,* 269, 14297, 1994.

59. Yoshimasa, Y., Seino, S., Whittaker, J., Kakehi, T., Kosaki, A., Kuzuya, H., Imura, H., Bell, G.I., and Steiner, D.F., Insulin-resistant diabetes due to a point mutation that prevents insulin prorecptor processing, *Science,* 240, 784, 1988.

60. Accili, D., Frapier, C., Mosthaf, L., McKeon, C., Elbein, S.C., Permutt, M.A., Ramos, E., Lander, E., Ullrich, A., and Taylor, S., A mutation in the insulin receptor gene that impairs transport of the receptor to the plasma membrane and causes insulin-resistant diabetes, *EMBO J.,* 8, 2509, 1989.

61. Longo, N., Langley, S.D., Griffin, L., and Elsas, L.J., Activation of glucose transport by a natural mutation in the human insulin receptor, *Proc. Natl. Acad. Sci. U.S.A.,* 90, 60, 1993.

62. Flier, J.S., Moller, D.E., Moses, A.C., O'Rahilly, S., Chaiken, R.L., Grigorescu, F., Elahi, D., Kahn, B.B., Weinreb, J.E., and Eastman, R., Insulin-mediated pseudoacromegaly: clinical and biochemical characterization of a syndrome of selective insulin resistance, *J. Clin. Endocrinol. Metab.,* 76, 1533, 1993.

63. O'Rahilly, S., Krook, A., Morgan, R., Rees, A., Flier, J.S., and Moller, D.E., Insulin receptor and insulin-responsive glucose transporter (GLUT 4) mutations and polymorphisms in a Welsh type 2 (non-insulin-dependent) diabetic population, *Diabetologia,* 35, 486, 1992.

64. Moller, D.E., Cohen, O., Yamaguchi, Y., Assiz, R., Grigorescu, F., Eberle, A., Morrow, L.A., Moses, A.C., and Flier, J.S., Prevalence of mutations in the insulin receptor gene in subjects with features of the type A syndrome of insulin resistance, *Diabetes,* 43, 247, 1994.

65. O'Rahilly, S., Choi, W., Patel, P., Turner, R.C., Flier, J.S., and Moller, D.E., Detection of mutations in insulin-receptor gene in NIDDM patients by analysis of single-stranded conformation polymorphisms, *Diabetes,* 40, 777, 1991.

66. Moller, D.E., Yokota, A., and Flier, J.S., Normal insulin-receptor cDNA sequence in Pima Indians with NIDDM, *Diabetes,* 38, 1496, 1989.

67. Cama, A., Patterson, A.P., Kadowaki, T., Kadowaki, H., Siegel, G., D'Ambrosio, D., Lillioja, S., Roth, J., and Taylor, S.I., The amino acid sequence of the insulin receptor is normal in an insulin-resistant Pima Indian, *J. Clin. Endocrinol. Metab.,* 70, 1155, 1990.

68. O'Rahilly, S., Trembath, R.C., Patel, P., Galton, D.J., Turner, R.C., and Wainscot, J.S., Linkage analysis of the human insulin receptor gene in type 2 (non-insulin-dependent) diabetic families and a family with maturity onset diabetes of the young, *Diabetologia,* 31, 792, 1988.

69. Elbein, S.C., Ward, W.K., Beard, J.C., and Permutt, M.A., Familial NIDDM: molecular-genetic analysis and assessment of insulin action and pancreatic beta-cell function, *Diabetes,* 37, 377, 1988.

70. McClain, D.A., Henry, R.R., Ullrich, A., and Olefsky, J., Restriction-fragment-length polymorphism in insulin receptor gene and insulin resistance in NIDDM, *Diabetes,* 37, 1071, 1988.

71. Raboudi, S.H., Mitchell, B.D., Stern, M.P., Eifler, C.W., Haffner, S.M., Hazuda, H.P., and Frazier, M.L., Type II diabetes mellitus and polymorphism of insulin-receptor gene in Mexican Americans, *Diabetes,* 38, 975, 1989.

72. Sten-Linder, M., Vilhelmsdotter, S., Wedell, A., Stern, I., Pollare, T., Arner, P., Efendic, S., Luft, R., and Luthman, H., Screening for insulin receptor gene DNA polymorphisms associated with glucose intolerance in a Scandinavian population, *Diabetologia,* 34, 265, 1991.

73. Oelbaum, R.S., Bouloux, P.M.G., Li, S.R., Baroni, M.G., Stocks, J., and Galton, D.J., Insulin receptor gene polymorphisms in type 2 (non-insulin-dependent) diabetes mellitus, *Diabetologia,* 34, 260, 1991.

74. Elbein, S.C., Borecki, I., Corsetti, L., Fajans, S.S., Hansen, A.T., Nerup, J., Province, M., and Permutt, M.A., Linkage analysis of the human insulin receptor and maturity onset diabetes of the young, *Diabetologia,* 30, 641, 1987.

75. Moller, D.E. and Flier, J.S., Detection of an alteration in the insulin-receptor gene in a patient with insulin resistance, acanthosis nigricans, and the polycystic ovary syndrome (type A insulin resistance), *N. Engl. J. Med.,* 319, 1526, 1989.

76. Shimada, F., Taira, M., Suzuki, Y., Hashimoto, N., Nozaki, O., Taira, M., Tatibana, M., Ebina, Y., Tawata, M., Onaya, T., Makino, H., and Yoshida, S., Insulin-resistant diabetes associated with partial deletion of insulin-receptor gene, *Lancet,* 335, 1179, 1990.

77. Krook, A., Kumar, S., Laing, I., Boulton, A.J.M., Wass, J.A.H., and O'Rahilly, S., Molecular scanning of the insulin receptor gene in syndromes of insulin resistance, *Diabetes,* 43, 357, 1994.

78. Wertheimer, E., Litvin, Y., Ebstein, R.P., Bennet, E.R., Barbetti, F., Accili, D., and Taylor, S., Deletion of exon 3 of the insulin receptor gene in a kindred with a familial form of insulin resistance, *J. Biol. Chem.,* 78, 1153, 1994.

79. Barbetti, F., Gejman, P.V., Taylor, S., Raben, N., Cama, A., Bonora, E., Pizzo, P., Moghetti, P., Muggeo, M., and Roth, J., Detection of mutation in insulin receptor gene by denaturing gradient gel electrophoresis, *Diabetes,* 41, 408, 1992.

80. **Hone, J., Accili, D., Al-Gazali, L.I., Lestringant, G., Orban, T., and Taylor, S.I.,** Homozygosity for a new mutation (Ile119 to Met) in the insulin receptor gene in five sibs with familial insulin resistance, *J. Med. Genet.,* 31, 715, 1994.

81. **Almind, K., Bjorbaek, C., Vestergard, H., Hansen, T., Echwald, S., and Pedersen, O.,** Aminoacid polymorphisms of insulin receptor substrate-1 in non-insulin-dependent diabetes mellitus, *Lancet,* 342, 828, 1993.

82. **Vaxillaire, M., Vionnet, N., Vigouroux, C., Sun, F., Espinosa, R., III, LeBeau, M.M., Stoffel, M., Lehto, M., Beckmann, J.S., DeTheux, M., Passa, P., Cohen, D., van Schaftigen, E., Velho, G., Bell, G.I., and Froguel, P.,** Search for a third susceptibility gene for maturity-onset diabetes of the young: studies with eleven candidate genes, *Diabetes,* 43, 389, 1994.

83. **Mueckler, M.,** The molecular biology of glucose transport: relevance to insulin resistance and non-insulin-dependent diabetes mellitus, *J. Diabetes Complications,* 7, 130, 1993.

84. **Baroni, M.G., Oelbaum, R.S., Pozzilli, P., Stocks, J., Li, S.R., Fiore, V., and Galton, D.J.,** Polymorphisms at the GLUT1 (HepG2) and GLUT4 (muscle/adipocyte) glucose transporter genes and non-insulin-dependent diabetes mellitus (NIDDM), *Hum. Genet.,* 88, 557, 1992.

85. **Li, S.R., Baroni, M.G., Oelbaum, R.S., Stock, J., and Galton, D.J.,** Association of genetic variant of the glucose transporter with non-insulin-dependent diabetes mellitus, *Lancet,* 2, 368, 1988.

86. **Li, S.R., Oelbaum, R.S., Bouloux, P.M., Stocks, J., Baroni, M.G., and Galton, D.J.,** Restriction site polymorphisms at the human HepG2 glucose transporter gene locus in Caucasian and West Indian subjects with non-insulin-dependent diabetes mellitus, *Hum. Hered.,* 40, 38, 1990.

87. **Baroni, M.G., Alcolado, J.C., Gragnoli, C., Franciosi, A.M., Cavallo, M.G., Fiore, V., Pozzoli, P., and Galton, D.J.,** Affected sib-pair analysis of the GLUT1 glucose transporter gene locus in non-insulin-dependent diabetes mellitus (NIDDM): evidence for no linkage, *Hum. Genet.,* 93, 675, 1994.

88. **Oelbaum, R.S.,** Analysis of three glucose transporter genes in a Caucasian population: no associations with non-insulin-dependent diabetes and obesity, *Clin. Genet.,* 42, 260, 1992.

89. **Kusari, J., Verma, U.S., Buse, J.B., Henry, R.R., and Olefsky, J.M.,** Analysis of the gene sequences of the insulin receptor and the insulin-sensitive glucose transporter (GLUT- 4) in patients with common-type non-insulin-dependent diabetes mellitus, *J. Clin. Invest.,* 88, 1323, 1991.

90. **Matsutani, A., Koranyi, L., Cox, N., and Permutt, M.A.,** Polymorphisms of GLUT2 and GLUT4 genes. Use in evaluation of genetic susceptibility to NIDDM in blacks, *Diabetes,* 39, 1534, 1990.

91. **Mueckler, M., Kruse, M., Strube, M., Riggs, A.C., Chiu, K.C., and Permutt, M.A.,** A mutation in the Glut2 glucose transporter gene of a diabetic patient abolishes transport activity, *J. Biol. Chem.,* 269, 17765, 1994.

92. **Tanizawa, Y., Riggs, A.C., Chiu, K.C., Janssen, R.C., Bell, D.S.H., Go, R.P.C., Roseman, J.M., Acton, R.T., and Permutt, M.A.,** Variability of the pancreatic islet beta cell/liver (GLUT2) glucose transporter gene in NIDDM patients, *Diabetologia,* 37, 420, 1994.

93. **Alcolado, J.C., Baroni, M.G., and Li, S.R.,** Association between a restriction fragment length polymorphism at the liver/islet cell (GluT 2) glucose transporter and familial type 2 (non-insulin-dependent) diabetes mellitus, *Diabetologia,* 34, 734, 1991.

94. **Janssen, R.C., Bogardus, C., Takeda, J., Knowler, W.C., and Thompson, D.B.,** Linkage analysis of acute insulin secretion with GLUT2 and glucokinase in Pima Indians and the identification of a missense mutation in GLUT2, *Diabetes,* 43, 558, 1994.

95. **Patel, P., Bell, G.I., Cook, J.T., Turner, R.C., and Wainscoat, J.S.,** Multiple restriction fragment length polymorphisms at the GLUT2 locus: GLUT2 haplotypes for genetic analysis of type 2 (non-insulin-dependent) diabetes mellitus, *Diabetologia,* 34, 817, 1991.

96. **Froguel, P., Vaxillaire, M., Sun, F., Velho, G., Zouali, H., Butel, M.O., Lesage, S., Vionnet, N., Clement, K., Fougerousse, F., et al.,** Close linkage of glucokinase locus on chromosome 7p to early-onset non-insulin-dependent diabetes mellitus, *Nature,* 356, 162, 1992.

97. **Patel, P., Lo, Y.-M.D., Hattersley, A., Bell, G.I., Tybjaerg-Hansen, A., Nerup, J., Turner, R.C., and Wainscot, J.S.,** Linkage analysis of maturity-onset diabetes of the young with microsatellite polymorphisms: no linkage to ADA or GLUT2 genes in two families, *Diabetes,* 41, 962, 1992.

98. **Magnuson, M.A.,** Glucokinase gene structure: functional implication of molecular genetics studies, *Diabetes,* 39, 523, 1990.

99. **Matschinsky, F., Liang, Y., Kesavan, P., Wang, L., Froguel, P., Velho, G., Cohen, D., Permutt, M.A., Tanizawa, Y., Jetton, T.L., Niswender, K., and Magnuson, M.A.,** Glucokinase as pancreatic β cell glucose sensor and diabetes gene, *J. Clin. Invest.,* 92, 2092, 1993.

100. **Hattersley, A.T., Turner, R.C., Permutt, M.A., Patel, P., Tanizawa, Y., Chiu, K.C., O'Rahilly, S., Watkins, P.J., and Wainscot, J.S.,** Linkage of type 2 diabetes to the glucokinase gene, *Lancet,* 339, 1307, 1992.

101. **Hager, J., Blanche, H., Sun, F., Vionnet, N., Vaxillaire, M., Poller, W., Cohen, D., Czernichow, P., Velho, G., Robert, J.-J., Cohen, N., and Froguel, P.,** Six mutations in the glucokinase gene identified in MODY by using a nonradioactive sensitive screening technique, *Diabetes,* 43, 730, 1994.

102. **Vionnet, N., Stoffel, M., Takeda, J., Yasuda, K., Bell, G.I., Zouali, H., Velho, G., Iris, F., Passa, P., Froguel, P., and Cohen, D.,** Nonsense mutation in the glucokinase gene causes early-onset non-insulin-dependent diabetes mellitus, *Nature,* 356, 721, 1992.

103. **Stoffel, M., Patel, P., Lo, Y.-M.D., Hattersley, A.T., Lucassen, A.M., Page, R., Bell, J.I., Bell, G.I., Turner, R.C., and Wainscot, J.S.,** Missense glucokinase mutation in maturity-onset diabetes of the young and mutation screening in late-onset diabetes, *Nat. Genet.,* 2, 153, 1992.

104. **Stoffel, M., Froguel, P., Takeda, J., Zouali, H., Vionnet, N., Nishi, S., Weber, I.T., Harrison, R.W., Pilkis, S.J., Lesage, S., Vaxillaire, M., Velho, G., Sun, F., Iris, F., Passa, P., Cohen, D., and Bell, G.I.,** Human glucokinase gene: isolation, characterization, and identification of two missense mutation linked to early-onset non-insulin-dependent (type 2) diabetes mellitus, *Proc. Natl. Acad. Sci. U.S.A.,* 89, 7698, 1992.

105. **Sun, F., Knebelmann, B., Pueyo, M.E., Zouali, H., Lesage, S., Vaxillaire, M., Passa, P., Cohen, D., Velho, G., Antignac, C., and Froguel, P.,** Deletion of the donor splice site of intron 4 in the glucokinase gene causes maturity-onset diabetes of the young, *J. Clin. Invest.,* 92, 1174, 1993.

106. **Velho, G., Froguel, P., Clement, K., Pueyo, M.E., Rakotoambinina, B., Zouali, H., Passa, P., Cohen, D., and Robert, J.-J.,** Primary pancreatic beta-cell secretory defect caused by mutations in glucokinase gene in kindreds of maturity onset diabetes of the young, *Lancet,* 340, 444, 1992.

107. **Shimada, F., Kanatsuka, A., Sakurada, M., Hashimoto, N., Sano, H., Hatanaka, Y., Miki, T., Makino, H., and Yoshida, S.,** Insulin response to intravenous glucose injection in a family with a glucokinase mutation, *Horm. Metab. Res.,* 26, 392, 1994.

108. **Katagiri, H., Asano, T., Ishihara, H., Inukai, K., Anai, M., Miyazaki, J.-I., Tsukuda, K., Kikuchi, M., Yazaki, Y., and Oka, Y.,** Nonsense mutation of glucokinase gene in late-onset non-insulin dependent diabetes mellitus, *Lancet,* 340, 1316, 1992.

109. **Stoffel, M., Bell, K.L., Blackburn, C.L., Powell, K.L., Seo, T.S., Takeda, J., Vionnet, N., Xiang, K.-S., Gidh-Jain, M., Pilkis, S.J., Ober, C., and Bell, G.I.,** Identification of glucokinase mutations in subjects with gestational diabetes mellitus, *Diabetes,* 42, 937, 1993.

110. **Gidh-Jain, M., Takeda, J., Xu, L.Z., Lange, A.J., Vionnet, N., Stoffel, M., Froguel, P., Velho, G., Sun, F., Cohen, D., et al.,** Glucokinase mutations associated with non-insulin-dependent (type 2) diabetes mellitus have decreased enzymatic activity: implications for structure/function relationships, *Proc. Natl. Acad. Sci. U.S.A.,* 90, 1932, 1993.

111. **McCarthy, M.I., Hitchins, M., Hitman, G.A., Cassell, P., Hawrami, K., Morton, N., Mohan, V., Ramachandran, A., Snehalatha, C., and Viswanathan, M.,** Positive association in the absence of linkage suggests a minor role for the glucokinase gene in the pathogenesis of type 2 (non-insulin-dependent) diabetes mellitus amongst South Indians, *Diabetologia,* 36, 633, 1993.

112. **Takekawa, K., Ikegami, H., Fukuda, M., Ueda, H., Kawaguchi, Y., Fujioka, Y., Fujisawa, T., and Ogihara, T.,** Early-onset type 2 (non-insulin-dependent) diabetes mellitus is associated with glucokinase locus, but not with adenosine deaminase locus, in the Japanese population, *Diabetes Res. Clin. Practice,* 23, 141, 1994.

113. **McCarthy, M.I., Hitman, G.A., Hitchins, M., Riikonen, A., Stengard, J., Nissinen, A., Tuomilehto-Wolf, E., and Tuomilehto, J.,** Glucokinase gene polymorphisms: a genetic marker for glucose intolerance in a cohort of elderly Finnish men, *Diabetic Med.,* 11, 198, 1994.

114. **Nishi, S., Hinata, S., Matsukage, T., Takeda, J., Ichiyama, A., Bell, G.I., and Yoshimi, T.,** Mutations in the glucokinase gene are not a major cause of late-onset type 2 (non-insulin-dependent) diabetes mellitus in Japanese subjects, *Diabetic Med.,* 11, 193, 1994.

115. **Laurino, C., Bertolini, S., and Cordera, R.,** Linkage analysis does not support a role for glucokinase gene in the aetiology of type 2 diabetes mellitus among North Western Italians, *Mol. Cell. Endocrinol.,* 104, 147, 1994.

116. **Froguel, P., Zouali, H., Vionnet, N., Velho, G., Vaxillaire, M., Sun, F., Lesage, S., Stoffel, M., Takeda, J., Passa, P., et al.,** Familial hyperglycemia due to mutations in glucokinase. Definition of a subtype of diabetes mellitus [see comments], *N. Engl. J. Med.,* 328, 697, 1993.

117. **Shulman, G.I., Rothman, D.L., Jue, T., Stein, P., DeFronzo, R.A., and Shulman, R.G.,** Quantitation of muscle glycogen synthesis in normal subjects and subjects with non-insulin-dependent diabetes by 13-C nuclear magnetic resonance spectroscopy, *N. Engl. J. Med.,* 322, 223, 1990.

118. **Groop, L.C., Kankuri, M., Schalin-Jantti, C., Ekstrand, A., Nikula-Ijas, P., Widen, E., Kuismanen, E., Eriksson, J., Franssila-Kallunki, A., Saloranta, C., and Koskimies, S.,** Association between polymorphism of the glycogen synthase gene and non-insulin-dependent diabetes mellitus, *N. Engl. J. Med.,* 328, 10, 1993.

119. **Lehto, M., Stoffel, M.G., Groop, L.C., Espinosa, R., LeBeau, M.M., and Bell, G.I.,** Assignment of the gene encoding glycogen synthase (GSY) to human chromosome 19, band q13.3, *Genomics,* 15, 460, 1993.

120. **Zouali, H., Velho, G., and Froguel, P.,** Polymorphism of the glycogen synthase gene and non-insulin dependent diabetes mellitus [letter to the editor], *N. Engl. J. Med.,* 328, 1568, 1993.

121. **Kadowaki, T., Kadowaki, H., and Yazaki, Y.,** Polymorphism of the glycogen synthase gene and non-insulin-dependent diabetes mellitus [letter to the editor], *N. Engl. J. Med.,* 328, 1568, 1993.

122. **Groop, L., Schalin-Jantti, C., and Lehto, M.,** Polymorphism of the glycogen synthase gene and non-insulin-dependent diabetes mellitus [letter to the editor], *N. Engl. J. Med.,* 328, 1569, 1993.

123. **Kuroyama, H., Sanke, T., Ohagi, S., Furuta, M., and Nanjo, K.,** Simple tandem repeat DNA polymorphism in the human glycogen synthase gene is associated with NIDDM in Japanese subjects, *Diabetologia,* 37, 536, 1994.

124. **Dent, P., Lavoinne, A., Nakielny, S., Caudwell, F.B., Watt, P., and Cohen, P.,** The molecular mechanism by which insulin stimulates glycogen synthesis in mammalian skeletal muscle, *Nature,* 348, 302, 1990.

125. **Chen, Y.H., Hansen, L., Chen, M.X., Bjorbaek, C., Vestergaard, H., Hansen, T., Cohen, P.T.W., and Pedersen, O.,** Sequence of the human glycogen-associated regulatory subunit of type 1 protein phosphatase and analysis of its coding region and mRNA level in muscle from patients with NIDDM, *Diabetes,* 43, 1234, 1994.

126. **Attardi, G. and Schatz, G.,** Biogenesis of mitochondria, *Annu. Rev. Cell Biol.,* 4, 289, 1988.

127. **Alcolado, J.C., Majid, A., Brockington, M., Sweeney, M.G., Morgan, R., Rees, A., Harding, A.E., and Barnett, A.H.,** Mitochondrial gene defects in patients with NIDDM, *Diabetologia,* 37, 372, 1994.

128. **van den Ouweland, J.M.W., Lemkes, H.H.P.J., Ruitenbeek, W., Sandkuijl, L.A., de Vijlder, M.F., Struyvenberg, P.A.A., van de Kamp, J.J.P., and Maassen, J.A.,** Mutation in mitochondrial tRNA Leu(UUR) gene in a large pedigree with maternally transmitted type II diabetes mellitus and deafness, *Nat. Genet.,* 1:368, 1992.

129. **Kadowaki, T., Kadowaki, H., Mori, Y., Tobe, K., Sakuta, R., Suzuki, Y., Tanabe, Y., Sakura, K., Awata, T., Goto, Y.-I., Hayakawa, T., Matsuoka, K., Kawamori, R., Kamada, T., Horai, S., Nonaka, I., Hagura, R., Akanuma, Y., and Yazaki, Y.,** A subtype of diabetes mellitus associated with a mutation of mitochondrial DNA, *N. Engl. J. Med.,* 330, 962, 1994.

130. **Reardon, W., Ross, R.J.M., Sweeney, M.G., Luxon, L.M., Pembrey, M.E., Harding, A.E., and Trembath, R.C.,** Diabetes mellitus associated with a pathogenic point mutation in mitochondrial DNA, *Lancet,* 430, 1376, 1992.

131. **Katagiri, H., Asano, T., Ishihara, H., Inukai, K., Anai, M., Yamanouchi, T., Tsukuda, K., Kikuchi, M., Kitaoka, H., Ohsawa, N., Yazaki, Y., and Oka, Y.,** Mitochondrial diabetes mellitus: prevalence and clinical characterization of diabetes due to mitochondrial tRNA Leu(UUR) gene mutation in Japanese patients, *Diabetologia,* 37, 504, 1994.

132. **van den Ouweland, J.M.W., Lemkes, H.H.P.J., Trembath, R.C., Ross, R., Velho, G., Cohen, D., Froguel, P., and Maassen, J.A.,** Maternally inherited diabetes and deafness is a distinct subtype of diabetes and associates with a single point mutation in the mitochondrial tRNALeu(UUR) gene, *Diabetes,* 43, 746, 1994.

133. **Ballinger, S.W., Shoffner, J.M., Hedaya, E.V., Trounce, I., Polak, M.A., Koontz, D.A., and Wallace, D.C.,** Maternally transmitted diabetes and deafness associated with a 10.4 kb mitochondrial DNA deletion, *Nat. Genet.,* 1, 11, 1992.

134. **Suzuki, S., Hinokio, Y., Hirai, S., Onoda, M., Matsumoto, M., Ohtomo, M., Kawasaki, H., Satoh, Y., Akai, H., Abe, K., and Toyota, T.,** Diabetes with mitochondrial gene tRNALYS mutation, *Diabetes Care,* 17, 1428, 1994.

135. **Pilz, D., Quarrell, O.W.J., and Jones, E.W.,** Mitochondrial mutation commonly associated with Leber's optic neuropathy observed in a patient with Wolfram syndrome (DIDMOAD), *J. Med. Genet.,* 31, 328, 1994.

136. **Rothschild, C.B., Akots, G., Hayworth, R., Pettenati, M.J., Rao, P.N., Wood, P., Stolz, F.-M., Hansmann, I., Serino, K., Keith, T.P., Fajans, S.S., and Bowden, D.W.,** A genetic map of chromosome 20q12-q13.1: multiple highly polymorphic microsatellite and RFLP markers linked to the maturity-onset diabetes of the young (MODY) locus, *Am. J. Hum. Genet.,* 52, 110, 1993.

137. **Bell, G.I., Xiang, K.-S., Newman, M.V., Wu, S.-H., Wright, L.G., Fajans, S.S., Spielman, R.S., and Cox, N.J.,** Gene for non-insulin-dependent diabetes mellitus (maturity-onset diabetes of the young subtype) is linked to DNA polymorphism on human chromosome 20q, *Proc. Natl. Acad. Sci. U.S.A.,* 88, 1484, 1991.

138. **Reynet, C. and Kahn, C.R.,** Rad: a member of the Ras family overexpressed in muscle of type II diabetic humans, *Science,* 262, 1441, 1993.

INDEX

A

Abiotic environmental factors, 65, see also specific factors
Absolute thyroidal uptake rate, 244
"Accurate pacemakers", 53
Acetylcholine (ACh), 126, 129, 182, 186, 209
Acetyl-coenzyme A, 77
N-Acetyl-5-methoxykynurenamine, 80
N-Acetyl-5-methoxytryptamine, see Melatonin
ACh, see Acetylcholine
ACTH, see Adrenocorticotropic hormone
Activity rhythms, 96
Additives, 61
Adenohypophyseal system, 160–161
Adenohypophyseal-thyroid axis, 131
Adenohypophysis, 45
Adenomas, 274–276, see also Cancer; specific types
Adipose tissue regulation, 174
Adrenal function, 136
Adrenal gland, 8–11, 63, 87
Adrenal hormones, 9
Adrenal hyperplasia, 320
Adrenal medulla, 44, 49, 87
Adrenocorticotropic hormone (ACTH), 10, 12–14, 45, 48, 142, 161, 163
    21-hydroxylase deficiency and, 320
    melatonin and, 87, 91
Adrenocorticotropin, see Adrenocorticotropic hormone (ACTH)
Advanced puberty, 96
Affinity, 32
AGD, see Antigonadotropic decapeptide
Aging, 53
AHO, see Albright's hereditary osteodystrophy
AIB, see Aminoisobutyric acid
Albright's hereditary osteodystrophy (AHO), 326
Alcohol, 59, 62, 64, 65
Alcohol-induced birth defects, 65
Aldosterone, 10, 87
Alkylating agents, 61, see also specific types
Ambient temperature, 56
Amine precursor uptake and decarboxylation (APUD) series, 240
Amino acids, 128, 129, 175, 186, see also specific types
alpha-Aminoisobutyric acid (AIB), 175
Amphotericin B, 61
Anabolic-androgenic steroids, 63, see also specific types
Analgesics, 61, see also specific types
Analysis of variance (ANOVA), 52
Anaplastic thyroid cancer, 240, 261, 264, 265
Anatomy, 230–232
    of hypothalamus, 159–162
    of parathyroid gland, 232
    of pineal gland, 70–76
Ancephaly, 64

"AND GATE", 79
Androgens, 25, 26, see also specific types
Anesthetic agents, 59, see also specific types
Anestrina, 77
Anestrous condition, 123
ANF, see Atrial natriuretic factor
Angiography, 249–250, 276
Angiotensin, 10, 15–16, 127, 209
Annual cycle, 55–58
Anorexia nervosa, 96
Anovulation, 57
Anovulin, 77
Anterior hypothalamus, 127, 128
Anterior pituitary function, 162-165
Antibiotics, 61, 62, see also specific types
Antibodies, 241, 304–305, see also specific types
Anti-CEA monoclonal antibodies, 241
Anticonvulsive activity of melatonin, 97
Antidiuresis, 48
Antifreeze, 64
Antigens, 291, see also specific types
Antigonadotropic decapeptide (AGD), 77
Antigonadotropic hormone, 89
Antigonadotropic substances, 76, see also specific types
Antigonadotropin, 77
Antihypercholesterolemic effect, 88
Antiknock mix, 64
Anti-stress effect of melatonin, 97
Antithyroid drugs, 254, see also specific types
Antitumor effect of melatonin, 97
APUD, see Amine precursor uptake and decarboxylation
Arginine vasotocin (AVT), 76
Arteriography, 230, 275
Aspartate, 128
Aspermia, 96
Astrocytomas, 98
Atmospheric pressure, 65
Atresia, 60
Atrial natriuretic factor (ANF), 17–18
Automobile coolant, 64
AVT, see Arginine vasotocin
Azathioprine, 63
Azoospermia, 64

B

Barbiturates, 96, see also specific types
Barium contrast esophagography, 249
Barium swallow, 258
Barometers, 64
Batteries, 64
Benzene, 64
Benzodiazepines, 94, 96, see also specific types
β-adrenergic agonists, 86, see also specific types
β-adrenergic blockers, 79, see also specific types
β-adrenergic receptors, 73, see also specific types